D0014218

The Oxford Dictionary of

Sports Science
and Medicine

The Oxford Dictionary of
Sports Science
and Medicine

Second Edition

Michael Kent

Oxford New York Tokyo
OXFORD UNIVERSITY PRESS
1998

Oxford University Press, Great Clarendon Street, Oxford OX2 6DP

Oxford New York

Athens Auckland Bangkok Bogota Bombay
Buenos Aires Calcutta Cape Town Dar es Salaam
Delhi Florence Hong Kong Istanbul Karachi
Kuala Lumpur Madras Madrid Melbourne
Mexico City Nairobi Paris Singapore
Taipei Tokyo Toronto Warsaw

and associated companies in
Berlin Ibadan

Oxford is a trade mark of Oxford University Press

Published in the United States
by Oxford University Press Inc., New York

A catalogue record for this book is available from the British Library

Library of Congress Cataloging in Publication Data
The Oxford dictionary of sports science and medicine
Michael Kent — 2nd ed.
(Oxford medical publications)
Includes bibliographical references.
1. Sports medicine—Dictionaries.   2. Sports sciences—Dictionaries.
I. Kent, Michael, Dr.   II. Series
[DNLM: 1. Sports Medicine—dictionaries.   2. Sports—dictionaries.
QT 13 098 1998] RC 1206.094 1998 617.1'027'03–dc21 97–41377

ISBN 0 19 .262845 3

Typeset by Alliance Phototypesetters, Pondicherry
Printed in Great Britain by Bookcraft (Bath) Ltd
Midsomer Norton, Avon

Preface
to the second edition

The disciplines of Sports Science and Sports Medicine have grown rapidly since the publication of the first edition of the *Oxford Dictionary of Sports Science and Medicine*. Sports Science has become an established part of the curriculum in schools and universities with many new and exciting courses being offered. Sports Medicine has gained general acceptance among medical practitioners as an important speciality. There is a general awareness among athletes and their coaches that a scientific understanding of sport can enhance performance. Everyone is becoming more aware of the importance of exercise as a cornerstone of preventative medicine. This upsurge of interest and activity in sports science and medicine has generated a wealth of new information which has necessitated a complete revision of the dictionary. New terms and illustrations have been introduced along with several appendices of useful information; obsolete terms have been removed, and established terms updated.

The revisions for this edition are my own and I must bear responsibility for any errors I may have introduced. However, it has been built on the foundation provided by the first edition, and I owe a great debt of gratitude to the original contributors and advisers (Dr Stuart Biddle, Dr Geoff Edwards, Dr Ken Fox, Dr Mike Hutson, Merryn Kent, Professor Greg McLatchie, Dr Andrew Sparkes and Bryan Woods) who did so much to make this book possible. I am also grateful to Professor Clyde Williams of Loughborough University for his continued support and encouragement.

Michael Kent
St Austell College, Cornwall
December 1997

Preface
to the first edition

Sports science includes any discipline which uses scientific methods to study sports phenomena. It is a relatively recent addition to the curriculum, but it is fast becoming an established area of study at schools, colleges, and universities in Britain and many other countries, and it forms the theory base for national coaching courses.

Sports medicine first emerged out of the growth of the modern Olympic movement and the search for methods of improving athletic performance. It was originally concerned with the prevention and treatment of sports injuries, especially in the élite athlete. But modern sports medicine has grown in response to the demands of the large number of people who take part in sport for pleasure and for health. Many sports authorities recognize the need for sports people of all abilities to have access to adequate medical and scientific support when and where they need it. Sports medicine has become accepted as an important aspect of preventative medicine and now takes its place among the other branches of medicine.

Sports science and medicine is truly multidisciplinary, covering topics such as anatomy, biomechanics, ergogenic aids, exercise physiology, nutrition, sport psychology, and sport sociology, as well as the cause and treatment of sports injuries. These topics have generated a wealth of specialist literature, each with its own language. The main aim of this dictionary is to make this literature more accessible to the non-specialist: to help explain words and expressions found in textbooks used by the student, coach, athlete, or medical professional, who has a need for multidisciplinary knowledge.

This dictionary contains over 7500 entries covering all the main areas of sports science and medicine. Most terms are defined in a few short sentences with some longer accounts. The entries are extensively cross-referenced so that the dictionary is as self-contained as possible.

The entries cover words and expressions in current use and explain the meanings attached to them in the context they were made. Sports Science and medicine is a very dynamic and relatively new subject. However, it has drawn on older, established disciplines and has adopted many of their terms. Therefore, the dictionary includes some terms which have become obsolete or fallen out of fashion, but which the student is likely to encounter in the older literature.

The inspiration for this dictionary came from work done with Michael Allaby on *The Concise Oxford Dictionary of Zoology* and *The Concise Oxford Dictionary of Botany*. Michael has offered advice and encouragement throughout the project. I would also like to express my thanks to Simon Nicholas, Head of Physical Education at St Austell College, for his encouragement and comments, and to William D. Stanish M.D. who made some helpful criticisms concerning the original headword list.

The dictionary has been compiled with the help of a team of eminent advisers and contributors. They have worked extremely hard and kept to very tight deadlines. Their enthusiasm and support for the project has been greatly appreciated. This book would have been impossible without their expert knowledge. Any mistakes that have occurred are the editor's.

I would also like to express my thanks to the librarians at the School of Education, Exeter University, who allowed me free access to the library, and to the staff of Oxford University Press for their support,

There is absolutely no doubt that this book would not have been completed without the staunch support and contribution of my wife, Merryn. Her work went far beyond the demands of the marriage vows.

Michael Kent
St Austell College,
Cornwall, January 1993

Contributors and advisors
to the first edition

....

Dr Stuart Biddle, Senior Lecturer, Exeter University; President, European Federation of Sport Psychology.

Dr Geoffrey P. L. Edwards, General Practitioner, The Health Centre, Wadebridge.

Dr Ken Fox, Lecturer, Exeter University; Fellow of the P.E. Association.

Dr Mike Hutson, Orthopaedic and Sports Physician, Park Row Clinic, Nottingham, and London Bridge Clinic.

Merryn Kent, MA (Oxon).

Dr Michael Kent, Senior Lecturer, St Austell College.

Greg R. McLatchie, MB, ChB, FRCS, Visiting Professor in Sports Medicine and Surgical Sciences, School of Health Sciences, University of Sunderland; Director of the National Sports Medicine Institute of the United Kingdom, St Bartholomew's Medical College.

Dr Andrew Sparkes, Senior Lecturer, Exeter University; Associate Director, Physical Education Association Research Centre.

B. D. Woods, Lecturer, Exeter University; Physiotherapist to the British Olympic Association.

Bibliography

Aldridge, J. A. and Pilgrim, N. (1984). *Prevention and rehabilitation of injury*. The National Coaching Foundation, Leeds.

American College of Sports Medicine (1971). *Encyclopaedia of sports sciences and medicine*. Macmillan, New York.

Armstrong, N. A. and Sparkes, A. (eds.) (1991). *Issues in physical education*. Cassell, London.

Arnold, P. (1968). *Education, physical education and personality development*. Heinemann, London.

Astrand, P. O. and Rodahl, K. (1986), *Textbook of work physiology*. (3rd edn.) McGraw Hill, New York.

Badewitz-Dodd, L. (1991). *Drugs and sport*. Media Medica, Chichester, Sussex.

Baumann. W. (ed.) (1983) *Biomechanics and performance in sport*. Karl Hofmann, Schorndorf, W. Germany.

Bean, A. (1993). *A complete guide to sports nutrition*. A. C. Black London.

Beashel, P. and Taylor, J. (1996). *Advanced studies in physical education and sport*. Nelson, Surrey, UK.

Berridge, M. E. and Ward, G. R. (1987). *International perspectives on adapted physical activity*. Human Kinetics, Champaign, Illinois.

Biddle, S. (ed.) (1987). *Foundations of health-related fitness in P.E.* Ling Publishing Co., London.

Blakey, P. (1992). *The muscle book*. Bibliotek Books, Stafford, UK.

Bull, R., Davis, R. J., Roscoe, D. A. and Roscoe, V. J. (1990). *Physical education and the study of sport*. Wolfe, London.

Bull, S. J. (1991). *Sport psychology: a self-help guide*. Crowood Press, Wiltshire, UK.

Burke, E. R. and Newsom, M. M. (1988). *Medical and scientific aspects of cycling*. Human kinetics, Champaign, Illinois.

Christina, R. W. and Corcos, D. M. (1988). *Coaches' guide to teaching sport skill*. Human Kinetics, Champaign, Illinois.

Cooper, J. M., Adrian, M., and Glassow, R. B. (1982). *Kinesiology*, (5th edn). C. V. Mosby, London.

Cooper, K. (1983). *The aerobics program for total well-being*. Evans, New York.

Corbin, C. B. and Lindsey, R. (1985). *Concepts of physical fitness with laboratories*. Wm. C. Brown, Dubuque, Iowa.

Cratty, B. J. (1981). *Social psychology in athletics*. Prentice-Hall, New Jersey.

Cox, R.H. (1994) *Sport psychology; concepts and applications*, (3rd edn). Wm. C. Brown, Dubuque, Iowa.

Davies, D. (1989). *Psychological factors in competitive sport*. Falmer Press, Basingstoke.

Davis, D., Kimmet, T., and Auty, M. (1986). *Physical education: theory and practice*. Macmillan, Melbourne.

de Vries, H. A. (1986) *Physiology of exercise*. Wm. C. Brown, Dubuque, Iowa.

Dick, F. W. (1989). *Sports training principles*. 2nd edn. A. and C. Black, London.

Dirix, A., Knuttgen, H. G., and Tittel K. (eds.) (1988). *The encyclopaedia of sports medicine*. Vol. 1. Blackwell, Oxford.

Dunning, E. (ed.) (1971). *The sociology of sport*. Frank Cass, London.

Dyson, G. H. G. (1986). *Dyson's mechanics of athletics*, (8th edn). revised by B. D. Woods and P. R. Travers, Hodder and Stoughton London.

Edwards, H. (1973). *Sociology of sport*. Dorsey Press, Homewood, Illinois.

Elias, N., and Dunning, E. (1970). *The sociology of sport*. Frank Cass, London.

Elias, N., and Dunning, E. (1986). *The quest for excitement*. Blackwell, Oxford.

Eriksson, B. O., Mellstrand, T., Peterson, L., Renstrom, P., and Svedmyr, N. (1990). *Sports medicine: health and medication.* Guinness Publishing, London.

Faria, I. E. and P. R. Cavanagh (1978). *The physiology and biomechanics of cycling.* John Wiley, New York.

Fleishman, E. A. (1964). *The structure and measure of physical fitness.* Prentice-Hall, New Jersey.

Fox, E. L. (1979). *Sports physiology*, (2nd edn). W.B. Saunders, Philadelphia.

Fox, E. L. and Mathhews, D. K. (1981). *The physiological basis of phyiscal education and athletics*, (3rd edn). W. B. Saunders, Philadelphia.

Gill, D. L. (1986). *Psychological dynamics of sport.* Human Kinetics, Champaign, Illinois.

Green, J. H. (1986). *An introduction to human physiology.* Oxford University Press, Oxford.

Greendorfer, S. L. and Yiannakis, A. (eds.) (1981). *Sociology of sport.* Leisure Press, New York.

Hall, S. J. (1995). *Basic biomechanics*, (2nd edn). Mosby. St. Louis.

Harries, M, Williams, C., Stanish, W. D., and Micheli, L. J. (1994). *Oxford texbook of sports medicine.* Oxford University Press. Oxford.

Harris, D. V. and Harris, B. L. (1984). *The athletes guide to sports psychology.* Human Kinetics, Champaign, illinois.

Harris, N., Lovesey, J., and Oram, C. (1982). *The sports health handbook.* Kingswood Press.

Hay, J. G. (1985). *The biomechanics of sports techniques*, (3rd. edn). Prentice-Hall, New Jersey.

Hazeldine, R. (1990). *Strength training for sports.* Crowood Press, Wiltshire.

Howley, E. T. and Franks, B. D. (1986). *Health/Fitness instructor' handbook.* Human Kinetics, Champaign, Illinois.

Humphreys, J. and Burke, E. (1982). *Fit to exercise.* Pelham, London.

Hutson, M. A. (1996). *Sports injuries: recognition and management.* Oxford Univeristy Press, Oxford.

Jary, D. and Jary, J. (1991). *Collins dictionary of sociology.* Harper Collins, London.

Jenkins, S. P. R. (1990). *Sports science handbook.* Sunningdale publications, Berks.

Katch, F. I. and McCardle, W. D. (1988). *Nutrition, weight control, and exercise.* Lea and Febiger, Philadelphia.

Kent, M. (1997). *Food and fitness: a dictionary of diet and exercise.* Oxford University Press.

Klavora, P. and Daniel, J. V. (eds.) (1979). *Coach, athlete, and the sport psychologist.* School of Physical and Health Education, Publications Division, University of Toronto.

Knapp, B. (1977) *Skill in sport.* Routledge and Kegan, London.

Krause, J. V. and Barham, J. N. (1975). *The mechanical foundations of human motion.* A programmed Text. C.V. Mosby, London.

Kreighbaum, E. and Barthels, K. M. (1985). *Biomechanics: a qualitative approach to studying Human Movement.* Burgess, Minneapolis.

Lamb, D. R. (1984). *Physiology of exercise.* Macmillan, New York.

Leunes, A. D. and Nation J. R. (1989). *Sport psychology: an introduction.* Nelson-Hall, New York.

Loy, J. W., Kenyon, G. S, and McPherson, B. D. (ed.) (1981). *Sport, culture and society: a reader on the sociology of sport.* Lea and Febiger, Philadelphia.

McArdle, W. D., Katch, F. I., and Katch, V. L. (1986). *Exercise physiology.* Lea and Febiger, Philadelphia.

MacDougall, J. D., Wenger, H. A. and Green, H. J. (eds.) (1991). *Physiological testing of the high performance athlete*, (2nd edn). Human Kinetics, Champaign, Illinois.

McPherson, B. D., Curtis, J. E., and Loy, J. W. (1989). *The social significance of sport: an introduction to the sociology of sport.* Human Kinetics, Champaign, Illinois.

Marieb, E. N. (1989). *Human anatomy and physiology.* Benjamin/Cummings, California.

Martens, R. (1988). *The coach's guide to sport psychology*. Human Kinetics, Champaign, Illinois.

Martin, E. A. (1996). *Concise colour medical dictionary*. Oxford University Press, Oxford.

McLatchie G. R. (1993). *Essentials of sports medicine*, (2nd edn). Churchill Livingstone, Edinburgh.

McLatchie, G. R., Harries, M., Williams, C., and King, J. B. (1995). *ABC of sports medicine*. BMJ, London.

Mellion, M. B. (1993). *Sports medicine secrets*. Hanley & Belfus, Philadelphia.

Micheli, L., and Jenkins, M. (1995). *The sports medicine bible*. Harper Collins, New York.

Morris, T., and Summers, J. (1995). *Sport psychology: theory, applications, and issues*. John Wiley & Sons, Queensland, Australia.

Mottram, D. R. (ed.) (1996). *Drugs in sport*, (2nd. edn), Chapman and Hall London.

National Coaching Foundation (1986). *The coach at work*. The National Coaching Foundation, Leeds.

National Coaching Foundation (1986). *Physiology and performance*. The National Coaching Foundation, Leeds

Newsholm,E., Leech, T., and Duester, G. (1994). *Keep on running: the science of training and performance*. John Wiley & Sons, Chichester.

Nideffer, R. M. (1985). *Athlete's guide to mental training*. Human Kinetics, Champaign, Illinois.

Noakes, T. D. (1991). *Lore of running*. Leisure Press, Human Kinetics, Champaign, Illinois.

Noakes, T. and Granger, S. (1990). *Running injuries*. Oxford University Press, Oxford.

Noble, B. J. (1986). *Physiology of exercise and sport*. Times-Mirror/Mosby College publications, St. Louis.

Ottaway, P. B. and Haigh, K. (1985). *Food for sport: handbook of sports nutrition*. Resource, Cambridge.

Page, R. L. (1978). *The physics of human movement*. Wheaton, Pergamon, Exeter.

Paish, W. (1979). *Diet in sport*. E. P. Publishing, Wakefield.

Peterson, J. and Renstrom, P. (1986). *Sports injuries, their prevention and treatment*. Martin Dunitz, London.

Pitt, V. H. (ed.) (1977). *Penguin dictionary of physics*. Penguin books, London.

Rasch, P. J., with contributions by Grabinier M. D., Gregor, R. J. and Garhammer, J. (1989). *Kinesiology and apllied anatomy*. Lea and Febiger, Philadelphia.

Rees, C. R. and Mirade A. W. (eds.) (1986). *Sport and social theory*. Human Kinetics, Champaign, Illinois.

Reilly, T. (1981). *Sports fitness and sports injuries*. Faber and Faber, Lond.

Reilly, T. Atkinson, G., and Waterhouse, J. *Biological rhythms and exercise*. Oxford University Press, Oxford.

Reilly, T., Secher, N., Snell, P., and Williams, C. (1990). *Physiology of sports*. Chapman and Hall, London.

Roberts, G. C., Spink, K. S., and Pemberton C. L. (1986). *Learning experiences and sport psychology*. Human Kinetics, Champaign, Illinois.

Roy, S. and Irving, R. (1983). *Sports medicine: prevention, evaluation, management and reha-bilitation*. Prentice-Hall, New York.

Rowett, H. G. Q. (1988). *Basic anatomy and physiology*. Murray, London.

Schmidt, R. A. (1988). *Motor control and learn-ing: a behavioural emphasis*. Human Kinetics, Champaign, Illinois.

Sharkey, B. J. (1984). *Physiology of fitness*. Human Kinetics, Champaign, Illinois.

Sharkey, B. J. (1986). *Coaches' guide to sport physiology*. Human Kinetics, Champaign, Illinois.

Sharp, C. (1985). *Developing endurance*. The National Coaching Foundation, Leeds.

Silva, J. M. and Weinber, R. S. (eds) (1984). *Psychological foundations of sport*. Human Kinetics, Champaign, Illinois.

Singer, R. N. (1982). *The learning of motor skills*. Macmillan, New York.

Singer, R. N. (1980). *Motor learning and human performance*, (3rd edn). Macmillan, New York.

Sperryn, P. N. (1983). *Sport and medicine*. Butterworths, London.

Straub, W. F. and Williams, J. M. (1984). *Cognitive sports psychology*. Sport Science associates, New York.

Strauss, R. H. (1987). *Drugs and performance in sports*. W. B. Saunders Co., Philadelphia.

Thompson, C. W. (1985). *Manual of structural kinesiology*, (10th edn). Times Mirror/Mosby College Publications, St. Louis.

Tucker, C. (1990). *The mechanics of sports injuries*. Blackwell, Oxford.

Tver, D. F. and Hunt, H. F. (1986). *Encyclopaedic dictionary of sports medicine*. Chapman and Hall, London.

Walder, P. (1994). *Mechanics and sport performance*. Feltham Press, London.

Wasserman, K., Hansen, J. E., Sue, D. Y., and Whipp, B. J. (1987). *Principles of exercise testing and interpretation*. Lea and Febiger, Philadelphia.

Watkins, J. (1983). *An introduction to mechanics of human movement*. MTP Press, Lancaster.

Weinberg, R. S. and Gould, D. (1995). *Foundations of sport and exercise psychology*. Human Kinetics, Champaign, Illinois.

Whitehead, N. (1985). *Conditioning for sport*. E.P. Publishing, Wakefield.

Williams, C., and Devlin, J. T. (1992). *Foods, nutrition and sports performance*. E & FN Spon, London.

Williams, J. M. (1993). *Applied sport psychology: personal growth to peak performance*, (2nd edn). Mayfield, California.

Williams, M. H. (ed.) (1983). *Ergogenic aids in sport*. Human Kinetics, Champaign, Illinois.

Williams, J. G. P. (1990). *A colour atlas of injury in sport*, (2nd edn). Wolfe, London.

Williams, J. G. P. and Sperryn, P. N. (1976). *Sports medicine*. Arnold, London.

Wilmore, J. H. and Costill, D. L. (1994). *Physiology of sport and exercise*. Human Kinetics, Champaign, Illinois.

Wirhed, R. (1984). *Athletic ability and the anatomy of motion*. Wolfe, London.

Wooton, S. (1988). *Nutrition for sport*. Simon Shuster, London.

Wooton, S., de Looy, A. and Walker, M. (1984). *Nutrition and sports performance*. The National Coaching Foundation, Leeds.

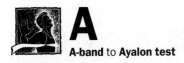

A

A-band to **Ayalon test**

A-band A dark band on electron micrographs of *striated muscle. Part of the A-band contains interdigitating *actin and *myosin filaments and is located towards the centre of a *sarcomere. *Compare* **I-band**. *See also* **H-zone**.

ABC of resuscitation A guide, produced by the Resuscitation Council (UK), to the initial management of a person who has collapsed (e.g., an athlete knocked unconscious on the field of play): A = airway (ensure that the airway is open); B = breathing (check that the patient is breathing, if not, commence expired air respiration); C = circulation (check pulse, if no pulse commence external chest compression).

ABCDE A mnemonic used as a guide for a step-by-step assessment of an athlete who collapses on the field of play. A represents Airway and cervical spine (ensure that the airway is clear, and suspect a cervical spine injury if the athlete becomes unconscious after an injury to the head or above the collar bone); B, Breathing (look and listen for spontaneous breathing); C, Circulation (check the carotid pulse for quality, rate, and regularity; if the pulse is absent, start external cardiac massage); D, Disability (for a limited neurological examination, use the AVPU mnemonic); E, Exposure (check extremities and other body parts for bleeding, fractures, and contusions).

abdomen Lower part of the trunk between the diaphragm and the pelvis, containing viscera which include the stomach, kidneys, liver, and intestines. The shape of a healthy abdomen varies. In children it often protrudes, but if this is too marked it may indicate a disease such as *kwashiorkor. In young adults, the abdomen should be slightly indrawn or only slightly prominent with the outline of the abdominal muscles visible.

abdominal Pertaining to the abdomen.

abdominal injury Physical damage to the abdomen and its contents. The abdomen is particularly vulnerable to direct blows during contact and collision sports. Most closed injuries are not serious and involve *winding or superficial bruising which requires application of an ice pack. A direct blow to the abdomen may, however, cause a serious injury by rupturing one of the internal organs. The liver and spleen are the organs most likely to be injured. Paradoxically, a serious injury is often undramatic with signs varying from mild discomfort to abdominal rigidity and shock. Any persistent abdominal pain (whether or not associated with a blow) should be treated very seriously as it is a symptom of several medical conditions which are potentially fatal if not properly diagnosed and treated. In such cases, medical advice should be sought, no medication or drinks given to the patient, and physical exertion avoided. A penetrating injury may damage any internal structure. The wound should be covered (preferably with an antiseptic dressing) and the casualty taken to hospital immediately. If the intestines are protruding, they should not be replaced but covered in moist dressing.

abdominal muscles Four pairs of muscles (the rectus abdominis, external oblique, internal oblique, and the transverus abdominis) often referred to as the stomach muscles, that support and protect the contents of the abdomen and contribute to forceful exhalation. Strong and healthy abdominal muscles support the back during lifting by stabilizing the vertebral column. If the muscles are weakened by lack of exercise they become pendulous, forming a 'pot-belly'.

abdominal pain *See* **abdominal injury**.

THE Ⓐ Ⓑ Ⓒ OF

Read the diagram in columns from left to right, and follow the black or grey lines, according to the patient's condition

APPROACH

DANGER
Establish there is no danger to yourself or the patient from outside elements; Electricity, Gas, Falling Masonry, Traffic etc.

IS THE PATIENT CONSCIOUS?
(Establish by gentle shaking & shouting)

No   Yes

PLACE IN RECOVERY POSITION
OBSERVE Ⓐ Ⓑ Ⓒ
CONTROL EXTERNAL BLEEDING

1. Establish there is no danger to yourself or the casualty. For instance the patient may be unconscious due to electric shock or gas leak, so check the relevant supply.
2. Establish consciousness of the casualty by shouting 'WAKE-UP' loudly 2-3 times and shaking the shoulder gently, remembering the possibility of a neck or other upper body injury.
3. Place casualty in recovery position.

Ⓐ AIRWAY

OPEN AIRWAY
1. Place patient on back
2. Clear mouth of obstructions
3. Tilt head to open airway
4. Support jaw & CALL FOR HELP

Tilt head
and Support jaw

IF THE CASUALTY IS UNCONSCIOUS
1. Open Airway
   Inspect the casualty's mouth and throat; Remove blood, vomit, loose teeth or broken dentures.
   Leave well fitting full dentures in place as it will assist in expired air respiration if this is necessary.
2. If there is any doubt whether the casualty is breathing adequately, tilt the head and support the jaw as shown in the diagram. This will open the airway. At this point check again to see if the casualty is breathing (see B Breathing).

RESUSCITATION

Ⓑ BREATHING

IS PATIENT BREATHING?

No | Yes

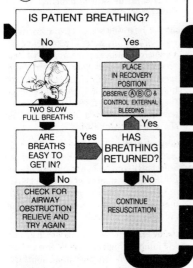

TWO SLOW FULL BREATHS

PLACE IN RECOVERY POSITION
OBSERVE Ⓐ Ⓑ Ⓒ & CONTROL EXTERNAL BLEEDING

ARE BREATHS EASY TO GET IN? — Yes → HAS BREATHING RETURNED? ← Yes

No

CHECK FOR AIRWAY OBSTRUCTION RELIEVE AND TRY AGAIN

No → CONTINUE RESUSCITATION

1. Look, listen and feel for breathing.
2. Kneel beside casualty, tilt his head back and raise the chin upwards thus opening the airway. Remember to clear the mouth of any obstructions and commence Expired Air Respiration. Open casualty's mouth and pinch his nose. Open your mouth, take a breath, seal his mouth with yours and breathe firmly into it. Breathe just firmly enough to raise the casualty's chest. Remove your mouth and allow his chest to fall.
3. As soon as the casualty's breathing returns place him in the recovery position. Vomiting often occurs when breathing returns and placing the casualty in the recovery position will prevent him from choking if vomiting does occur.
4. If there are no signs of life after two breaths, check if there is a pulse (see C Circulation).

Ⓒ CIRCULATION

IS THERE A PULSE?

No | Yes

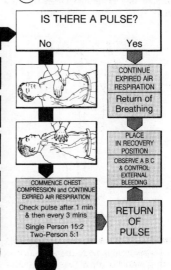

CONTINUE EXPIRED AIR RESPIRATION
Return of Breathing

PLACE IN RECOVERY POSITION
OBSERVE A B C & CONTROL EXTERNAL BLEEDING

COMMENCE CHEST COMPRESSION and CONTINUE EXPIRED AIR RESPIRATION
Check pulse after 1 min & then every 3 mins
Single Person 15:2
Two-Person 5:1

RETURN OF PULSE

1. Check for the presence of the Carotid pulse in the neck.
2. To commence External Chest Compression (E.C.C.) place the casualty flat on his back. Apply interlocked hands two finger breadths above the lower end of the breastbone and commence chest compression. Keep your hands on the chest at all times, this will minimise chest damage.
3. The rates for E.C.C. are as follows: *Working alone:* 15 Cardiac compressions (rate approximately 80 compressions per minute) followed by 2 inflations. *With assistance:* 5 Cardiac compressions (rate 60 compressions per minute) followed by 1 inflation.
4. If spontaneous pulse does not return, prepare to continue E.C.C. until skilled help arrives.
5. External bleeding should be controlled by direct pressure over the wound, using a clean dressing such as a handkerchief. When a pulse is detected, elevation of both lower legs on a suitable support will reduce the severity of shock.

abdominal rigidity An extreme tension of the abdominal muscles over an area of localized tenderness or irritation. It may be due to an underlying pathological condition, such as appendicitis, but in sport it is commonly caused by poor conditioning, poor protective gear, or a direct blow.

abdominals *See* **abdominal muscles**.

abduction Movement of a body segment (e.g., arm or leg) away from the midline of the body. The term also refers to the movement of fingers or toes when they are spread apart. *Compare* **adduction**.

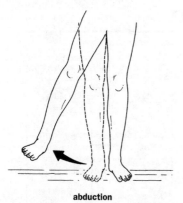

abduction

abductor digiti minimi A muscle originating on the pisiform bone in the wrist and inserting onto the ulnar base of the proximal phalanx of the fifth digit. Its primary actions are abduction and flexion of the fifth metacarpophalangeal joint.

abductor pollicis brevis A small muscle crossing the wrist. It helps to straighten the thumb and move the thumb away from the fingers. It is attached proximally to the trapezium and scaphoid bones (origin), and distally to the base of the first phalanx of the thumb (insertion).

abductor pollicis longus A muscle deep in the forearm. It helps to move the forearm sideways from the trunk. Its other actions include *abduction and extension of the thumb. It is attached proximally to the posterior surface of the ulna and radius (origin), and distally to the base of the first metacarpal (insertion).

abductor A muscle that moves a part of the body away from the midline, or spreads the fingers or toes apart.

abilities-to-skill transfer The effect of practising an ability on the learning and performance of a skill. For example, there is likely to be some positive transfer when a gymnast who has developed the abilities of balance, coordination, and flexibility, engages in the skill of dancing. *See also* **transfer of training**.

ability A relatively stable characteristic or trait which contributes to proficiency in a number of skills. For example, *balance, *coordination, and *flexibility are abilities used in the skill of trampolining. Abilities are largely inherited. Unlike skills, they are not learned but they may be extended and developed by experience. *See also* **general motor ability**.

ability-orientation The tendency of an individual to emphasize circumstances which reflect highly on his or her ability while belittling circumstances which reflect badly (for example, when a sportsperson attributes team success to him or herself, but failure to poor officials).

Ablakov test A *power test in which an athlete jumps as high as possible from a half-squat position. An automatic stop-tape, one-end attached to the athlete's waist and the other fixed to the floor, records the height reached by the athlete.

able-bodied athlete An athlete who has no physically challenging disabilities.

abnormal quadriceps pull A lateral pull of the quadriceps muscle on the patella which may result in *overpronation, excessive internal rotation of the tibia, and associated knee problems. It is caused by an abnormally large angle of insertion of the quadriceps tendon (*see* **Q-angle**).

abrasion (graze) An acute injury resulting from shearing forces between the skin surface and another surface (e.g. road surface, football pitch, mat, or skin). The skin surface is broken but there is no complete tear throughout its depth. Abrasions are common in sport and are often viewed by athletes as being trivial. Consequently, they are often inadequately treated and become infected with disease-producing organisms. Treatment includes thorough and immediate cleansing of the abrasion with soap and water, thorough irrigation, followed by application of a sterile dressing. A useful mnemonic of the treatment is SID: S = Soak, soap, scrub; I = Irrigate, irrigate, irrigate; D = Dressing.

absence A transient lessening of consciousness that may occur, for example, as a result of a physical blow.

absolute Not relative; independent of other objects or factors. In sport, it often relates to units of strength, work, or energy which are not adjusted for individual differences such as age, weight, and gender.

absolute angle Angular orientation of a body segment measured consistently in the same direction with respect to a single, fixed line of reference, either vertical or horizontal. *Compare* **relative angle**.

absolute dose The amount of drug taken up by the body. Most drugs are designed to be swallowed and absorbed into the bloodstream through the intestinal wall. Usually, not all of the drug ingested is absorbed.

absolute error The average deviation of a set of scores from a target value. Absolute error is a measure of overall error and does not take into account the direction of the deviation.

absolute humidity *See* **humidity**.

absolute load The total resistance to a movement, irrespective of an individual's body size. *Compare* **relative load**.

absolute outcome *See* **outcome**.

absolute refractory period A brief period following the stimulation of a nerve cell or muscle fibre during which the nerve cell or muscle fibre remains completely unresponsive no matter how strong a stimulus is applied.

absolute strength The maximum force an athlete can exert with his or her whole body or part of the body, irrespective of body size or muscle size. *Compare* **relative strength**.

absorption The process by which a drug passes from its point of administration into the blood. *See also* **intestinal absorption**.

abstinence syndrome A group of unpleasant symptoms produced by the abrupt termination of drug taking. These symptoms, called withdrawal symptoms, include anxiety, muscle weakness, nausea, vomiting, tremor, and a rapid heart beat. They are usually reversed rapidly when the drug is readministered.

abstracting The process of discerning common elements in situations which are otherwise different. Abstracting is particularly useful in team games when a player is said to have the ability to 'read a situation'.

academic sport psychology The traditional form of *sport psychology which focuses on the research-oriented aspects of the subject. *Compare* **applied sport psychology**.

acceleration The rate of change in *velocity or the change in velocity occurring over a given time interval. It is usually expressed as metres per second squared (ms^2).

acceleration due to gravity Acceleration of a mass towards the centre of the Earth. *See also* **acceleration of free fall**.

acceleration of free fall Constant acceleration of a body falling freely under gravity, in a vacuum, or when air resistance is negligible. It varies slightly in different geographical locations as a result of differences in the distance from the centre of mass of the Earth. The standard accepted value, usually abbreviated as g, is 9.80 665 metres per second per second, or 32.17 feet per second per second. Sky divers are sometimes said to be in free fall, but this is not strictly true because their downward velocity is reduced by air resistance.

acceleration, law of Newton's second law of motion which states that when a body is acted on by a *force, its resulting change in *momentum takes place in the direction in which the force is applied, is proportional to the force causing it, and inversely proportional to its mass. The relationship can be expressed as: $a = f/m$ or $f = ma$, where a represents acceleration; f represents force, and m represents mass. Thus, a football, for example, tends to travel in the direction of the line of action of the force of a kick, at a speed directly proportional to the force and inversely proportional to the mass of the football.

acceleration sprint A special form of sprint-training in which running speed is gradually increased from jogging to striding and finally to sprinting at maximum pace. Each component is usually about 50 metres long. Acceleration sprints are a good form of anaerobic training. They are particularly effective in emphasizing and maintaining the technical components of the sprint action as speed increases. The progressive nature of acceleration sprinting reduces the risk of muscle injury.

acceleration–time curve A graphical representation of acceleration plotted against time. It is used in the analysis of an athlete's performance at different phases of a run, cycle, swim, etc.

accelerometer A device that measures the acceleration of a system.

acceptance 1 A phase of *hypnosis during which the subject accepts the idea, judgement, or belief suggested. **2** A coping strategy used by athletes to deal with social and psychological stress, such as a serious sports injury or involuntary retirement from a sport. See also **social death**.

access 1 The extent to which facilities, including participation in a sport, are available to people, whatever their social category (e.g. ability, ethnicity, colour, gender, or sexual orientation). **2** The ability of a researcher to gain entry and acceptance to a social situation to gather data.

accessory bone A bone, such as the *os trigonum, which is not present in all people.

accident-prone Applied to a person who suffers more than the usual number of accidents. An accident is sometimes defined as 'an injury with no apparent cause'. Each year, thousands of exercisers are injured sufficiently badly to require medical attention. Although athletes subject themselves to more mechanical stresses and strains than sedentary people, most of their so-called accidents are preventable, and are due to lack of fitness, insufficient warm up, poor technique, or lack of skill. The very young and very old are particularly accident prone. The young because their bones are not fully developed, and the old because their bones are often fragile (see **osteoporosis**). Sports that impose high impact forces (e.g., distance running), are especially risky for these groups.

acclimation A reversible adaptation to changes in a single environmental factor (e.g. temperature). Acclimation is applied most commonly to physiological experiments conducted in a laboratory under controlled conditions. Compare **acclimatization**.

acclimatization A reversible physiological adaptation to environmental changes (e.g. a change of altitude or climate). See also **altitude acclimatization**; and **heat acclimatization**.

accommodation 1 Process by which the shape of the lens in the eye changes so that distant or near objects can be brought into focus. Accommodation, with pupillary constriction and convergence, enables an individual to retain an object in focus as it approaches. This ability is particularly important for ball players. **2** An effect produced on sense organs by continuous and unvarying stimulation, so that eventually no sensation is experienced (see **habituation**). **3** A social process, sometimes encouraged by sporting links, in which different racial or political groups adjust to each other and coexist without necessarily resolving underlying differences. **4** A social process, analogous to biological adaptation, by which a society or individual adjusts to its environment. **5** In Piaget's theory, a mechanism by which a child develops from one stage to the next.

accommodation principle A principle which states that training should progress from the general to the specific. Initial concern should be with improving overall body condition and strength. Skills and specific fitness components should be improved only after attaining a good level of general fitness.

accommodation to competition Response of an individual to frequent exposure to competitive situations. If accommodation is positive, the individual will have optimal levels of arousal so that performance can be maximized.

acculturation 1 A process occurring when different cultural groups are in contact Acculturation leads to the acquisition of new cultural patterns by one or more of the groups, with the adoption of some or all of another's culture. Many argue that sport makes a major contribution to acculturation; this is possibly one reason for support of national teams by governments. **2** Any transmission of culture between groups, including different generations. *See also* **enculturation**; and **socialization**.

accumulated feedback A form of *feedback in which information is presented to a performer after he or she has made a series of responses. The information represents a summary of all the responses, enabling the performer to determine how successful he or she has been.

accuracy 1 The ability to hit a target. **2** Ability of a performer, such as an ice-skater, to repeat movements successfully. **3** The ability to perform without making any errors. **4** The reliability of a measurement often expressed in terms of the deviation (+ or −) of the measurement from its true value. *Compare* **precision**.

acetabular fossa A rounded depression which serves as the attachment point of the *ligamentum teres from the femur onto the acetabulum. It is perforated by numerous small holes.

acetabular labrum Horseshoe-shaped rim made of fibrous cartilage which deepens the acetabulum and makes the hip joint more stable.

acetabulum Deep cup-like socket on the lateral surface of each hip bone (*see* **coxal bone**) into which the ball-shaped head of the femur fits.

acetaminophen The name used in the USA for *paracetamol.

acetazolamide A *diuretic drug on the International Olympic Committee list of *banned substances, misused by athletes to reduce weight artificially. It is also a component of medicines used to treat a number of conditions including oedema and *altitude sickness (it is a carbonic anhydrase inhibitor which probably acts as a respiratory stimulant).

acetic acid (ethanoic acid) A colourless liquid; the main acid in vinegar. Strong acetic acid is corrosive and an irritant poison, but low dilutions are used to treat excessive sweating. When sponged over the skin, acetic acid reduces perspiration and produces a cooling sensation. *See also* **acetylcholine**.

acetylcholine (ACh) A *neurotransmitter synthesized in the synaptic knobs of some nerve-endings from acetic acid and choline. It is released by all neurones which stimulate skeletal muscles, and neurones of the *parasympathetic nervous system. ACh elicits action potentials in nerve and muscle cells by making them more permeable to sodium ions. Its effect is short-lived because it is destroyed by acetylcholinesterase. Acetylcholine was the first neurotransmitter to be identified.

$$H_3C - \overset{\overset{\displaystyle O}{\|}}{C} - O - CH_2 - CH_2 - \overset{+}{N} - (CH_3)_3$$

acetylcholine

acetylcholinesterase An enzyme that breaks down acetylcholine (ACh) into choline and acetic acid. Acetylcholinesterase is released onto the *sarcolemma of muscle fibres and destroys ACh after the ACh has combined with receptors on the muscle fibre. Thus, acetylcholinesterase prevents continued muscle contraction in the absence of additional nervous stimulation.

acetyl CoA *See* acetyl coenzyme A.

acetyl coenzyme A (acetyl CoA) An important intermediate in the *aerobic metabolism of carbohydrates, fats, and proteins. When oxygen is available, pyruvic acid (formed from glucose during glycolysis), fatty acids (from lipids), and amino acids (from proteins) form acetyl coenzyme A which acts as the common entry point into the *Krebs cycle in a *mitochondrion.

acetylsalicylic acid (aspirin) A white crystalline powder which is a *nonsteroidal anti-inflammatory drug (NSAID), used as an antipyretic to treat headaches and as a mild analgesic to relieve pain. It is also widely used to treat muscle and joint injuries, arthritis, and cardiovascular disorders. It tends to increase clotting time and therefore increases the tendency of a person to bleed. Consequently, it can be harmful to individuals with stomach or duodenal ulcers. A few individuals are allergic to aspirin; if they ingest it they could go into an anaphylactic shock. Aspirin is a permissible drug, not on the *International Olympic Committee list of banned substances.

achieved status A high social status acquired by individual effort or open competition (for example, through winning at sport) rather than from the status the person is born with. *Compare* ascribed status.

achievement 1 The level of performance attained by an athlete, particularly in a standardized series of tests. **2** In sociology, the acquisition of social position or status as the outcome of personal effort in open competition with others e.g. in the Olympic Games.

achievement behaviour Behaviour in achievement situations. High achievers tend to select challenging tasks of intermediate risk, and perform better when evaluated. Low achievers tend to avoid challenging and risky situations, and perform worse when evaluated.

achievement goal A personal target that a performer sets himself or herself to achieve. Achievement goals are subjective and are based on what the individual regards as being successful outcomes. *See also* goal.

achievement goal theory The theory that three main factors interact to determine *achievement motivation: *achievement goals, *perceived ability, and *achievement behaviour.

achievement motivation A motivation predisposing an athlete to engage in or avoid competition. It is a fundamental drive that can motivate athletes to commit large proportions of their lives to achieve particular personal goals. It is associated with a number of behaviour characteristics of an athlete during a sporting situation, such as the effort applied, the ability to continue trying, the choice of action possibilities (e.g., decision to approach or avoid achievement situations), and the performance outcomes. Achievement motivation is affected by a number of factors, including an individual's desire for success and fear of failure. *See also* **achievement need**; **motive to avoid failure**; **motive to avoid success**.

achievement need A drive related to how hard an athlete tries to gain success and his or her capacity to experience pride in accomplishments. In sport, success may be self-evaluated or externally evaluated; it may be viewed in terms of winning a contest, improving the quality of a performance, or gaining approval from people whose views the performer values. Athletes with a high achievement need may require constant information and reassurance about their performance. *See also* **achievement motivation**.

achievement orientation The motive state of an athlete in an *achievement situation; for example, whether the athlete is motivated out of a fear of failure or from a desire to succeed. Achievement orientation is influenced by a number of factors, including the individual's emotional state, the specific task being undertaken, and the environment in which the task is being performed.

achievement situation A situation in which an individual believes that his or her performance will be evaluated. *See also* **competition**.

achievement test A test measuring what has been accomplished as in a sargent jump or Ablakov test; it contrasts with tests of potential such as aptitude tests.

Achilles bursitis (heel bursitis) An inflammation of either the deep retrocalcaneal bursa lying between the Achilles tendon and the calcaneus (in which case it is sometimes called retrocalcaneal bursitis), or the superficial bursa lying between the Achilles tendon and the skin (in which case it is sometimes called postcalcaneal bursitis). Retrocalcaneal bursitis is characterized by tenderness and redness involving the posterior and superior aspects of the heel. The symptoms are often absent if the patient goes barefoot. Achilles bursitis is often caused by excessive compensatory pronation.

Achilles tendinitis An *overuse injury characterized by inflammation, pain, and tenderness in and around the Achilles tendon. It is common in runners who train over long distances on hard surfaces and those who increase their training intensity too quickly. Women distance runners who usually wear high-heeled shoes are at particular risk because their everyday shoes effectively shorten the Achilles tendon over a period of years. When they adopt the more flat footed position during running, their tendons are subjected to more stress than they are used to. Training shoes with a high back also increase the risk of injury. Treatment usually includes rest, medication, such as *acetylsalicylic acid (aspirin) to reduce the swelling, and appropriate physiotherapy. Relief may be obtained by using a heel pad to restrict the range of movement. In severe cases, surgery may be required. An acute inflammation of the Achilles tendon, if not treated properly, can develop into a chronic condition which is very difficult to resolve.

Appropriate stretching reduces the risk of this injury.

Achilles tendon A large *tendon at the back of the ankle which connects the calf muscles (gastrocnemius and soleus) to the heel bone (calcaneus). The tendon is very susceptible to injuries. An Achilles tendon weakened by lack of exercise may rupture if the calf muscle contracts suddenly, for example, when a badminton player suddenly changes from a backward to a forward motion or when a jogger misjudges a curb and lands too far forward on his or her foot. A rupture is often accompanied by a loud crack and the victims often think that they have been struck viciously behind the heel. In extreme cases, the tendon may be completely ruptured, leaving the victim incapacitated and requiring surgery. Less severe than a complete rupture, but more common is *Achilles tendinitis.

achyllodonia A pain felt in and around the attachment of the Achilles tendon in the heel-bone.

acid A substance which dissolves in water and, in solution, liberates hydrogen ions (protons). An acid reacts with a base to give salt and water only.

acidaemia A condition in which the concentration of hydrogen ions in the blood plasma is higher than normal. *See also* **acidosis**.

acid–base balance The relatively stable relationship between the concentration of acids and bases in the body. An equilibrium is usually maintained by buffering, but this may be disrupted, for example by heavy exercise and hyperventilation. An acid–base imbalance can affect some body functions adversely, such as muscle actions and the conduction of nerve impulses.

acidosis An abnormally high acidity of the blood and tissue fluids. It can reduce the efficiency of metabolic reactions, interfere with muscle actions, and may lead to fatigue. There are two main types of acidosis: metabolic acidosis and respiratory acidosis. Metabolic acidosis may be caused by loss of bases, ingestion of highly acidic foods, or the production of excessive amounts of acids in the body (e.g., during severe exercise when large amounts of both lactic acid and carbon dioxide are produced). Respiratory acidosis results from a failure to exhale carbon dioxide from the lungs as quickly as it forms in respiring tissues. Carbon dioxide accumulates in the blood and tissues where it forms carbonic acids. Sufferers of acidosis usually breathe very heavily in order to flush out excess carbon dioxide from the body and eliminate excess acids (a process called compensatory hyperventilation). Some athletes use sodium hydrogen carbonate (baking soda) as a performance enhancer in the expectation that it decreases acidity and reduces the risk of acidosis. *Compare* **alkalosis**.

acquired Applied to a condition contracted after birth and not due to an inherited disease.

acquired ageing The possession of characteristics commonly associated with ageing but that are, in fact, caused by other factors, such as lack of mobility. *See also* **hypokinetic disease**. *Compare* **time-dependent ageing**.

acquired immune deficiency disease A disease caused by a blood-borne virus (called human immunodeficiency virus or HIV) that disrupts the body's normal immune responses. HIV is transmitted via body fluids primarily through sexual relationships, transfusion of infected blood and plasma products, and injections of drugs through contaminated needles. The general medical consensus is that the risk of infection is very low in groups exercising together or participating in a sport. However, the risk is increased during activities, such as boxing, in which blood contact may occur. Standard common-sense precautions and adherence to basic principles of hygiene should always be followed if any bleeding occurs to prevent infection with HIV or other disease organisms such as the hepatitis viruses. Exercise usually has a beneficial effect on HIV-infected individuals. If started when the individual is still healthy, it can play an important role in the management of the disease while improving the quality of life.

acquired motivation (secondary motivation) A *motivation which is not inborn and does not satisfy a basic physiological need. An example of an acquired motivation would be the desire to win an Olympic medal.

acromial Pertaining to the point of the shoulder.

acromiale (acromial point) **1** An anatomical landmark at the superior and external border of the acromion process of a subject standing erect with arms relaxed. **2** The most lateral point on the inferior border of the acromion process.

acromial point *See* **acromiale**.

acromial spur A bony projection from the acromion.

acromioclavicular joint A small, irregular joint between the *acromion process of the scapula and the distal end of the clavicle. With the *sternoclavicular joint, it forms the pectoral (shoulder) girdle. The acromioclavicular joint permits limited motion in all three planes. The deltoid muscles attach to the anterior of the joint and the trapezius to its posterior.

acromion process A projection of bone from the scapula (shoulder blade); it combines with the clavicle to form the acromioclavicular joint.

acropodion (akropodion): An anatomical landmark at the most anterior point on the toe (the first or second phalanx) of the foot of a subject standing erect. The subject's toe-nail is sometimes clipped before making the measurement.

ACSA *See* **anatomical cross-sectional area**.

actin A contractile, fibrous protein that is the main constituent of the thinner of the two types of filaments in muscle fibres (the other type consists of myosin). *See also* **sliding-filament theory**.

actin filament The thinner of the two filaments in a muscle fibre. It consists of *actin, *tropomyosin, and *troponin. One end of each actin filament is attached to a z-line. *See also* **sarcomere**.

actinic dermatitis *See* **sunburn**.

actin–myosin cross bridge *See* **cross bridge**.

action 1 Any unit or sequence of social activity or behaviour. The term is sometimes restricted to social activities which are intentional and involve conscious deliberation rather than merely being the result of a behavioural reflex. **2** In biomechanics, the product of work and time. *Compare* **power**. **3** *See* **muscle action**.

action knowledge Knowledge which has practical applications; for example, knowledge acquired by applied sport scientists which can be used to improve the performance of an athlete.

Action Pact A programme devised in Southern Australia to improve the physical fitness, self-confidence, and self-esteem of primary school children in relation to physical activity. The programme includes self-awareness, goal-setting, self-monitoring strategies, and relaxation techniques using guided imagery.

action plan Plan of a specific action that helps to achieve a particular *goal. For example, an athlete who has set himself or herself the goal of running one mile in less than four minutes, might select two immediate action plans: to train one extra morning per week, and to do hill sprints on Thursdays.

action point During a muscle stretch, the point at which you begin to feel tension but no pain.

action potential A transient feature of the cell surface membranes of neurones and muscle fibres during which the electrical potential inside the membrane becomes temporarily positive with respect to the outside. This depolarization conforms to the *all-or-none law and lasts about one millisecond, after which the resting potential is re-established. The action potential at one membrane site provides a stimulus to adjacent sites, resulting in conduction of the action potential through the cell.

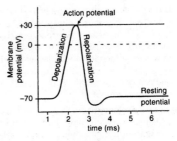

action potential

action research A methodology used in a number of disciplines, including physical education, sport psychology, and sport sociology, which has the dual aims of action (e.g., application of an intervention strategy by a sport psychologist) and research.

action theory A method of sociological analysis which regards the purposive social actions of individuals as the basis on which to seek explanations for social reality.

activation The state of readiness of an individual to respond to a stimulus. It is an internal state which occurs immediately prior to an activity. Activation may be elicited by exposing an athlete to an audience, by verbal exhortation, or by exposure to competitive situations. *See also* **arousal**.

Activation Deactivation Adjective Checklist A questionnaire that measures *state anxiety.

activation system Body systems, such as the sensory system, memory, and perception, which effect *activation.

active assisted stretching A stretch performed by the subject alone until a limit is reached, at which point a partner assists to gain a further stretch. This type of stretching should be performed with care. The partner must be competent and well trained, and must have established good communication and trust with the subject to prevent overstretching.

active force A force due to movement entirely controlled by muscular activity.

During walking and running, active forces reach their maximum value at least 50 ms after the foot strikes the ground. Active forces are responsible for all the movements of an individual who, when standing on both feet, bends his or her knees and returns to the upright position. *Compare* **impact force**.

active insufficiency The inability of a muscle which spans two or more joints to exert enough tension and shorten sufficiently to cause a full range of movement in all joints at the same time. *See also* **passive insufficiency**.

active mobility exercise Movements, totally under the control of the exerciser, that improve mobility.

active recovery *See* **exercise recovery**.

active rest A type of treatment sometimes prescribed for *overuse injuries. Active rest involves performing light exercises (often swimming or cycling) that stimulate the recovery process without imposing undue stress on the injured body part. *See also* **rest**.

active stability That part of *joint stability provided by muscle actions.

active state Condition of a muscle immediately before and during a muscle action. A muscle in the active state is nonextensible. The active state is due to *myosin cross bridges attaching to *actin filaments in the muscle fibres.

active stretching Stretching by actively contracting antagonistic muscles (i.e. the muscles on the side of the joint opposite the joint structures to be stretched). *Compare* **passive stretching**.

active transport The net movement of a substance across a cell membrane against a concentration gradient (i.e., from a region of lower to a region of higher concentration). Active transport requires the expenditure of energy provided by the breakdown of ATP.

activity-induced anorexia *See* **anorexia nervosa**.

activity fragmentation The breakdown of a *skill into components in such a way that

the meaningful relationship between components is lost.

activity theory A theory which proposes that as people age they substitute the roles they lose for other roles so that their total activity is maintained. It also suggests that high activity and maintenance of roles during ageing are positively related to *self-concept and life satisfaction.

actomyosin A protein formed by the coupling of *actin and *myosin during muscle actions. *See also* **sliding-filament theory**.

actor (social actor) Any person involved in a social *action. The person may or may not be playing a role. *See* **role theory**.

actual leader behaviour The behaviour a coach or other leader exhibits, irrespective of the norms or preferences of those who are led.

actual productivity *See* **Steiner's model**.

actuarial age Age in years nearest to the subject's past or next birthday. It is used by many insurance companies, and in the CP-index.

acupuncture An ancient Chinese system of healing in which symptoms are relieved by inserting anywhere from 3 to 20 thin needles through the skin and muscle at certain points in the body. The points are plotted along the body on lines determined by tradition. Selected points are stimulated by rotating the needle or by passing an electric current through it. The precise mechanism of acupuncture is unknown, but it is thought that the needles act as an external stimulus which encourages the release of chemicals, natural painkillers called *endorphins, that are believed to initiate self-healing within the body. Acupuncture is used in the Far East as an alternative to anaesthesia for some major operations. It is gaining popularity in the West to relieve the pain associated with some sports injuries.

acute Applied to a condition which develops rapidly and which is usually of brief duration.

acute injury An injury with a rapid onset. An acute injury usually responds well to early treatment, but if left untreated can develop into a chronic condition that is much more difficult to treat.

acute muscle soreness A pain felt in muscles during and immediately following exercise. It is probably due to an inadequate flow of blood to active muscle, resulting in the accumulation of metabolic waste products such as protons (hydrogen ions) or lactate from lactic acid.

acute reaction phase The response of the immune system to muscle cell damage 1–4 days after the damage has occurred during severe exertion or heavy exercise. During this phase, an increase of *C-reactive protein activates the complement system and initiates cell-damaging and inflammatory reactions necessary for resolving and repairing tissue damage.

acute response A physiological response (e.g., change in heart rate) of the body to an individual bout of exercise, such as running on a treadmill. *Compare* **chronic adaptation**.

acyclic activity An activity in which body movements are not regularly repeated. Maximal strength sports, such as weightlifting, are generally acyclic. *Compare* **cyclic activity**.

adaptability The ability to adjust to different conditions. It is applied to athletes who can modify their playing style to suit a number of different playing situations.

adaptation 1 The process by which a person's body responds positively over a period of time to the effects of exercise so that he or she can cope with higher workloads. In a well-designed training programme, it is important to increase the workloads gradually as adaptation takes place, to ensure that there is a sufficient training stimulus (*see* **overload principle**). **2** In sociology, the manner in which any social system, such as a sports club or sporting body, responds to its environment in order to survive. **3** Sensory adaptation; a decline in the transmission of a sensory impulse when a receptor is stimulated continuously with a constant stimulus strength.

adaptation energy A hypothetical measure of an individual's capacity to resist *stress. Each person is believed to have a finite amount of adaptation energy which is used to cope with different types of stress. Energy expended to cope with one type of stress, such as staying up late, results in less being available for other stresses, such as training. When adaptation energy is low, a person is more likely to suffer from stress-related diseases and conditions known as *burnout and *rundown.

adapted physical exercise Exercise and sport performed by people with physical disabilities and/or learning difficulties. Many disabled athletes train on a daily basis. They train, often with weights, for flexibility, strength, speed, power, endurance, and to develop specific skills. The training principles for the disabled are the same as those for the able-bodied, but disabled athletes have the additional challenge of developing an individual style that takes their specific disability into account, but which allows them to use their abilities to the maximum. Sports participation offers disabled people a powerful incentive to become fitter, and there is no doubt that it plays an important part in both the psychological and physical rehabilitation of the disabled.

adaptive achievement pattern Patterns of behaviour in which success is achieved through adapting to the environment. This is accomplished by developing new ways of coping with challenging situations; by actively seeking challenges and persisting in overcoming them; and through satisfaction felt in taking challenges. Hence an adaptive achievement pattern of behaviour is an important factor in making an athlete successful.

adaptive learning *See* **adaptive training**.

adaptive training (adaptive learning) A form of training which progresses from easier to more difficult tasks as the learner improves. Adaptive training may use equipment designed to provide automatic adjustments of task difficulty according to the learner's level of performance, with the learner's errors maintained at a constant level as difficulty varies.

adaptogen An *ergogenic aid derived from Siberian ginseng (*Eleutherococcus senticosus*) which, it is claimed, heightens resistance to stress, enhances stamina, and accelerates recovery from heavy training.

addiction A state of physiological dependence produced by habitually taking drugs such as morphine, heroin, or alcohol. The term is also applied to a state of psychological dependence produced by drugs such as barbiturates.

addiction to exercise (exercise addiction; exercise dependence) Physiological or psychological dependence on a regular regime of exercise, characterized by unpleasant symptoms if withdrawal from exercise occurs. The addiction may be for any exercise, but is most commonly associated with distance running. The term is often used in a pejorative sense and implies that the individual has an uncontrollable craving for exercise which can damage his or her functioning in other ativities. *See also* **exercise adherence**.

Addison's disease A metabolic disorder caused by degeneration of the adrenal cortex and a failure to secrete adequate amounts of certain vital hormones, such as *cortisol. The disease is characterized by an inability to maintain blood pressure when standing, depression, progressive weight loss, and severe physical incapacitation. It has been suggested that athletes who overtrain for long periods (months and even years) may develop this disease. Overtrained athletes do exhibit an abnormally low cortisol response to stress, but this is probably due to disturbance of the *hypothalamus rather than the *adrenal gland itself.

additive principle The notion in sports psychology that *intrinsic motivation and *extrinsic motivation combine to create the need for achievement (*see* **achievement motivation**). *Compare* **multiplicative principle**.

adduction Movement of a body segment closer to the midline of the body; or move-

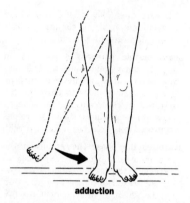

adduction

ment of the fingers or toes towards each other after being spread apart.

adductor brevis One of three adductor muscles in the thigh. The adductor brevis is a short muscle in the medial compartment which has its origin on the main body and lower border of the pubis, and its insertion on the linea aspera above the insertion of the adductor longus. The adductor brevis adducts and laterally rotates the thigh.

adductor longus The most anterior of the three adductor muscles in the thigh. The adductor longus has its origin near the *pubic symphysis and its insertion on the *linea aspera. Its main actions are to adduct, flex, and laterally rotate the thighs.

adductor magnus A thigh adductor muscle. It has two origins on the pelvic girdle: one on the pubis and the other on the *ischial tuberosity. It has a broad insertion on the *linea aspera and the adductor tubercle of the femur. Its anterior portion adducts, laterally rotates, and flexes the thigh. Its posterior part acts as a synergist of the hamstrings during thigh extension.

adductor muscle 1 Any muscle that causes *adduction. **2** One of the three anterior thigh muscles (adductor brevis, adductor longus, and adductor magnus) which move the thigh towards the midline of the body.

adductor pollicis A muscle with its origin on the capitate (the largest bone of the wrist)

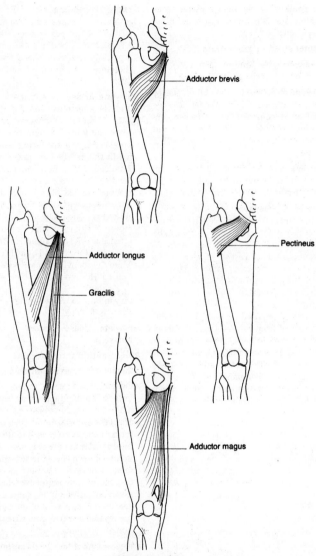

Adductor brevis

Pectineus

Adductor longus

Gracilis

Adductor magus

adductor muscles

and the second and third metacarpals. Its insertion is on the ulnar proximal phalanx of the thumb. Its primary actions are adduction of the carpometacarpal joint of the thumb.

adductors 1 Any muscles which cause adduction. **2** The three anterior thigh muscles (adductor brevis, adductor longus, and adductor magnus) which pull the knees and thighs together. Groin strains are common with these muscles. They become too tight with overuse and often tear when stretched.

adductor strain *See* **groin strain.**

adenohypophysis (anterior pituitary) The anterior part of the pituitary gland.

adenosine diphosphate (ADP) A high-energy compound occurring in all cells. It is the nucleotide (consisting of a nitrogen containing base, adenine, a ribose sugar, and two phosphate groups) from which ATP is formed.

adenosine triphosphatase (ATPase) An enzyme that catalyses the following reversible reaction: ATP + H_2O ↔ ADP + Pi.

adenosine triphosphate (ATP) A high-energy compound found in every cell in the body. It is the only form of energy which can be used directly by a cell for its activities. ATP is a nucleotide consisting of adenine (an organic base), ribose (a pentose sugar), and three phosphate groups. It is formed when ADP is phosphorylated (i.e. when another phosphate group combines with ADP). The energy required for phosphorylation is obtained from the respiration of food. ATP is stored in cells, especially muscle cells. The hydrolytic breakdown of each molecule of ATP to ADP and inorganic phosphate is accompanied by the release of a relatively large amount of free energy (34 kJ at pH 7) which is used to drive

energy-demanding metabolic activities. An active cell requires more than 2 million ATP molecules per second. The store of ATP in a human body is sufficient to satisfy a person's needs for only a few seconds, therefore, the store needs to be continuously replenished.

adenylate kinase An enzyme which catalyses the interconversion of ATP, ADP, and AMP. It forms an enzyme system (the adenylate kinase system) that is able to provide ATP rapidly during intense activity. In the presence of adenylate kinase, 2 molecules of ADP are converted to 1 molecule of ATP and 1 molecule of AMP. The reaction can take place in both directions, but formation of ATP is favoured if there is an excess of free ADP and the AMP is removed, a situation which occurs during intense activity. The amount of free ADP in muscles is limited and quickly consumed when the adenylate kinase system is functioning. This system, therefore, is regarded as a reserve energy system used during very intense exercise or when muscle glycogen is depleted.

adenylate kinase system *See* **adenylate kinase.**

ADH *See* **antidiuretic hormone.**

adherence *See* **exercise adherence.**

adhesion An abnormal union of separate tissues, commonly resulting from inflammation or haemorrhage. Adhesions may affect the synovial membranes of joints or form in and around muscle after a sports injury. *Manipulation is often necessary to breakdown the adhesion and prevent loss of normal function. Many sports doctors advocate aggressive rehabilitation involving early mobilization (e.g., by using continuous passive motion exercises on the injured joint) to minimize the formation of adhesions.

adhesive capsulitis *See* **frozen shoulder.**

adipocyte A cell containing a glistening oil droplet composed almost entirely of *fat. The droplet occupies most of the cell's volume, compressing other components such as the nucleus to one side. Mature adipocytes are among the largest cells of

NH₂

Adenine

H

$$O^- - P - O - P - O - P - O - H_2C$$

Phosphate groups ionized under physiological conditions in the cell

OH   OH
Ribose

adenosine triphosphate

the body. Although they can get plumper by taking up more fat or become more wrinkled by losing fat, they are fully specialized for fat storage and have a restricted ability to divide. The number of fat cells within an adult does not usually change, except when a high percentage of the cells are completely full of fat. However, an appropriate diet and exercise programme can be effective at reducing the size of adipocytes.

adipose tissue Fairly loose connective tissue containing large numbers of fat-storing cells (*see* **adipocyte**) which make up 90 per cent of the tissue. Adipose tissue has a rich blood supply and has a high metabolic activity. It may develop anywhere, but tends to accumulate beneath the skin where it can act as a shock-absorber and insulator. Women tend to have more adipose tissue than men. *See also* **android fat distribution**; **brown fat**; and **gynoid fat distribution**.

adipostat A hypothetical mechanism which works like a thermostat, keeping an individual's amount of body fat within a narrow range despite considerable variations in diet and activity. *See also* **set point theory**.

adiposis *See* liposis.

adolescence The period between childhood and adulthood. Adolescence begins after the secondary sexual characteristics (e.g., pubic hair) appear and continues until complete sexual maturity. It is a period during which bones are still growing and there is a high risk of skeletal injuries. Physical changes are accompanied by important psychological ones relating particularly to the way the adolescent perceives himself or herself (*see* **self-concept**). Parents and others, especially sports coaches and teachers, who work with adolescents must be very sensitive to both the physical and the psychological changes taking place during this period. It is unwise for adolescents to take part in exercises which put undue strain on the growth regions of their bones. This is one reason why they are usually excluded from taking part in long-distance running events, such as the marathon.

adolescent growth spurt Period during adolescence of rapid growth rate, usually expressed as the age of peak height velocity (peak body mass velocity usually occurs some months later). Most girls have their adolescent growth spurt between the age of 12 and 13 years; the growth spurt of most boys occurs between the age of 14 and 15 years. During the growth spurt, young people are particularly prone to sports injuries because a discrepancy between bone matrix formation and bone mineralization diminishes bone strength. In addition, the growth plates are extremely vulnerable to external forces. Repetitive, moderate to high-intensity activities (e.g., distance running and baseball pitching) can easily overload the musculoskeletal system causing injuries such as Osgood–Schlatter disease and little leaguer's elbow.

ADP *See* adenosine diphosphate.

adrenal cortical hormones Hormones secreted by the cortex of the adrenal gland. They include aldosterone, cortisol (hydrocortisol), and testosterone.

adrenal cortex The outer part of the adrenal glands.

adrenal glands Endocrine glands located above each kidney. The inner part of the adrenal gland (the medulla) secretes epinephrine (adrenaline) and norepinephrine (noradrenaline); its activity is controlled by the sympathetic nervous system. Regular endurance training increases the secretory capacity of the adrenal medulla causing 'sports adrenal medulla', characterized by an exaggerated response to various stimuli (e.g., hypoglycaemia, glucagon, and caffeine), and, possibly, an increase in the size of the adrenal medulla. The outer part (cortex) secretes adrenocorticoid hormones; its activity is controlled by adrenocorticotrophic hormone (*see also* **adrenal shock**).

adrenaline (epinephrine) A *hormone secreted by the adrenal medulla. It has wide-ranging effects on muscles, the circulatory system, and carbohydrate metabolism, preparing the body for action or what is commonly referred to as the 'flight or fight' response. Adrenaline increases heart rate, depth and rate of breathing, metabolic rate, and the conversion of glycogen to glucose. It also improves the force of muscle actions and delays the onset of fatigue. Adrenaline is a stimulant on the International Olympic Committee list of *banned substances.

$$OH$$

$$OH - \bigcirc - CH (OH) CH_2 NH CH_3$$

adrenaline

adrenal medulla The central part of the adrenal gland which secretes adrenaline and noradrenaline.

adrenal shock Failure of the *adrenal cortex and reduction of cortical hormone secretion. Lack of aldosterone disrupts the regulation of potassium and sodium ions, and lack of cortisol disrupts the regulation of water and carbohydrate stores. Adrenal shock develops as a result of impairment of blood flow to the adrenal glands. For example, during prolonged physical activity (e.g., a marathon or ultramarathon) when an athlete becomes overheated and dehydrated the blood pressure falls, reducing blood flow to the adrenal cortex. Adrenal shock can be exacerbated by psychological stress and is often associated with a decrease in the effectiveness of the immune system, increasing vulnerability to infections.

adrenal virilism Condition found in females with hyperactive *adrenal glands producing male hormones at a concentration high enough to give rise to male characteristics (see **masculinization**). Compare **testicular feminizing syndrome**.

adrenergic A drug that exerts the same effect as *adrenaline.

adrenergic agonist See **adrenergic stimulant**.

adrenergic antagonist A drug (an alpha blocker or beta blocker) which blocks or inhibits the activity of adrenoceptors.

adrenergic stimulant (adrenergic agonist; sympathomimetic amine): A drug, such as *adrenaline, noradrenaline, and isoprenaline, that stimulates adrenoceptors. Adrenergic stimulants are sometimes called stress hormones because they prepare the body for action in the presence of environmental stressors (e.g., when danger threatens or before a competition). Their effects improve the blood supply to skeletal muscle.

adrenocorticotrophic hormone (ACTH) A hormone secreted by the front lobe of the pituitary gland. It stimulates the secretion of other hormones such as hydrocortisone from the cortex (outer part) of the *adrenal gland. ACTH secretion is increased when a person is in a stressful condition.

adult onset diabetes See **obesity**.

advancement The surgical detachment of a muscle or tendon and its reattachment further forward.

aerobic Applied to conditions or processes occurring in the presence of or requiring oxygen.

aerobic capacity See **maximal oxygen consumption**.

aerobic endurance (aerobic fitness; cardiorespiratory endurance) The capacity to continue prolonged physical activity and withstand *fatigue. The level of aerobic endurance is reflected by the length of time an aerobic exercise involving large muscle groups (e.g., running, cycling, and swimming) can be performed. It depends on the ability of the lungs and heart to take in and transport adequate amounts of oxygen to working muscles, and on the ability of the muscles to extract and use the oxygen efficiently. Most sports scientists regard *maximal oxygen uptake (VO_2 max) as the best objective laboratory indicator of aerobic endurance.

aerobic energy system (oxidative system) The generation of ATP by the breakdown of food with the aid of oxygen. See also **aerobic metabolism**.

aerobic exercise Exercise of relatively low intensity and long duration that uses large muscle groups and depends on the aerobic energy system. As exercise intensity decreases and duration increases, fat becomes more important as a fuel. Aerobic exercise increases the body's demand for oxygen, thereby adding to the workload of the heart and lungs, and raising the heart rate. Such exercise, if performed regularly over a period of months or years, strengthens the cardiovascular system, and helps develop *aerobic endurance. Aerobic exercises include walking, jogging, swimming, cycling, and cross-country skiing.

aerobic fitness *See* aerobic endurance.

aerobic glycolysis *See* glycolysis.

aerobic high intensity training Training designed to improve *maximal oxygen uptake so that an athlete is capable of exercising at high levels of intensity for prolonged periods of time. During aerobic high intensity training, an athlete exercises intermittently at different intensities with an average heart rate of about 180 beats per minute. This type of training is especially suitable for players of sports such as soccer and hockey.

aerobic interval training A form of interval training in which short bouts of moderate- to high-intensity activity lasting from 30 s to 5 min are separated by brief periods of rest (10 to 15 s). The brevity of the rest periods ensures that respiration is mainly aerobic.

aerobic low intensity training Training designed to improve endurance. It consists of exercising either continuously or intermittently with a mean heart rate around 160 beats per minute. Work periods, even in intermittent training, should be longer than 5 minutes.

aerobic metabolism (cellular respiration) A process that uses oxygen to produce energy in the form of ATP. Aerobic metabolism of glucose consists of *glycolysis, the *Krebs cycle, and respiratory chain (including the electron transport system).

aerobic points (Cooper points) A system devised in the 1960s by Dr Kenneth C. Cooper to score the beneficial effects of different aerobic exercises on the heart, lungs, and circulatory system. Each exercise is awarded points dependent on the type of exercise, its frequency, intensity, and duration. For example, a two mile walk completed in under 30 minutes, performed five times a week, scores 25 points; four sessions of aerobic dance classes per week scores 36 points. Dr Cooper proposed that in order to develop cardiovascular fitness a person needs to earn at least 30 aerobic points each week. Cooper's proposition that you have to expend a certain amount of energy to be healthy is generally supported, but the scientific validity of his point system has been questioned.

aerobic power (aerobic work capacity) The maximum amount of energy that can be produced from the aerobic energy system per unit time (i.e. the rate of ATP production by aerobic metabolism). Aerobic power depends on the ability of tissues to use oxygen to breakdown metabolic fuels, and the combined abilities of various systems (pulmonary, cardiac, vascular, and cellular) to transport oxygen from the air to mitochondria. Aerobic power is usually measured in terms of oxygen consumption (*see* **maximal oxygen uptake**).

aerobic respiration *See* aerobic metabolism.

aerobic training Training that improves the cardiorespiratory system and the efficiency of *aerobic metabolism. Aerobic training can be divided into three overlapping types: *aerobic low intensity training, *aerobic high intensity training, and recovery training. The minimum training intensity which will usually result in significant improvements require an oxygen uptake of at least 50–55 per cent maximal oxygen uptake. This corresponds to approximately 70 per cent maximum heart rate. The most effective training intensities are usually between 90–100 per cent maximal oxygen uptake, but sessions of long duration and low intensity can be as effective as those of shorter duration and high intensity. *See also* **aerobic training zone**.

aerobic training adaptations Physiological adaptations associated with regular, vigorous aerobic exercise include: enlargement and strengthening of heart muscle, improving the ability to pump blood; improvement of coronary blood supply, reducing the risk of heart attack; lowering of resting heart rate; lowering of heart rate needed to perform given workload, reducing stress on heart; improvement of lung ventilation; strengthening of respiratory muscles (e.g., intercostals); enhancement of pulmonary blood supply; improvement of ability to extract oxygen from lungs; thickening of articular cartilage and bones with weight-bearing aerobic exercises; increase of plasma volume; increase of total number of red blood cells, improving oxygen transport; increase of high density (beneficial) lipoproteins while low density (harmful) lipoproteins reduced, cholesterol level lowered, and arterial blood pressure lowered, reducing tendency for blood to clot spontaneously; skeletal muscles used during the exercise enlarged and made stronger; increase in the size (but probably not the proportion) of slow-twitch muscle fibres; increase of the total number of capillaries and the number of capillaries per unit area of muscle; muscle glycogen and fat (triglyceride) content increased improving fuel supply; improved ability to utilize fatty acids, sparing muscle glycogen stores; mitochondria size and density increased; myoglobin content increased, improving muscles' ability to use oxygen; mental alertness improved; depression and anxiety reduced; ability to relax and sleep improved; stress tolerance improved; lean-body mass increased; ·metabolic rate increases, reducing tendency to suffer from obesity or diabetes mellitus. Individuals vary in their response to aerobic training, but if performed properly with due regard for individual abilities, it has a positive effect on many components of health and fitness.

aerobic training threshold The minimum intensity of aerobic training below which there is no observable training effect. The aerobic training threshold is usually expressed as a percentage of a person's maximum oxygen uptake or, more conveniently, as the heart rate which corresponds approximately to this percentage. Karvonen suggested the following formula to estimate the heart rate at which the aerobic threshold is reached: THR = 0.7 (max HR − resting HR) + resting HR; where THR is the training heart rate at the aerobic threshold; max HR is the maximum heart rate (assumed to be 220− age); and resting HR is the heart rate at rest.

aerobic training zone The range of training intensities between aerobic training threshold and anaerobic threshold.

aerobic work capacity *See* **aerobic power**.

aerobics 1 A form of *aerobic exercise popularized by Kenneth C. Cooper in the 1960s. He evaluated the demands of particular exercises for oxygen and their subsequent effects on the heart and lungs. He then devised exercise programmes, giving them points according to their duration, frequency, and intensity. To develop cardiovascular fitness, a person is expected to earn at least 30 points per week. **2** A type of aerobic exercise consisting mainly of continuous callisthenics performed to music.

aerodynamic drag force *See* **air resistance**.

aerodynamic force A force acting on a body due to the relative motion of the air and the body.

aerodynamics The mathematical and physical study of forces affecting the motion and control of a body (e.g., a javelin or human body) in the air.

aerofoil (foil) A body shaped so that it can generate lift as a fluid flows over it. A typical aerofoil is the wing of an aeroplane, but projectiles such as javelins also share this property.

aerosol administration 1 The application of a coolant spray from a pressurized can to treat soft tissue injuries. The spray contains volatile compounds which evaporate on contact with the skin surface causing rapid chilling which may reduce inflammation. **2** A method of administering drugs in extremely small liquid or solid particles in a pressurized spray which is inhaled. Aerosol administration is commonly used by asthmatics. It enables a drug, such as salbutamol, to be applied directly to the bronchi and bronchioles, thus reducing the risk of unwanted side-effects which may accompany systemic therapy.

aesthetic activity An activity, such as ice-skating, dance, and gymnastics, which has elements related to pure beauty.

aetiology A branch of medicine dealing with the study of the cause or causes of a disease or injury.

affect An individual's emotional response to a situation. In sport psychology, it is often used synonymously with emotion.

affective characteristics The emotional and temperamental characteristics, such as confidence, which influence an individual's responses to a situation. They also include characteristics such as the desire to learn which are important in acquiring a skill.

affective disorders Disorders of mood or emotions such as overanxiety and depression.

affective response The emotional response to a situation. For example, the feeling of pride and satisfaction a person obtains when winning, or the feeling of disappointment on losing.

affective sport involvement The emotional involvement of an individual in a sport which he or she does not play (e.g., sports fans who experience mood changes when their teams win or lose).

affiliation incentive Any factor that motivates an individual to join a group. Affiliation incentives include opportunities to make friends and to satisfy the need to feel wanted. Much of the success of sports clubs depend on their ability to satisfy the affiliation incentive of their members.

affirmations Statements that promote positive attitudes or thoughts about oneself. Vivid, believable affirmations (e.g., 'I perform well under pressure.') can be effective at improving athletic performance.

aflatoxins Complex organic poisons produced by the fungus *Aspergillus flavus*. The fungus grows on peanuts, wheat, corn, beans, and rice stored for a long time in a moist warm atmosphere. Aflatoxins are suspected carcinogens and may damage the liver if eaten in large amounts.

after discharge The continued contraction of a muscle for a second or more after cessation of the stimulus from an afferent neurone. An afferent neurone has a network of connections with a number of interneurones which transmit impulses along different routes to the motor neurones which serve a muscle. After a strong stimulus, impulses arrive at the neuromuscular junction at different times, resulting in the muscle having a prolonged contraction.

after hyperpolarization The condition of a neurone immediately following an *action potential when the potential difference across the cell surface membrane becomes more negative than the normal resting potential.

age 1 The period of time a person has lived. **2** A period or state of the human life cycle. *See* **actuarial age**; **biological age**; **chronological age**.

ageing process A process that accompnies chronological ageing. Ageing is often associated with degenerative processes which include a reduction in muscle strength, bone weakening (*see* **osteoporosis**), longer reaction times, an increased difficulty in breathing, an increased tendency towards *obesity, and a decrease in both anaerobic capacity and aerobic fitness (*see* **percentage change in maximal aerobic power**). However, since we tend to become more sedentary with age, it is often difficult to differentiate between the natural irreversible deterioration in physiological function that accompanies ageing and the harmful effects of physical inactivity. It is generally agreed that regular physical activity can retard the degenerative processes.

ageism 1 Any process or expression of ideas in which stereotyping of and/or discrimination against people occurs by virtue of their age. Ageism applies particularly to such actions directed against older people, but the term may also be employed to refer to unreasonable discrimination against anyone where this occurs because of the person's chronological age. **2** Values, beliefs, and norms that support the proposition that the value and capability of an individual is determined by the age group to which he or she belongs. Ageism also refers to the practices which support these beliefs and leads to reduced expectations and opportunities for some age groups.

agency In sociology, a human action which is purposive and intentional, and carried out at the volition of the individual or group concerned and not because of constraints imposed by a social structure.

aggregate A collection of individuals with no internal social structure or basis for persistence. *Compare* **group**.

aggression Behaviour intended to harm a person either physically or mentally. It includes physical attacks and verbal abuse. The aggression may be against another person (extropunitive behaviour) or against oneself (intropunitive behaviour). It does not include unintentionally harming another person or doing destructive violence to an inanimate object. *Compare* **assertive behaviour**. *See also* **hostile aggression**; and **instrumental aggression**.

aggression–approval proposition A proposition which suggests that aggressive behaviour and the results of such behaviour become more valuable the more they are rewarded. When an aggressive person receives rewards he or she expects, or does not receive the punishment he or she expects, the person will be more likely to repeat the behaviour.

aggressive rehabilitation Rehabilitation which encourages the early mobilization of injured athletes. Although complete immobilization may be necessary in the initial stages of an injury, prolonged immobilization can result in loss of muscle strength and chronic joint stiffness. Early mobilization, on the other hand, accelerates recovery by promoting tissue healing. It also helps the injured athlete maintain coordination and sports-related motor skills.

agility The ability to change body position rapidly and accurately without losing *balance. It is important in sports and activities in which opponents or obstacles have to be avoided (e.g., slalom events). It is a basic component of physical fitness. Its exact nature has not been determined, but it does depend on muscular power, reaction time, coordination, and dynamic flexibility. *See* **Illinois agility test**.

agility and skill drills An advanced stage of rehabilitation in which an athlete performs basic skills directly related to the sport or activity he or she wishes to resume. The drills are performed progressively from the simple to more complex so that the athlete undergoes a process of progressive motor learning and relearning. *See also* **rehabilitation programme**.

agonal contest A ritualized contest in which an individual or a team attempts to establish physical superiority over the opposition. Agonal contests offer the means of determining social rank, recognizing excellence, and according honour to an individual, an institution or, even, a nation. For example, the success of a national team in a world championship or the Olympic Games is held by many to reflect national character and to serve as an index of moral superiority. All sports are to some extent agonal contests, but the amount of honour won depends on many factors, including the status and ability of the opponents, the importance of the contest to the peer group of the participants, and the value of the prize.

agonist 1 (prime mover) A muscle primarily responsible for a given movement. Some muscles are agonists for more than one action on two or more joints. The *biceps brachii, for example, is an agonist for elbow flexion, radioulnar supination, and several movements of the shoulder joint. **2** A drug that interacts positively with receptors to produce a response in a tissue or organ.

AIDS *See* acquired immune deficiency syndrome.

aiming A skill-orientated ability in which a person aims a body part (e.g., a boxer jabbing with his fist) or a projectile at a target. Aiming underlies tasks where the subject attempts to hit a target with a pencil or stylus using very quick movements. Such tasks have often been used to study motor control.

airfoil *See* aerofoil.

air pollutants Substances, such as carbon monoxide in vehicle exhaust fumes and sulphur dioxide in airborne industrial wastes, which reduce the quality or life-supporting capacity of the environment. High pollution levels adversely affect athletic performances in endurance events, but little is known about the effects of air pollutants on performances in power events.

air resistance (aerodynamic drag force) A frictional force which tends to remove the speed of a body moving through air and cause the body to fall to the ground before it has completed its parabolic flight path. Air resistance increases with speed and lightness of the body. It is also increased by motions, such as the quivering of an arrow, the spinning of a ball, or the flapping of shoe laces, when the motions are in a direction other than that of the whole body. Air resistance is affected by the surface covering and shape of the body (*see* **streamlining**). *See also* **drafting**; **drag**; and **fluid resistance**.

airways Body structures through which air enters and leaves the lungs.

akropodion *See* acropodion.

ala (pl. alae) Wing-like portion of the *ilium. Its thickened margin is called the iliac crest.

alactacid phase The phase immediately after exercise during which extra oxygen

is consumed to restore muscle phosphagen stores (ATP and PC). This phase lasts only a short time (the processes have a half reaction time of about 15 minutes) and requires about 2–3 litres of extra oxygen. *Compare* **lactacid phase**.

alactic anaerobe system *See* ATP–PCr system.

alanine A relatively insoluble amino acid which occurs in two forms: one form (laevorotatory-alanine) is involved in the metabolism of glucose and glycogen; the other form (beta-alanine) is a component of coenzyme A which plays an important role in aerobic metabolism. Alanine production is increased in exercising muscle. Some body-builders and weight-lifters take alanine supplements to increase muscle glycogen levels and improve their muscular endurance and strength-training ability. Alanine, however, is a non-essential amino acid that can be made from other amino acids. A deficiency should not occur in people who eat a well-balanced diet. Research on amino acid supplementation shows no beneficial effects on strength, power, or muscle growth.

albumins Water-soluble, simple globular proteins abundant in body fluids, including blood plasma and synovial fluid. Albumins transport materials and help maintain the osmotic pressure of the blood.

alcohol Any of a large group of organic compounds derived from hydrocarbons in which a hydrogen atom has been replaced by a hydroxyl (-OH) group. The alcohol commonly used in drinks is ethyl alcohol or ethanol (C_2H_5OH), a colourless, tasteless liquid formed during the fermentation of yeast. In medicine, alcohol is used as a solvent and as an antiseptic. As a drink, it is rapidly absorbed into the bloodstream from the buccal cavity and stomach. After absorption, alcohol acts as a depressant of the central nervous system, reducing feelings of *fatigue but also adversely affecting judgement, self-control, and concentration. Reactions are slowed and muscular coordination impaired.

Alcohol is broken down in the liver to acetate, a potential source of fuel for cardiac and skeletal muscle, which has an energy value of about 7 kcalg$_{-1}$. Alcohol interacts harmfully with some drugs, including *antihistamines and many *analgesics. A moderate intake of alcohol may reduce the risk of coronary heart disease, but excessive chronic use may result in cirrhosis of the liver and damage to the kidneys and heart. In sport, alcohol has been used as a mild tranquillizer by archers, and as an energy source for cyclists. However, it interferes with the release of *antidiuretic hormone, causing the body to excrete more urine and increasing the risk of *dehydration when performing in hot environments. In cold environments, alcohol may increase the risk of *hypothermia by causing blood vessels in the skin to dilate. Alcohol is banned from some sports venues (such as Scottish soccer grounds) because of its association with crowd violence. It is not on the International Olympic Committee list of banned substances, but acceptable breath or blood alcohol levels may be set by governing bodies of particular sports and it is *banned in certain sports including the modern pentathlon, fencing, and shooting. It is generally accepted that heavy drinking is not compatible with serious sport participation.

aldosterone A mineralocorticoid hormone secreted by the *adrenal cortex, which regulates salt balance. Aldosterone increases reabsorption of sodium and secretion of potassium by the kidney tubules. It also has an important role in controlling the volume of body fluids. Aldosterone secretion is increased during and after exercise.

alertness Awareness of environmental stimuli and the ability to respond quickly to those stimuli. Alertness is reflected by an increase in electrical activity of the *reticular formation and *cerebral cortex in the brain.

Alexander technique A technique that corrects established defects of posture, particularly with regard to the back when lying, sitting, standing, or walking.

According to its deviser, the Australian therapist F. M. Alexander, the technique promotes relaxation and can help eliminate aches, pains, and other disorders associated with muscle tension and poor posture.

algorithm of reflexes A set of reflexes established in the central nervous system after a period of training which can produce a *movement pattern.

alimentary canal (gut) The tubular passage extending from the mouth to the anus that has regions specialized for ingestion (mouth and buccal cavity), digestion (mainly stomach and small intestine), absorption (mainly the small intestine for food-stuffs and the large intestine for water), and egestion (rectum and anus).

alkalaemia Reduction in the hydrogen ion concentration (pH) in the blood. *See also* **alkalosis**.

alkali A substance that has a high pH (pH>7) when in solution and which tends to neutralize acids.

alkaline excess *See* **base excess**.

alkalinizer A substance, such as sodium bicarbonate, used to boost the alkali reserve artificially. Alkalinizers have also been used by some athletes to avoid drug detection. By raising the pH, they reduce the excretion of metabolic by-products of some stimulant drugs, thereby masking them.

alkali reserve (standard bicarbonate) The amount of alkali available in the body to act as a *buffer, moderating changes in pH. Most of the alkali is in the form of bicarbonate ions. A high alkali reserve is particularly important for those involved in high-intensity activities lasting up to three minutes (e.g., 800 metre run). The bicarbonate ions help to neutralize lactic acid produced during anaerobic respiration. Some athletes boost their alkali reserve artificially by ingesting extra amounts of sodium bicarbonate (a process called bicarbonate loading).

alkaloid A member of a group of nitrogen-containing compounds that include *cocaine, morphine, and *nicotine.

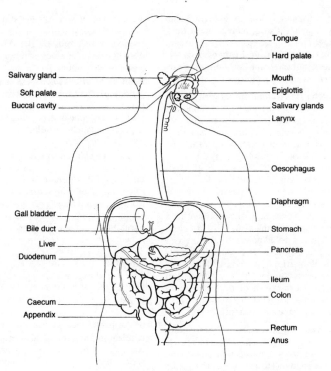

alimentary canal

alkalosis Abnormally high pH in the blood or tissue fluids (pH > 7.45). Excess alkali can make muscles overreact, causing them to go into cramp-like spasms. There are two forms of alkalosis. Respiratory alkalosis usually results from hyperventilation (heavy breathing) which reduces carbon dioxide levels in the body fluids. It can also occur at high altitudes where the air is thin and oxygen levels are low. Metabolic alkalosis often results from ingesting excessive amounts of alkalinizers, or from losing large amounts of acid (for example by, vomiting the acidic stomach contents).

allele (allelomorph) One of two or more different forms of the same gene, only one of which is carried on a single chromosome.

allelomorph *See* **allele**.

allergen A substance, foreign to the body, that provokes an immune response. *See also* **allergy**.

allergic contact dermatitis A skin disorder caused by an allergic reaction to any number of factors, including certain types of sports equipment, the rubber in swimming goggles, the adhesive used in tape and strapping, and deodorants. Symptoms usually develop within a day to a week of contact. They include itching, redness, swelling, and an oozing rash. In all cases of dermatitis, medical advice should be sought to prevent a chronic condition. Treatment may include the application of topical corticosteroids.

allergy An abnormal condition of the skin or mucous membranes resulting from an overzealous immune response and heightened sensitivity to a substance that is, in normal amounts, innocuous to the majority of people. Causes include house dust, fungi, and drugs. Of particular interest in sport is the hypersensitivity of some athletes to adhesive tape (*see* **allergic contact dermatitis**) and **antibiotics**.

allometry The relationship between the rate of growth of one body-part with another part or the whole body. The relationship may be described by allometric equations which have been used to compare athletic abilities and physiological functions of individuals of different size. In Huxley's allometric equation ($\log Y = a - b \log X$), for example, structural variables such as mass or stature, are usually represented in the equation by X, with Y representing a functional variable, such as strength, maximal aerobic power, or another performance measure. The value a represents the allometric constant (unity for isometric growth). The obtained b values are then compared to the theoretical expectancy (e.g., for a geometrical system in which size and shape are constant).

all-or-none law A law stating that certain structures, such as a neurone or a muscle fibre, either responds completely (all) or not at all (none) to a stimulus. There is no partial nerve impulse in a neurone, or partial contraction of a muscle fibre. *Compare* **graded potential**.

alpha-actinin A muscle protein, associated with the Z-line of *sarcomeres, which holds thin filaments in place. Z-lines of slow fibres have more alpha-actinin than fast ones.

alpha blocker (alpha antagonist, alpha adrenoceptor blocker) A drug (e.g., indoramin, phentolamine, phenoxybenzamine, prazosin, and tolazoline) used to treat high blood pressure and other vascular disorders. Alpha blockers inhibit alpha receptors.

alpha motor neurone A large efferent neurone that innervates *extrafusal fibres of striated muscle.

alpha receptor (alpha adrenoceptor) An adrenoceptor which may be either an alpha$_1$ receptor which when stimulated causes vasoconstriction, or an alpha$_2$ - receptor which inhibits the release of noradrenaline from postganglionic sympathetic nerve fibres.

altered state of consciousness A mental condition different from the normal state of being awake. It may be induced by hypnosis, drugs, a peak experience, fatigue, hypoxia, metabolic disorders, and trauma (especially to the head).

alternate aerobic–anaerobic metabolism The type of metabolism required by those taking part in alternate or mixed sports (the majority of team sports, e.g., basketball, soccer, and water polo) in which the energy demands vary in intensity and duration. Participants of alternate sports benefit from having the capacity to produce high levels of muscular power, the capacity for quick recovery after a performance, and the capacity to repeat the same performance after a short time-interval.

alternate and shuttle test A modified shuttle test to evaluate the specific fitness of those who take part in mixed sports requiring high racing speeds and quick recovery. The test consists of nine series of sprints, each consisting of four repetitions over a distance of 9 m (covered therefore four times backwards and forwards). The interval between each series is 20 s. The total time reflects the subject's anaerobic power and the achievement of steady results over the nine series reflects the special aerobic fitness and ability to recover.

alternate sports *See* **alternate aerobic–anaerobic metabolism**.

alternate test A test of alternate aerobic–anaerobic metabolism. It consists of 12 series of jumps, performed with countermovement, with a 20 s rest between one jump and the next, except that between the third and fourth, sixth and seventh, and ninth and tenth jumps, the rest time is 30 s. During the extra rest period, a blood sample may be taken from the ear lobe for *blood lactate analysis. Evaluation is based on height of the jumps, work and power output, and (if blood sample taken) lactate production.

altitude The vertical distance above sea level. Medium altitudes are between 1829 m and 3048 m above sea level; high altitudes are higher than 3048 m above sea level. As altitude increases, the barometric pressure decreases and oxygen partial pressures become lower, reducing *maximal oxygen uptake. In addition, temperature drops at a rate of 1 °C for every 150 m. Maximal oxygen uptake decreases as altitude increases above 1600 m, consequently, both medium and high altitude can adversely affect performance in endurance activities, particularly in those who normally live at sea level. *Short-term anaerobic performance capacity is not adversely affected by medium altitude. On the contrary, the rarified atmosphere can be beneficial to sprinters, throwers, and jumpers. *See also* **altitude acclimatization**; and **altitude training**.

altitude acclimatization Reversible physiological adaptations to high altitudes. Although a number of environmental factors change with altitude, the adaptations are mainly in response to lower oxygen partial pressures. Early adaptations include hyperventilation and increases in submaximal heart rate which raise the *cardiac output. Major long-term adaptations improve the oxygen-carrying capacity of the blood by increasing the haemoglobin content and haematocrit, polycythaemia, and a decrease in plasma volume. Muscles develop more capillaries, and their myoglobin content and 2,3-diphosphoglycerate content increases with altitude. Acclimatization at medium altitudes (greater than 1829 m above sea level) takes about two weeks, but it may take much longer at higher altitudes. Effects persist for about three weeks on return to sea level.

altitude hypoxia Breathlessness and respiratory distress caused by low oxygen partial pressures at high altitudes.

altitude sickness (mountain sickness) Sickness characterized by shortness of breath, fatigue, headache, rapid pulse, loss of appetite, insomnia, and nausea, which occurs at high altitudes due to lack of oxygen. In extreme cases the patient may lose consciousness and, if untreated, altitude sickness can be fatal. Individuals differ in their susceptibility, but nearly everyone suffers at altitudes higher than 4900 m above sea level. Usually, symptoms are lost rapidly on return to lower altitudes. Typically, altitude sickness develops between 6 and 96 h after reaching high altitudes. Some climbers and skiers develop acute altitude sickness when ascending too quickly above 2100 metres. The sickness usually lasts several days. *See also* **high altitude cerebral oedema**; and **high altitude pulmonary oedema**.

altitude training Training undertaken at moderately high altitudes to acquire the benefits of altitude acclimatization and to improve performance in endurance activities. It is used especially by athletes accustomed to low altitude conditions who are going to compete at high altitudes. To be effective, the training must take place 1500 m or higher above sea level and for a period of not less than three weeks, with the first week consisting of light exercise. Training effects are usually lost three to six weeks after living at sea level. Altitude training is used by many athletes to improve performances in endurance events at low altitudes. Opinion is divided as to its effectiveness, but most physiologists believe that it is of little benefit to sea-level competition. Long-term altitude training, over a period of months, can lead to a loss of body weight and a reduction of muscle mass.

altruism Concern for the welfare of others rather than oneself.

alveolar–arterial oxygen partial pressure difference The difference between the partial pressure of oxygen in the *alveolus and the mean arterial pressure of oxygen, measured in mmHg or kPa. It indicates the efficiency of gaseous exchange in the lungs. During heavy exercise, the alveolar–arterial oxygen partial pressure difference increases 2.0 to 2.5 times the resting levels.

alveolar–capillary membrane The membrane separating the *alveolus from the pulmonary capillaries. It is the site of *gaseous exchange in the lungs.

alveolar ventilation The volume of air entering the alveoli for *gaseous exchange. It is usually expressed as volume per minute and is given by the folowing equation: alveolar ventilation = (tidal volume – anatomical dead space) × respiratory frequency.

alveolus A microscopic air-filled sac at the end of the finest divisions of the bronchioles through which gaseous exchange takes place. The wall of an alveolus is one cell thick and lined on the outside with capillaries. Millions of alveoli occur in each lung to provide a very large surface area.

ambient Pertaining to the surrounding environment.

ambivalence A state of experiencing two opposing emotions at the same time. It may be produced by being pulled psychologically in opposite directions by two significant others. For example, a coach may encourage an athlete to win at all costs, while a parent encourages the athlete to believe that taking part and developing good sporting behaviour is the most important consideration.

ambivert An individual who has neither pronounced *introvert or *extrovert characteristics.

ambyopia Poor vision not correctable with lenses. It may be due to an inability to focus with both eyes simultaneously, a condition known as lazy eye.

amenorrhoea Absence of menses (blood flow during the menstrual cycle) for at least 3 months, or less than 2 menstrual cycles in a year. Women over 18 years of age who have never started to menstruate are said to have primary amenorrhoea; those whose normal menstrual function has been lost for months or even years are said to have secondary amenorrhoea. Although its exact cause is not known, secondary amenorrhoea has been linked to stress and low body fat. It is common in middle- and long-distance runners who train intensively, and in athletes of appearance sports and weight-classification sports who restrict their diet. It was once regarded as a harmless variation of the gonadal rhythm since its effects appear to be reversed when training is reduced and food intake increased, and it does not affect long-term fertility (in fact, even amenorrhoeic athletes can become pregnant). However, failure to menstruate for long periods may lead to hormonal alterations, decreasing oestradiol secretions and increasing the risk to stress fractures and osteoporosis. Many questions still remain to be answered about the long-term effects of amenorrhoea on the skeletal integrity of female athletes.

AMI *See* **Athletic Motivation Inventory**.

amine hypothesis The hypothesis that increased secretion of amine neurotransmitters (e.g., norepinephrine, serotonin, and dopamine) is related to improved mental health. Exercise is thought to have a positive effect on psychological mood by stimulating the production of these amines.

amino acids The chemicals which form the building blocks of protein. They have an amine group $(-NH_2)$ and a carboxyl group (-COOH). There are about 80 naturally occurring amino acids, but only about 20 are used in proteins. Some of the amino acids can be obtained only from the diet; these so-called essential amino acids can then be used to manufacture the others. Amino acids may be used as an energy source during endurance activities, but they probably supply no more than 10 per cent of the body's demands. Some amino acids, such as gamma-aminobutyric acid and glutamate function as neurotransmitters, acting as chemical intermediaries during the transmission of nerve impulses. The essential amino acids are histidine (essential for children only), isoleucine, leucine, lysine, methionine, phenylalanine, threonine, tryptophan, and valine. The non-essential amino acids are alanine, arginine, aspartic acid, cysteine, cystine, glutamic acid, glutamine, glycine, hydroxyproline, ornithine, proline, serine, and tyrosine.

amino acid

amino acid supplements (protein supplements) Dietary supplements which come in the form of tablets, capsules, or powders containing a particular concoction of amino acids usually claimed by the manufacturers to have special properties. Most amino acid supplements are sold as anabolic agents to help in body-building; arginine and ornithine, for example, are frequently promoted as 'natural steroids'. Since amino acids are the building blocks of protein, the main component of muscle, many people believe that just by taking extra amino acids they can develop larger muscles. But a muscle grows only in response to extra physical demands placed on it. Excess amino acids not needed for growth or repair of body tissues are broken down and excreted as urea, converted into glucose and used as an energy source, or converted to body fat. Amino acid supplements may be beneficial when there is a natural stimulus to increase muscle bulk, for example during the initial stages of training. There is little support for the claims that amino acid supplements improve strength, power, muscle growth, or work capacity. Most sports nutritionists agree that a normal, healthy person eating a well-balanced diet need never consume amino acids supplements. Over-consumption may lead to health risks. Many amino acids are toxic when taken in excess.

aminophylline A water-soluble drug belonging to the methyl xanthines and related to caffeine. It is a derivative of theophylline and has been used as a bronchodilator to relieve asthmatic attacks. It is not on the International Olympic Committee's list of *banned substances although it can have harmful side-effects on the cardiovascular system.

ammonia A colourless, pungent gas, extremely soluble in water. Ammonia is produced during intense exercise, causing its concentration to be increased in the blood. This may occur when, during aerobic metabolism, muscles generate adenosine triphosphate (ATP) from adenosine diphosphate (ADP) and form adenosine monophosphate (AMP), which is subsequently broken down to inosine monophosphate (IMP) and ammonia.

ammonium salts (smelling salts) A group of salts derived from ammonia. They are used as mild *diuretic drugs and *stimulants. In the past, they have been used to revive an unconscious or dazed semi-conscious athlete, but it is generally agreed that this practice should stop and that ammonium salts should play no role in the treatment of head-injured athletes. Instead, controlled verbal arousal should be used with precautions taken in case of spinal injury until the athlete becomes sufficiently coherent to give a personal assessment of injuries.

amnesia Loss of memory. Amnesia can occur after a blow to the head during a contact or collision sport. The duration of post-traumatic amnesia (the duration of memory loss from the moment of injury to the onset of continuous memory) is used as a clinical measure of the extent of diffuse brain damage. A duration of up to about 10 minutes is quite common. Longer than this probably indicates structural damage. However, it should be recognized that any alteration of consciousness, however transient, is serious and requires a thorough medical investigation.

amortization phase The phase during locomotion in which a limb is being forced to yield prior to the amortization point. The duration of the amortization phase is critical to the efficient contribution of the combined forces from contractile and elastic components of the limb.

amortization point The point during the locomotory movement of a limb (such as that of the take-off leg in a jump) at which an *eccentric action stops prior to a *concentric action.

AMP *See* **adenosine monophosphate.**

amphetamines A group of drugs belonging to the *stimulants banned by the International Olympic Committee. Amphetamines include dextroamphetamine, methamphetamine, methyl phenidate, and phenmetrazine. Although their effects are inconsistent, amphetamines mimic the action of the sympathetic nervous system (hence, they are also known as sympathomimetic amines), acting as powerful stimulants on the central nervous system producing feelings of euphoria, aggression, and alertness which may be achieved at the expense of judgement and self-criticism. They suppress feelings of hunger and are components of some slimming pills. Amphetamines tend to increase metabolic rate, cardiac output, blood pressure, blood glucose levels, and arousal. Claims that they improve athletic performance have not been supported by unequivocal scientific evidence. They are potentially very harmful. Administration may be followed by severe bouts of depression and dependence. Several fatalities have been attributed to the ability of amphetamines to suppress feelings of fatigue, permitting individuals to overexert themselves to the point where they suffer *heat stroke and cardiac failure.

$$NH_2$$
$$H — C — CH_3$$
$$CH_2$$

amphetamine

amphiarthrosis A cartilaginous joint which permits only slight movement; examples are vertebral joints in which *intervertebral discs allow movement, the pubic symphysis, and the sacroiliac joint.

amygdala One of the *basal ganglia in the limbic system of the brain thought to control motivation and emotion. It may also contain the memory of recent events.

anabolic steroids A class of synthetic drugs related in structure and activity to the male hormone *testosterone, but which have less androgenic effects (*compare* **androgenic steroid**). Anabolic steroids are usually taken in tablet form or by intramuscular injection to improve muscle strength, power, and size. They encourage retention of nitrogen, potassium, and phosphate, increase protein synthesis, and decrease amino acid breakdown, but their effects are dose dependent. They may also increase tolerance to hard training by improving tissue repair and delaying fatigue. Doped athletes may also feel stronger, more aggressive, and more confident. Among teenagers and children, the use of anabolic steroids can adversely affect skeletal growth, leading to premature fusion of the *epiphyses. In adults, anabolic steroids may produce psychological changes (e.g., the so-called 'roid rage'), and damage the liver and heart. In males, excessive levels of testosterone may reduce the size of the testes and affect sperm - production. In females, they may cause masculinization. Anabolic steroids are responsible for much drug abuse in sport. They are on the International Olympic Committee list of *banned substances.

anabolism Chemical reactions in the body which synthesize large molecules from smaller ones as in body building, growth, and repair. Anabolism requires energy. It is the constructive form of metabolism. *Compare* **catabolism.**

anaemia A condition in which the amount of haemoglobin in the blood or the number of blood cells is below the normal range for a healthy population of comparable age and sex. The standard varies from country to country, but in women the haemoglobin content is normally greater than 12 grams per decilitre and in men greater than 13.0 grams per decilitre. Anaemia reduces the oxygen carrying capacity of the blood and is characterized by tiredness, shortness of breath, and headaches. *See also* **athletic pseudoanaemia;**

iron-deficiency anaemia; sickle-cell anaemia.

anaerobic Applied to conditions or processes not requiring oxygen; in the absence of oxygen.

anaerobic capacity The total amount of energy obtainable from the anaerobic energy systems (the combined capacity of the ATP–PCr and lactacid systems).

anaerobic capacity test A test of the ability to undertake anaerobic exercise using the ATP–PCr system and *lactic acid system. See also **intermediate anaerobic test**; **long-term anaerobic test**; **short-term anaerobic test**.

anaerobic energy systems Metabolic systems which manufacture ATP without using oxygen. See **ATP–PCr system**; and **lactic acid system**.

anaerobic exercise Exercise usually of short duration and high intensity that uses anaerobic metabolism of carbohydrates (especially muscle glycogen) as the main energy sources. Anaerobic exercises include sprinting, throwing, and weight-lifting.

anaerobic glycolysis (oxygen-independent glycolysis) The incomplete breakdown of carbohydrate to form pyruvic acid. During anaerobic glycolysis, there is a net production of only two molecules of ATP for each molecule of glucose. See also **lactic acid system**.

anaerobic metabolism Cellular respiration that uses glucose as a substrate to produce energy in the form of ATP, without using oxygen. See **ATP–PCr system**; and **lactic acid system**.

anaerobic power The maximum amount of energy that can be generated by the anaerobic energy systems per unit time.

anaerobic power test A test, such as the *Margaria staircase test and the *sargent jump test, which measures explosive power.

anaerobic respiration See anaerobic metabolism.

anaerobic threshold The level of activity at which the *aerobic energy system cannot meet all of the body's demands for ATP. As the intensity of activity increases above the threshold, energy supply becomes increasingly dependent on the anaerobic metabolism. A number of methods have been used to determine anaerobic threshold, including ventilatory breakpoint (see **minute ventilation method**) and *lactate threshold. However, no method is completely satisfactory. The lactate threshold, for example reflects anaerobic threshold under most conditions, but the relationship is not perfect.

anaerobic training Training that improves the efficiency of anaerobic metabolism and which can increase muscular power. Regular anaerobic training increases tolerance to acid–base imbalances during high intensity activity, and improves the ability to recover after the activity. Anaerobic training can be divided into *speed endurance training and *speed training.

anaerobic training adaptations Physiological adaptations associated with regular anaerobic training that require near maximal force production. These adaptations include increased muscular strength and speed of action; improved muscle buffering capacity and greater tolerance of changes of tissue fluid pH during intense activity; and increased activity of enzymes involved in the ATP–PCr energy system and glycolysis. Anaerobic training at speed also improves efficiency of movement.

anaerobic training zone A range of training intensities, commonly taken as being above the *anaerobic threshold, for developing cardiovascular fitness and power using anaerobic exercises.

anaesthetic A substance that produces partial or complete loss of sensation either in a restricted area (regional and local anaesthetics) or in the whole body (general anaesthetic). Use of certain injectable local anaesthetics (e.g., porocaine, xylocaine, and carbocaine, but not cocaine) are permitted by the International Olympic

Committee when medically justified. Details (including diagnosis, dose, and route of administration) must be submitted to the International Olympic Committee Medical Commission. There is no ban on the topical use of local anaesthetics.

analeptic A drug used to stimulate the nervous system and restore consciousness to a patient in a coma or a faint. Analeptics act mainly on the cardiac and respiratory control centres in the brain. They include adrenaline, caffeine, camphor, ephedrine, and strychnine.

analgesia Reduced sensitivity to a normally painful stimulus with no loss of consciousness. Analgesia can be induced by a number of treatments (*see* **acupuncture**, **hypnosis**, and **drugs**).

analgesia system A pain control system in the brain. Opiate substances, such as encephalins and endorphins act on receptors in the system to help reduce pain.

analgesic Drug used as a painkiller. Analgesics are classified into narcotic analgesics (e.g., morphine) and nonnarcotic analgesics (e.g., aspirin and paracetamol).

analogue A drug which differs in minor aspects of molecular structure from its parent drug. Analogues may be synthesized so that they have more potent effects, less side-effects, or are more difficult to detect than the parent drug.

analyser The left cerebral hemisphere of the brain which, in sport, is concerned with learning new skills, correcting flaws in technique, and developing strategy. The term is based on the oversimplified idea that the cerebral hemispheres exhibit a division of labour between the left and right sides. *Compare* **integrator**.

analysis An explanation of a process or phenomenon in terms of its component parts. Analysis of chemicals, such as drugs, involves breaking down the substance in order to determine the type of constituents (qualitative analysis) or the amount of each constituent (quantitative analysis).

analysis of variance (ANOVA) A statistical technique to analyze the total variation of a set of observations as measured by the *variance of the observations multiplied by their number. Analysis of variance is used to determine whether the differences between the means of several sample groups are statistically significant.

anamnesis (case-history) A statement of the past history of a particular person's injuries or diseases. Anamnesis acts as an important starting point in the diagnosis of many sports injuries.

analphylactic shock An immediate overreaction of the immune system to a drug or other agent in an individual who has previously encountered the agent and has produced antibodies to that agent. Anaphylactic shock is characterized by nausea, lowered blood pressure, irregular heart beat, vomiting, and difficult breathing. It may lead to coma or death. *See also* **anaphylaxis**.

anaphylaxis A condition which occurs in individuals who are hypersensitive to some substance (e.g., a bee sting) to which they have an abnormal allergic reaction. Histamine, a powerful *vasodilator, is released from tissues causing either local or widespread reactions. A severe, widespread reaction can be life-threatening. It is characterized by nausea, lowered blood pressure, irregular heart beat, vomiting, and respiratory distress. *See also* **exercise-induced anaphylaxis**.

anastomosis (pl. anastomoses) **1** A union or joining together of blood vessels or other tubular structures. Anastomosis usually refers to the direct connection between arteries, veins, venules, and arterioles without any intervening capillaries. If an anastomosis is present when an artery is blocked with a blood clot, the anastomosis forms a collateral circulation enabling other arteries to take over the blocked artery's work. If no anastomosis is present, the tissue beyond the clot is likely to die. Endurance training may increase anastomoses of coronary arteries, reducing the effects of a coronary thrombosis. **2** A surgical union of two tubular structures, usually by sutures or staples.

anatomical cross-sectional area (ACSA) For an individual muscle, the largest cross-sectional area along the length of that muscle. Cross-sectional areas may be measured non-invasively by magnetic resonance imaging techniques which reconstructs three-dimensional images of individual muscles. *Compare* **physiological cross-sectional area**.

anatomical dead space (respiratory dead space) The volume of air that remains in the respiratory passages (nose, buccal cavity, pharynx, trachea, bronchi, and bronchioles) during ventilation and which does not participate in gaseous exchange. A typical resting value for the anatomical dead space is 150 ml. *See also* **dead space**.

anatomical joint angle The angle through which a joint has to move to take it from the anatomical position to another position. *See also* **strength curve**.

anatomical position (neutral position) Position of an individual standing erect with feet slightly separated, arms hanging relaxed by the side with palms facing forward and thumbs pointed away from the body. The anatomical position is the reference position in the definition of body movement terms.

anatomical reference axis One of three axes that describes human motion. Each axis is oriented perpendicular to one of the three *cardinal planes of motion. *See also* **anteroposterior axis**; **longitudinal axis**; and **transverse axis**.

anatomical reference plane *See also* **cardinal plane**.

anatomical short leg Condition in which one leg is shorter than the other. As with functional short leg, it can cause complications, such as low back pain and joint dysfunctions.

anatomical snuff box The triangular area formed between the thumb and index finger. When the thumb is extended, it is defined laterally by the raised tendons of the abductor pollicis longus and the extensor pollicis brevis, and medially by the extensor pollicis longus.

anatomical task analysis The analysis of the role of different muscle groups in a specific movement or motor skill.

anatomy A branch of science dealing with the form and arrangement of body parts.

anchored racket exercises Controlled resistance exercises of racket stroke motions performed with a racket attached by an elastic band to a solid object. These exercises often form part of the rehabilitation programme for injured racket players.

anconeus Short, triangular arm muscle closely associated with the distal end of the *triceps brachii on the posterior surface of the humerus. Its origin is on the lateral epicondyle of the humerus, and its insertion is on the lateral aspect of the olecranon process and posterior ulna. The anconeus abducts the ulna during forearm pronation and it acts as a *synergist of the triceps brachii during elbow extension.

androcentrism A tendency towards male bias in institutions or a tendency to disregard the female contribution to society and culture.

androgen Any substance, such as testosterone and some steroid drugs, which promotes the development of male secondary sexual characteristics.

androgenic Pertaining to an androgen.

androgenic steroid A *steroid drug having a strong masculinizing effect (*see* **masculinization**).

androgenital syndrome *See* **masculinization**.

androgyny A category derived from *Personal Attribute Questionnaires in which subjects are scored according to their levels of masculinity and femininity. Androgynous individuals have high scores for both *masculinity and *femininity.

android fat distribution The distribution of adipose tissue mainly within and around the abdominal cavity. When excess fat is distributed in this way it can lead to 'apple-shaped' obesity. It is far more common in males than females. Regardless of the level of obesity, this type of fat storage is associated with an increased risk of diabetes and heart disease. *Compare* **gynoid fat distribution**.

androstane A *steroid drug closely related to *testosterone. The structure of androstane is used as a reference when naming compounds closely related to or derived from testosterone.

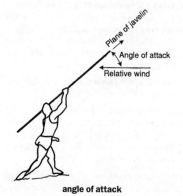

androstane

aneurine *See* **vitamin B$_1$**.

ANF *See* **atrial natriuretic factor**.

anger self-report test A questionnaire that uses a Likert-type scale to yield separate scores for awareness of anger, expression of anger, guilt, condemnation of anger, and mistrust.

angina pectoris A pain in the chest which sometimes extends down the left arm. It is induced by an increase in physical exertion and relieved by rest. The pain usually lasts about 15 minutes. Angina results from an inadequate oxygen supply to heart muscle and is a symptom of *coronary artery disease. A controlled programme of physical activity can benefit those with angina, provided it is performed under medical supervision and is at a safe level. The appropriate level is usually determined by an exercise stress test.

angiotensin A protein derived from a plasma protein and released by the action of *renin from the kidneys. It increases the output of *aldosterone from the adrenal cortex. It can also cause blood vessels to constrict thus raising blood pressure.

angle The space between two intersecting lines or planes. It is measured in degrees or radians.

angle of approach 1 The angle, with reference to the horizontal plane, between the paths taken by two bodies before they collide. *Compare* **angle of incidence**. **2** The direction of approach of an athlete about to perform a jump. For high-jumpers, the recommended angle of approach is about 20–30°. An angled approach (that is, one which is not at right angles to the bar) has the advantage of allowing the free leg to swing through a great range of movement at take-off, and enables the jumper to throw a body-part over the bar before the *centre of gravity reaches its maximum height. At very acute angles, the effective spring may be reduced and the jumper travels too far along the bar, increasing the risk of knocking off the bar.

angle of attack The angle between the primary axis (usually the longitudinal axis) of a body moving through a fluid and the direction of fluid flow. The angle of attack affects both lift and drag. No angle of attack combines maximum lift and minimum drag. A zero angle produces minimum drag but zero lift. Lift is increased as the angle of attack increases until a critical angle is reached when drag exceeds lift and the object stalls (*see* **stall angle**). *See also* **lift:drag ratio**.

angle of attack

angle of entry The angle between the path of a body before impact and the surface with which it collides. Theoretically, it equals the *angle of rebound.

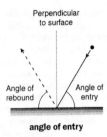

angle of entry

angle of fibre pinnation The angle between the line of orientation of muscle fibres and the line of muscle action (i.e. the line of pull of the tendon). *See also* **physiological cross-sectional area**.

angle of force application *See* **muscle force**.

angle of gait During locomotion, the angle formed between a line drawn from the midpoint of the calcaneus (heel bone) to the midpoint of the second toe of the same foot, and the line of direction of movement.

angle of impact The angle between the tangent to the flight path of a projectile at the point of impact, and the plane tangent to the struck surface at the point of impact.

angle of incidence For colliding bodies, the angle formed by the direction in which a body is travelling before impact with a surface, and the line perpendicular to that surface at the point of impact. *Compare* **angle of reflection**.

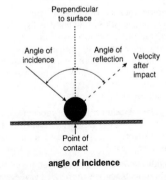

angle of incidence

angle of projection *See* **angle of release**.

angle of pull The angle formed between the line of pull of a muscle and the longitudinal axis of the bone on which the muscle is acting. The line of pull is usually indicated by the joint angle. It affects the strength of muscle action: at only certain angles of pull can a muscle exert maximal tension. Variable resistance exercise machines compensate for variations in muscular tension at different joint angles.

angle of rebound The horizontal angle between the surface with which a body collides and the path of rebound. It is theoretically equal to the *angle of entry.

angle of reflection For colliding bodies, the angle that the direction of velocity makes with the perpendicular to the surface at the point of impact. When applied to the behaviour of a ball, the angle formed by the direction in which the ball is travelling after impact with a surface, and the line perpendicular to that surface at the point of impact. The angle of reflection is equal to the angle of incidence.

angle of release (angle of projection; angle of take-off) The angle, relative to the ground, at which a body is projected into the air. The angle of release is an important factor affecting the flight path of a projectile. For any given speed of release, the angle of release which produces maximum horizontal displacement is 45°, assuming a constant relative projection height, and that there is no spin or air resistance. In sport, the best angles of release

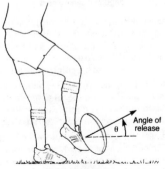

angle of release

are usually between 35° and 45° because of aerodynamic effects.

angle of stall *See* stall angle.

angle of take-off *See* angle of release.

angular acceleration The rate at which angular velocity changes with respect to time. Angular acceleration = (final angular velocity – initial angular velocity)/ time.

angular displacement The difference between the initial and final angular position of a moving body. It is measured in *radians. Angular displacement has both magnitude and direction. Conventionally, clockwise movements are described as positive (+) and anticlockwise movements as negative (−). Angular displacements of human body segments also usually indicate the type of joint movement (e.g., flexion or extension).

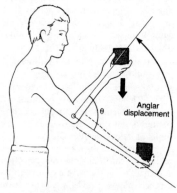

θ   Anglar displacement

angular displacement

angular distance 1 The sum of all the angular changes that occur during the rotation of a body. **2** The distance between two bodies measured in terms of the angle subtended by them at the point of observation.

angular impulse A change in *angular momentum of a system equal to the product of *torque and the time interval during which the torque acts. *See also* **impulse**.

angular momentum A measure of the *angular motion that a particular body possesses. It is the product of the *moment of inertia of a rotating body, or a system of

bodies, about the axis of rotation and the angular velocity about that axis (i.e. angular momentum = moment of inertia × angular velocity, measured in kgm^2.s^{-1}). It is a vector quantity, possessing both magnitude and direction. The angular momentum of a system tends to remain constant (*see* **conservation of angular momentum**), therefore, if the moment of inertia is changed, the rate of rotation, indicated by the angular velocity, also changes. Angular momentum is an important concept for analysing turning movements in sport.

angular motion Rotation of a body or body part about a fixed point or line in space (the axis of rotation) so that all parts of the body travel through the same angle, in the same direction, in the same time. The axis of rotation may be internal or external (i.e. it may or may not pass through the body itself. *Compare* **linear motion**.

angular movement A movement which increases or decreases the angle between two bones. An angular movement can occur in any plane and includes *flexion, *extension, *abduction, *adduction, and *circumduction.

angular speed A measure of how fast a rotating body is changing its angular position. The average angular speed (w) is obtained by dividing the *angular distance through which the body rotates by the time taken: $w = θ/t$, where $θ$ = angular distance, and t = time taken in seconds.

angular velocity The rate of *angular displacement of rotating body in a specified direction (either clockwise or anticlockwise as determined by the *right-hand thumb rule). Angular velocity is measured in degrees, radians, or revolutions per unit time. Average angular velocity = angular distance/time.

angular vibration A form of motion which occurs along the arc of a circle, such as the motion of a gymnast during a giant swing on a high-bar.

angulus inferior The inferior angle of the shoulder blade. It is the origin of the *teres major muscle.

anisotropic Applied to a material, such as bone, that exhibits different mechanical properties in response to forces acting on it from different directions.

anhydrosis Absence or an abnormally low level of sweating.

animal starch *See* glycogen.

ankle Region of the lower limb which includes three joints: that between the tibia and fibula (distal tibiofibular joint), the tibia and talus (tibiotalar joint), and the fibula and talus (fibulotalar joint). All three articulations are enclosed in a *joint capsule. Most motion is about the tibiotalar hinge joint. The ankle is supported by a number of strong ligaments.

ankle extension *See* plantar flexion.

ankle flexion *See* dorsiflexion.

ankle fracture A crack, break, or complete shattering of a bone in the ankle. It usually involves the bottom end of the fibula when the athlete rolls over on the ankle. Signs and symptoms are similar to an ankle sprain. Confirmation that a swollen, painful ankle is fractured often requires an X-ray examination. Treatment will depend on the severity of the fracture. A splint may be applied if there is no displacement, but surgical replacement and fixing of the bones may be necessary if there is displacement. Recovery time varies, but it usually takes at least 4 months before an athlete can return to full activity.

ankle injuries Ankle injuries are the single most common sports injury. The ankle is particularly susceptible to sports injuries since the stresses and strains of balancing, checking, turning, and running are all focused there. When diagnosing an ankle injury, it is important to distinguish between injuries to the *Achilles tendon and other tendons, dislocation, sprains, and fractures. Tendinitis is typically of gradual onset and is usually precipitated by an increase in training. Pain and swelling is usually localized. Sprains, involving disruption of the medial and/or lateral ligaments, are the most common ankle injury. They are usually caused by a single trau-

matic event, for example, when the foot rolls over on the outside of the ankle. Fractures are also associated with a single event. They may produce an obvious deformity of the ankle with displacement of the foot in relation to the leg. Swelling associated with tenderness over the bone also indicates a fracture, requiring referral to hospital and an X-ray examination. Overuse injuries in the ankle include *stress fractures to the distal tibial bone, the tarsals, and the fibula. Stress fractures are associated with a gradual onset of pain accompanied by tenderness, but little swelling or bruising.

ankle instability A predisposition for fractures, dislocations, and sprains in the ankle. Chronic instability is thought to be due to repeated injuries stretching the ligaments, weakening muscles, compromising proprioception, and impairing coordination. The ankle becomes lax and 'gives way' more easily. To improve stability after an ankle injury, rehabilitation should include exercises which strengthen the muscles of the lower leg, and training on an unstable surface, such as a wobble board, to regain proprioception and coordination.

ankle joint mortice The articular surface of the ankle joint formed by the tibia and fibula engaging with the talus.

ankle sprain Disruption of the medial and/or lateral ligaments in the ankle. An ankle sprain usually occurs when the foot rolls over on the outside of the ankle. When this happens, the ligament most commonly damaged is the anterior talofibular ligament. In many cases, the calcaneofibular ligament is disrupted at the same time. Ankle fractures are caused by the same type of event that can cause a sprain. Any ankle that is severely swollen and painful should be X-rayed to rule out a fracture. The main treatment for an ankle sprain is rest, ice, compression, and elevation (*see* **RICE**). Modern rehabilitation techniques involve an aggressive approach which emphasizes early mobilization of the joint (for example, by wearing a splint that prevents the ankle from rolling over, but allows up and down movements) to accelerate recovery. *See also* **sprain**.

ankylosing spondylitis A back disorder in which the vertebrae become squared and connected by fibrous tissue causing the spine to become rigid (known as bamboo spine). Ankylosing spondylitis usually begins in the sacroiliac joints and progresses up the spine. It is a disease which mainly affects men between 20 and 40 years. It is characterized in the early stages by low back pain (especially morning stiffness) which is relieved by exercise and non-steroidal anti-inflammatory drugs, and is aggravated by rest. Physiotherapy combined with good posture constitutes an essential part of the treatment.

ankylosis Loss of movement in a joint, usually from *arthritis but also from sports injuries such as fractures which involve joint surfaces. During healing of the fracture, the moving parts may fuse with the broken parts. Prolonged immobility may also cause ankylosis.

annulus fibrosus The thick outer ring of fibrous cartilage that forms the external surface of an intervertebral disc. The annulus fibrosus is composed of bands of collagen fibres arranged in such a way that they are more sensitive to rotational forces than compression, shear, or tension.

anomie A situation, affecting individuals or society, in which a lack of moral or social direction leads to a loosening of the moral framework which governs that individual or society.

anorexia nervosa An eating disorder (usually abbreviated as anorexia, and sometimes called self-starvation syndrome) characterized by loss of appetite and desire for food, a refusal to maintain body weight over minimal weight for age and height, an intense fear of becoming fat or gaining weight, a distorted body image, and amenorrhoea. A persistent anorexic may suffer serious medical complications and the condition can be fatal. Anorexia nervosa occurs in males and females, but is most frequent in adolescent girls. Gymnasts, cheerleaders, and dancers may be particularly prone to anorexia because of the pressures on them to remain slim. The illness requires medical treatment and may respond to psychotherapy. *See also* **eating disorder**.

anorexiant drug (anorectic agent) A drug that reduces the appetite through an action on the central nervous system. Anorexiants, such as *amphetamines and other sympathomimetic amines, are sometimes included in slimming tablets. They should be used only under strict medical supervision (dexfenfluramine has been used successfully as an anorexiant to treat obesity).

ANOVA *See* **analysis of variance**.

anoxia A state in which there is no supply of oxygen to body tissues. *Compare* **hypoxia**.

anoxic Applied to conditions in which there is no oxygen.

anserine bursa A *bursa in the lower limb which lies deep to the pes anserinus (combined tendons of the sartorius, gracilis, and semitendinosus).

anserine bursitis Inflammation of the anserine bursa. The bursitis may result from overuse and cause a nagging ache on the medial aspect of the knee. Treatment is with localized anti-inflammatories.

antagonist 1 A muscle that opposes an agonist (prime mover) for a given movement. Antagonists play a protective role, preventing overstretching of the agonist. They also help to control a movement by slowing or stopping the action of the agonist. The opposing action between agonists and antagonists produces muscle tone. **2** A drug that interacts negatively with receptor sites (for example, at neuromuscular junctions) to inhibit a response in a tissue or organ.

antagonist co-contraction The simultaneous contraction of *antagonists and *agonists (prime movers) during the performance of a movement. It is often assumed that antagonists are inhibited during a movement (*see* **reciprocal inhibition**), but antagonist co-contraction is quite common during strong and/or rapid movements, and when precise movements are required. Antagonist co-contraction would appear to be counterproductive, especially for strength tasks. However, the ability of antagonist co-contraction to limit, by *reciprocal inhibition, the action of agonists may be a protective mechanism in activities involving strong or rapid contractions. Antagonist co-contraction may also contribute to joint stability during forceful movements.

antebrachial In anatomy, pertaining to the forearm.

antebrachium *See* **forearm**.

antecubital Pertaining to the front (anterior) of the elbow.

anterioposterior plane *See* **sagittal plane**.

anterior (ventral) The front of a person, organ, or part of a body. *See also* **directional terms**.

anterior apprehension test A clinical test for assessing instability of a painful shoulder. The problem shoulder of a supine or sitting patient is passively abducted and rotated then fully stressed, while the examiner studies the patient's face for apprehension and examines the shoulder muscle for muscle spasm. The normal shoulder is manipulated in the same way and the two sides compared to detect loss of passive movement. The test needs to be performed carefully by an expert because of the danger of provoking an anterior dislocation in a very unstable shoulder.

anterior compartment A muscle compartment of the lower leg which contains the tibialis anterior, extensor digitorum longus, external hallucis longus, and peroneus tertius muscles.

anterior compartment syndrome (anterior tibial syndrome) A potentially dangerous overuse injury of the lower leg characterized by feelings of pressure or severe pain and burning in the shins during exercise. The symptoms abate during rest. Its exact cause is uncertain, but it probably results from muscle hypertrophy. The anterior tibial compartment is bounded medially by the tibia, laterally by the fibula,

posteriorly by the posterior interosseous membrane, and anteriorly by the deep fascia. All of these are relatively inflexible structures. During exercise, increased blood flow raises the pressure in the compartment, pressing muscles and other internal structures against the compartment walls; this can lead to ischaemia. Anterior compartment syndrome may require radical treatment: cessation of activity, elevation, compression (bandages and massage), and anti-inflammatory and diuretic drugs to increase urine flow and reduce swelling. Unless the condition is managed properly, it can deteriorate and become so severe that pressure in the compartment permanently damages nerves. Surgery may be necessary to divide muscle fascia and give the enlarged muscle more space. Surgery may also be required in cases of anterior compartment syndrome resulting from heavy bleeding inside the muscles caused by a traumatic accident (e.g., a fracture or when the leg is severely bruised after a kick).

anterior cruciate ligament *See* **cruciate ligament**.

anterior drawer test A clinical test commonly used to determine ligamentous laxity in a sprained ankle or knee. When examining the ankle, the tibia and fibula are stabilized with one hand while the other hand, holding the foot in 20° plantar flexion, applies a posterior to anterior force in an attempt to move the talus forward in the ankle mortice. The amount of movement reflects the degree of injury to the ligaments. A similar procedure is used to assess the degree of instability of the tibia on the femur associated with a knee injury. The test is performed at 90° knee flexion with gentle pressure behind the tibial plateau to draw the tibia forward on the femur.

anterior fascial compartment of the forearm An anatomical compartment in the forearm which contains muscles acting on the wrist and fingers. The muscles are the brachioradialis, flexor carpi radialis, flexor carpi ulnaris, flexor digitorum profundis, flexor digoitorum superficialis, flexor pollicis longus, pronator quadratus, and the pronator teres.

anterior horn of spinal cord Area of *grey matter in the spinal cord containing bundles of motor neurones.

anterior pituitary See adenohypophysis.

anterior–posterior chest depth In *anthropometry, the depth of the chest at the mesosternale level (an anatomical landmark on the *sternum).

anterior–posterior plane See sagittal plane.

anterior superior iliac spine A blunt process on the anterior aspect of the *iliac crest. It is an important anatomical landmark which can be felt easily through the skin and may be visible.

anterior talofibular ligament The external lateral *ligament of the ankle, between the *fibula and *talus. It prevents the foot from slipping forward on the tibia. It is the most commonly damaged ligament in the ankle.

anterior tibial syndrome See anterior compartment syndrome.

anteroposterior axis See sagittal axis.

anthropometer An instrument for measuring the dimensions of the human body.

anthropometric tape A special nonextensible but flexible tape for the very accurate measurement of parts of the human body.

anthropometry The measurement of the size and proportions of the human body and its different parts. Exact anthropometrical studies have identified ideal values for the body dimensions of athletes in different sports. However, athletes who deviate from the ideal are still able to excel in competitions because factors other than physical attributes affect athletic performance.

antibiotic A substance that inhibits the growth of microorganisms or kills them. The best-known is penicillin, originally obtained from the fungal mould Penicillium notatum. It kills some bacteria by preventing cell-wall synthesis. Some antibiotics (e.g., ciprofloxacin) have been used as a prophylactic treatment of traveller's diarrhoea by elite athletes travelling abroad to important competitions, but physicians are loath to encourage the widespread use of antibiotics for fear of the development of resistant microorganisms.

antibody A type of protein formed in the body that attacks foreign substances. Antibodies are produced by B-lymphocytes, usually in response to specific antigens. Antibodies inactivate viruses, and mark foreign cells and cancer cells so that they can be eliminated by other cells of the immune system.

antibruise cream A cream containing an anti-inflammatory drug to reduce inflammation. Most antibruise creams are not very effective.

anticholinergic A drug, such as *atropine, that inhibits the function of cholinergic neurones (e.g., neurones in the parasympathetic nervous system, and motor neurones supplying skeletal muscle) by blocking the action of acetylcholine. Anticholinergics are used to treat stomach ulcers and gastritis. They can cause temporary visual impairment, reducing the ability to judge distances which can be a serious disadvantage in many sports.

anticipation The ability to look forward and judge correctly what is going to happen next. Anticipation is a skill; thus a sportsperson can learn what to anticipate team mates or opponents are about to do in certain situations. See also **elective attention**; **perceptual anticipation**; and **receptor anticipation**.

anticipatory socialization A process in which an individual tries to change his or her social behaviour in the expectation of joining, and being accepted by, another social group which may or may not have a higher social status or class than that which the individual currently occupies. See also **socialization**

antidiuretic hormone (ADH) A hormone produced in the *hypothalamus and secreted by the posterior pituitary gland. ADH stimulates reabsorption of water through the distal convoluted tubules and collecting ducts of the kidney, resulting in less water being excreted in the urine, thus conserving water. Intense exercise is usually associated with an increase in ADH secretion so that plasma volume levels may be maintained, minimizing the risk of *dehydration during periods of heavy sweating.

antigen A substance (usually a protein or carbohydrate) that is identified by cells in the immune system as being foreign to the body, and which induces an *immune response.

antigravity muscle A muscle which acts, often through the *stretch reflex, to counterbalance the pull of gravity and to maintain an upright posture. Many antigravity muscles have a high proportion of slow-twitch muscle fibres and are often called tonic muscles.

antihaemorrhagic vitamin See vitamin K.

antihistamine A drug which counteracts the effects of *histamine and relieves the symptoms of some allergic reactions, such as hay fever, but not others, such as asthma. According to the International Olympic Committee's 1993 treatment guidelines, antihistamines for treatment of hayfever are permitted for use by athletes. However, it is recommended to use only preparations which are associated with a low incidence of sedation.

antihypertensive A drug reducing blood pressure and used to treat *hypertension. Beta blockers are antihypertensives.

anti-inflammatory A drug which reduces a tissue's inflammation response. Anti-inflammatories include *nonsteroidal anti-inflammatory drugs, enzymes (e.g., *hyaluronidase and heparinoid ointment), and *steroids.

antinaturalism In sociology, an approach to analysis opposed to the sole use of models drawn from the physical sciences to explain or study human social actions.

antioxidant A compound, usually organic, that prevents or retards oxidation by molecular oxygen of materials such as food. Some antioxidants, such as *beta carotene, *selenium, and *vitamin C, may provide some protection against cancer because they neutralize *free radicals.

antipsychotic A drug, such as *dopamine, which reduces *aggression.

antipyretic A drug, such as *acetylsalicylic acid (aspirin), which can reduce an elevated body temperature.

antirachitic factor See **vitamin D**.

antiseptic A substance that counteracts putrefaction. Antiseptics are usually applied to the body to prevent infection of wounds.

antispasmodic A drug which relieves *spasms of *smooth muscle.

antispastic A drug which relieves *spasms of striated or skeletal muscle.

antisterility factor See **vitamin E**.

antithrombin A substance in the blood plasma that inhibits *coagulation by inactivating thrombin.

antitussive A drug which suppresses coughing either by a local soothing action or b y depressing the cough centre in the central nervous system. Great care must be taken by athletes when purchasing a cough or cold remedy because many contain antitussives, such as *sympathomimetic amines and *narcotic analgesics, which are on the International Olympic Committee list of *banned substances.

anxiety A subjective feeling of apprehension and heightened physiological tension. The term is often used synonymously with *arousal, but anxiety is usually restricted to high arousal states which produce feelings of discomfort. The condition is closely associated with the concept of fear, but is more a feeling of what *might* happen rather than a response to an obvious fear-provoking situation. Anxiety can be viewed as an enduring personality trait (*see* **trait anxiety**) and also as a temporary state (*see* **state anxiety**). Anxiety in sport may be affected by the *objective competitive situation and the *subjective competitive situation. Generally a high level of pre-competitive anxiety depresses the level of performance by its affects on selectivity and/or the intensity of attention. The detrimental effect may be due to *cognitive state anxiety (also known as task irrelevant cognitive activity or tica) impairing a person's ability to discriminate between relevant and irrelevant information, resulting in the person wasting time doing irrelevant tasks. There is evidence that regular exercise may reduce anxiety levels.

anxiety blocking *See* **relaxation methods**.

anxiety hierarchy A person's ranking of a class of situations from least to most anxiety-producing, which may then be used as a basis of systematic *desensitization.

anxiety-prone athlete An athlete who is highly susceptible to anxiety and has a predisposition towards responding to competitive situations with elevated *state anxiety.

anxiety–stress spiral The downward-spiral effect of *anxiety causing poor performance which results in even more anxiety. The anxiety–stress spiral can be reversed by reducing anxiety and tension, for example, by using *relaxation procedures.

anxiolytic A drug that reduces *anxiety.

aorta The major *artery in the body. It carries blood from the left ventricle of the heart.

aortic body A receptor area in the wall of the aortic arch near the heart, sensitive to levels of carbon dioxide, oxygen, and pH in the blood. Information from the aortic body is conveyed by sensory neurones to the *respiratory centre.

aortic valve Semilunar valve that prevents backflow of blood from the aorta to the left ventricle of the heart.

apartheid An institutionalized discriminatory system of restricted contact between races, as occurred in the Republic of South Africa when the population was separated and defined by law into 'whites', 'blacks', 'coloured', and 'mixed racial'. This separation was reflected in restrictions on sport participation.

apex The highest point in the trajectory of a projectile.

Apley test A test used to assess a knee injury. With the patient lying in the prone position and the thigh firmly anchored, the knee is flexed to 90°. Using the patient's foot as a lever, the lower leg is rotated internally and externally, first with distraction and then with compression. Pain on distraction suggests ligamentous injury: pain on compression or 'grinding' indicates a meniscus tear.

apnoea Cessation of the breathing impulse (e.g., through hyperventilation).

apneusis Condition characterized by prolonged inspiratory spasms.

apneustic centre *See* **inspiratory centre**.

apocrine gland *See* **sweat gland**.

aponeurosis flattened ribbon-shaped or sheet-like tendinous connective tissue which replaces a *tendon in muscles which are flat and have a wide attachment area.

apophyseal joint A *synovial joint between the arches of vertebrae. Such joints are not supplied with nerves therefore an injury may provide no warning pain and the damage may go unnoticed.

apophysis A prominent process projecting from the surface of a bone upon which it has never been able to move, and from which it has never been separated (*compare* **epiphysis**). Apophyses often act as attachment sites for tendons.

apophysitis Inflammation of an *apophysis. Common sites of apophysitis are the calcaneus (*see* **Sever–Haglund disease**) and the tibial tubercle at the site of the patellar tendon attachment (*see* **Osgood–Schlatter disease**).

apophysitis calcanei *See* **Sever–Haglund disease**.

apoplexy *See* **stroke**.

appendicular skeleton The bones of the limbs and limb girdles attached to the *axial skeleton.

apperception The perception of a situation in terms of past experience rather than in terms of the stimuli which are immediately present. In sport, apperceiving may result, for example, in a teamplayer misreading a situation and making inappropriate anticipatory movements.

appetite A psychological desire to eat. Unlike hunger, it is probably a learned response associated with pleasant-tasting and satisfying foods. It is an agreeable sensation undoubtedly necessary for good digestion, and is accompanied by secretion of saliva and digestive juices. It also provides the desire to eat enough food to maintain the body and supply it with sufficient energy to carry out its functions. However, as with other body functions, disorders of appetite occur. Excessive appetite can lead to *obesity, while a chronic diminished appetite is a sign of many illnesses and may be a manifestation of *stress. *See also* **amphetamines; anorexia nervosa**; and **bulimia**.

applicability The degree to which experimental data acquired by a *naturalistic approach may be applied to other studies and situations.

applied sport psychology A branch of sport psychology. It focuses on identifying and understanding psychological theories so that they can be applied to sport and exercise to enhance the performance and personal development of athletes and other sport participants. *Compare* **academic sport psychology**.

appositional growth Process by which bones increase in thickness rather than length.

apprehension test A test used to diagnose some sports injuries. It involves passively manipulating an injured joint into a particular position and examining the patient for signs of apprehension. *See also* **anterior apprehension test**.

approach–approach conflict A situation in which an individual is confronted with a choice between equally attractive alternatives. *Compare* **approach-avoidance conflict**.

approach–avoidance conflict A situation in which an individual is confronted with a single object or event which has both attractive and aversive features. When two or more such objects or events are involved, the situation is called double approach–avoidance conflict.

approximations, method of A procedure in *operant conditioning, which may be adopted as a coaching strategy, by which an individual learns a certain behaviour in a step-by-step manner, each step involving a response slightly more complex than the one preceding it. The correct behaviour at each step is reinforced until that step is mastered, then the next step which is still closer to the final criterion is reinforced, and so on. *See* **learning methods**.

apraxia Disorder of the *cerebral cortex which results in an inability to make precise skilled movements.

aptitude The capacity to learn readily and to achieve a high level of skill in a specific area, such as horseriding, football, or gymnastics. Aptitude refers to an individual's potential rather than actual accomplishment. *See also* **ability**.

arachidonic acid A 20-carbon, straight-chained, polyunsaturated fatty acid formed from *linoleic acid. Arachidonic acid is found in low concentration in free form throughout the body, but most of the acid occurs as a form bound with phospholipids on cell membranes. Following an injury, arachidonic acid is released from damaged cells. Biologically active substances (e.g., *leukotrienes and *prostaglandins) involved in the inflammation response are derived from it.

arc, flattening of A movement pattern of the arm which improves accuracy when throwing or hitting a projectile. It involves flattening the centre of the arc of the curve in which the arm is travelling and in the direction in which the projectile is to follow.

arches Three curved structures, arch-like in profile, which span the foot. The three arches (a medial longitudinal and a lateral longitudinal arch, and an anterior transverse arch) are formed by the tarsal and metatarsal bones. Together the arches form a half-dome shape which is essential for efficient load-bearing and locomotion. The arches distribute about half our standing and walking weight to the heel-bones and half to the heads of the metatarsals. The shape is maintained by the combined action of foot-bones, the *plantar fascia, strong ligaments, and the tension of some muscles. Healthy arches reduce the energy cost of walking and running by storing mechanical energy in their elastic structures during the weight-bearing phases and releasing the energy in the push-off phase.

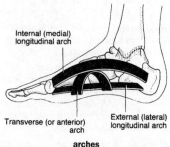

Internal (medial) longitudinal arch

Transverse (or anterior) arch

External (lateral) longitudinal arch

arches

Archimedes' principle A physical principle which states that a body wholly or partly submerged in a fluid is buoyed up by a force equal to the weight of the displaced fluid.

archival research Research based on recorded information; for example, research on aggression based on information recorded by official scorers during a game.

arch sprain Disorder characterized by pain in the arches of the foot. There are two main types of arch sprain: static and traumatic. Static arch sprain is marked by pain and tenderness along the plantar ligament and is commonly caused by prolonged stress on the feet which may be precipitated by changing footwear (e.g., from flat training shoes to spiked track shoes). Traumatic arch sprain is due to overstretching the ligaments supporting the arches.

arch support Extra material placed inside a training shoe which provides mechanical support for the arches. *See also* **orthoses**.

areolar tissue Connective tissue which has a loose arrangement of fibres within a semifluid ground substance formed mainly of hyaluronic acid. It provides a reservoir of water and salts for surrounding body tissue. If extracellular fluid accumulates in the areolar tissue, the affected area swells and becomes puffy, contributing to *oedema.

argot A specialized language or jargon, shared by members of a *subculture.

arithmetic mean *See* **mean**.

arm Region of the body extending the length of the *humerus.

arm movements Movement of the *humerus about the glenohumeral (shoulder) joint. Coordination of humeral movements with motions of the scapula enable a much greater range of motion than when the scapula is fixed.

arm abduction Movement of the arm away from the midline of the body.

arm abductors Muscles which effect *arm abduction. The major abductors of the humerus are the middle deltoid and supraspinatus.

arm adduction Movement of the arm towards the midline.

arm adductors Muscles which effect *arm adduction. The main adductors of the humerus are the sternal pectoralis major, the latissimus dorsi, and the teres major. The rhomboideus, serratus anterior, and trapezius act as fixators.

arm ergometer *See* **ergometer**.

arm extension An angular, backward, and downward movement of the arm about the glenohumeral (shoulder) joint.

arm extensors Muscles which effect *arm extension. The main extensors of the humerus are the sternal pectoralis major, latissimus dorsi, and teres major.

arm flexion An angular, forward, and upward movement of the arm about the glenohumeral (shoulder) joint.

arm flexors Muscles which effect *arm extension. The main flexors of the humerus are the clavicular pectoralis major, the anterior fibres of the deltoids, and the coracobrachialis.

arm–hand steadiness A skill-oriented ability which underlies tasks such as archery and riflery. It is believed to exist within the movement control area.

arm horizontal abduction *See* **arm horizontal extension**.

arm horizontal abductors *See* **arm horizontal extensors**.

arm horizontal adduction *See* **arm horizontal flexion**.

arm horizontal adductors *See* **arm horizontal flexors**.

arm horizontal extension (arm horizontal abduction) Movement of the arm from the front horizontal position to the side horizontal position.

arm horizontal extensors Muscles which effect *arm horizontal extension. The main arm horizontal extensors are the middle and posterior fibres of the deltoids, the infraspinatus, and the teres minor.

arm horizontal flexion (arm horizontal adduction) Movement of the arm from a side horizontal position to a front horizontal position.

arm horizontal flexors (arm horizontal adductors) Muscles which effect *arm horizontal flexion. The main arm horizontal flexors are the sternal pectoralis major, the anterior fibres of the deltoid, and the coracobrachialis.

arm inward rotation (arm medial rotation) Movement of the arm around its axis towards the midline of the body. It is effected by the anterior fibres of the deltoids and the latissimus dorsi assisted by the teres major, while the rhomboideus acts as a fixator of the scapula.

arm lateral rotation *See* **arm outward rotation**.

arm medial rotation *See* **arm inward rotation**.

arm outward rotation (arm lateral rotation) Movement of the arm around its axis away from the midline of the body. The prime movers are the posterior fibres of the deltoids and infraspinatus, with the rhomboideus acting as a *fixator.

arm preference A person's tendency to favour the use of one arm rather than the other when performing a task. *See* **handedness**

arousal The state of general preparedness of the body for action. It varies along a continuum ranging from deep sleep to extreme excitement. The term arousal is sometimes used synonymously with alertness and interchangeably with anxiety, although the latter is more correctly confined to situations of high arousal accompanied by unpleasant sensations. Arousal involves the activation of various organs under the control of the autonomic nervous system. The degree of arousal, therefore, is reflected by a number of physiological indicators including blood pressure, EEG brain wave patterns, galvanic skin reaction, heart rate, muscle tension, and respiration rate. Biochemical indicators include concentrations of adrenaline and noradrenaline in the blood. There is not a perfect correlation between these indicators. Different sports have different optimal arousal levels. The relationship between arousal and performance is often described by the *inverted U-hypothesis. This hypothesis is based on the assumption that arousal is unidimensional, but there is evidence that there are two or more arousal systems in the brain. Some workers distinguish between psychological arousal (the readiness of an individual to respond to stimuli) and physiological arousal (as indicated by heart rate, sweating etc). *See also* **catastrophe theory**.

arousal reaction A reaction which occurs when an individual is confronted with sudden, usually threatening environmental situations which stimulate the *reticular activating system. Other brain structures are then activated along with the sympathetic nervous system, resulting in large quantities of *adrenaline and noradrenaline being released into the blood stream.

arrested progress (plateau) A period during training (or learning a skill) when there is no apparent improvement in performance; the usual trend towards further gains ceases even though practice continues. Because this period is so demoralizing, it has been called the 'plateau of despond'. However, if an athlete perseveres and continues the training effort for long enough, the period invariably passes and it is often followed by accelerated improvement. *See also* **physiological limit**.

arrhythmia An irregular heartbeat. It may be produced by various heart diseases which affect the mechanism controlling the rhythm of the heartbeat. Sinus arrhythmia is a normal deviation in the rhythm of the heart beat which accelerates during inspirations.

artefact In the microscopic preparation of tissues, a structure which is not present in the natural state but which appears during preparation or examination of the material.

arterial Pertaining to the arteries.

arterial and tidal pCO2 differences The difference between the *mean arterial pressure of carbon dioxide and the *end-tidal carbon dioxide partial pressure.

arterial plaque Deposits of fatty substances (e.g., cholesterol) on arterial walls; it can lead to *atherosclerosis.

arteriosclerosis A pathological condition involving thickening, hardening, and loss of elasticity of arteries. *See also* **atherosclerosis**; and **hypokinetic disease**.

arteriovenous anastomosis A small blood vessel with a relatively thick muscular coat which provides a direct connection between an artery and vein, thus bypassing capillaries. Arteriovenous anastomoses play an important role in shunting.

arteriovenous oxygen difference The difference between the oxygen content of arterial blood and *mixed venous blood. It may be expressed as millilitres of oxygen per 100 millilitres of blood. The value represents the extent to which oxygen is removed from the blood as it passes through the body. Usually, the arterial oxygen concentration is measured in blood from the femoral, brachial, or radial artery, and the oxygen content of mixed venous blood is measured from blood withdrawn from the pulmonary artery. At rest, the average arterial–venous oxygen difference is about 4 to 5 ml per 100 ml of blood, but it increases progressively during exercise reaching up to 16 ml per 100 ml of blood, indicating that more oxygen is extracted from the blood by active muscles. The maximum arteriovenous oxygen difference of a trained athlete usually exceeds that of an untrained person. The training effect may be due to adaptations in the mitochondria, increased myoglobin content of muscles, or improved muscle capillarization.

artery A large, muscular blood vessel conveying blood away from the heart.

arthalgia Pain in or around a *joint.

arthritis A term which covers a number of conditions characterized by inflammation of the joints. The most common is osteoarthritis which results from degeneration and wearing away of articular cartilage. This may gradually progress to affect underlying bones. Osteoarthritis may result from trauma, incorrect loading of the joint, or disease. Knees and hips are the most common sites affected. Athletes who repeatedly injure their joints may accelerate the onset of arthritis. Those with arthritis should choose physical activities which put the least stress on the affected joint. Cycling and swimming are often suitable if the hip is affected, for example. Severe arthritis may preclude participation in sport. *See also* **rheumatoid arthritis**.

arthrodesis The surgical fusion of bones across a *joint which eliminates movement of that joint.

arthrodial joint *See* **gliding joint**.

arthrogram An image of a *joint produced on a photographic plate using *arthrography.

arthrography An X-ray technique for examining joints, using air and/or a dye injected

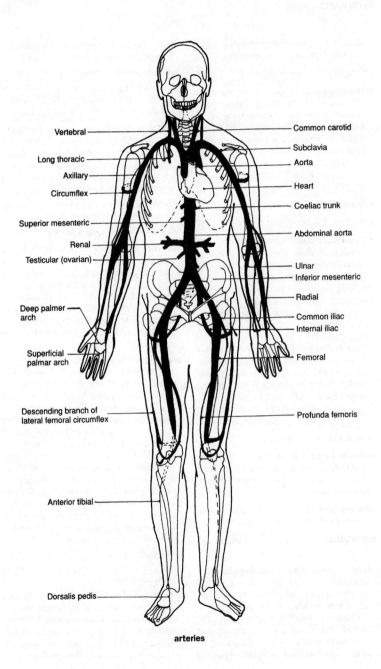

Vertebral

Long thoracic

Axillary

Circumflex

Superior mesenteric

Renal

Testicular (ovarian)

Deep palmer arch

Superficial palmar arch

Descending branch of lateral femoral circumflex

Anterior tibial

Dorsalis pedis

Common carotid

Subclavia

Aorta

Heart

Coeliac trunk

Abdominal aorta

Ulnar

Inferior mesenteric

Radial

Common iliac

Internal iliac

Femoral

Profunda femoris

arteries

into the joint, which enables defects, such as a torn cartilage, to be detected.

arthropath A disease or disorder of a *joint.

arthroscopy A technique that enables a surgeon to see directly into a *joint through a special microscope, called an arthroscope. A small incision is made in a joint through which the arthroscope can be inserted. A fibre optic system allows the surgeon to look around corners and into small crevices for any signs of injury. Arthroscopy is mainly used to examine the knee.

arthrosis *See* gliding joint.

articular capsule *See* joint capsule.

articular cartilage A protective layer of firm, flexible cartilage over the articulating ends of bones. It provides a smooth surface for joint movement, protecting the ends of long bones from wear at points of contact with other bones. It also helps to absorb shock and distribute forces. Articular cartilage contains collagen fibres continuous with those of the bone below. Although the cartilage lacks blood vessels, it plays an important role in the nourishment of the underlying bone. Synovial fluid is forced in and out of the cartilage with changes of pressure produced by movements. The fluid penetrates into the bone supplying it with nutrients.

articular discs *See* menisci.

articular fibrocartilage Discs (*see* **intervertebral discs**) or partial discs (*see* **menisci**) made of fibrocartilage present in some synovial joints.

articular surface Surface of a bone which meets another bone in a *joint.

articulation A *joint; a point where two bones meet.

artificial resuscitation (cardiopulmonary resuscitation; CPR) Restoration of normal breathing and pulse, usually by mouth-to-mouth (or mouth-to-nose) respiration and rhythmical compression of the chest. The ability to carry out artificial resuscitation effectively should be a prerequisite for sports coaches and officials, especially those involved in water sports, collision sports, and contact sports.

ascorbic acid *See* vitamin C.

ascribed status Status in society which depends on the position into which an individual is born. *Compare* **achieved status**.

aseptic techniques Procedures free from disease-causing organisms. When open wounds are being treated in hospital, for example, the air is filtered, instruments are autoclaved (sterilized by heat), and operators wear protective clothing.

asocial Applied to a person who is unconcerned about the welfare of others.

aspartates *See* aspartic acid salts

aspartic acid salts (aspartates) Salts of aspartic acid, an amino acid which takes part in the *ornithine cycle. Aspartic acid and aspartates are used as ergogenic aids in the belief that they delay the onset of fatigue by accelerating the conversion of ammonia to urea. Experimental results provide conflicting evidence of their usefulness.

asphyxia (suffocation) A term which means loss of pulse, but which is applied to a whole series of conditions which occur when breathing and the heartbeat stops. If not treated quickly, asphyxia deprives tissues of oxygen which may lead to loss of consciousness and death. It can be caused by inhaling water and passing food (especially chewing gum) or equipment into the trachea. Any athlete who has lost consciousness because of a blow to the head or fainting is in danger of asphyxiation if he or she is not in the correct position (*see* **recovery position**) since the tongue may fall back and block the airway, or the athlete may choke on his or her own vomit.

aspiration Withdrawal of fluid from the body, for example, from a swollen joint (*see* **joint aspiration**).

aspirational level (level of expectation) Expectancy of success or failure. Aspirational level acts as an important motivation determining actual performance. Athletes with high aspirational levels expect to succeed and often perform well, while those with low aspirational levels expect to fail and often perform badly.

aspirin *See* acetylsalicylic acid.

assertive behaviour In sport, the use of legitimate, acceptable physical force and the expenditure of an unusually high degree of effort to achieve an external goal, with no intent to injure (although another person may be injured accidentally). The goal may be offensive and designed to acquire a valued resource, such as yardage in American football; or it may be defensive. There is considerable confusion between the terms *aggression and *assertion. Sometimes assertive behaviour has been labelled *instrumental aggression, adding to the confusion.

assessment of performance Measurement of the qualitative and/or quantitative value of a performance. In sports science, the phrase often relates to physiological measurements of an individual's ability to perform physical tasks. To be meaningful, assessments of performance should be conducted with the same rigour as other scientific investigations and follow the same rules of experimental design.

assimilation 1 In physiology, the incorporation of new materials into the internal structure of an organism. **2** In sociology, a process in which a minority group adopts the values and behaviour patterns of a majority group and eventually become absorbed into the majority group. *Compare* **accommodation. 3** A cognitive process in which children incorporate new experiences into their present interpretation of their world. The new experiences become part of the child's current *conceptual schema which therefore becomes fuller and more elaborate. If the new experiences cannot be assimilated, then the conceptual schema is changed (*see* **accommodation**).

assistant movers Muscles which, by virtue of their small size or disadvantageous angle of pull, are not prime movers but may by their actions contribute to the effectiveness of a particular movement.

assisted active exercise An exercise in which the muscle action of the exerciser is assisted by an external force to produce a desired movement which the subject cannot produce alone.

association 1 An *attentional style which is consistent with internal focus. It is illustrated by some distance runners who tend to be very aware of their own emotions and internal body sensations, for example how their legs feel during performance. Compare dissociation. **2** Used synonymously with correlation in descriptive statistics. **3** A form of learning which establishes the relationship between different events. The basic elements of association learning are connections between the stimulus and response, and the strength of an association is influenced by the frequency with which these events are presented together. An association area in the anterior of the cerebral cortex is assumed to integrate previously stored information with incoming information. *See* **conditioning**.

association area *See* association processes.

association neurone *See* interneurone.

association process A cognitive process which establishes relationships between or among events and which enables *association to occur. An association area in the anterior of the cerebral cortex is assumed to integrate previously stored information with incoming information.

associative coping style A technique for managing *stress where the subject focuses internally on thoughts and body sensations, but ignores external stimuli. For example a golfer may focus on the muscle groups required to execute the swing while ignoring the noise from the crowd in the gallery.

associative stage A stage in learning motor skills when the learner refines movements by detecting and correcting errors.

associative strategy A method of focusing on internal body sensations and thoughts which enables athletes to monitor their internal condition continuously.

associator An individual who internalizes or adopts a narrow attentional focus. Elite marathoners tend to be associators focusing on physiological sensations while running and so allowing for self-regulation. *Compare* **dissociators**.

A-state A temporary state of *anxiety evoked by a particular situation (*see* **state anxiety**).

asthma A respiratory disorder characterized by recurrent attacks of difficult breathing, particularly on exhalation, due to an increased resistance to airflow through the respiratory bronchioles. Asthmatics are usually hypersensitive to a variety of stimuli which cause the airways to narrow by contraction of their smooth muscle, by a swelling of the mucous membrane, or due to an increased mucus secretion. All asthmatics wheeze upon exercise, but some seem to be particularly sensitive to exercise (*see* **exercise-induced asthma**). Sports vary in their tendency to induce asthma with running having a high tendency, cycling a moderate tendency, and gymnastics and swimming a low tendency. Paradoxically, many asthmatics gain relief from their bronchospasms by regular exercise, and exercise is now regarded as important in the management of asthma. Many drugs help to control asthma, but some are on the International Olympic Committee list of *banned substances (e.g., those containing *sympathomimetic amines such as ephedrine). Several athletes, including the 400 m men's freestyle swimming champion of the Olympic Games in 1972, have been disqualified because of pre-race administration of an oral anti-asthmatic drug. According to guidelines based on the 1993 International Olympic committee Doping Classes, asthmatic athletes are allowed to use salbutamol and terbutaline inhalers but their use must be declared to the relevant medical authority.

Astrand–Rhyming test A *cycle ergometer test of *aerobic fitness. The subject cycles at 50 rev. min^{-1} for six minutes at a work load set at a level related to the sex and condition of the subject (unconditioned males, 50–100 watts, unconditioned females 50–75 watts, conditioned males 100–150 watts, and conditioned females 75–110 watts). The subject's heart rate is taken in the last ten seconds of each of the two final minutes of exercise. The average of these two figures, corrected for the subject's age, is used to estimate *maximal oxygen uptake (VO_2 max). The estimate is based on the assumption that subjects of the same age have a similar *maximal heart rate.

astringent A drug which shrinks cells. Astringents may be used to harden and protect the skin.

ataxia The shaky movements and unsteady gait of a person lacking muscle coordination. Ataxia may be due to a failure of the cerebellum to regulate posture and movements.

ataxiagraph *See* ataxiameter.

ataxiameter An instrument that evaluates balance by measuring the anterior to posterior and lateral movements of the head. Where a graph record is obtained, the instrument is called an ataxiagraph.

atherosclerosis A type of *arteriosclerosis characterized by the accumulation of

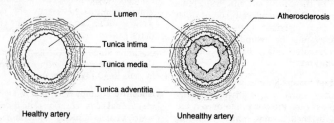

Healthy artery   Unhealthy artery

atherosclerosis

fatty materials within arterial walls. This results in a progressive narrowing of the arteries and reduced blood flow which can encourage the formation of a blood clot and may lead to a stroke or heart attack. Atherosclerosis is not, as some people believe, a disease of the aged. It starts in childhood, with its progress depending on heredity and lifestyle choices. Regular, aerobic exercise may retard the onset of atherosclerosis.

athlete An individual who, by virtue of special training or natural talent, is fit to compete in a physically demanding sport. The term athlete is derived from the Latin word 'athleta' which referred to a person who competed in physical exercises for a prize.

athlete profile A table or other representation which outlines important aspects of an athlete's characteristics. These may include personal details such as age, sex, weight, as well as details of athletic performance and achievements in physiological tests. A profile can be used by a coach to monitor progress, to modify a training programme, and to identify an athlete's strengths and weaknesses. Special psychological and medical profiles may also be constructed to help a coach. *See* **iceberg profile**.

athlete's foot (tinea pedis) A contagious infection caused by the fungus *Tinea pedis* and characterized by peeling skin and an itchy, sometimes sore, feeling between the toes. It may be rampant where there is poor hygiene and communal washing, such as in changing rooms. The condition can be avoided by taking scrupulous care in washing feet and the use of antifungal ointments and powders.

athlete's heart A nonpathological enlargement of the heart which is a physiological adaptation to training, especially endurance training. The heart enlarges as a result of an increase in the volume of the chamber of the left ventricle and, as revealed by magnetic resonance imaging, a thickening of the muscular wall of the left ventricle. Athlete's heart is usually associated with *bradycardia but there is no evidence that the condition is detrimental to health.

athlete's kidney An abnormality of the kidney associated with repeated episodes of microtrauma, as might be caused by boxing or other contact sports. It is characterized by recurrent haematuria (blood in the urine) and structural changes in the kidney.

athletic amenorrhoea Failure to menstruate (*see* **menstrual cycle**).

athletic identity The degree to which a person is identified as being an athlete. Athletic identity is a social construct, greatly influenced by the opinion of friends, family, coaches, and the media. Those with a very strong athletic identity tend to interpret events, such as an injury, in terms of how it affects their athletic involvement. Strong athletic identity tends to increase an individual's commitment to sport, but those with an exclusive athletic identity (i.e. whose only role in life is perceived to be that of an athlete) tend to have emotional difficulties when their athletic careers end.

athleticism Devotion to, or emphasis on, physical fitness. Athleticism and an enthusiasm for sporting activities was a component of so-called 'muscular Christianity': a loosely knit movement at the end of the nineteenth century which aimed to instil into youth Godliness, patriotism, and physical fitness which were seen to be, in some way, connected.

athletic motivation inventory (AMI) An inventory designed to measure *personality traits thought to be related to athletic ability. These traits include aggression, coachability, conscience development, determination, drive, emotional control, leadership, mental toughness, responsibility, self-confidence, and trust. Although the inventory is much used, its ability to predict athletic success has been seriously questioned.

athletic neurosis A form of *neurosis in athletes who develop an extreme psychological dependence on athletic activity because it becomes an essential mechanism for coping with their neurotic fears of illness.

athletic pseudoanaemia A false anaemia associated with regular and vigorous aerobic exercise. During the exercise the blood plasma volume is lowered by sweating, the production of metabolites, and an increase in arterial pressure. The body adapts to these changes by conserving water and salt between bouts of exercise. This results in an increase in the base plasma volume, diluting the red blood cells and decreasing the haemoglobin concentration. The absolute amount of haemoglobin (i.e. the total red cell mass) is usually higher than in a sedentary person and, unlike true *anaemia, the oxygen carrying capacity of the blood of a person with athletic pseudoanaemia is not impaired. *See also* **iron-deficiency anaemia**.

athletic pseudonephritis (jogger's nephritis) The occurrence of protein and white and red blood cells in the urine due to strenuous physical activity, such as regular long-distance jogging. These signs and symptoms mimic those of a very serious kidney disease, glomerulonephritis. However, athletic pseudonephritis is a transient condition that clears completely within 3 days of rest. Differential diagnosis is difficult, but in athletic pseudonephritis there is an absence of sepsis, anaemia, and hypertension, and there is usually a normal white blood cell count.

atlantoaxial joint The *synovial joint between the atlas and axis, which allows rotation of the head.

atlas The first *cervical vertebra that articulates with the occipital bone of the skull and the atlas. It has no centrum and no spinal process.

atmosphere 1 Gases enveloping the Earth at sea level consisting of approximately 78% nitrogen, 20.95% oxygen, and 0.36% carbon dioxide, and variable amounts of water vapour. **2** Unit of pressure; one normal atmosphere equals 101 325 newtons per square metre.

atony A condition in which muscles are flaccid and lack their normal elasticity.

atopy Form of allergy in which there is a hereditary or constitutional predisposition to develop hypersensitivity to allergens (e.g., atopic eczema and allergic asthma).

ATP *See* **adenosine triphosphate**.

ATPase *See* **adenosine triphosphatase**.

ATP–PCr system (phosphagen system) An *anaerobic energy system in which the generation of ATP is coupled with the exergonic breakdown of phosphocreatine stored in muscle cells. The breakdown frees inorganic phosphate which then combines with ADP to form ATP. The ATP–PCr system is the quickest source of ATP for muscle actions. Athletes in power events lasting up to 10 seconds (e.g., 100 m sprint) derive most of their ATP from this system.

A-trait An enduring personality factor indicating an individual's predisposition to experience *anxiety under stress.

atrial natriuretic factor (ANF) A polypeptide isolated from the atrium of the heart, and also present in the brain. ANF is thought to act as a hormone, helping to regulate the volume of extracellular fluid and electrolytes; for example, it increases renal sodium excretion. The concentration of atrial natriuretic factor increases during exercise, but the significance of this is not yet understood.

atrial systole Contraction of the atria of the heart forcing blood into the ventricles during the *cardiac cycle.

atrioventricular node A specialized area of tissue located in the right atrium of the heart which acts as a second pacemaker. It receives the impulse to contract from the sinoatrial node and transmits it through the atrioventricular bundle to the ventricles.

atrioventricular bundle (bundle of His) Specialized fibres in the heart which transmit the wave of contraction from the atrium to the ventricles.

atrium 1 Either of two upper chambers of the heart; also known as the auricle. The right atrium receives deoxygenated blood from the body via the venae cavae, and the left atrium receives oxygenated blood from the lungs via the pulmonary veins. **2** An anatomical passage or chamber, such as the terminal saccule of the bronchioles associated with the alveoli in the lungs.

atrophy Reduction in size or wasting away of an organ or tissue from lack of use or disease. Atrophy begins very quickly if training is stopped or if a muscle is immobilized. During the first week of muscle immobilization, strength decreases averaging 3 per cent to 4 per cent each day are associated with muscle atrophy. Muscle atrophy can be avoided if training is reduced, as in a maintenance programme, rather than stopped.

atropine A drug extracted from belladonna (the juice of the deadly nightshade) which blocks the action of acetylcholine (ACh). Since ACh is the main neurotransmitter of the parasympathetic nervous system, atropine puts this system out of action leaving the sympathetic nervous system to function unopposed. Thus, atropine mimics some actions of the sympathetic nervous system and *adrenaline. Small doses of atropine cause a marked increase in heart rate. Belladonna is used in some cold-remedies for bronchitis and whooping cough.

attending Readiness to perceive, as in looking or listening for relevant stimuli. Focusing of the sense organs is involved.

attention The selection of information so that the mind can concentrate on one out of several simultaneously presented objects or trains of thought. Attention involves withdrawal from some things in order to deal effectively with others. It enables a person to concentrate on the task in hand. Information processing models hypothesize that a selective filter in the brain restricts the amount of information that can be attended to at any one time. Attention can be measured by the extent to which interference occurs between two tasks which a person is performing simultaneously (*see* **structural interference** and **capacity interference**). In the early stages of skill acquisition, more attention is required than when the skill is fully learnt. *See* **attentional style**.

attentional focus The ability to focus attention on cues in the environment which are relevant to the task in hand. Athletes with good attentional focus are able to narrow or broaden attention according to the situation (*see* **focus**). It also refers to the ability to maintain concentration over the course of a game or event.

attentional narrowing *See* **narrowing**.

attentional skills Cognitive processes affecting attention which can be developed and improved by training. The types of attentional skills which can be learnt for specific sports include the ability to select the correct stimuli to attend to; the ability to shift attention, when appropriate, from one set of stimuli to another; and the ability to sustain attention. These skills are needed for success in most sports.

attentional style An athlete's characteristic manner of attending to stimuli. Sport psychologists often refer to a two-dimensional model of the direction (external to internal) and the width (broad to narrow) of attention. *See also* **broad internal**; **broad external**; **external overload**; **focus**; **internal overload**; **narrow focus**; **reduced focus**; **scan**.

attentional wastage Misdirection of an athlete's concentration to irrelevant cues. Attentional wastage can reduce the effectiveness of an athletic performance, and can retard the learning process during skills training.

attention arousing device A small countdown timer that can be attached to an athlete's belt or pocket, set to vibrate at any time interval from one minute to twenty-four hours. The vibrations remind the athlete to focus for a short time on controlling concentration and attention, for example, in competition or training.

attention control training A complex training process that enables an athlete to control *attention. It involves developing intervention strategies that help athletes avoid undue stress by controlling their attention and to focus it more effectively. The training includes learning to recognize different attentional styles; learning to understand individual attention strengths and weaknesses; and learning to identify the specific attentional demands of a given sport, and to identify factors that can affect attention (e.g., competitors and spectators).

attention span The period of time a person is able to sustain *attention on selected stimuli.

attenuation A weakening of the strength of a stimulus.

attitude 1 A relatively stable characteristic that predisposes an individual to certain behaviours. Attitudes, unlike personality traits, are not general dispositions, but rather are directed towards specific objects, people, events, or ideas. In addition to behavioural components, attitudes have cognitive and affective components. Thus, they may include beliefs, such as agreeing with the proposition that jogging is good for health; and they may involve having negative or positive feelings, such as liking or disliking, a person. A coach may have a great influence on the attitudes of an athlete. A particular attitude may be acquired by direct instruction, classical conditioning, and modelling. However, once an attitude is established, it may be very difficult to change. Attitudes can be measured by using an attitude scale. *See also* **belief, conviction, opinion, prejudice, view**. **2** The orientation of the axis of a projectile in relation to a particular plane or the direction of motion. *See also* **attitude angle**.

attitude angle The angle formed between the main plane of projectile and the horizontal ground. *Compare* **angle of attack**.

attitude scale A method of measuring attitudes based on the assumption that holding an *attitude leads to consistent responses to particular persons, objects, or ideas. The scale presents statements about the topic of interest (for example, 'drugs should be banned in sport') and the

respondent states his or her degree of agreement or disagreement with the statement. *See also* **Guttman scale, Likert scale, Osgood semantic differential scales**; and **Thurstone scales**.

attraction, law of *See* **gravitation, law of**.

attribution *See* **variable**.

attributions The perceived causes of events and behaviours, such as the outcome of a performance. Attributions may be internal or external. *See* **attribution theory** and **locus of control**.

attribution model A model which posits that attributions are formulated to enhance self-esteem, gain social approval, and serve other social and psychological functions.

attribution theory (causal attribution theory) A theory of *motivation which postulates that individuals make common sense explanations of their own behaviour which can affect future behaviour. Inherent in the theory is the belief that an athlete is not a passive performer but actively processes information about a performance and constantly reflects on why he or she is losing or winning. The attributions that athletes select to explain their performance outcomes may reveal much about their motivation. Attribution theory assumes that athletes postulate reasons for their success or failure in a performance which influences their future level of performance. These reasons, or attributions, may be arranged on several scales, including attributions which are internal or external to the athlete (*see* **locus of control**); and causes that are stable (such as ability) or unstable (e.g., effort). It is generally agreed that successful athletes tend to attribute success to relatively stable, internal causes. *See* **cognitive theory**.

Atwater factor The energy value per unit weight of food expressed as kilocalories per gram.

audience In sport, passive observers or spectators of an athletic event. *See also* **coaction**; and **hidden audience**.

audience anxiety A feeling of *anxiety brought about by the presence or the anticipated presence of an audience. *See also* **audience effect**.

audience density The number of spectators in relation to the capacity of a stadium or sports arena into which they are crowded.

audience effect The effect of an audience on the performance of an athlete. The relationship between audience and the performer is complex, and is determined by the interaction of the particular factors pertaining in any specific sporting situation. The general effect of an audience is to raise the *arousal levels of participants and improve their performance, but for some competitors the audience will be a source of considerable stress and can cause anxiety.

audience hostility The level of ill-feeling that an audience expresses towards officials and the visiting team.

audience intimacy The closeness of the audience to the performers. The psychological presence of an audience tends to increase with audience intimacy.

audience size The number of spectators in an audience. *Compare* **audience density**. *See also* **audience intimacy**.

audience sophistication The level of knowledge members of an audience have about the sport they are watching. An audience with high levels of knowledge tend to have a beneficial effect on performance.

audiograph A graph of the minimal level of sound that a person can hear at various frequencies. During hearing tests, separate audiographs are obtained for each ear.

audiometer An instrument for measuring the level of human hearing.

audition The act or power of hearing. Sounds can provide important *feedback, for example the sound of a ball against a cricket bat may indicate how well the ball was hit.

auditory acuity Keenness or acuteness of hearing. Auditory acuity may refer to the ability to perceive sounds of low intensity; the ability to detect differences between two sounds on a characteristic such as frequency or intensity; or the ability to

recognize the direction from which a sound proceeds.

auditory canal *See* **Eustachian tube**.

auditory discrimination *See* **auditory acuity**.

Auerbach's plexus A network of motor nerves forming a nerve ganglion between the longitudinal and circular muscles of the intestines.

augmented feedback (extrinsic feedback) *Feedback which athletes would not normally receive as a natural consequence of their performance. Augmented feedback is added to the intrinsic feedback which is typically received in the task and it is provided by a source (such as a coach, team mate, or videotape) external to the athlete.

augmenter An individual who tends to exaggerate the intensity of incoming stimuli. This makes augmenters hypersensitive and easily distracted by extraneous stimuli. They also tend to have low pain tolerances.

auricle 1 The pinna or flap of the ear. **2** *See* **atrium**.

auricular haematoma Accumulation of blood in the auricle of the ear which can cause swelling and pain. It often results from physical injury which, if repeated, can disfigure the external ear. The blood supply to the cartilage is impaired and new cartilage forms in the space made by the haematoma (a condition known as cauliflower ear). Urgent treatment, consisting of draining the haematoma of blood, injection of hyaluronidase in a local anaesthetic, and application of a firm pressure bandage, is needed to prevent permanent deformity. The ear can be protected from further damage by covering it with a few layers of two-way stretch strapping wrapped around the head.

authoritarian leadership A *leadership style which is best explained in terms of *initiating structure. A coach exhibiting authoritarian leadership will expect strict obedience of athletes to the training regime that he or she lays down. *See also* **autocratic leadership**.

authoritarian personality The *personality of someone who prefers or believes in a system in which some individuals control, while others are controlled. Those with an authoritarian personality usually exhibit deference to those with higher authority, and hostility to those with lower authority. The term applies particularly to the personalities of some sports officials, coaches, and PE teachers.

authority 1 The established ruling body, for example, of a sport, which can legitimately exert power. **2** The power or right to control and judge the actions of others. This may be through the personal authority of a strong leader (charismatic authority); the established authority (known as traditional authority), for example, of governing bodies of individual sports which can impose and enforce their own rules and regulations; or legal authority, for example of the state.

autoconditioning *See* **biofeedback training**.

autocratic behaviour Coaching behaviour which involves independent decision-making and stresses the personal authority of the coach but not of the athlete.

autocratic leadership A task-structured form of leadership that discourages coach--athlete interaction. Autocratic leadership tends toward behaviour which is best explained in terms of *initiating structure. *See also* **authoritarian leadership**.

autocrine Applied to a secretion of a cell that affects that cell itself. For example, insulin-like growth factor secreted within a muscle cell has growth-promoting actions on that cell.

autogenic inhibition Reflex inhibition of a *motor unit in response to excessive tension in the muscle fibres it supplies. The tension is monitored by the *Golgi tendon organs. Autogenic inhibition is a protective mechanism, preventing muscles from exerting more force than the bones and tendons can tolerate. *Deinhibition training is designed to reduce or counteract the inhibitory impulses, allowing muscles to exert greater forces.

autogenic training A relaxation technique, involving self-suggestion, in which an athlete learns to associate a series of verbal cues and visual images with feelings of warmth and cold in different parts of the body; and with certain physiological responses, such as heart rate, and depth and rate of breathing. Once learnt, these responses can be self-generated when required. Autogenic training has been found to be particularly useful in reducing anxiety before competition.

autohypnosis Hypnosis of oneself as opposed to being hypnotized by another person.

automaticity The extent to which *automatic processing can be used to perform a task. Strong automaticity refers to processing which is almost entirely automatic and can be carried out without *attention. Partial automaticity refers to processing that can be performed without conscious control, but which is performed better with attention.

automatic processing The activation of a learned sequence of elements or behaviours in the permanent memory. A task performed using automatic processing is fast, effortless, does not require conscious control, and can also be carried out without attention. Some sport psychologists believe that once a skill has been automated, applying conscious attention to the skill can disrupt performance.

autonomic arousal *See* **physiological arousal**.

autonomic nervous system (involuntary nervous system; visceral nervous system) A division of the peripheral nervous system that controls what are normally involuntary activities, such as heart rate, respiration, body core temperature, blood pressure, and urinary output. The autonomic nervous system includes the *sympathetic nervous system and the *parasympathetic nervous system which innervate cardiac muscle, smooth muscles, and glands.

autonomic restructuring A method of mental training in which athletes learn to think positively about autonomic physiological responses that are often interpreted negatively. For example, by using positive thoughts, an athlete can learn to interpret an increase in heart rate before competition as an important preparation for a good performance rather than as an indicator of nervousness.

autonomous stage A late stage in the learning of a skill when performance is habitual and requires little *attention.

autoregulation The automatic adjustment of blood flow to a particular body region in response to its current requirements. *See also* **shunting**.

autosuggestion The acceptance by an individual of a suggestion arising in the individual's own mind.

autotraction Traction using a person's own body weight or muscle strength.

autotransfusion *See* **blood doping**.

auxology The study of growth.

auxotonic muscular activity The neuromuscular pattern of activity which dictates the correct sequence and strength of different muscle actions for a given sports technique.

avascular Applied to body structures that do not have blood vessels.

avascular necrosis Interruption of the blood supply to a structure causing it to 'die' or disintegrate. In children, a *stress fracture to the top of the thigh bone can lead to avascular necrosis in the ball of the hip joint. Avascular necrosis can also occur after a fracture to the scaphoid bone in the wrist, due to absence of blood supply to the proximal pole of the bone.

AV block Delayed or blocked transmission of impulses from the atria to the ventricles in the heart.

AV bundle *See* **atrioventricular bundle**.

average A vague term which refers to the normal or typical amount. It sometimes refers specifically to the arithmetic mean. *See also* **measures of central tendency**.

average angular velocity The arithmetic mean of all *instantaneous angular veloc-

ities obtained by a rotating body during a given period of time.

average speed The distance travelled by a body divided by the time taken: $s = l/t$, where s = average speed, l = distance travelled, and t = time taken.

average velocity The displacement of a body divided by the time taken: $v = d/t$, where v = average velocity, d = displacement in a specified direction, and t = time taken.

aversion therapy A type of behaviour modification which relies on negative reinforcement. The subject learns that by doing something or behaving in a certain way, an unpleasant consequence can be avoided. The reinforcer is the avoidance of pain or unpleasantness.

aversive event A stimulus resulting in behaviour which terminates the stimulus.

AV node *See* **atrioventricular node**.

avocational sport subculture A group of people, including players, coaches, and spectators, pursuing a sporting interest that they value highly, but which they do not pursue as an occupation. *Compare* **occupational sport subculture**; *see also* **deviant sport subculture**.

avoidance–avoidance conflict A situation in which an individual is confronted by two unattractive alternatives.

AVPU A mnemonic used for a limited grading of the neurological responsiveness of an injured athlete on the field of play. A: Alert; V: responsiveness to Vocal stimuli; P: responsiveness to Painful stimuli; U: Unresponsive. *See also* **Glasgow coma scale**.

avulsion fracture A fracture in which a tendon or ligament pulls off a portion of a bone. Explosive jumping and throwing movements can result in avulsion fractures of the ankle bone and humerus.

awareness The state of being fully conscious of pertinent stimuli and really experiencing a task or situation. Awareness requires the ability to totally focus *attention on a task. An aware athlete is conscious of subtle fluctuations in a performance or contest and is able to exert more control over situations than an athlete who lacks awareness.

axial skeleton Part of the skeleton consisting the skull, vertebrae, sternum, and ribs, that forms the central, longitudinal axis of the body. *Compare* **appendicular skeleton.**

axial force A force directed along the longitudinal axis of a body.

axilla The space between the upper part of the arm and the side-wall of the chest, commonly called the armpit. The axilla is enclosed by the pectoral muscles in front, and the latissimus dorsi and teres major muscles behind.

axillary In anatomy, pertaining to the *axilla or armpit.

axillary nerve (circumflex nerve) A nerve which runs close to the shoulder. It supplies the deltoid and teres minor muscles. After a glenohumeral injury to the *rotator cuff or glenoid labrum, the shoulder may become unstable and the axillary nerve can become trapped as it crosses anteriorly across the humeral head to the deltoid muscle; this is a common cause of *entrapment neuropathy among racket players.

axis 1 The second *cervical vertebra. It has a vertical superior process called the odontoid process, around which the atlas rotates. **2** *See* **axis of rotation.**

axis of rotation (axis) An imaginary line perpendicular to the plane of rotation and passing through the centre of rotation about which a given system rotates.

axolemma The cell surface membrane of an *axon.

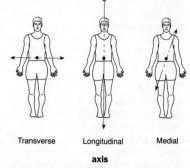

Transverse   Longitudinal   Medial

axis

axon A single, long, relatively unbranched process projecting from a cell body of a neurone which transmits *nerve impulses away from the cell body.

axon hillock The cone-shaped region of an *axon close to the cell body.

axon terminal (terminal fibril) One of numerous branched endings of an *axon.

axonotmesis An injury causing disruption of the *axon and *myelin sheath of a nerve. It results from degeneration of the axon distal to the point of injury, but regeneration is usually spontaneous.

Ayalon test A test of explosive power consisting of measuring the time required to perform a half pedal turn of 180° with the left leg on a pedal of a cycle ergometer, braked by a load which can be set at either 2.9 kg or proportional to the subject's body-weight. Power is estimated as the product of the force (equal to the resistance applied to the half circumference of the pedal) and the distance (equal to half the circumference of the pedal), divided by the time taken to perform the half pedal turn.

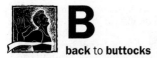

B

back to **buttocks**

back Region of the body consisting mainly of the vertebral column and the lateral and posterior parts of the ribs, the iliac bones and the sacrum. The bones, are covered by thick and powerful muscles, the chief of which are the *erector spinae. Muscles also pass upwards to support the head, and downwards into the lower limbs.

backache Pain in the back which may result from a number of causes. Many backaches are the result of mechanical injuries. In a small percentage of cases, pain may be referred to the back from diseased, deep-seated organs. In the UK and USA, more working days are lost because of chronic backache than from any other single cause. Backache may be due to congenital anatomical abnormalities, overuse (especially repetitive forward and backward bending), and degenerative processes associated with ageing, however, most complaints are due to poor posture, lack of fitness (including poor flexibility, especially in the hamstrings, and lack of strength in the abdominal muscles which support the back), and inappropriate load-carrying techniques.

backbone *See* vertebral column.

back injuries Physical damage to structures in the back. As a result of our bipedal gait, we are very prone to injuries which cause backache. Mechanical stresses imposed on the back during exercise, especially high impact activities, can cause muscle tenderness and ligament strains, fractures of the spine, prolapsed discs, sciatica, and spondylosis. Acute injuries involving the spinal column and spinal cord are very serious. Any injury that causes the loss of sensation, numbness, or weakness in the lower extremities requires immediate emergency medical attention.

back pain *See* backache.

back region 1 The private part of a social organization which is not freely accessible to nonmembers (e.g. a team changing room). **2** *See* back.

backspin Angular rotation of a projectile, such as a ball, in which the top of the ball travels backwards and the bottom forwards relative to its centre. A backspin is produced by an implement such as bat or racket, being brought downwards and forwards across the path of the projectile. On hitting another surface, the backspin tends to make the ball slow down and to increase its *angle of reflection.

backward chaining method A method of learning a complex skill consisting of several actions. The actions are learnt in reverse order with the final action being learnt first, and so on. It is a variant of the *part-method of learning. *Compare* **chaining**.

Baker's cyst A *bursitis or *hernia that usually forms a mass at the back of the knee. It is relatively common in athletes and may or may not reduce mobility.

balance 1 The ability to maintain a stable and specific orientation in relation to the immediate environment. Static balance refers to the ability to hold a stationary position; dynamic stability is the ability to maintain equilibrium while moving. Balance is maintained by multiple reflexes involving the eyes, semi-circular canals and other structures in the ear, pressure receptors in the skin (particularly on the soles of the feet), and muscle proprioceptors. Good balance is a feature of successful performance in many sports, especially those such as gymnastics which require sudden changes in movement. **2** The harmonious development of physical, mental, and spiritual aspects of a person. Balance was a philosophical ideal of the ancient Greeks who thought that sport played a key role in the acquisition of balance. **3** A device that measures weight.

balanced diet A diet which provides all the essential nutrients in sufficient quantity and in the correct proportions to promote good health. The six main classes of nutrients are *carbohydrate, *fat (lipid), *protein, *vitamins, *minerals, and *water. For the general population, health professionals suggest that a healthy, balanced diet is one which provides at least 50 per cent of energy from carbohydrate, 35 per cent from fat, and 15 per cent from protein. Many sports nutritionists suggest that a balanced diet for athletes should include more carbohydrates with at least 60 per cent of energy coming from this source, 30 per cent or less from fat, and 10 to 15 per cent from protein. The precise optimal quantities of each nutrient will vary with age, sex, and activity. Vitamins and minerals are required in relatively small amounts. In addition to nutrients, *fibre is a necessary component of a healthy diet. In the past, athletes in training ate large amounts of protein, such as eggs, steaks, and milk, but it is now recognized that carbohydrate, not protein, is the best source of energy. Pasta parties have become almost a ritual for runners on the eve of a marathon race (*see* **carbohydrate loading**).

balanced tension theory A theory related to social behaviour which suggests that a degree of stress between groups can be productive if it is controlled and channeled. *See also* **channelled aggression**; *compare* **conflict theory**.

balance tests Methods of evaluating the ability to maintain a stable equilibrium. One of the simplest involves testing the subject's ability to stand still on two feet with eyes open or closed. This may be combined with an ataxiameter which quantifies head movements. More elaborate tests include the stick-lengthwise test in which the subject stands with the ball of the foot or length of one foot on a stick measuring 1 inch by 1 inch by 12 inches (2.54 cm by

2.54 cm by 30.5 cm). Some investigators increase the difficulty of the test by raising the stick above the floor. In addition to these tests, teeter boards are often used to measure static balance. *See also* **blind stork test**; and **posturography**.

ball-and-socket joint A *synovial joint (e.g., the hip joint and the glenohumeral joint in the shoulder) in which the ball shaped head of one bone articulates with the concave, cup-shaped socket of another. Such joints are sometimes called universal joints because they allow movement along three axes (i.e., they allow abduction, adduction, circumduction, extension, flexion, and rotation).

ballistic mobility exercise (kinetic mobility exercise) A mobility exercise in which subjects use their own body movements to extend joint range. Arm swings (e.g., windmills) and leg swings are forms of ballistic mobility.

ballistic movement A forced movement initiated by muscle actions but continued by the *momentum of the limbs. Ballistic movements have three main phases: an initial phase of *concentric action which starts the movement, a coasting phase which relies on the momentum generated in the initial phase, and a deceleration phase accompanied by *eccentric actions. *See also* **ballistic stretching**.

ballistic response A task accomplished by a movement so quick that, once initiated, it cannot be voluntarily changed except for minor adjustments. The fast movement usually takes less than 0.2 s. The ballistic response explains why there is not much point in a player keeping his or her eye on a ball during the last quarter second before hitting or catching it, as the movement is already committed. Of course, the player may still miss the ball.

ballistics The study of the flight path of projectiles.

ballistic strength *See* **dynamic strength**.

ballistic stretching (dynamic stretching) A potentially injurious type of stretching in which an individual performs quick, bouncing actions which force muscles to lengthen. The lengthened muscle reflexively contracts (*see* **stretch reflex**), thus shortening and increasing the risk of muscle tears. The momentum generated by the movements may also damage tissue by carrying joints beyond their maximum range of motion. *Compare* **static stretching**.

ballistocardiograph An instrument which records the displacement of the body produced by the pumping action of the heart. The recording may be altered by disease.

balneotherapy The science of treating disease and injury with baths. *See also* **baths**; and **contrast baths**.

bamboo spine *See* ankylosing spondylitis.

bandage A pad or strip of material which may be wrapped around an injured or diseased body part to stop bleeding or to hold a dressing or splint in place. An elastic bandage (called a compression bandage) is used to exert pressure, for example on a swollen joint. The bandage is wrapped distally to proximally, with approximately one half of the width of the bandage being overlapped on each turn. Enough pressure is applied to reduce swelling, but it is vital that the bandage is not wrapped so tightly that it restricts blood flow. *See also* **RICE**.

bandaging *See* taping.

Bandura's self-efficacy theory A theory of situation-specific self-confidence which proposes that *self-efficacy is fundamental to initiating certain behaviours necessary for competent performance. According to the theory, self-efficacy is enhanced by four factors: successful performances, vicarious experiences, verbal persuasion, and emotional arousal. Successful performance, which can be achieved by *participatory modelling, is regarded as the most important factor.

Bankart lesion A detachment of the *glenoid labrum and capsule from the anterior glenoid rim, for example, as a result of repetitive forceful throwing by a baseball pitcher. The detachment sometimes includes a fragment of bone from the glenoid rim. A Bankart lesion is often associated with recurrent anterior dislocations of the shoulder.

Bankart operation An operation which stabilizes a shoulder after a *Bankart lesion by reattaching the glenoid labrum and shortening the capsule and subscapularis tendon. Although the operation takes a long time, it is designed to allow early range of movement and little if any restriction in external rotation.

banned substance A performance-enhancing drug which is subject to doping controls. The International Olympic Committee list of banned substances is accepted by the governing bodies of most sports. The 1994 list includes the following doping classes and methods: I Doping classes: (A) stimulants; (B) Narcotics; (C) Anabolic agents; (D) Diuretics; (E) Peptide hormones and analogues. II Doping methods: (A) Blood doping; (B) Pharmacological, chemical, and physical manipulation. III Classes of drugs subject to certain restrictions: (A) Alcohol; (B) Marijuana; (C) Local anaesthetics; (D) Corticosteroids; (E) Beta blockers. It is not a comprehensive list of individual drugs; the ban applies to all compounds related to those in the list. This has the advantage that new drugs, some of which may be especially designed as ergogenic aids, are also banned. In addition, some sports federations have their own list of banned substances.

bar Unit of pressure equivalent to 0.986923 atmospheres, 100 000 Nm^{-2} (pascals), or 1 000 000 dynes per square metre.

barbell A long bar with adjustable weights at each end, used as free weights in weight-training.

barbiturates Drugs derived from barbituric acid. Barbiturates are depressants of the central nervous system and have powerful anxiolytic and sedative properties. They have been commonly used in sleeping pills. Their effects are likely to disrupt the performance of complex motor skills. Habitual use of barbiturates can result in a true addiction.

bar chart (bar graph) Diagrammatic representation of information such as frequency distributions. Bars of equal width are drawn to represent different categories, with the length of each bar being proportional to the number or frequency of occurrence of each category. *Compare* **histogram**.

bar graph *See* **bar chart**.

baroreceptor Receptor consisting of nerve-endings, mainly in the *carotid sinus and aortic arch, which are sensitive to changes of blood pressure.

barotrauma A tissue injury caused by pressure changes (e.g., during diving or after the discharge of a gun). Any part of the body can be affected, but the eardrum, sinuses, and lungs are particularly vulnerable. A torn eardrum can lead to infection and deafness; burst lungs can be fatal.

Barr body Particles found in the nucleus of certain non-dividing cells in the buccal epithelium of females. The particles are probably derived from the inactive X chromosome, therefore there is one less Barr body than X chromosomes. Females usually have one Barr body; males usually have none. Presence of Barr bodies in a buccal smear was introduced by the International Olympic Committee Medical Commission as a sex determination (gender verification) test in 1968. This test, known as the Barr test or buccal smear sex test, was responsible for excluding about one female competitor in 400 from international competition. Six female competitors failed the test in the 1984 Los Angeles Olympic games. At the 1992 Barcelona Olympics, the Barr test was replaced by the polymerase chain reaction test.

barrier In psychology, an insurmountable obstacle which interferes with the satisfaction of a need. The barrier may be environmental or within an individual.

Barr test *See* **Barr body**.

basal ganglia (basal nuclei) Clusters of nerve cells in the base of the *cerebral cortex of the brain. Basal ganglia help control voluntary movements at a subconscious level.

They appear to be particularly important in initiating slow, sustained, stereotyped movements, such as arm-swinging during walking. The ganglia are also involved in maintaining muscle tone and posture. They form important relay stations between the cerebral cortex, the thalamus, and groups of nerve cells in the brain stem.

basal metabolic rate (BMR) The minimal rate of *metabolism in an individual at complete rest, at normal body temperature who is not digesting or absorbing food. BMR represents the lowest rate of energy use that can sustain life. It is usually expressed in units of energy per unit surface area per unit time. BMR is estimated when the subject is resting quietly in a laboratory under optimal conditions, after at least 8 hours sleep and 12 hours since the last meal. BMR for adults is between 1200 and 1800 kcal day^{-1}. It is relatively constant for a particular individual (although it may be increased by regular intensive exercise) but varies widely among different people. Factors affecting BMR include age, body size, body composition (especially the relative amount of fatty and lean body mass), and sex.

basal nuclei *See* **basal ganglia**.

base 1 A proton (hydrogen ion) acceptor. **2** In *anthropometry, a firm horizontal surface on which the subject stands during body measurements. *See also* **base of support**.

baseball finger An injury resulting from a hard, moving object impacting the tip of an extended finger, suddenly stretching its distal end or middle interphalangeal joint, sometimes tearing the collateral ligament. The injury causes swelling, immobility, and pain. It occurs commonly in baseball, cricket, volleyball, and other ball games.

base excess (alkaline excess) A parameter which indicates the *acid–base balance in the body. Base excess is affected by *blood lactate, with which it has a high correlation, and organic acids which accumulate during and after exercise. It may, therefore, reflect adaptation to exercise.

Normal base excess values are between −2.3 and +2.3 mmol l^{-1}

baseline A level of performance or fitness prior to training which is used as a standard to evaluate the effects of the training.

base of support The region bounded by body-parts in contact with a support surface or surfaces, such as the ground, that exerts a counterforce against the body's applied force. The outline of a foot is the base of support when standing on one leg.

base training High volume, low intensity training designed to improve overall physical condition in preparation for intensive training that is specific to a particular sport. Base training usually includes long-slow-distance running, swimming, or cycling which improves the cardiovascular system and aerobic capacity. The training is purposely slow to reduce the risk of injury, but the speed and distance are increased gradually as fitness improves. Many coaches recommend between 6 months to 1 year of base training for those unused to exercise before they start intensive, anaerobic training.

basic movement (basic skill, fundamental skill) A movement or skill, such as walking, running, hopping, stretching, and twisting which forms the basis of other, more complex skills.

basic skill See **basic movement**.

basic skills training A component of *psychological skills training in which a range of techniques (e.g., stress management techniques, positive self-talk, and attention control training) is used to develop essential psychological skills, such as self-confidence and arousal control.

basking in reflected glory phenomenon See BIRG phenomenon.

baths Form of treatment used as a relaxant after activity and as a therapy for some sports injuries. There are many types of baths, but they all act by either extracting heat from or adding heat to the body. See also **contrast baths**.

B complex Water soluble chemicals that include *vitamin B.

BCAA See **branched-chain amino acids**.

B-cell (B-lymphocyte) A *lymphocyte formed in bone marrow. After stimulation by a particular antigen, a specific type of B-cell divides to produce identical daughter cells all of which can produce the same *antibody that attacks the antigen.

bee pollen A mixture of bee saliva, plant pollen, and nectar. Bee pollen is taken by some athletes as an *ergogenic aid, but claims that it boosts performance have not been supported by scientific evidence. Bee pollen can cause allergic reactions in some people.

behaviour 1 The alteration, movement, or response of an object, person, or system acting within a particular context. **2** The externally observable response of a person to an environmental stimulus. In sociology, an important distinction is made between automatic forms of behaviour which can be analysed in terms of reflexes, and intended action, where social meaning and purposes are also involved. The behaviour of sportspersons can involve a complex mixture of both.

behavioural anxiety A form of *anxiety reflected by a person's overt behaviour such as avoidance of social contact.

behavioural coaching A coaching strategy which emphasizes the use of *positive feedback. Typically, the coach breaks down a motor skill into specific parts which are then modelled for the athlete to copy. The coach then supports and encourages the athlete during and after the athlete's attempts to perform the skill.

behavioural contract A written agreement between two individuals (e.g., a coach and athlete) referring to desired behavioural changes and the consequences of those changes. The contract usually includes a description of the behaviour that is to be changed, the punishment for breaking the contract, the reward for successful completion of the contract, the names and signatures of the contract partners, and the date. Behavioural contracts can be very effective in changing a wide range of behaviour, including excessive aggression.

behavioural kinesiology The study of the structures and processes of human movement and how they are modified by inherent factors, by environmental events, and by therapeutic intervention.

behavioural orientation An approach to sport psychology which views the environment (especially reinforcement) as the primary determinant of behaviour as coming from the environment. *Compare* **psychophysiological orientation**; and **cognitive-behavioural orientation**.

behavioural sciences The discipline concerned with the scientific study of the behaviour.

behaviour checklist A means of categorizing and recording behaviours of interest as they occur during an activity. The behaviours are usually clear and specific. The observer records the frequency and/or timing of the behaviours, such as incidents of fighting in a game of soccer.

behaviourism A school of psychology which stresses an objective natural science approach to psychological questions. Behaviourists usually study the principles of learning, for example, through animal experiments, then apply these principles to understanding and manipulating human behaviour. The main tenet of behaviourism is that only observable behaviour can be scientifically studied. Although this observable behaviour may include verbal behaviour which expresses thoughts, behaviourists tend to ignore mental functions; they concentrate their studies on stimulus–response relationships and the circumstances under which conditioning takes place. Behaviourism has influenced sports psychology in procedures such as *behaviour modification and the use of rewards and punishments in coaching.

behaviouristic leadership A style of *leadership adopted by coaches which applies the principles of psychology to training. It assumes a close relationship between an athlete's behaviour and performance.

behaviour modification The intentional alteration of human behaviour by various psychological techniques. For example, certain kinds of behaviour may be rewarded when they occur, with the result that these rewarded behaviours are repeated and unrewarded behaviours dropped. Sports coaches have varied opinions about behavioural modification. Some see it as a major method of motivation; others are very opposed and view it as a corrupt means of manipulating people; yet others see it as a useful tool to be used only in certain situations.

behaviour therapy A technique for changing problem behaviour, including relaxation procedures requiring the subject to approach a feared situation gradually while maintaining physiological arousal at a low level.

belief 1 An attitude based subjectively on emotions rather than on objective evidence. There are many beliefs in sport, particularly concerning diet, ergogenic aids, training, and injury. Some of these beliefs are based on empirical evidence, others are based on superstition or misunderstood theory. An important task of the sports scientist is to examine these beliefs; to support those which are beneficial and have scientific validity, and to give rational explanations that lead to the abandonment of those that are harmful or useless. **2** A socially constructed and shared view about what should or should not be, or what is, was, or will be. Beliefs have been classified as either a descriptive belief or a normative belief. A descriptive belief is concerned with what is, or was, or will be; a normative belief is concerned with what should be or ought to be.

belief systems The entire body of knowledge and beliefs which exist in a particular society or culture. The term may be used to describe patterns of belief and values in sport, and the central principles underlying these which give distinctiveness and coherence to the attitudes towards sport within a society or culture. The belief system of a culture has important implications for the development of sport within that culture.

belladonna The poisonous substance obtained from deadly nightshade (*Atropa belladonna*) from which atropine is obtained.

belly 1 The fleshy, middle part of a muscle which forms the main, actively contractile part. **2** Applied colloquially to the abdomen or abdominal cavity.

Bem Sex-Role Inventory (BSRI) An inventory in which subjects indicate on a seven-point scale how well each of sixty masculine, feminine, and neutral items describes them. On the basis of the responses, the subjects receive a masculinity, femininity, and undifferentiated score. Subjects scoring low in both femininity and masculinity are labelled undifferentiated, whereas those high in both are labelled androgynous or flexible in their sex-role (*see* **androgyny**). There is a close relationship between *competitive A trait and a person's sex and gender role classification. Females who endorse a feminine gender role have significantly higher competitive state anxiety than males who endorse a masculine gender role. This may be one reason why females tend to avoid competitive situations.

bench A step used in tests of cardiovascular efficiency. The height of the bench and rate of stepping determines the effort intensity.

bending force A force that produces tension on one side of an object and compression on the other side.

bending moment The algebraic sum of the moments of all vertical forces to one side of any point on a loaded lever.

bends Pain in the joints and limbs resulting from a rapid reduction in atmospheric pressure which causes bubbles of nitrogen gas to accumulate in different parts of the body. *See also* **caisson disease**.

benign Applied to a condition, such as a tumour, that is not malignant or harmful.

benign hypermobility A condition characterized by generalized *hypermobility which is not associated with increased risks of musculoskeletal complaints. *Compare* **hypermobile joint disease**.

Bennett's fracture dislocation A fracture or fracture dislocation of the metacarpal at the base of the thumb. It is a common hand injury in boxing caused by forceful backward bending of the thumb that tears off a portion of bone. It is usually the result of poor punching technique because the thumb has its own compartment in the boxing glove and should be protected. The injury is treated by manipulation and/or internal fixation followed by immobilization (e.g., in plaster-of-Paris) for about 4 weeks. If there are no complications, recovery time is about 6 to 8 weeks.

Benson's relaxation response A relaxation technique that includes an attention control element whereby the subject sits in a comfortable position and concentrates on slow and rhythmic breathing. With each breath, the subject repeats a single meaningless word to achieve a state of focused relaxation.

benzodiazepines Widely prescribed and therefore easily obtainable mild tranquillizers and *anxiolytics. Benzodiazepines have been used by sportspeople for their calming effects, to overcome jetlag, and treat insomnia. They have a low toxicity and low incidence of serious side-effects. They are not, at present, on the International Olympic Committee list of *banned substances. However, care should be taken in prescribing benzodiazepines to athletes, as long-term use may foster dependence and tolerance of the same medication.

beriberi Deficiency disease caused by lack of *thiamin (vitamin B1). Beriberi leads to a decreased appetite; gastrointestinal disturbance; peripheral nerve changes indicated by weakness of legs, cramping of calf muscles, numbness of feet; heart irregularities, including tachycarditis; and mental confusion.

Berkowitz's reformulation A modification of the *frustration–aggression hypothesis which states that although frustration creates a readiness for aggression, aggressive responses can be modified by learning.

Bernoulli effect An effect due to the relationship between relative velocity and relative pressure which acts on an object as it moves through a fluid. The pressure exerted on the object by the fluid decreases as the velocity of the fluid increases. Thus regions of relative high velocity fluid flow are associated with regions of relative low pressure, and conversely regions of relative low velocity fluid flow are associated with regions of relative high pressure. The Bernoulli effect acts on balls and other projectiles in flight. When a region of relative high pressure is created on the under surface of a projectile and a region of relative low pressure on the upper surface, the result is a lift force directed perpendicular to the projectile from the high pressure side to the low pressure side.

beta-adrenergic receptors: Receptors in the heart and lungs which respond to catecholamines (e.g., adrenaline).

beta adrenergic blockers *See* **beta blockers**.

beta$_1$ agonist$_s$ Drugs which stimulate beta$_2$ receptors, increasing the rate and force of contraction of heart muscle.

beta$_2$ agonists Drugs belonging to the sympathomimetic amines which stimulate beta$_2$ receptors. Selective beta$_2$ agonists are potent bronchodilators. They are used to treat asthma and other respiratory ailments. The use of certain types of beta$_2$ agonists (specifically, salbutamol and terbutaline) in aerosol form is permitted by the IOC, but only after a written notification has been made to the relevant medical authority by the team physician and the appropriate authority given. All oral forms are banned.

beta blockers (beta-adrenergic blockers) **1** A class of pharmacological agents which block-beta adrenoceptors, acting as beta-antagonists, preventing adrenaline and noradrenaline from exerting their beta-receptor mediated effects. Beta blockers are used clinically to treat a variety of conditions, including cardiac arrhythmias, glaucoma, high blood pressure, and angina. Because of the drug's ability to reduce anxiety and muscle tremor, beta blockers can enhance performance in certain sports (e.g., archery, bobsleigh, diving, and shooting). Consequently, to discourage abuse, beta blockers are on the International Olympic Committee's list of banned substances and they are tested for in those sports where they are likely to enhance performance.

beta carotene A nutrient converted by the body to vitamin A. Valuable sources include orange fruits and vegetables such as apricots, canteloupes, and carrots, as well as leafy green vegetables, such as broccoli and spinach. Beta carotene lacks the toxicity of vitamin A.

beta cells Cells in the Islets of Langerhans of the pancreas which secrete insulin.

beta oxidation The first step in the aerobic metabolism of fatty acids. The acids are broken down into acetic acid which is then converted into acetyl coenzyme A before entering the *Krebs cycle.

beta receptor Adrenoceptors which are subdivided into beta$_1$ receptors and beta$_2$ receptors. Stimulation of beta$_1$ receptors increase the rate and force of contraction of heart muscle, increasing cardiac output. Stimulation of beta$_2$ receptors causes bronchodilation and vasodilation of blood vessels in skeletal muscle. Stimulation of these receptors is blocked by inhibiting drugs called beta blockers.

between-play routines A performance routine, developed by *psychological skills

beta carotene

training, that is designed to help an athlete focus *attention appropriately during breaks in the action of games such as golf, tennis, basketball, and baseball.

biacromial breadth In anthropometry, the distance between the most lateral points of the two acromion processes in a subject standing upright with arms hanging loosely at the sides. It is a measure of shoulder width. *See also* **body breadths**.

biacromial: biiliocristal ratio The ratio of shoulder width (*see* **biacromial breadth**) to hip width (*see* **biiliocristal breadth**). The biacromial:biiliocristal ratio is an indicator of trunk build. Males tend to have higher ratios than females.

biarticulate muscle A muscle which spans two joints.

bias 1 In research, the distortion of data or findings by the research method employed, or by the researcher's suppositions. Bias results in a loss of *accuracy, *reliability, and *validity of the research. **2** In statistics, a difference between the hypothetical 'true value' of a variable in a population and that obtained in a particular sample.

biased sample In statistics, a population sample which is not a true reflection of the parent population.

biaxial joint A synovial joint which permits motion around two axes of rotation (e.g., condyloid joint).

biaxial movement Movement in two planes.

bicarbonate Ions formed as a by-product of carbonic acid. Bicarbonate ions are the main form by which carbon dioxide is transported in the blood.

bicarbonate loading Ingestion of bicarbonate (hydrogen carbonate) ions as an ergogenic aid. It is claimed that the ions increase the *alkali reserve and help neutralize lactic acid, thereby delaying the onset of fatigue during strenuous, prolonged exercise.

biceps A two-headed muscle. *See also* **biceps brachii**; and **biceps femoris**.

biceps brachii A two-headed fusiform muscle which bulges when the forearm is flexed. The long head originates from the upper rim of the *glenoid cavity; the short head originates from *coracoid process of the *scapula. The long head and short head insert via a common tendon onto the tuberosity of the radius. The primary actions of the long head and short head are flexion and supination of the arm about the elbow. The long head also assists with abduction about the shoulder; the short head assists with flexion, adduction, medial rotation, and horizontal adduction about the shoulder.

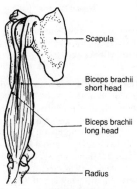

Scapula

Biceps brachii
short head

Biceps brachii
long head

Radius

biceps brachii

biceps femoris The most lateral of the *hamstring muscles. The biceps femoris is two-headed: the origin of the long head is on the lateral ischial tuberosity and that of the short head is on the *linea aspera and distal part of the femur. It has a common insertion on the posterior lateral condyle of the tibia and the head of the fibula. The primary action of the long head is extension of the thigh. The primary actions of the short head are flexion and lateral rotation about the knee.

biceps groove *See* **bicipital groove**.

bicipital groove (biceps groove; intertubercular groove) A deep groove in the upper part of the humerus separating the greater tubercle from the lesser tubercle. The groove guides the long tendon of the

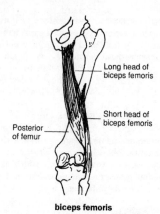

Long head of
biceps femoris

Short head of
biceps femoris

Posterior
of femur

biceps femoris

*biceps brachii to its point of attachment onto the rim of the glenoid cavity. It is also the insertion point for the *latissimus dorsi.

bicipital tendinitis Inflammation of the long tendon of the biceps. The tendon is particularly susceptible to injury because it has to pass through a narrow groove in the upper arm (the bicipital groove). Bicipital tendinitis is caused by repetitive overarm motions. Consequently, racket players, golfers, swimmers, gymnasts, and athletes in throwing sports are most at risk. The tendinitis often occurs in conjunction to an *impingement syndrome. Typical symptoms include a gradual onset of discomfort over the front of the shoulder. Pain increases when the arm is held at right angles (as when looking at the face of a watch on the top of the wrist), and there is often crepitus (a crackling sound) over the top of the shoulder when the glenohumeral joint is bent or straightened. Mild cases respond well to rest and ice. If untreated, it can develop into a chronic condition with the tendon tending to slip out of the groove repeatedly. This may require surgical treatment which involves translocating the tendon from the top of the shoulder to the front of the shoulder. Recovery of mild cases may occur in a week but chronic cases may require more than three months of rehabilitation after surgery.

bicondylar breadth In anthropometry, the distance between the distal *condyles of the femur; a measure of breadth across the knee.

bicuspid valve The heart valve preventing back flow of blood from the left ventricle to the left atrium.

bicycle ergometer *See* cycle ergometer.

bicycler's palsy *See* handlebar palsy.

bigeminy Alternating normal and premature ventricular *systole, as revealed by an electrocardiogram.

Big Fish Little Pond Effect The effect on *self-confidence of the type of individuals against which an athlete compares his or her performance. Low self confidence tends to occur when athletes compare themselves with more able athletes; high self-confidence tends to be exhibited when they compare themselves with less able athletes.

bilateral Pertaining to both sides of the body or body-part.

bilateral deficit A situation occurring during a movement that requires simultaneous activation of both limbs, when the total force exerted by two limbs is less than the sum of the forces produced by the left and right limbs acting alone. The bilateral deficit varies according to the type of movement and between individuals. For example, bilateral deficit tends to be greater for cycling than rowing, and it may even be absent in athletes who train with bilateral movements. Some elite rowers actually perform better in the bilateral condition than unilateral condition.

bilateral integration The simultaneous co-ordination of both sides of the body to perform a smooth movement.

bilateral transfer Transfer of a skill learned on one side of the body to the other side. For example, the acquisition of a particular skill involving the left hand is accelerated if that skill has already been learnt for the right hand. *See also* **transfer of training**.

bile A greenish-yellow or brownish fluid produced in the liver containing cholesterol, inorganic salt, and bile pigments (bilirubin and biliverdin, breakdown products of red blood cells). Bile is stored in the gall bladder and released into the small intestine where it aids the digestion and adsorption of fats through its alkaline, emulsifying action.

bile salts The sodium salts (sodium taurochlorate and sodium glycholate) secreted in bile. They help to emulsify fats in the intestine.

biliocristal breadth The distance between the most lateral points of the right and left *iliac crest; it is a measure of hip width.

bioassay A technique in which the presence of a chemical is quantified by comparing its effects on living organisms with the effects of a known standard.

bioavailability The proportion of a drug that reaches its site of action in the body.

biochemistry The study of the chemistry of living organisms.

bioelectric impedance A method of estimating body composition in which an electric current is passed through tissues (typically, electrodes are attached at the ankle, the foot, wrist, and back of the hand). Conductivity is greater in fat-free tissue than fatty tissue so the resistance to current flow through the tissues reflects the relative amount of fat in the tissues.

bioenergetics The study of energy transformations in living organisms.

biofeedback Continuous visual or auditory information supplied to a subject concerning his or her physiological responses, such as heart rate and blood pressure, at the same time as they occur. *See also* **biofeedback training**.

biofeedback training (autoconditioning) A relaxation technique which depends on the subject receiving a continuous and immediate flow of information about some of his or her physiological functions that are commonly considered involuntary. The subject then attempts to modify these functions by a conscious effort; the results of the attempt are feedback to the subject. For example, an athlete may be presented with a visual display of heart rate and muscle action potentials, indicating muscle tension, and learns progressively to control these variables.

biogenic amines Biologically active amines (organic chemicals derived from ammonia) which can function as neurotransmitters or hormones. They include *catecholamines and *indolamines.

bioinformational theory A theoretical explanation for how *imagery improves athletic performance. It assumes that the mental image created by the subject is stored in the long-term memory of the brain as an organized set of stimulus propositions linked to response propositions. Stimulus propositions describe the stimulus content of the image (e.g., the feel of the ball, the sound of the crowd when imagining taking a basketball shot), and response propositions describe the response to the stimuli in the imagined situation (e.g., the muscle tensions when making a shot and the exhilarating feeling when the ball goes through the net). It is suggested that performance can be enhanced by repeatedly recalling response propositions for a particular stimulus situation and modifying these responses to represent perfect control and execution of a skill. When a perfect response can be imagined, repeating the imagery is thought to strengthen the links between the stimulus propositions and response.

biological rhythm Cyclical changes that recur regularly over a given length of time and are related to underlying physiological processes. In humans, the length of a cycle (known as the period) varies from a fraction of a second to months. Rhythms with periods less than a day are called ultradian, and those more than a day are called infraradian. Rhythms associated with the solar day are called circadian. *See also* **biorhythm**.

biomechanics The application of mechanical principles to the study of the movement of organisms. In sport, biomechanics is especially concerned with how the human body applies forces to itself and to other bodies with which it comes into contact, and how the body is affected by external forces. A sound knowledge of biomechanics enables a coach or athlete to choose appropriate training techniques, and to detect faults that may arise in their use. The biomechanics of human movement is a subdiscipline of *kinesiology.

biophysics The study of the properties of matter and energy in living organisms.

biopsy See **muscle biopsy**.

biorhythm Sometimes used as a synonym for biological rhythm, but often referring to specific types of cycles of human biological activity. According to this concept, each person has negative and positive periods within a 23-day physical cycle, a 28-day emotional cycle, and a 33-day intellectual cycle. Advocates of the concept suggest that an athlete's performance can be predicted by compiling biorhythm charts which plot the cycles. Although there are wide individual differences, there is a poor correlation between changes of athletic performance and these biorhythm cycles. These biorhythms, which have little scientific foundation, should not be confused with biological rhythms which are well-documented in the scientific literature. See also circadian rhythm.

biotin (vitamin H) A member of the vitamin B complex. Biotin acts as a coenzyme involved in the metabolism of fatty acids, and the movement of pyruvic acid into the *Krebs cycle. Deficiency causes mental and muscle dysfunction, fatigue and nausea. Food sources include liver, eggs, and yeast. Some biotin is synthesized by intestinal bacteria. There is insufficient information to set recommended levels.

bipennate See **pennate muscle**.

BIRG phenomenon (Basking In Reflected Glory phenomenon) An individual's positive identification with a successful sports team in order to escape from a normally mundane lifestyle.

bit A unit of information used in computers. The term is derived from binary ('bi') digit ('t'). One bit is the amount of information required to reduce the original amount of uncertainty by half.

black box model A model of information processing in which an individual is considered to be a black box into which information flows from the environment. The information is processed in various ways inside the box until it is expressed as observable behaviour (the output). Researchers using this model focus mainly on what goes into the box (the information or stimuli) and the behavioural output. Nothing of the structure of the box is known beyond what can be deduced from the behaviour.

black bulb thermometer A thermometer placed in a black globe to measure radiant energy or solar radiation; one of the three temperatures required to complete the *Wet Bulb Globe Thermometer (WBGT) index.

black eye (periorbital haematoma) Bruising of the eye producing discoloration. The area around the eye is well supplied with blood therefore a blow to the eye or surrounding structures can cause internal bleeding. It is usually not serious and resolves itself spontaneously in a few days, but careful examination is required because it may be linked to a more serious injury, such as a fractured cheek bone.

black heel See **calcaneal petechiae**.

black nail (runner's toe; soccer toe; subungual haematoma) Blackening of the toenail near its base. It may be very painful and accompanied by swelling. Black nail is commonly caused by the patient's shoe being too short or too wide so that the foot slides forwards and jams against the end of the shoe, especially on dry, artificial turf. Black nail may also be caused by a direct blow to the toe. The nail later dies and grows out, with the black area growing away from the nail bed and eventually dropping off. Black nail can be prevented by wearing well-fitted shoes. It can be treated by inserting a heated, sterilized pin (or the end of a paper clip) through the nail to create a hole which releases the blood. See also **turf-toe syndrome**.

blackout A temporary loss of consciousness. This has many causes, including a direct blow to the head (*see* **concussion**). *See also* **weight-lifter's blackout**.

bleeding nose *See* **nosebleed**.

blind stork test (stork stand test) A test of *balance. The subject with eyes closed stands upright for as long as possible on a firm surface, hands on hips, weight supported on the stronger leg, and the sole of other foot resting against the knee of the supporting leg. Balancing ability is reflected by how long the subject can maintain the one-legged stance without moving the supporting foot.

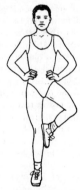

blind stork test

Bliss–Boder hypothesis An early, largely unsubstantiated hypothesis, that *attention devoted to well-practised movements will result in their disruption.

blister An injury to the skin in which the top layer is detached from the underlying layer; the gap between the layers becomes filled with a watery fluid lost from damaged cells. The blister is usually painful because the thick outer epidermis is lifted away, exposing nerve endings. Blisters are usually caused by friction between the skin and another surface. They are common in athletes who train or compete in new shoes which have not been worn-in properly. The prophylactic application of surgical spirits is a time-honoured tradi-

tion which may help prevent blisters. A blister can be treated by releasing the fluid with a sterilized needle and then applying a sterile dressing. The roof of the blister should not be removed because it acts as biological dressing and accelerates healing.

block rotation Simultaneous lateral rotation of the trunk and pelvis.

blocked practice Practice within a single period in which each component of a multi-task skill is practised completely before moving on to the next component. *Compare* **random practice**.

blocker's exostosis Deposition of bone in the muscle of the upper arm. Its name derives from the relatively high incidence of the injury in American Football defensive blockers who suffer blows to the arm. *See also* **myositis ossificans**.

blood Connective tissue consisting of red blood corpuscles, white blood cells, and blood platelets in a liquid matrix called the plasma. Blood is the main transport medium in the body. *See also* **lymph**.

blood–brain barrier The layer of fatty cells covering the capillaries of the brain which acts as a barrier to the passage of some chemicals (including some drugs) from the blood to brain tissue.

blood chemistry tests Blood tests that measure the levels of chemicals in the blood (e.g., glucose, lactate, or performance-enhancing drugs).

blood clotting *See* **coagulation**.

blood doping Any artificial means of increasing the total number of blood cells in the body, other than as a legitimate medical treatment. Blood doping is carried out because it can significantly increase maximal oxygen uptake (VO_2 max) and therefore improve endurance. Blood doping is usually accomplished by transfusion of blood either previously donated by the individual (an autotransfusion or autologous transfusion), or by transfusion of blood of the same blood type from someone else (homologous transfusion). In autotransfusions of athletes, the blood (about 900 ml or more) is usually extracted 5 to 6 weeks before a major competition so that the body has an opportunity to replace the lost blood. The blood is frozen for storage to minimize destruction of the cells Then the stored blood is transfused back immediately prior to the competition to boost the red cell count. In addition to contravening the ethics of medicine and sport, the procedure carries a number of risks. These include the possibility of increased blood viscosity which may put an extra strain on the heart, the transmission of infectious diseases, kidney damage, and overload of the circulatory system. Blood doping is banned by the International Olympic committee. *See also* **erythropoietin**.

blood flow Volume of blood flowing through a vessel or organ at a particular time. *See also* **shunting**.

blood glucose Concentration of glucose in the blood. Too much causes *hyperglycaemia, too little causes *hypoglycaemia; both conditions are harmful. Blood glucose concentration is controlled mainly by the interaction of hormones: insulin tends to reduce blood glucose; glucagon, adrenaline, and glucocorticoids tend to increase blood glucose levels.

blood lactate Lactate dissolved in blood. Blood lactate concentration is used as a biochemical measure of the effects of endurance training and a means of monitoring muscle adaptations. Normal resting values are between 0.7 and 1.8 mmol l^{-1}. As a result of training, blood lactate concentrations become lower for the same amount of work.

blood lipids Lipids, such as triacylglycerols (triglycerides) and cholesterol, carried in the blood.

blood oxygen-carrying capacity The maximum amount of oxygen the blood can transport. It depends mainly on the haemoglobin content of the blood.

blood pH A measure of the acidity, neutrality, or alkalinity of blood (*see* **pH**). At rest, blood pH is slightly alkaline (about pH 7.4).

At exercise intensities above 50 per cent maximal aerobic capacity, the blood becomes more acidic as respiration becomes more dependent on anaerobic metabolism. At first the decrease in pH is gradual, but it becomes rapid near the point of exhaustion. Blood pH values of less than 7.0 have been recorded following maximal sprint-type exercise. *See also* **blood lactate**.

blood plasma *See* **plasma**.

blood platelets (platelets; thrombocytes) Disc-like components of the blood. Platelets are non-nucleated fragments of large bone marrow cells. They play an important role in blood clotting.

blood pressure The force exerted by blood against a unit area of blood vessel. A blood pressure gradient from the arteries leaving the left ventricle to the veins entering the right atrium enables blood to circulate the body. The magnitude of the blood pressure is determined by the amount of blood pumped out of the heart per beat (stroke volume) and the resistance the blood encounters as it passes through the blood vessels (peripheral resistance). Usually two measurements of blood pressure are made: systolic and diastolic pressures, traditionally expressed as two figures in millimetres of mercury (mmHg), e.g., 130/80 mmHg (or 130 over 80) The first figure is always the highest. It refers to the systolic blood pressure, obtained when the blood is ejected into the arteries from the heart. In children, systolic pressure is about 100 mmHg; in young adults, 120 mmHg; thereafter it tends to rise with age as arterial walls thicken. The second figure is the diastolic pressure. It is obtained when the blood drains from the arteries. Blood pressure varies according to the subject's body position (*see* **postural hypotension drop**). It is difficult to define precisely what is 'normal' blood pressure, but there is general agreement that a desirable blood pressure is less than 140/90 mmHg. *See also* **hypertension**.

blood pressure cuff *See* **sphygmomanometer**.

blood retransfusion *See* **blood doping**.

blood serum Blood plasma from which *fibrinogen has been removed.

blood transfusion The intravenous administration of red blood cells or related blood products that contain red blood cells. *See also* **blood doping**.

blood vessel *See* **artery**; **capillary**; and **vein**.

blood volume The volume of blood in the circulatory system, typically about 5 litres.

blow-out fracture A fracture of the orbital wall of the eye. The rim of the eye is not fractured so a blow-out fracture is not palpable. Clinical features include enophthalmus (i.e. the eye appears sunken in the orbit) and diplopia (double vision). This injury is caused by a sudden increase in intraorbital pressure, such as when a squash ball or fist hits the rim of the eye.

B-lymphocyte *See* **B-cell**.

BMI *See* **body mass index**.

BMR *See* **basal metabolic rate**.

board-and-scale method (reaction board method) A method of calculating the *centre of gravity of a person by weighing the person in different positions on a large reaction board and applying principles of static equilibrium in the calculation. Typically, the reaction board is supported on two thin edges, one of which rests on a block of wood and the other on a platform consisting of a set of scales.

bobo doll An inflatable plastic doll used in the research of *aggression. The doll provides reinforcement for acts of physical aggression against it; when punched, the eyes light up and marbles are dispensed from the doll's stomach.

body 1 The human body. **2** In biomechanics, a term referring to both animate objects (e.g., the human body) and inanimate objects (e.g., a projectile or other item of sports equipment). In some cases it is convenient to consider the human body in its entirety; in other cases it is better to consider it as a system comprised of separate bodies (*see* **body segment**s).

body awareness The recognition of different parts of one's own body, their relative position during movement, and their relationship to the environment. Body awareness is dependent on sensory information from the muscles and joints and is essential for smooth, coordinated movement. *See also* **kinaesthesis**.

body breadths Measurements of the linear extent from side to side of part of the human body (*see* **biacromial breadth**, **biliocristal breadth**, **femur width**, and **transverse chest width**).

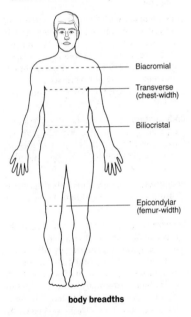

body breadths

body build *See* **somatotype**.

body building A form of exercise and competitive sport in which the primary aim of participants is to develop muscularity and body mass, and to produce symmetry and harmony between different body parts. In addition, body-builders try to achieve definition so that muscles can be separated from each other. During competition, body-builders are judged while posing in specific body positions. Weight-training for body-building usually incorporates 'split' systems (a few selected muscles or muscle groups are exercised in each session) which have a low risk of serious injury. The training does not improve maximal aerobic power or endurance capacity, but it does seem to have some health-promoting effects (e.g., steroid free male and female body-builders tend to have favourable lipoprotein–lipid profiles, reducing the risk of coronary heart disease). Well-trained body-builders are characterized by having lean and muscular bodies with enhanced muscular strength and power.

body composition The relative amounts of different components in the body. Sports scientists often divide the body into two main components: fat-free mass (consisting of all the body tissue which is not fat) and fat mass (usually expressed as the percentage of the total body mass composed of fat).

body culture An emphasis on a particular type of personal appearance that reflects the prevailing cultural preferences or fashions of society (e.g., the cult of slenderness).

body density The weight of the body per unit volume, usually expressed as kg l^{-1} or gcm^{-3}.

body fat The amount of fat in a human body. It is usually expressed as a percentage of total body weight. An average adult male has about 15–17 per cent body fat; and an average female has about 25 per cent body fat. Athletes, especially those involved in vigorous activities, tend to have low body fat. Body fat can be measured directly by *cadaver dissection analysis, but it is usually estimated from body density, for example, by using the Siri equation: percentage body fat = (495/body density) −450. Other methods of estimating body fat include *skinfold measurements, ultrasound, computerized tomography, and magnetic resonance imaging. The absolute body fat is the total weight of fat in the body. It is the product of percentage body fat and total body weight.

body fluids The watery solutions in the human body. They include intracellular fluid, tissue fluid, blood, and lymph. Body fluids make up more than half the body weight of an individual. Most metabolic reactions take place in the body fluids.

body fuel stores (metabolic fuels) Food stores which can be used as a source of energy to generate ATP for the body's activities. The primary body fuels for athletic activity are muscle glycogen and free fatty acids. Protein is also used as an energy source during exercise, but it contributes less than 10 per cent of total energy production except under extreme conditions (e.g., carbohydrate depletion).

body girths Measurements of the circumference of different parts of the human body. Body girths are commonly used in anthropometry (see **chest girth, gluteal girth, neck girth, relaxed-arm girth, thigh girth, waist girth**, and **wrist girth**).

body heights (body lengths) Measurement of the human body from the bottom of a structure to the top of the same structure, or a measurement taken at standardized points which indicate body stature. A number of different measurements of body height are used in anthropometry (see **dactylion height, radial height, spinale height, stylion height, tibial height**, and **trochanterion height**).

body image (body schema) The perception, both conscious and unconscious, of one's own body and physical dimensions. *See also* **self-concept**.

body language A form of non-verbal communication using movements and positioning of body parts. *See also* **kinesics**.

body length *See* **body heights**.

body mass In anthropometry, the mass of the human body measured to the nearest tenth of a kilogram when the subject is nude, or with clothing of known mass so that a correction for nude mass can be made.

body mass index (BMI; Quetelet index) An estimate of body composition used extensively as an indicator of obesity. BMI = weight in kg/(height in metre)^2. The index has insignificant correlations with stature, but has a strong positive correlation with *skinfold measurements. The assumption that the index is always a good reflection of body fat is not always true. Lean but heavy individuals, such as weight-lifters, may have a high BMI but they are not obese.

body mechanics Application of physical laws to the human body at rest or in motion. Body mechanics once referred to postural activities only. Generally, the term has been replaced by *biomechanics.

body of vertebra See **centrum**.

body part identification The ability to name different parts of the body in response to a label. A component of body *awareness.

body schema See **body image**.

body segments The division of the body into regions. There are eight main body segments: the head, trunk, arms, forearms, hands, thighs, legs, and feet.

body size The height and mass of a body. It is often expressed as the ponderal index: body height divided by the cube root of body weight.

body sway The slight postural movements made by an individual in order to maintain a balanced position. It is also called postural sway.

body temperature The temperature of the human body as measured with a clinical temperature. See also **core temperature**.

body volume Body mass divided by body density. It may be measured by hydrostatic weighing.

body weight The gravitational force that the Earth exerts on a human body at or near the Earth's surface. Body weight is the product of *body mass (in kg) and acceleration due to gravity (9.81 ms^{-2}) measured in newtons (N).

Bohr shift A shift to the right of the *oxygen–haemoglobin dissociation curve due to an increase in carbon dioxide or acid in the blood. At most partial pressures of oxygen in the body, this results in a reduced affinity of haemoglobin for oxygen so that oxygen can be unloaded more efficiently from active tissues.

boil See **furuncle**.

bomb calorimeter A thick-walled container in which organic material is burned completely in an oxygen-rich atmosphere to estimate the energy content of the material. Bomb calorimetry is used to measure the calorific value of food. Food of known mass is placed in the chamber and ignited with an electric spark. Combustion of the food liberates heat which changes the temperature of water surrounding the chamber. The energy content of the food can be calculated from these temperature changes.

bond That which links or holds one person to another.

bonding Establishing a close inter-personal relationship; for example, the attachment process that occurs between an infant and parent.

bone The hardest connective tissue in the body. Bone consists of hard calcified matrix (mainly calcium phosphate) and collagen fibres. Over 200 bones make up the human skeleton. Bone is living material and is very well vascularized (see **Haversian system**). Bones support and protect soft body parts; they act as levers for muscles during locomotion; they store calcium and fats; and they are involved in the production of blood cells. Bones fall into four main categories according to their size and shape (see **flat bones, irregular bones, long bones, and short bones**). Bone may also be classified according to its density and porosity as either smooth, dense compact bone, or less dense, porous spongy bone.

bone atrophy A decrease in bone mass. Bone atrophy may result from inactivity when calcium is withdrawn from the bone making it less dense, weaker, and more susceptible to fractures. This bone demineralization may also increase the risk of kidney stones.

bone growth See **ossification**; and **bone hypertrophy**.

bone hypertrophy Increase in bone density. Bone hypertrophy occurs in response to physical activity. The bones in the throwing arm of a baseball pitcher and the racket arm of a tennis player are denser and thicker than the other arm. In addition, physical activity increases bone density throughout the skeletal system, not only in the bones being stressed. Bone hypertrophy is stimulated more by the magnitude of the skeletal loading than by the frequency of loading. Consequently, it appears to be greater in weight-lifters than runners. Although it is greatest in weight-bearing exercises, it also occurs to a lesser extent in response to some nonweight bearing exercises such as cycling. Swimmers who spend much time in the water, however, may have a lower bone mineral density than that of sedentary individuals. Bone hypertrophy reduces the risk of *osteoporosis. *Compare* **bone atrophy**.

bone injury Common bone injuries in sport include *epiphysitis, *fractures, and *stress fractures. Although bone is made of a hard material, it is relatively rigid making it strongest in resisting compression and weakest in resisting shear forces. Sensation is confined to the *periosteum so unless this structure is damaged, disorders of the bone can be painless. However, pain is severe if the periosteum is even slightly damaged (e.g., by a stress fracture).

bone marrow Modified vascular tissue found in long bones and some flat bones. Bone marrow fills the tiny spaces between the *trabeculae of spongy bone and in the medullary cavity of the shaft of long bones. It is red between the trabecullae and yellow in the medullary cavity.

bone remodelling The ability of bone to respond to the mechanical demands placed on it by changing its size, shape, and structure; the process involved in bone formation and destruction in response to hormonal, nutritional, and mechanical factors. Bones have to be mechanically stressed to remain healthy. They become heavier and stronger if gravity and muscle actions impose forces on them. Inactivity results in *bone atrophy. *See also* **Wolff's law**.

bone scan A technique for producing pictures of the internal structure of bones using a radioactive tracer (such as technetium-99 complexed with a diphosphonate derivative) in conjunction with a scintillation counter (a process known as scintigraphy). The differential distribution of the tracer is used in the diagnosis of sports injuries, such as *stress fractures, which are difficult to diagnose using X-radiography.

bone spur An abnormal projection from a bone due to bone overgrowth. In some cases, surgery is required to remove a bone spur.

bony thorax (thoracic cage) Bones that form the framework of the thorax (ribs, sternum, and thoracic vertebrae).

boredom Condition characterized by wandering attention, impaired physical and mental efficiency, and low levels of arousal. It is sometimes confused with physiological fatigue, but boredom is usually the result of lack of stimulation, motivation, and interest. It is commonly caused in sport by monotonous training routines.

born athlete Term commonly applied to an individual who exhibits great proficiency in a range of physical activities, apparently after very little practice. *See also* **genetic endowment**.

Borg scale A numerical scale for rating perceived exertion, devised by the Swedish physiologist, Gunnar Borg (*see* **Rating of Perceived Exertion**).

Bosco jump test (ergo jump test) A test which estimates the *anaerobic power generated during a jump. Using an instrumented landing pad, the exact time spent in the air is measured during a series of repeated maximum jumps, standardized with respect to the amount of knee and hip flexion. The average power generated (W) is calculated from the test duration (T_s, from 15 to 60 s), the number of jumps (n), total flight time (F_t), so that: $W = (F_t \, T_s \, g^2)/4n(T_s{-}F_t)$, where g is the acceleration due to gravity.

bottleneck In structural models of *attention, a certain point in the central nervous system through which the passage of information is restricted.

bounce jumping A test which indicates maximal power production during jumping. The subject, hands on hips, makes a series of repeated jumps as high as possible. Both contact time and flight time are recorded.

bouncing breast syndrome A condition in females who run with breasts not fully supported. Running causes the breasts to move, damaging the suspensory ligaments. It can lead to a form of mastitis (breast inflammation). A simple preventative procedure is to wear a well-fitted sports bra.

boundary layer The layer of fluid immediately adjacent to a body in a fluid. Adhesion between fluid particles and the body surface create viscous stresses (*see* **viscosity**) which increase *drag.

boundary layer separation point The point at which the boundary layer of a fluid passing over a body separates from the surface of the body. It often coincides with the point of eddy formation, the breakdown of laminar flow, and the development of turbulence.

boutonniere injury A finger injury caused by a sudden flexion force tearing the central slip of the extensor digitorum communis muscle over the back of a proximal interphalangeal joint. Treatment includes splinting the interphalangeal joint in extension 24 hours a day for 4–6 weeks, with the distal joint left free for flexion. During the early stages of the injury, lateral bands of the muscle enable the finger to be extended, but if the injury is untreated these bands slip forwards so that the finger can no longer be fully extended. A flexion curvature develops with the joint coming through the lateral bands like a button through its hole (the so-called boutonierre deformity).

boutonniere deformity *See* **boutonniere injury**.

bow legs *See* **genu varum**.

bowler's hip A condition characterized by chronic deep pain in the hip. It is caused by inflammation of the *iliopsoas tendon (iliopsoas tendinitis) and the bursa at the attachment point of the tendon on the inner part of the femur just below the hip. Bowler's hip may occur in any sports person, but is common in those who couple repeated hip extensions with twisting actions of the lower back. It can be an extremely frustrating injury to resolve if it is not treated in the early stages (e.g., with rest and anti-inflammatories).

bowler's thumb An injury to the tendon or ulnar nerve at the base of the thumb. It can lead to a thickening and scarring of the connective tissue around the nerve. Bowler's thumb is common in tenpin bowlers who attempt to spin the ball by retaining the thumb in the thumbhole until the last possible moment before release. This action puts great strain on the tendons and ulnar nerve. It may be a transient condition which resolves itself after a rest from bowling, but it can result in permanent damage to the nerve. Bowler's thumb can be avoided by widening the thumb hole, changing technique, or padding the thumb.

boxer's arm An injury resulting from a direct blow to the arm detaching a small spur of bone which develops just above the elbow in some boxers. After extended rest, the bone usually reattaches itself.

boxer's fracture *See* **Bennett's fracture dislocation**.

boxer's knuckle An injury of the soft tissue of the knuckle which commonly occurs in boxers who have their outstretched hands bandaged before a fight. This results in the bandage being too tight when the hand is flexed to make a fist, damaging the underlying tissue. The damage may result in a *bursitis over the metacarpal head or a *distraction strain of the intermetacarpal ligaments.

boxer's muscle *See* **serratus anterior**.

Boyle's law A gas law that refers to the relationship between pressure and volume of a perfect gas. It states that at a constant temperature, the volume (V) of a given quantity of gas is inversely proportional to the pressure (*P*) acting on the gas; that is, *V* is proportional to 1/*P*. Thus, increasing the pressure of a gas causes a proportional decrease in its volume. Conversely, decreasing the pressure, causes an increase in the volume of the gas (e.g., when a diver rises to the surface, the gases within the lungs expand). *See also* **caisson disease**.

brace An external hinged support made of metal or a prefabricated material. Braces are used as an alternative to taping to support ankles and knees. There are three main types. A prophylactic brace is designed to reduce the risk of sustaining an injury, but their use is very controversial; some sports doctors believe they actually increase the risk of injury. A rehabilitative brace is designed to protect a joint after an injury; for example, it prevents lateral movements which would put stress on the knee, but allows controlled bending and straightening of the knee to accelerate healing. A functional brace is designed to compensate for unstable joints by improving the relationship between the articulating structures and the loads acting on them. Most sports doctors agree that the best way to prevent joint injuries is to follow an appropriate conditioning programme to develop a natural 'brace' provided by strong muscles around the joint.

brachial In anatomy, pertaining to the arm.

brachialis A strong muscle lying immediately below the *biceps brachii in the upper arm. Its origin is on the anterior lower half of the humerus and it inserts onto the anterior coronoid process of the ulna. Its primary action is elbow flexion, especially when the forearm is midway between full flexion and full extension.

brachial plexus A complex set of nerves (four cervical nerves and one thoracic nerve) at the base of the neck that serve the shoulder muscles. It is also the origin of three major nerves (the radial, ulnar, and median nerves) that travel down the arm to the hand.

brachial plexus neurapraxia (burner; cervical nerve stretch syndrome; stinger): A

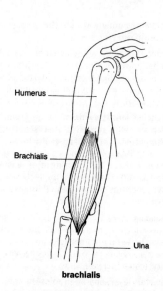

Humerus

Brachialis

Ulna

brachialis

neurological injury common in contact and collision sports such as football and wrestling. It is usually caused by stretching, pinching, or compressing the *brachial plexus when the head is hit and forcefully bent sideways and downward. The condition is characterized by pain and a burning or tingling sensation in the neck, shoulder, and down the affected arm. There is also usually a slight weakness and/or a loss of sensation in the arm or hand of the injured side. Symptoms are usually transient and sports participants with a simple burner return to play when asymptomatic. However, if the symptoms persist for more than 5 minute, medical advice should be sought in order to differentiate between the common stinger or burner and a more serious cervical spine injury.

brachioradialis A superficial arm muscle which has its origin on the lateral supracondylar ridge of the humerus and its insertion on the styloid process of the radius. The primary action of the brachioradialis is elbow flexion.

brachium The arm, especially between the shoulder and elbow.

bracketed morality In sport, the suspension during competition of the high level of ethical morality necessary for everyday life.

bradycardia A slow resting heart rate (less than 60 beats per minute). It may be due to a pathological defect in the cardiovascular system. Highly trained endurance athletes, however, often develop low resting heart rates (Miguel Indurain, the professional cyclist, had a resting pulse rate of 28 beats per minute when he won the Tour de France). This is an advantageous adaptation and does not indicate a pathological defect.

bradykinin A potent, pain eliciting chemical produced wherever body tissue is damaged. Bradykinin triggers the production of other chemicals such as *histamines and *prostaglandins. Some researchers believe that bradykinin attaches to pain receptors, causing them to send impulses to the central nervous system. During exercise, bradykinin may be released in response to the increased acidity which occurs in active muscle, causing vasodilation in the tissues and promoting sweating. It probably also contributes to the inflammation response, particularly in the early stages.

brain The part of the central nervous system contained within the skull. *See also* **cortex, cerebellum, and medulla oblongata**.

brain stem Part of the brain situated between the cerebrum and spinal cord. It includes the midbrain, the pons, and the medulla oblongata. It contains the major autonomic regulatory centres (*see* **autonomic nervous system**) that control the respiratory and cardiovascular systems.

branched-chain amino acids (BCAA) A group of three essential amino acids: isoleucine, leucine, and valine. They may be important in promoting muscle growth, particularly after strenuous training. They are the main amino acids used as fuel by exercising muscles. Claims that BCAA supplements reduce feelings of fatigue are still being tested. Sports drinks containing BCAAs may reduce perceived exertion, but appear to have little effect on performance.

breast bone *See* **sternum**.

breaststroker's knee A knee injury characterized by tenderness on the medial

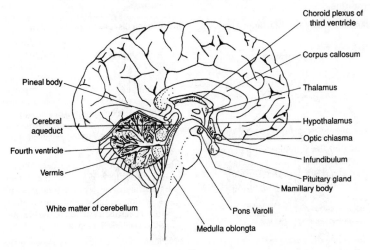

brain

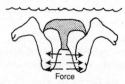

breakstroker's knee

(inner) side of the knee. It is often caused by the hydrodynamic forces produced by swimmers using a breaststroke action. In the propulsive phase, the knee extends and rotates medially while the foot is pronated. Hydrodynamic forces tend to abduct the leg at the knee. The tender spot often coincides with the adductor tubercle (an attachment point of the *adductors on the femur) and the associated medial collateral ligament. It is likely that swimmers who perform whip-kicks are more prone to the condition because of extensive abduction–adduction at the hip. Strong contraction of the stabilizers, the quadriceps, and hamstrings, may limit abduction and adduction of the lower leg and reduce the risk of this injury.

breathing External respiration; the process by which air is drawn into and expelled from the alveoli in the lungs. *See also* **respiration**.

breathing reserve *See* **ventilatory reserve**.

breathlessness An inability to breathe easily. Breathlessness may indicate a pulmonary or cardiac malfunction if it occurs with mild exertion. *See also* **exercise-induced asthma**.

breathplay method A modification of the normal method of breathing which involves active expiration with attempts at passive inhalation. It is claimed that it improves pulmonary function, but its effectiveness in athletic competition awaits a full scientific analysis.

BREG shoulder therapy kit A kit designed for rehabilitation exercises following a shoulder injury. The kit comprises a collapsible bar, an overhead pulley which can be mounted onto a door, and three different thicknesses of extremely flexible surgical tubing with which to do rehabilitation exercises.

Bristow repair *See* **Bristow–Helfet procedure**.

Bristow–Helfet procedure (Bristow repair) A procedure for repair of recurrent shoulder dislocations. The coracoid process is detached along with its tendons (the coracobrachialis and short head of the biceps) and transferred to a roughened area on the scapula.

brittle-bone disease *See* **osteoporosis**.

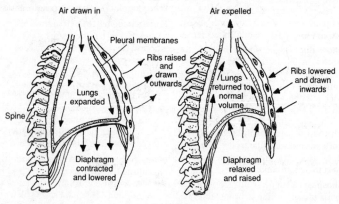

breathing

Broadbent model A model of selective *attention based on the proposition that irrelevant stimuli are eliminated before they reach the memory. Therefore, most information received by the senses is gated out (ignored) and never analysed. *Compare* **pertinence model; and Triesman model.**

broad cross-fibre stroke A massage administered with the thumb slowly stroking across a muscle at 90°. This massage stretches the muscle across its breadth.

broad external An *attentional style in which an individual is able to deal effectively with many external stimuli at the same time. *Compare* **external overload.**

broad internal An *attentional style in which an individual is able to integrate several ideas at the same time. *Compare* **internal overload.**

bronchial tree *See* **respiratory tree.**

bronchiole A small terminal branch of the bronchus in the lungs. It lacks cartilage, and is lined with smooth muscle which controls the lumen size.

bronchitis Inflammation of the bronchi resulting in restricted air flow to the lungs. It is marked by a hacking cough which attempts to clear the tubes. Acute bronchitis is due to a viral or bacterial infection, and is aggravated by physical activity. Chronic bronchitis is associated with tobacco smoking. A planned programme of aerobic exercise, particularly in those who give up smoking, can improve pulmonary function and is used to manage the illness.

bronchodilator A drug which relaxes the smooth muscle in a *bronchiole, thereby dilating its lumen and making it easier for air to pass in and out of the lungs. Bronchodilators are used to treat asthma. Many are sympathomimetic drugs which act as beta$_2$ agonists. These drugs are on the IOC list of banned substances but the use of some bronchodilators (e.g., salbutamol) by asthmatic athletes is permitted, subject to certain conditions.

bronchospasm A sudden contraction of the smooth muscle lining a bronchiole, restricting airflow in and out of the lungs. It

may be induced by an allergen, as in asthma, or it may be associated with bronchitis.

bronchus (pl. bronchi) One of the pair of tubes leading from the trachea into the lungs. Each bronchus is reinforced with an incomplete ring of cartilage to prevent it from collapsing. It is lined with ciliated glandular epithelial tissue which propels small solid particles, such as dust, towards the mouth.

brown adipose tissue *See* **brown fat.**

brown fat A layer of special heat-producing fat cells found mainly around the shoulder blades and kidneys. It is more abundant in infants than adults. Brown fat cells have a high density of mitochondria. The mitochondria contain large amounts of pigmented cytochromes which enables them to generate large amounts of heat which is transported quickly by the good blood supply. The metabolic activity of brown fat is stimulated by ingestion of food and by noradrenaline. Brown fat makes up less than 1 per cent of adult body weight and is generally regarded as unimportant in adults. However, it has been suggested that some forms of obesity may be linked with a lack of brown fat cells.

Brozec formula A formula for determining the percentage body fat from body density: percentage body fat = (4.570/body density − 4.142) &mult; 100.

Bruce protocol *See* **Bruce's treadmill test.**

Bruce's treadmill test A treadmill test much used in the USA for testing cardiac function. In this test, the speed and gradient of the treadmill are increased every third minute, starting at 1.7 miles per hour at a 10 per cent gradient and rising at stage seven to 6 miles per hour at a 22 per cent gradient (the Bruce protocol). Generally, heart rate is monitored with an ECG and the test continues until exhaustion or a predetermined heart rate is reached.

bruise (contusion) Bleeding in soft tissue resulting from a direct blow with a blunt object. A bruise is usually associated with swelling and *oedema. A severe blow or an aggravated bruise can result in dramatic pooling of blood in the area of the bruise (*see* **haematoma**). A bruise changes colour, first to blue as the red pigment of haemoglobin loses its oxygen, and then to brown or yellow as the haemoglobin is broken down and reabsorbed. Prevention of effusion of blood from small bruises can be achieved by applying a firm pressure for 3–5 minutes, followed by a cold compress.

BSRI *See* **Bem Sex-Role Inventory**.

B-TAIS A test of attentional and interpersonal styles designed specifically for baseball and softball players. It is derived from the general TAIS but its sport-specific questions give it greater validity for use with baseball and softball players than the general test.

buffer A chemical that combines with either an acid or a base to minimize changes in *pH. Many proteins, including haemoglobin, are good buffers. *See also* **renal buffering**; and **ventilatory buffering**.

bulimia nervosa An eating disorder characterized by recurrent episodes of excessive eating (diagnostically, at least two binge eating episodes a week for three months) followed by strict dieting, self-induced vomiting, excessive exercise, or some other means of losing weight (the condition is sometimes known as the 'binge–purge syndrome'). Bulimics are over-concerned about their own appearance and often commonly suffer depressive moods. *See also* **eating disorder**.

bundle of His *See* **atrioventricular bundle**.

bunion (hallux valgus) A deformity at the base of the toe commonly caused by ill-fitting shoes. The skin over the big toe is thickened and the head of a metatarsal bone becomes unduly prominent; normally the big toe is angled outwards by ten degrees, but in a bunion the displacement is greater. Friction from footwear can cause a growth of cartilage or bone (an exostosis) to develop over the bone where the angle is greatest. A painful *bursitis can also develop over the exostosis. Treatment may involve simple *orthoses or the use of a spongy pad to straighten the big toe. Occasionally, surgery is needed. This involves cutting into the first metatarsal, straightening it, then pinning it back in place.

bunionette A deformity that affects the little toe, similar in other respects to a *bunion.

buoyancy The upward, vertical thrust exerted upon a body which is wholly or partially immersed in a fluid. The thrust is equal to the weight of the fluid displaced by the body. Therefore, a body weighs less in water, for example, than in air; the apparent loss in weight being equal to the weight of water displaced (*see* **Archimedes' principle**). In humans, buoyancy is affected by body composition and the air in the lungs. If buoyancy exceeds the weight in air, the body will float.

bureaucracy 1 An administrative organization based on a hierarchical structure and governed by written rules and established procedures. The authority attached to an official and the position of an official within the hierarchy depends on the office held, rather than the personal attributes and status of the incumbent. **2** A term used pejoratively to describe any official process which is deemed inefficient or unnecessarily obstructive.

burner *See* **brachial plexus neurapraxia**.

burnout A complex psychophysiological syndrome characterized by feelings of anxiety, tension, mental fatigue, physical exhaustion, and a loss of concern for the people with whom one is living and working. It appears as a result of chronic stress. Burnout comprises the complex interaction of a number of physiological and psychological components. It has been conceptualized as an imbalance between the psychological resources of an individual and the demands being made on those resources. It has been used with reference to a decrease in the psychological capabilities of athletes, coaches, and managers to deal with stressful situations.

burns Damage to the skin or other tissue as a result of excessive heat. In sport, burns are seldom caused by direct heat (except sunburn). They are usually caused by friction when the skin rubs against another surface. A burn should be cooled immediately with tap water or an ice pack. The pain of a minor burn may be relieved with an analgesic. Extensive burns require hospitilization. The ability of a burns sufferer to participate in sport is determined largely by the extent and location of the burns. Even with minor burns, activities which involve the risk of friction against the affected areas should be avoided. In the case of more severe burns, activities which could lead to infection should be avoided. *See also* **blister**; and **mat burn**.

bursa A small fibrous sac lined with *synovial membrane and containing synovial fluid. Bursae usually separate tendon from bone, acting as a cushion between the two structures and reducing friction during joint motion. Some bursae, such as the one in the elbow (the olecranon bursa) separate bone from skin.

bursitis An inflammation of a *bursa which results in a form of internal blistering causing the bursal sac to become inflated with fluid. Bursitis may be caused by repeated mechanical irritation (frictional bursitis), substances formed as a result of inflammation or degeneration of tissue (chemical bursitis), or bacterial infection (septic bursitis). Treatment may include diathermy and the topical application of anti-inflammatory drugs. Chronic bursitis may require surgical excision.

Buss aggression machine (shock box) A machine that allows an experimenter to record a subject's level of state *aggression in terms of the duration and intensity of an electric shock that the subject is prepared to give an accomplice. No shock is actually given, but the accomplice behaves as if he or she has received a shock. Such research has declined in recent years because of the risk of psychological damage to the subject.

Buss–Durkee hostility scale A pencil and paper questionnaire designed to measure a subject's *aggression. It includes the measurement of seven aspects of hostility: assault, indirect hostility, irritability, negativism, resentment, suspicion, and verbal hostility.

butterflies An uncomfortable feeling in the stomach associated with high levels of arousal and arising from excessive muscular tension. Butterflies may be distracting and worrying, and therefore detrimental to performance. They can be controlled by *relaxation techniques. *See also* **visceral reactions**.

buttocks The two prominences at the lower posterior part of the trunk formed mainly by the flesh-covered gluteal muscles and fat.

 # C

cable tensiometer to **cytosol**

cable tensiometer A device designed to measure the tension of aircraft cables, which has been adapted to measure muscle tension during static muscle actions.

cadaver dissection analysis A method of measuring body composition by dissecting a fresh, dead human body, and determining the percentage fat in each body part.

cadence Stride rate during locomotion.

caecal slap syndrome A condition characterized by diarrhoea and a stitch-like pain in the right side of the abdomen. It is common in distance runners and is thought to be due to the posterior wall of the caecum slapping against the anterior wall, producing bleeding and bruising.

caecum A blind-ending sac, between the small intestine and the large intestine, from which the appendix arises.

caffeine A mildly addictive central nervous system stimulant. It is a constituent of many common products including chocolate bars, coffee, tea, and cola-type drinks. A cup of ordinary percolated coffee contains about 100 to 150 mg of caffeine. Low to moderate caffeine consumption is permitted by the IOC, but a urinary concentration exceeding 12 micrograms per millilitre is regarded as a positive indicator of doping. Caffeine may enhance the performance of endurance activities by improving the mobilization of fatty acids, enabling the more efficient use of fat as fuel and sparing glycogen reserves. The caffeine also lowers an endurance athlete's perception of effort at a given work rate, potentially enabling the athlete to work harder for the same perceived effort. Caffeine also enhances physical performances requiring speed and strength. It improves reaction times and alertness immediately after it is taken, but these improvements may be followed by feelings of mild fatigue and depression. Caffeine consumed before a physical activity acts as a *diuretic drug, increasing the risk of dehydration, but its diuretic effect seems to be absent when the caffeine is taken during the activity. Chronic, excessive caffeine intake can lead to insomnia, diarrhoea, fluid and weight loss, stomach irritation, ulcers, and hypertension.

caffeinism A medical condition resulting from excessive *caffeine consumption. A daily intake greater than 600 mg may produce symptoms which characterize the condition. These include anxiety, depression, mood changes, sleep disruption, and other psychological and physiological abnormalities. Abstinence following high intake can lead to withdrawal symptoms. Caffeine intoxication is a recognized medical condition in the USA.

caisson disease A syndrome occurring in people breathing air at high pressure. It was common in those who worked deep underwater in caissons, watertight chambers open at the bottom and containing air at high pressure. On returning to the surface and normal atmospheric pressure, nitrogen dissolved in the bloodstream forms bubbles which can cause pain if trapped in the joints (*see* **bends**). They can also block the circulation to the brain and elsewhere (decompression sickness). Symptoms are relieved by returning the patient to a high pressure.

cal Abbreviation for calorie.

Cal Abbreviation for Calorie or kilocalorie.

calcaneal In anatomy, pertaining to the heel.

calcaneal apophysitis *See* Sever–Haglund disease.

calcaneal petechiae (black heel) A heel blackened with specks of blood which have seeped out of dermal capillaries ruptured by shear forces. Black heel is common in participants of sports such as badminton, basketball, and soccer, who repeatedly sprint short distances and stop suddenly. No treatment is required, except reassurance. However, it is important to distinguish black heel from a malignant melanoma.

calcaneofibular ligament An ankle ligament which runs between the calcaneus and the fibula. The talar tilt or inversion stress test is used to assess the instability of the calcaneofibular ligament in a suspected ankle sprain.

calcaneum *See* calcaneus.

calcaneus (calcaneum; heel-bone) The large ankle bone that projects from the heel. It

caffeine

forms part of the tarsus, articulating with the talus and cuboid bones. The *Achilles tendon attaches onto the calcaneus.

calciferol *See* vitamin D.

calcific bursitis *See* calcification shoulder.

calcification The deposition of calcium salts in tissue. Calcification is important in bone formation.

calcification shoulder (calcific bursitis) A chronic inflammation of the shoulder, with calcium deposition in the subacromial bursa. Calcification shoulder may result from impingement of the subacromial bursa between the acromion and the supraspinatus tendon on the shoulder blade. It is associated with repetitive overarm motions that trap the subacromial bursa between the rotator cuff tendons and the underside of the shoulder blade. Degeneration of the tendons associated with ageing, may contribute to this condition. Calcified *rotator cuff tendons usually require surgical treatment.

calcitonin A polypeptide *hormone secreted by the thyroid gland which is a major regulator of calcium-ion concentration in the blood of children. It inhibits bone degradation and stimulates the uptake of calcium and phosphate by bone.

calcium A mineral essential for normal development of bone and teeth, and for the maintenance of overall health. Calcium is required for blood clotting, muscle and nerve activity, and cell permeability. It is the most abundant mineral in the body (over 1 kg is contained in the average adult). In the UK, the daily adult Reference Nutrient Intake is 700 mg, with more being recommended for pregnant or lactating women. The US daily Recommended Dietary Allowance (1989) is 1200 mg. Sources of calcium include milk, meat, fish, poultry, legumes, nuts, and wholegrains. Its absorption is aided by vitamin D. About one third of the dietary intake of calcium is lost in the faeces. Losses in urine and sweat increase during vigorous activity. These extra losses are used to justify the use of calcium supplements by some elite athletes, but studies indicate that

supplementation is of no value to athletes whose dietary intake equals the recommended levels. Excess calcium depresses neural and motor functions and can lead to the development of kidney stones. Calcium deficiency can retard growth and cause *rickets in children. Deficiencies may lead to *osteomalacia and *osteoporosis in adults.

calcium antagonist (calcium channel blocker) A drug which reduces the inflow of calcium ions into cardiac muscle and smooth muscle, thereby reducing the strength of contraction of these muscles. Calcium antagonists are administered to treat *angina pectoris and *hypertension. There is no restriction by sport governing bodies, such as the International Olympic Committee, on the use of these drugs to treat these disorders.

calcium channel blocker *See* calcium antagonist.

calf Region at the back of the lower leg formed mainly of the skin-covered *soleus and *gastrocnemius muscles.

calf girth Maximum circumference of the *calf of an individual standing upright with legs slightly apart and weight distributed on both feet.

calf muscle The *gastrocnemius and *soleus muscles, which have a common insertion on the *calcaneus.

calf strain A stretch, tear, or complete rupture of muscle fibres in the calf. It usually occurs at the point where the *gastrocnemius joins the *Achilles tendon. The strain is often caused by a massive contraction of the calf muscles, especially when an athlete stops quickly by planting the foot on the ground, then suddenly straightens the leg. Calf strains are common in squash and tennis players, particularly those who are unfit. Initial treatment involves rest, ice, compression, and elevation (*see* **RICE**). This should be followed by a rehabilitation programme of stretching and strengthening exercises. Surgery is rarely necessary, even in severe cases. However, if a calf strain is not properly rehabilitated, the muscle may become more pliable and more susceptible to injury.

calibration The determination of the accuracy of an instrument by measuring its variation from a known standard.

California Psychological Inventory (CPI) A questionnaire-type inventory which measures interpersonal behaviour in normal subjects. It has eighteen classes divided into four categories: Class 1 measures poise, ascendancy, self-assurance, and interpersonal adequacy; Class 2 measures socialization, maturity, responsibility, and intrapersonal structuring values; Class 3 measures achievement potential and intellectual efficiency; and Class 4 measures intellectual and interest modes.

callisthenics Systematic, rhythmic, light exercises, such as abdominal curls and push-ups, that utilize the weight of the body as resistance. Callisthenics are designed to tone and strengthen muscles, and to promote general fitness.

calliper A two-pronged instrument for measuring diameters.

callosity (callus) A thickening and hardening of the outer horny layer of skin. A callus protects the skin from rubbing, but it can crack and become painful (*see* **spinner's finger**). The tightening of the skin that accompanies callus formation may also cause pain. In the early stages, calluses can be gently filed down with a pumice stone. A thick callus that causes pain should be dealt with by a doctor who might pare off the excess skin with a blade or use some other technique (e.g., a salicylic acid plaster) for removing the hardened skin.

callus 1 Tissue containing blood and bone cells that form around bone following a fracture. Callus formation is an essential part of healthy bone repair. **2** *See* **callosity**.

calorie (cal) Unit of *work and *energy. One calorie is the amount of heat required to raise the temperature of 1 g of water by $1°$. Although it has been replaced by the joule in the SI system, calories are still widely used, especially in describing energy values of food and exercise expenditure. Physiologists tend to use the kilocalorie (equal to 1000 calories), sometimes referred to as the Calorie (Cal) to distinguish it from the calorie.

calorific balance A condition reached when the energy intake from food and drink equals energy expenditure by body activities.

calorific equivalence *See* **heat equivalence**.

calorimeter A device that measures heat production. In exercise physiology, a calorimeter is sometimes used to measure energy expenditure; a technique called direct calorimetry. The subject is supplied with air in an insulated, hermetically sealed chamber surrounded by copper tubing through which water is circulated. Heat production is estimated from changes in the temperature of the surrounding water. *See also* **bomb calorimeter**.

calorimetry Measurements of energy production and energy consumption in terms of heat. *See also* **direct calorimetry**; and **indirect calorimetry**.

Canadian home-fitness test A safe, simple, self-administered fitness test, the purpose of which is motivational rather than to define fitness levels accurately. The subject completes a questionnaire prior to the test to ensure basic fitness. Then, after warming-up, the subject climbs two steps of a standard staircase (each step is 8 inches or 20.3 cm high) at a rhythm set according to the age and sex of the subject for one or two periods of 3 minutes. The stepping rate approximates to 70 per cent maximum aerobic capacity. A fitness score is obtained from the duration of the exercise and heart rate.

canaliculis A very fine tubular channel, for example, found in the liver and in the *Haversian system of bone. Bone canaliculi contain fluid which transports nutrients and oxygen to bone cells and waste products away from them.

cancellous bone *See* **spongy bone**.

cancer A group of diseases characterized by uncontrolled growth of abnormal cells which have the ability to spread through the body or body-parts. Several studies have shown that physically active people are less likely than those who have sedentary lifestyles to develop certain types of cancer (e.g., breast and colon cancer).

cannabis *See* **marijuana.**

capacitance A measure of how easily blood flows through a vessel; it is the inverse of *peripheral resistance.

capacitance vessels Vessels, mainly veins, capable of holding and storing blood. Between 60 and 70 per cent of the body's blood volume is usually contained in the veins.

capacity The maximum amount something can contain, absorb, or produce independent of time (*compare* **power**). The term is used in relation to the total amount of ATP that can be produced by an energy system.

capacity interference Interference between two or more tasks performed at the same time, caused by limitations of attention. That is, there is competition for the limited information-processing capacity of the brain. *See also* **structural interference.**

capacity model A model of *attention based on the notion that each person has a limited space in the central nervous system for information processing.

capillarization The development of a capillary network to a part of the body. Aerobic training improves the capillarization of heart and skeletal muscle, by increasing the absolute number of capillaries and the capillary density (number of capillaries for a given cross-sectional area of muscle).

capillary The smallest type of blood vessel located between arterioles (small arteries) and venules (small veins). A capillary wall consists only of an *endothelium which, because of its permeability, allows gases, nutrients, and waste products to move relatively easily between the tissue fluid and blood.

capillary bed An area where there is a high density of capillaries forming a network.

capillary-to-fibre ratio The number of capillaries to each muscle fibre. A high capillary-to-fibre ratio allows the blood to more fully perfuse muscle tissue. Trained athletes have a significantly higher capillary-to-fibre ratio (up to 1.6) than untrained individuals (averaging about 1.0).

capitate The largest bone of the wrist which articulates with the trapezoid and hamate laterally and medially; the second, third, and fourth metacarpals in front; and the scaphoid and lunate bones behind (*see* **carpus**).

capitellum The lateral, ball-like *condyle at the elbow end of the humerus which articulates with the radius.

capitulum A small, rounded end of a bone which articulates with another bone.

capsular ligament A localized thickening in the capsule of a *synovial joint which encases the joint like a sleeve.

capsulitis Inflammation of a *joint capsule.

carbaminohaemoglobin An organic compound made by carbon dioxide binding to *haemoglobin. It plays a small part in the transport of carbon dioxide in the blood.

carbohydrate An organic compound composed of carbon, hydrogen, and oxygen, with the general chemical formula of $C_x(H_2O)_y$. Carbohydrates are major sources of energy, each gram yielding approximately 4 kilocalories of energy. During a short-duration exercise of maximal effort, energy is supplied almost exclusively by carbohydrates. Carbohydrates include simple sugars, glycogen, and starches. Sugars are simple carbohydrates. Starches are complex carbohydrates found in legumes, potatoes, and other vegetables. Carbohydrates are classified according to the number of sugar-units they contain. Monosaccharides have one sugar-unit, disaccharides two, oligosaccharides a few, and polysaccharides many. The body stores of carbohydrate are mainly in the form of *glycogen in the liver and skeletal muscle. The stores are limited to less than 2000 kcal; only enough energy for about a 32 km (20 mile) run. Without an adequate intake of dietary carbohydrate, muscle and brain cells can be deprived of their main energy source.

carbohydrate loading (carboloading; glycogen loading) A procedure followed by some athletes to raise the *glycogen content of skeletal muscle artificially by following a special diet, usually combined with a special exercise regime. One carbohydrate loading procedure proposed by the famous sport physiologist Per-Olof Astrand is based on the assumption that depletion of muscle glycogen stores stimulates the body to take up and store more glycogen than normal. For a marathoner, the procedure starts seven days before a race when the athlete depletes the muscle of glycogen by running a long distance, usually about 32 km (20 miles). For the next three days, the athlete eats a high protein, low carbohydrate diet and continues exercising to ensure glycogen depletion and sensitization of the physiological processes which manufacture and store glycogen. For the final three days before the race, the athlete eats a high carbohydrate diet and takes little or no exercise. Even though it can more than double muscle glycogen content, most athletes find this procedure difficult to follow. They cannot train fully during the low carbohydrate stage. They often feel irritable and tired and sometimes suffer muscle weakness, insomnia, and diarrhoea. An alternative procedure proposed by Sherman and his co-workers consists of reducing training intensity a week before competition and eating a normal mixed diet from which carbohydrates provide 55 per cent of the calories. Three days before the competition, training is reduced to a warm-up and about 15 minutes of activity, and the athlete eats a carbohydrate-rich diet. Both procedures can raise muscle glycogen levels to 200 mmol per kg of muscle which should enable the athlete to delay muscle fatigue and perform much better in long-distance events. However, carbohydrate loading also has its negative aspects: it results in more water being stored (with each gram of glycogen stored,

there are about 2.7 g of water), sometimes making the athlete feel heavy and stiff; and regular carbohydrate loading may lead to *myoglobinuria, chest pains, and heart irregularities.

carboloading *See* carbohydrate loading.

carbon dioxide A colourless gas which makes up about 0.04 per cent of the atmosphere. It is denser than air. It is toxic only above about 6 per cent concentration, but it does not support respiration or combustion. It is excreted as a waste product of *aerobic metabolism, and is carried to the veins, mainly as hydrogen carbonate (bicarbonate) ions. Expired air contains about 4 per cent carbon dioxide. Increases in carbon dioxide levels stimulate the *vasomotor centre to increase the ventilation rate so that more carbon dioxide can be eliminated from the lungs.

carbon dioxide output The volume of carbon dioxide expired from the lungs into the atmosphere. It is usually expressed as litres per minute (VCO_2). Under steady state conditions, carbon dioxide output equals carbon dioxide production by aerobic metabolism.

carbon dioxide transport The transport of carbon dioxide from tissues to the lungs. Between 60–80 per cent is carried in the plasma as hydrogen carbonate ions, formed from carbonic acid in a reaction catalysed by carbonic anhydrase. A small percentage of carbon dioxide is transported in solution and as carbamino-haemoglobin. A series of chemical reactions enables carbon dioxide to be unloaded from the blood at the lungs. The carbon dioxide then diffuses into the alveoli along a concentration gradient and is expired into the atmosphere.

carbonic anhydrase An enzyme that catalyses the interconversion of carbon dioxide, water, and carbonic acid.

carbonic anhydrase inhibitor A chemical that interferes with the action of carbonic anhydrase. *See also* **acetazolamide**.

carbon monoxide A poisonous, odourless gas that occurs in the atmosphere as a result of incomplete combustion of carbon and carbon compounds. It is a common constituent of vehicle exhaust fumes and tobacco smoke. Carbon monoxide enters the blood stream rapidly and combines with haemoglobin to form carboxyhaemoglobin, a relatively stable compound which reduces the oxygen-carrying capacity of the blood. The affinity of haemoglobin for carbon monoxide is about 230 times its affinity for oxygen, so carbon monoxide binds preferentially to carbon monoxide. High blood carbon monoxide levels reduce the ability to perform aerobic activities and impair attention.

carboxyhaemoglobin See **carbon monoxide**.

carcinogen Any substance capable of causing a *cancer.

cardiac Pertaining to the heart.

cardiac arrest Cessation of the effective pumping action of the heart. During a cardiac arrest, the heart may be beating rapidly without pumping any blood, or it may stop beating completely. Cardiac arrest is marked by an abrupt loss of consciousness and absence of breathing or pulse.

cardiac arrhythmia A loss of rhythm of the heart beat which becomes irregular.

cardiac centre A mass of nerve cells in the *medulla oblongata which regulate the force and rate of the heartbeat to meet the varied demands of the body.

cardiac concussion Damage to the heart resulting from a blunt trauma to the chest which does not cause any internal bleeding, but which may disturb the heartbeat, occasionally causing lethal arrhythmias such as ventricular fibrillation. The existence of this injury is a subject of dispute among cardiologists. See also **cardiac contusion**.

cardiac contusion A haemorrhage of the heart caused by a blow to the chest with a blunt object, for example, resulting from a collision between players in a contact sport or when a hard ball hits the sternum. It is difficult to diagnose but should be

suspected after trauma to the chest wall causes bruising. Cardiac dysrhythmias are most likely to occur within the first 24 hours of the trauma (if they occur at all). They can be fatal. Anyone experiencing heart irregularities or chest pain after a chest trauma should be admitted to hospital for a thorough investigation.

cardiac cycle The sequence of events which take place during a single heartbeat. See **diastole**; and **systole**.

cardiac diastole See **diastole**.

cardiac dysrhythmia An abnormal rhythm of the heart beat which may lead to, or be a symptom of, severe cardiac problems. Regular aerobic exercise can reduce susceptibility of the heart to rhythm disturbances.

cardiac failure See **heart failure**.

cardiac fatigue A decrease in stroke volume attributed to a decrease in the contractility of cardiac muscle. It has been implicated as one of the causes for an increase in basal resting pulse rate which is a characteristic feature of overtraining.

cardiac hypertrophy Increase in size of the heart. In athletes, it is characterized by large ventricular cavities and normal thickness of ventricular walls, enhancing stroke volume capability. It is also associated with an increased capillarization of the heart (see **athlete's heart**). In non-endurance athletes who regularly perform intense resistance training and isometric training, cardiac hypertrophy is characterized by normal sized ventricular cavities and thickened ventricular walls; the *stroke volume is not affected. In nonathletes, cardiac hypertrophy may be the result of a number of pathological conditions including heart valve disease.

cardiac imaging The production of an image of the heart which can be used to study cardiac function and to diagnose heart disorders. Noninvasive methods of cardiac imaging include magnetic resonance imaging and echocardiography. Invasive methods include nuclear cardiology. This involves injecting a radioisotope to label red blood cells and using a nuclear camera to produce an image of the heart. A traditional invasive technique involves injecting a contrast medium directly into the heart via arterial and venous catheters.

cardiac impulse An electrical impulse which originates in the pacemaker region (sinoatrial node) of the heart and initiates contractions of cardiac muscle.

cardiac index Cardiac output divided by the estimated body surface area; an index which relates *cardiac output to body size.

cardiac massage *See* **external cardiac massage**.

cardiac minute volume The volume of blood pumped out of the heart per minute.

cardiac muscle Muscle found only in the heart. The cells are striated, contain a single nucleus, and branch so that they fit together tightly at junctions called intercalated discs. Although cardiac muscle is *myogenic, it has a contractile mechanism similar to that of striped muscle (*see* **sliding-filament theory**). However, cardiac muscle does not fatigue and it cannot tolerate lack of oxygen.

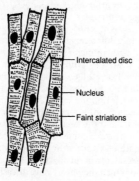

— Intercalated disc

— Nucleus

— Faint striations

cardiac muscle

cardiac output (Q) The volume of blood pumped out of the left ventricle of the heart in one minute. Cardiac output is the product of *heart rate and *stroke volume (i.e., $Q = SV \& mult; HR$). The average cardiac output at rest is 5–6 litres; during exercise it can exceed 30 litres in a trained endurance athlete.

cardiac rate The number of heartbeats per minute. *See also* **heart rate**.

cardiac rehabilitation programme A course of treatment designed to help patients who have suffered a heart attack to return to normal activity without additional health problems. Exercise is an integral part of many programmes. It appears that controlled aerobic exercise substantially reduces the risk of death from a subsequent heart attack, but has relatively little effect on reducing the risk for the recurrence of a nonfatal attack.

cardiac systole *See* **systole**.

cardinal plane One of three rectangular anatomical reference planes, each of which bisect the mass of body. For an individual in the anatomical position, the three cardinal panes intersect at a single point known as the *centre of mass. *See also* **frontal plane**; **sagittal plane**; and **transverse plane**.

cardiology The study of the heart and its functions.

cardiomyopathy *See* **hypertrophic cardiomyopathy**.

cardiopulmonary resuscitation *See* **artificial resuscitation**.

cardiopulmonary index An index of cardiorespiratory endurance which uses seven parameters, expressed in the following equation: $CPI = VC + MBH + MEP + age/SP + DP + PR$; where CPI is the cardiopulmonary index; VC = vital capacity in 100 ml units (i.e. 4400 ml is recorded as 44); MBH = maximum breath holding time in seconds; MEP = maximum expiratory pressure; age = age in years to nearest birthday; SP = systolic blood pressure; DP = diastolic blood pressure, PR = resting pulse rate per minute (all pressures are measured in mmHg). CPI scores range from 0.8 in healthy nonathletes to more than 1.8 for Olympic athletes. Those with heart disease may score less than 0.4. The CPI can also be used to indicate the level of fitness by recording the time required to restore all the parameters back to the normal resting level after a standardized exercise.

cardiorespiratory endurance *See* aerobic endurance.

cardiorespiratory endurance capacity *See* maximal oxygen uptake.

cardiorespiratory endurance test Any test of the ability of the heart and lungs to supply oxygen to large muscle groups, thereby allowing them to sustain activity for long periods. Some tests, such as the *cardiopulmonary index, are quite simple, while others are very complicated and may use formulae with up to 100 physiological indicators (*see* **Cureton's tables**). All the tests involve comparing physiological measurements during rest with those directly after exercise, and after a specified recovery period.

cardioselective beta blockers Drugs which selectively inhibit the action of beta₁ adrenoceptors (*see* **beta receptor**). The heart is a major site of these receptors, therefore cardioselective beta blockers exert a strong inhibitory action on the heart.

cardiovascular Pertaining to the heart and blood vessels.

cardiovascular deconditioning *See* deconditioning.

cardiovascular disease A disease of the heart and blood vessels. Risk factors include *hypertension, *obesity, *smoking, psychological stress, and lack of exercise.

cardiovascular drift (circulatory drift) A drifting upwards of heart rate when exercise is performed at a constant work rate over a prolonged period or in a hot environment. The cardiovascular drift is associated with sweating and a redistribution of blood so that peripheral circulation is increased. Body fluids are lost, reducing the volume of blood returning to the heart causing a decrease in stroke volume (*see* **Starling's law**). The heart rate increases in an attempt to compensate for the lower stroke volume and maintain a constant *cardiac output.

cardiovascular endurance The ability to sustain a large blood flow to active muscles.

cardiovascular fitness The ability of the heart and blood vessels to supply nutrients and oxygen to tissues (including muscles) during sustained exercise.

cardiovascular system A system in the body consisting of the heart, blood vessels, and blood that delivers nutrients to the body's various cells and removes waste products.

carnitene A coenzyme involved in the transport of fatty acids into mitochondria for metabolism by *beta oxidation.

carnitine A compound formed in the kidneys and liver and found in muscles where it plays an essential role in fatty acid metabolism. It transports fatty acids into mitochondria where they are used to generate energy by aerobic metabolism. It has been suggested that supplementation may result in more fatty acids being transported into the mitochondria so that energy production by fat metabolism is increased, sparing the metabolism of muscle glycogen, thus delaying fatigue. However, the evidence which supports the use of carnitine supplementation to improve endurance capacity is disputed, as there appears to be an excess of endogenous carnitine. Present evidence is insufficient to judge the effect of supplementation on high intensity exercise.

carotenes A group of yellow substances designated alpha-, beta-, and gamma-carotene, which are converted in the intestines and liver into vitamin A. Carotenes are present in a wide variety of foods, but concentrations are especially high in carrots, parsley, and green leafy vegetables. Carotenes are important *antioxidants.

carotid artery The main artery in the neck supplying oxygenated blood to the head.

carotid body A small mass of tissue in the carotid arteries which contains chemoreceptors sensitive to changes in carbon dioxide, hydrogen ion, and oxygen concentrations in the blood. Its main function is to control breathing so that an adequate supply of oxygen is maintained to all tissues of the body.

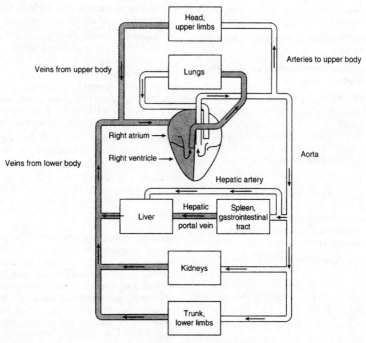

cardiovascular system

carotid pulse Pulse taken by pressing fingers gently against one of the carotid arteries. Simultaneous pressure against both carotid arteries is dangerous as it may stop blood flowing to the brain. *See also* **carotid sinus**.

carotid sinus A small swelling in the wall of each artery containing sensory nerve-endings which respond to changes in blood press0.ure. It is involved in maintaining a constant blood pressure to the brain. Squeezing the sinuses (e.g., in a wrestling strangle hold) causes the blood pressure to fall and the heart to slow by a reflex action, possibly resulting in the victim losing consciousness. Conversely, compression of the carotid artery below the sinus, produces a fall of pressure within the sinus, a reflex rise in blood pressure, and an acceleration of heart rate.

carpal Pertaining to the wrist.

carpal bones (carpals) Eight marble-shaped short bones (the scaphoid, lunate, triquetral, pisiform, trapezium, trapezoid, capitate, and hamate bones) closely united by ligaments to make up the wrist. The carpus as a whole is flexible, but movement between individual bones is restricted to gliding.

carpals *See* **carpal bones**.

carpal tunnel A narrow passageway between the carpal bones and the flexor retinaculum on the palm of the hand through which tendons and the median nerve pass from the wrist to the hand.

carpal tunnel syndrome A swelling which compresses the median nerve as it passes through the carpal tunnel in the palm of the hand. Symptoms include pain, pins-and-needles and numbness in the thumb and first three fingers. It can be caused by arthritis, an acute injury, or a chronic injury. Activities which involve repeated forceful wrist flexions can cause the syndrome. If the compression is not relieved, the muscles supplied by the median nerve can weaken and atrophy. Most cases respond to rest and hydrocortisone treatment, but sometimes surgical relief is required.

carpometacarpal joint A *synovial joint between the carpals and metacarpals of the four digits (fingers and thumbs). The carpometacarpal joint of the thumb is a saddle joint allowing a large range of motion similar to that of a ball and socket joint. The other carpometacarpal joints are gliding joints.

carponavicular fracture (scaphoid fracture) A fracture of the scaphoid bone in the wrist. It is caused by a fall onto the outstretched arm, forcibly bending the hand upward and backward. The impact drives the scaphoid back into the radius. Clinical signs are often conspicuous by their absence, but pain is usually felt in the 'snuffbox' area defined by the tendons near the thumb. This injury is quite common among young participants of contact sports and activities which have a high risk of falling. A carponavicular fracture is sometimes misdiagnosed as a wrist sprain and goes untreated. X-ray diagnosis is required to distinguish a wrist sprain from a carponavicular fracture. If a fracture is untreated, the bone will probably not heal properly, resulting in long-term wrist problems. The initial treatment of a suspected fracture or wrist sprain includes putting the forearm and wrist in a splint, gently applying ice, and obtaining medical assistance. Subsequent treatment of a confirmed fracture includes immobilization and, for a displaced bone, surgical repositioning. Recovery time is quite long: it may take up to four months for a displaced fracture to heal, and it is generally advised to protect the wrist during sports for a further three months.

carpus The Latin word for wrist, the proximal part of the hand consisting of carpal bones firmly joined together with liga-

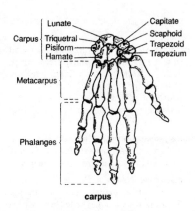

carpus

ments, but capable of some gliding movements over one another.

cartilage Tough and flexible connective tissue which forms the skeleton of an embryo and much of the skeleton of infants. As a child grows, much of the cartilage is converted to bone. Cartilage is characterized by rounded cartilage cells (called chondrocytes) surrounded by mucopolysaccharide matrix (chondrin) which is rich in collagen. Cartilage has no nerves or blood vessels and heals slowly when damaged. There are three main types: hyaline cartilage, fibrocartilage, and white fibrocartilage. The pieces of semi-lunar cartilage found in the knee are called *menisci.

Cartwright's model of team cohesion A model which proposes that there are forces, referred to as determinants, which strengthen team cohesion and certain outcomes, referred to as consequences, associated with effective team cohesion.

case history See anamnesis.

case study The study of a single example of something for its own sake (e.g., the study of the life of a famous sportsperson) or as an exemplar or paradigm of a general phenomenon.

CAT See computerized tomography.

catabolism Chemical reactions which take place in the body that result in the breakdown of large molecules into smaller ones. It is the destructive form of metabolism.

catalase An iron-containing enzyme found in all cells, but particularly abundant in active cells, such as those of the liver and muscles. Catalase helps to break down hydrogen peroxide, a poisonous byproduct of *aerobic metabolism, into water and oxygen.

catalyst Substance that increases the rate of a chemical reaction without itself being changed by the reaction. *See also* **enzymes**.

catastrophe theory A theory based on a mathematical model, developed by the French mathematician René Thom, which shows how through the interaction of various factors a small change in one of the factors can produce catastrophic changes. Sport psychologists use catastrophe theory to show that the *stress an athlete experiences in competition results from a complex interaction between physiological arousal (as reflected by changes in heart rate, sweating, and adrenaline secretion) and cognitive anxiety (i.e., mental anxiety). When athletes are subjected to a small increase in stress above a critical level, they may experience a huge and sudden loss of performance. *Compare* **inverted-U hypothesis**.

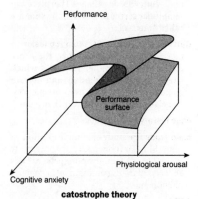

catostrophe theory

catastrophic injury In sport, there are three main types of very serious injury: nonfatal, serious, and fatal. A nonfatal catas-trophic injury is one in which there is a permanent severe neurological disability (e.g., a vertebral fracture that results in partial or complete quadriplegia). A severe catastrophic injury is one in which there is a transient but not permanent functional neurological disability (e.g., a fractured vertebra with no permanent paralysis). A fatal catastrophic injury may result directly from participation in the skills of sport, or indirectly from a systemic failure as a result of exertion while participating in a sport (e.g., heart failure). *See also* **sudden death**.

catecholamines A group of chemicals known as biogenic amines which can act as *neurotransmitters and *hormones. They include *adrenaline (epinephrine), *dopamine, and *noradrenaline (norepinephrine).

Catell 16PF An inventory that uses factor analysis to measure sixteen source traits of *personality. Many personologists have adopted the Catell 16PF for the personality assessment of athletes.

catharsis 1 The purging of emotions by evoking pity or fear. **2** A psychoanalytical method incorporating free association by which repressed emotions are brought to consciousness.

catharsis hypothesis 1 The suggestion that play affords an opportunity to discharge natural impulses, such as *aggression. **2** The suggestion that pent-up emotions, anger, and frustrations can be purged by expressing one's feeling's through aggression. *See also* **instinct theory**; *compare* **circular effect of aggression**.

catheter A long, slender flexible hollow tube which can be inserted into a body cavity or blood vessel to extract fluid, administer drugs, or monitor blood pressure.

catheterization The use of a *catheter to administer drugs or extract body fluids. Catheterization can be used to alter the integrity of urine so that banned substances may escape detection in dope tests of urine samples. This type of physical manipulation is on the International Olympic

Committee Medical Commission's list of banned doping classes and methods. For example, a male athlete on drugs may inject drug-free urine into his bladder via a catheter inserted into his penis.

cauda equina The bundle of coccygeal, lumbar, and sacral nerve roots that descend from the spinal cord to pass through openings in the vertebrae.

caudal *See* **inferior**.

cauliflower ear A permanent deformity of the external ear produced by repeated injury to the ear, common in many contact sports. *See also* **auricular haematoma**.

causal attribution model A model used to describe how a performer attributes outcomes to particular causes. The model has at least three dimensions (depending on the researcher's preference) with one dimension referring to stable–unstable causes, another to whether the locus of causality is internal or external, and a third to whether the causes are controllable or not. Therefore causes may be internal, stable, and controllable (e.g., ability), internal, unstable, and controllable (e.g., effort), and so on.

causal attribution theory *See* **attribution theory**.

Causal Dimension Scale A scale which assigns attributions to one of three dimensions: *locus of causality, *stability, and *controllability. The causal dimension scale has been used by athletes to determine what they believe are the causes for the success or failure of a performance. The athletes rate each perceived cause relative to nine questions, three for each dimension.

Causal Dimension Scale II A modified causal dimension scale in which the controllability dimension is divided into external control and personal control.

causal explanation An explanation which identifies an immediate precipitating cause or causes of a particular occurrence. Causal explanations usually depend on a number of assumptions concerning

physical laws. *See also* **cause-and-effect relationship**.

causalgia A very unpleasant burning pain felt in a limb in which a peripheral nerve has been traumatized.

causality 1 The relating of causes to the effects they produce. **2** The presumption that the occurrence or presence of an event or phenomenon is necessarily preceded, accompanied, or followed by the occurrence or presence of another event or other events. *See also* **cause-and-effect relationship**.

causal model A theoretical model of the causal relationship between variables used in causal modelling. *See also* **cause-and-effect relationship**.

causal modelling A method used in sport sociology and statistics to test the relationships underlying correlations between a number of variables. Causal modelling involves formulating and testing different theoretical models of the causal relationships between the variables and selecting the model which best fits the data. *See also* **path analysis**; and **log-linear analysis**. *Compare* **experimental method**.

causal relationship *See* **cause-and-effect relationship**.

causal schema A person's relatively permanent set of beliefs concerning the relationship between observed events and what the person perceives as causing the event.

cause A person, thing, or event which produces an effect. *See also* **cause-and-effect relationship**.

cause-and-effect relationship (causal relationship) A relationship between one variable and another or others such that a change in one variable effects a change in the other variable. A cause-and-effect relationship is claimed where the following conditions are satisfied: the two events occur at the same time and in the same place; one event immediately precedes the other; the second event appears unlikely to have happened without the first event having occurred. Many phenomena exhibit close association, but they may not have a cause-and-effect relationship. *See also* **correlation**.

cause variable *See* **independent variable**.

cavus foot (clawfoot; high arches; pes cavus) Condition characterized by rigidity of the foot, decreased mobility of the subtalar joint, and a decrease in internal rotation of the tibia during locomotion. After the foot strikes the ground, the heel remains everted, the longitudinal arch remains high and rigid, and the midtarsal joint does not unlock. During running, the foot remains inflexible so that it cannot conform easily to the underlying running surface. Therefore, the foot absorbs the full force of ground impact. Athletes with cavus foot are susceptible to a number of injuries including *stress fractures of the foot, *plantar fasciitis, and *Achilles tendinitis. The permanently high longitudinal arch may also cause problems on the top of the foot if footwear is not cut high enough or laces are tightened too much so that the foot becomes constricted during running.

CBAS *See* **Coaching Behaviour Assessment System**.

ceiling effect A limitation that places a maximum level to the score that a performer can achieve in a task. The ceiling effect is imposed either by the scoring system or by physiological and psychological limitations. As an individual's level of performance improves towards the ceiling, it becomes more difficult to improve. For example, in a sport which gives 10 marks for a 'perfect' performance, it is easier to improve a score from 6.5 to 7.0 than from 9.5 to 10.0.

cell The structural and functional unit of living organisms. Typical cell components include a nucleus and cytoplasm enveloped by a cell surface membrane. The cytoplasm contains a number of membrane-bound organelles, including mitochondria, the sites of *aerobic metabolism.

cell body An enlarged region of a nerve cell. It contains a nucleus.

cell membrane A selectively permeable biological membrane enveloping a cell (the cell surface membrane) or within a cell. Cell membranes consist of a bilipid layer with a variable amount of protein. They separate one structure from another and act as selective barriers, regulating the movement of materials in and out of the cell or its organelles. Conjugated proteins in cell surface membranes are involved in antigen–antibody reactions and distinguishing between self and nonself (usually foreign) cells.

cell nest A group of *chondrocytes within the matrix of *hyaline cartilage.

cell surface membrane *See* **cell membrane**.

cellular respiration The breakdown of food within a cell to release energy in the form of ATP. *See also* **aerobic metabolism**; and **anaerobic metabolism**.

cellulite A term adopted by the diet industry to describe the bulged, rippled, and waffled appearance associated with subcutaneous fat on hips, thighs, and buttocks. It occurs almost exclusively in women. Cellulite is merely an effect created by connective tissue filled with fat, and it can be reduced by diet and exercise.

cellulitis Bacterial infection of the skin which becomes inflamed but does not block blood vessels.

cellulose A fibrous, unbranched polysaccharide that is the main structural component of plant tissues and constitutes most of the *fibre in the diet.

central fatigue *See* **central inhibition**.

central group member A member of a group who has a pivotal role in the success of the group. The central group member of a sports team is usually very concerned about the team's success, highly motivated, highly talented, and plays in a position where he or she is involved in much of the action of the game.

central inhibition (central fatigue) Fatigue due to a change of neuronal activity in the central nervous system. Unlike subjective fatigue, central inhibition occurs even when an athlete is strongly motivated.

Athletes exhibit central inhibition when performing differently in nearly identical situations where biochemical factors are likely to be very similar. For example, in tests of fatigue, athletes tend to perform significantly less voluntary muscle contractions in stressful conditions (e.g., in an unfamiliar environment or when being observed by the experimenter) than in less stressful conditions. The reasons for central inhibition are unclear, but mental stress may change the distribution of blood in the brain, altering the supply of chemicals to neurones involved in physical activity.

centrality The degree to which a spatial position of a team member occupies the centre of the team formation. It is argued that central positions (such as quarter back in American football, or sweeper in soccer) are more highly interactive than those on the periphery, or those in positions which have independent tasks. A high proportion of managers and coaches are recruited from players of central positions.

central nervous system (CNS) The main mass of nervous tissue, lying between sensory receptors and effectors, which acts as an integrating centre. The CNS comprises the brain and spinal cord and consists of more than one hundred thousand million neurones.

central pattern generator (pattern generator; spinal generator) A hypothesized complex neural circuitry in the central nervous system containing a set of commands which, when activated, produce a coordinated movement sequence. The central pattern generator is thought to govern rapid motor actions and genetically determined actions. It is capable of producing a rhythm or oscillation in the output from motor neurones to the different muscles involved in a movement pattern. Experiments on spinal cord preparations of cats have shown that this oscillatory output first activates motor neurones to the flexors of the leg, and then to activate the extensors, then flexors again, in a pattern similar to that displayed in locomotion. *See also* **motor program**.

central tendency *See* **measure of central tendency**.

centre of buoyancy (centre of volume) The point at which the buoyant force acts on an immersed body, and the point around which a body's volume is equally distributed in all directions. It is the *centre of gravity of the water displaced by the body. In a symmetrical body, the centre of buoyancy coincides with the body's centre of gravity, but in an assymetrical body they may not coincide. In the human body, for example, the centre of buoyancy tends to be at chest level which is higher than the centre of gravity.

centre of gravity The point at which the whole weight of an object can be considered to act and, therefore, at which all parts of an object are in balance. The position of the centre of gravity varies according to the shape of the object. In objects with a regular shape, the centre of gravity coincides with its geometric centre. In objects with an irregular and variable shape (as in the human body), the centre of gravity cannot be defined easily and it changes with every change in position of the body; it may not even lie within the physical substance of the body. The centre of gravity of a projectile in flight follows a fixed path, but body movements may raise or lower the body parts around the centre of gravity. In this way it is possible to jump different heights even though the centre of gravity reaches the same height. *See also* **sacral promontory**.

centre of inertia *See* **centre of mass**.

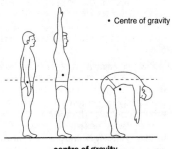

• Centre of gravity

centre of gravity

centre of mass (centre of inertia; mass centroid) The point at which the mass of a body may be considered to be concentrated and the sum of the *moments of inertia of all the components of the body is zero.

centre of oscillation The point on a pendulum, on the line through the point of suspension and centre of mass, which moves as if all the mass of the pendulum was concentrated at that point.

centre of percussion The point on a striking implement that produces fewest vibrations on hitting another object. A ball hit at the centre of percussion of a bat will produce fewer vibrations, and more force will be transferred to the ball, than if it was hit at another point. The centre of percussion on a bat, racket, or golf club, is also known as the sweet spot.

centre of pressure (centre of surface) The point at which the resultant of *lift and *drag acts on a body immersed in a fluid. For a projectile, the centre of pressure changes with the *angle of attack. If the centre of pressure is in front of the *centre of gravity, the projectile experiences a torque, known as the pitching moment, that rotates the leading edge upwards, resulting in a stall (*see* **stall angle**).

centre of rotation The point about which a body rotates.

centre of surface *See* **centre of pressure**.

centre of volume *See* **centre of buoyancy**.

centric force *See* **direct force**.

centrifugal force An outwardly directed force acting on a body rotating around a central point. It is a reaction force which is equal in magnitude but opposite in direction to the centripetal force acting on the body.

centring procedure A procedure adopted by athletes to help them focus on relevant stimuli, ignore irrelevant stimuli, and control physiological arousal. Centring involves consciously altering breathing and tension levels so that body weight coincides as closely as possible to *centre of mass (e.g., by breathing from the abdomen

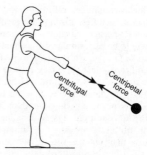

centrifugal force

instead of the chest, and relaxing neck and shoulder muscles). The performance of a centring breath is usually timed to coincide with an important action which requires total concentration (e.g., serving at tennis). *See also* **refocusing**; **thought stopping**.

centripetal force An inwardly directed force acting on a system rotating around a central point. The centripetal force acting on a body with a mass m moving in a circular path with radius r and with a velocity v is equal to mv^2/r.

centrum The main weight-bearing part of a vertebra.

cephalic In anatomy, pertaining to the head.

cerebellum Part of the brain behind the medulla and the pons. It has numerous connections with other parts of the brain and plays a crucial part in many aspects of locomotion. It is involved in the control of *posture and *muscle tone, and it helps to produce smooth, coordinated, locomotory movements. The cerebellum continuously and subconsciously integrates information from the *primary motor cortex, other motor areas of the brain, and sensory receptors, especially *proprioceptors.

cerebral cortex The outer, surface layer of *grey matter in the cerebral hemispheres of the forebrain. The cerebral cortex contains motor areas which control complex motor skills and some involuntary movements; sensory areas, which receive information from the sense organs; and association areas, which are responsible for thought, learning language, and personality. *See also* **prefrontal cortex**; **premotor cortex**; and **primary motor cortex**.

cerebral dominance There are two cerebral hemispheres, the left and the right. Cerebral dominance refers to the side which has the main responsibility for the development of language. In 90 per cent of people, it is the left hemisphere, while the right hemisphere is usually concerned with other tasks, such as motor activities, visual–spatial skills, intuition, and emotion. Most individuals with left cerebral dominance are also right-handed. *See also* **handedness**.

cerebral hemispheres *See* **cerebrum**.

cerebral perfusion imaging A scanning method that involves the injection of small amounts of a radioactive tracer into the blood. A special camera is used to view blood flow through the cerebrum to assess functional damage. This very sensitive technique has been used to monitor brain damage in boxers.

cerebral spinal fluid Fluid formed from blood plasma which circulates in the spaces of the brain and spinal cord. Cerebral spinal fluid, unlike blood plasma, has few cells and little protein. The fluid supports, cushions, helps nourish the brain and spinal cord, and removes metabolic wastes.

cerebrotonic trait A psychological characteristic of temperament which is said to be strongly correlated with being an *ecto-morph. Cerebrotonics tend to be solitary and adverse to crowds. They also tend to have an overfast reaction time and to be hyperactive.

cerebrovascular accident *See* **stroke**.

cerebrum Part of the forebrain consisting of a pair of large cerebral hemispheres. The surface of the hemispheres is a highly folded layer of *grey matter and is called the cerebral cortex. Underneath the cortex is *white matter which includes the *basal ganglia. The right hemisphere appears to be mainly concerned with sensory and motor functions on the left side of the body, and the right with those on the left side of the body. The hemispheres are interconnected by a band of nervous tissue (the corpus callosum). It is believed that this band transfers information from one side of the brain to the other so that memory can be duplicated in both hemispheres.

cervical Pertaining to the neck.

cervicale An anatomical landmark located on the most posterior point of the neural spine of the seventh vertebra.

cervical nerve stretch syndrome *See* **brachial plexus neurapraxia**.

cervical radiculitis A pinched nerve in the neck often associated with *cervical spondylosis and caused by repetitive impact and bending of the neck. Treatment is usually nonsurgical, and may include cervical traction, anti-inflammatories, and wearing a cervical collar.

cervical spondylosis A degenerative condition accelerated by repetitive impact and bending, common in contact sports such as rugby football. Cervical vertebrae lose their height and plumpness so that they move closer together, forming spurs where they come into contact. The spurs may grow and impinge on nerves in the neck (*see* **cervical radiculitis**).

cervical rib A short extra rib which sometimes occurs on the seventh cervical vertebra. It may cause problems if it presses against a nerve or artery.

cervical vertebra One of seven bones, identified as C1–C7, which are the smallest and lightest of the vertebrae. Each cervical vertebra has a transverse process containing a foramen through which the large vertebral arteries ascend to the neck to reach the brain. The first two cervical vertebrae are the atlas and axis.

chafing (intertrigo) Abrasion caused by mechanical friction where two areas of skin rub together (e.g., in the groin) causing redness and tenderness of the skin. Chafing which results from movements during exercise can be reduced by applying petroleum jelly to areas which are likely to rub together (e.g., the inner thighs and nipples of runners).

chaining 1 A concept that suggests that in a movement consisting of a number of components occurring in a sequence, termination of early components results in sensory feedback which acts as a stimulus initiating the next component, and so on until the movement is completed. **2** A method of learning a skill consisting of several actions linked in a series in which the completion of each action initiates the next action, for example a floor routine in gymnastics. The components are learnt in the same sequence as they are performed. *Compare* **backward chaining method**.

challenge 1 An invitation to engage in a contest. **2** A demanding or stimulating situation.

channel capacity A concept based on the idea that information has to pass through channels of limited capacity as it is processed in the brain. It is suggested that the channels act as bottlenecks restricting the amount of information going from the sense organs to the brain, and limiting the ability to attend to environmental stimuli (*see* **attention**).

channelled aggression Feelings of *aggression which are diverted into positive, productive actions in sport.

character 1 The personality structure or relatively fixed traits of an individual. **2** Attributes of *personality deemed culturally valuable or appropriate by society, for example determination and will to succeed. Sport is often said to develop character, but data supporting this assumption are sparse.

charismatic authority Authority based on the special personal qualities claimed by and for an individual which make the individual attractive to, and capable of influencing, large numbers of people. Originally used purely in a religious context, the term is now applied to individuals in many spheres including sport.

Charles's law A law which states that a gas at constant pressure will expand by 1/273 of its volume at 0 °C for each 1 °C rise in temperature. Thus the volume of a fixed mass of gas at constant pressure is proportional to absolute temperature.

charley horse (quadriceps haematoma) A muscle *haematoma of the *quadriceps femoris muscle, marked by severe and prolonged pain. It is caused by direct trauma and is a common injury in contact sports such as American Football. In its mild form it is well known as a 'dead leg'. This usually resolves itself within a week. In its severe form, a charley horse can cause much internal swelling and is sometimes linked with the development of calcium and bone in the muscle (*see* **myositis ossificans**). The term has also been used for similar hamstring injuries.

cheating A weight-training technique that enables a trainee to lift a load he or she could not otherwise lift. The ability to lift a weight at constant speed is limited by the strength of the muscle at its weakest point, commonly called the sticking point. Cheating is a slight assistance movement, such as bouncing the barbell and raising the hips during a bench press, that accelerates the bar beyond the sticking point.

chest girth The circumference of the thorax, around the mesosternale (an anatomical landmark in the sternum).

chest pain Discomfort and soreness in and around the chest. In sport, chest pains commonly result from an impact with another object (e.g., a ball), and physical over-exertion straining a chest muscle (e.g., the *intercostals used in breathing). A persistent pain in the centre or left side of the chest, especially if felt down the arm, neck, or back, requires urgent medical attention, particularly if the pain is combined with shortness of breath, cold sweat, and fatigue. Such pains may be associated with a heart disorder. A stabbing pain in the chest may be caused by a lung infection. *See also* **cardiac concussion**.

Cheyne–Stokes breathing An irregular pattern of breathing characterized by a few shallow breaths followed by increasingly deep breaths which then fall off rapidly. Breathing may then cease for a few seconds and the pattern repeated. The incidence of Cheyne–Stokes breathing increases with altitude, occurring 24 per cent of the time at 2440 m and 100 per cent of the time at altitudes above 6300 m. The interrupted breathing interferes with relaxation and normal sleep patterns. This type of breathing is also seen in terminal illness.

childhood onset obesity Obesity which first develops during childhood. It usually results in the development of an excessive number of adipocytes (fat cells) which gives a predisposition to obesity in later life.

chiropractic The treatment and correction of bodily ills by mechanical means. The spine is regarded by many chiropractors as the nerve centre of the body so that many ailments, such as headaches, can be treated successfully by correcting a badly aligned backbone. The established medical profession in western countries has expressed reservations about chiropractic treatment, especially if it is performed by someone who is not medically qualified.

chi-square Value obtained from *chi-squared test; a statistical test comparing observed frequencies with the frequencies expected from a given hypothesis. The larger the difference between observed and expected frequencies, the more likely it is that a statistically significant difference exists between the categories.

chi-squared test Statistical routine which is a test of significance comparing the observed results of an experiment or sample against the numbers expected from a theory of prediction. The test produces a value called *chi-square. It can be used only with data which falls into discrete categories.

chlorine Chlorine is an element distributed throughout the body fluids. It is required by the body to maintain the correct acid–base balance in the blood. It is also used to synthesize hydrochloric acid in the stomach. In the UK, the daily Reference Nutrient Intake of chlorine as chloride for adults is 2500 mg; in the USA, the daily Recommended Dietary Allowance is not established.

choice reaction time The reaction time for a task in which a performer has to make one of two or more choices. The performer may have to respond to one of several different stimuli (for example, the time it takes to choose which ball to hit with a racket when confronted with several balls at the same time), or may have to choose one of several responses to the same stimulus (for example, the time it takes to choose which shot to attempt in a racket game when the stimulus, a returned ball, is the same each time).

choking 1 Difficulty in breathing due to any interference of the airway causing partial or complete blockage. The condition may be due to internal causes, such as emotional disturbance, or external causes, such as a direct blow to the throat. **2** Colloquially applied to athletes whose performance deteriorates under stress, such as before an important competition. Such athletes may feel as if they are physically choking because their bronchial muscles tighten. An athlete who chokes may be one who, through poor pacing or excessive enthusiasm, develops a significant anaerobic effort too early in a competition. Consequently, the accumulation of lactic acid induces hyperventilation and an uncomfortable tightening of the airway. Alternatively, the fear of competition may induce excessive hyperventilation.

cholecalciferol *See* **vitamin D**.

cholecystokinin A peptide which acts as a *metabotropic neurotransmitter in the cerebral cortex of the brain.

cholesterol A lipid-related compound found in tissues and manufactured in the liver. Cholesterol has a number of essential functions: it is important for body tissue repair; it is a constituent of cell membranes which it helps strengthen; it forms the starting point of steroid manufacture, and is involved in the formation of several hormones; it forms bile salts; and it is the raw material for vitamin D. Dietary sources of cholesterol include animal products such as eggs, meat, and cheese. A high-fat diet can increase blood cholesterol levels, and nicotine (from tobacco smoking) increases deposition of cholesterol in arterial walls, but hereditary factors are also important determinants of blood cholesterol levels. High blood cholesterol levels are associated with cardiovascular diseases. Blood cholesterol levels can be decreased by taking regular aerobic exercise and eating a low-fat diet. A deficiency of cholesterol is rare. *See also* **high-density lipoproteins; low-density lipoproteins**.

choline A compound important for the synthesis of lecithin and other phospholipids, and of *acetylcholine. Choline is also involved in the transport of fat in the body. Deficiency is rare because choline can be synthesized in the body, but when it does occur, deficiency may lead to liver damage. Choline is sometimes classified as a vitamin but it is not a true vitamin because it can be made in the body.

cholinergic Applied to nerve and muscle fibres which use *acetylcholine as a neurotransmitter.

chondroblast Actively dividing cell which develops into *cartilage.

chondrocyte A specialized, mature non-dividing cartilage cell which secretes chondrin, the matrix of cartilage.

chondromalacia Roughening of cartilage (e.g., chondromalacia patellae).

chondromalacia patellae Deterioration and softening of the articular cartilage lining the undersurface of the kneecap. The damage is usually caused by repetitive rubbing of the kneecap on the femur. It sometimes, but not always, causes a patellofemoral pain. However, it should not be assumed that all such pain is due to chondromalacia patellae (*see* **patellofemoral pain syndrome**). Treatment of chondromalacia patellae includes *nonsteroidal anti-inflammatory drugs (NSAIDS) to reduce inflammation, and strengthening and stretching exercises to improve the structures around the knee.

chordae tendinae String-like tendinous cords which prevent the atrioventrcular valves of the heart from turning inside out.

chorionic gonadotrophin *See* **human chorionic gonadotrophin**.

chromatography A technique for separating and analysing the components of a mixture of liquids or gases. Chromatography depends on the selective absorption of the different components in a column of powder (column chromatography) or on a strip of paper (paper chromatography). Chromatography is one of the techniques used to identify specific drugs in a urine sample.

chromium A metallic element essential for efficient glucose metabolism. Chromium is readily available in a variety of foods, including liver, meat, cheese, wholegrains, brewer's yeast, and wine. There is no Reference Nutrient Intake in the UK, but a safe daily intake is set at 25 micrograms. In the USA, the Recommended Dietary Allowance is 50–200 micrograms.

chromium picolinate A substance claimed by some to act as an anabolic agent. It has been suggested that chromium picolinate supplementation increases lean body mass because of the ability of chromium to boost protein metabolism through its potentiating effect on *insulin. The results of at least one study appear to support the claim. However, further studies are necessary before any clear assessment of the effects of chromium picolinate supplementation on athletes can be made.

chromosome Coiled structure in the nucleus of cells, consisting of DNA and proteins.

chromosome test A test used for determining sex. It involves staining a thin scraping from inside the cheeks (a buccal smear) using a nuclear dye and a fluorescent compound. The former stains a dense body (the *Barr body) on the X chromosomes, while the latter reveals the Y body associated with the Y chromosome. *See also* **sex determination**.

chronic Applied to conditions which are long-lasting and are usually slow to develop. *Compare* **acute**.

chronic adaptation A physiological adaptation to repeated bouts of exercise; for example, enlargement of the muscles lining the heart. *Compare* **acute response**.

chronic arousal The basic *arousal level of an individual. It is thought by some to be a function of *personality: for example, *extroverts generally have low chronic arousal levels so they often seek out exciting or stimulating situations; *introverts tend to have high chronic arousal levels and avoid risk-taking situations.

chronic cerebral injury *See* **encephalopathy, traumatic**.

chronic electrical stimulation An experimental procedure for simulating the effects of a maximal endurance training stimulus on muscle. Experiments in which a rabbit anterior tibial muscle was subjected to a continuous train of electrical pulses showed that skeletal muscle has a remarkable capacity for adaptation to the extreme metabolic demands of chronic stimulation. After 5–6 weeks of chronic stimulation, the muscle changed from containing predominantly fast fibres (about 94 per cent) to containing only slow-twitch fibres. In addition, the muscle became significantly less fatiguable, and there was an increase in the number of blood capillaries per unit of muscle cross-sectional area.

chronic fatigue syndrome A disorder characterized by persistent fatigue, typically lasting at least 6 months, without neurological signs. Commonly associated features are muscle weakness and pain, psychiatric symptoms (anxiety and depression), and viral infections. There is much controversy surrounding the possible cause of chronic fatigue syndrome, with some believing that it is of organic origin (a virus, such as the Coxsachie virus, has been implicated), while others believe that it is of functional origin. Many doctors believe that chronic fatigue syndrome is a heterogeneous group of disorders. Whatever the cause, the syndrome is of major importance to sportspeople because the symptoms of muscle weakness and pain, headaches, forgetfulness, irritability, sore throat, poor concentration etc., are often severe enough to impair athletic performance. Where the cause cannot be identified, treatment is directed to the relief of symptoms. It is also important that doctors and coaches convey a positive and optimistic outlook towards the outcome, and provide support and reassurance during the gradual return to full activity. Sportspeople with chronic fatigue syndrome should be encouraged to exercise within their tolerance levels and to increase their activity gradually. There is no evidence to support the concept of total rest.

chronic fibrosis Persistent scarring which may occur after repeated damage to connective tissue.

chronic hypertrophy *See* **hypertrophy**.

Chronic Obstructive Lung Disease (COLD) A respiratory disease characterized by breathlessness and wheezing due to chronic obstruction of the airways. It is often associated with emphysema and is common among smokers. Those with COLD find exercise difficult and many become inactive. This results in a progressive decline in cardiovascular and musculoskeletal fitness. Aerobic exercise at 70–85 per cent predicted maximum heart rate combined with a warm-up, flexibility training, cool-down exercises gives some relief from the symptoms of COLD: it enhances mobility, increases oxygen uptake, and reduces anxiety, depression, and social isolation. However, exercise may increase the risk of cardiac arrhythmias in COLD patients.

chronobiology The scientific study of biological rhythms such as circadian rhythms.

chronological age 1 Actual age from birth regardless of development level. Chronological age is a measure of the time a person has spent out of the womb interacting with the environment. It is inseparably associated with biological growth and experience. Since individual growth rates vary widely, children of the same chronological age show marked differences in strength, motor proficiency, etc. **2** In anthropometry, the difference between the date of observation and the date of birth in years, months, and days.

chronometric approach An approach to the study of *information processing which concentrates on temporal aspects, considering the duration of the various processes. The approach makes extensive use of the study of reaction times.

chronoscope A device that measures speed of reaction.

chunking Grouping units of information into larger units or chunks in order to facilitate memorizing them. For example, if there are 15 different telephone numbers to learn they could be placed together in groups of three giving, in effect, five numbers to learn; the three letters C A T could be grouped into one word, CAT, which also has a meaning attached to it. Chunking has been used to improve learning, memory, and retrieval and recognizes the fact that the human brain can process only a limited amount of information at any one time.

circadian rhythm A biological rhythm associated with the solar day, which has a period of approximately 24 hours. Circadian rhythms have been demonstrated in humans for changes in heart rate, metabolic rate, wakefulness, and flexibility. Rectal temperature shows a distinct circadian rhythm, with temperatures being at their lowest at about 4 a.m., increasing during the day with a peak in the afternoon. Levels of sports performances also follow a circadian rhythm. Runners, cyclists, and swimmers tend to perform better in the afternoon and early evening than in the morning for both aerobic and anaerobic activities of short to moderate duration. The peak probably corresponds to the time when body temperature is highest since muscles work better when warm. Fencers tend to perform best in the middle of the day, perhaps because their sport depends on mental skills which

peak about that time. Studies of endurance athletes have not revealed any clear circadian rhythm, although some endurance athletes peak later in the day. There appear to be individual differences among athletes of all sports, with the phasing of circadian rhythms being affected by personality types. Those with a preference for early morning work have been called 'larks', and those with a preference for evening work have been called 'owls'.

circatricial Pertaining to scar tissue.

circuit training Training that involves performing selected exercises or activities at a series of stations (typically 6–10). The stations form a circuit through which a person progresses either as quickly as possible or in a predetermined time. Most circuit training produces modest improvements in *aerobic endurance and major improvements in strength, muscular endurance, and flexibility. Aerobic endurance can be emphasized by completing the circuit as quickly as possible with minimum rest, and by placing the stations further apart.

circuit resistance training A combination of *circuit training and *resistance training. Typically, it involves working at 40 per cent to 60 per cent of maximum strength for 30 s with a 15 s recovery. Circuit resistance training improves strength, muscular endurance, and flexibility. It can also increase muscle mass and decrease body fat content. Its beneficial effects on aerobic endurance are slight.

circular effect of aggression The notion that aggression begets aggression. Compare catharsis hypothesis.

circular motion The motion of a body about a circle; or, more precisely, a movement that traces an arc at a fixed distance (the radius) from a fixed point or line (the axis). See also **angular motion**.

circulation 1 The flow or motion of a fluid in or through a given system. **2** The flow or motion of blood through the blood vessels.

circulatory drift See **cardiovascular drift**.

circumduction A circular movement which combines flexion, extension, abduction,

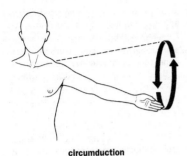

circumduction

and adduction so that the movement of the body-part describes a cone shape. The distal end of the limb moves in a circle while the proximal end remains stationary.

citrate synthase (CS) An enzyme, the level of which is commonly used in exercise physiology as a measure of the capacity of the *Krebs cycle.

citric acid cycle *See* **Krebs cycle**.

civilizing process The historical process by which people have acquired a greater capacity for controlling their emotions. Associated with the civilizing process has been a lower tolerance of anti-social behaviour such as football hooliganism. This may explain why, although football-associated violence has a long history, it has received increased attention in recent times.

Clarke's sign A clinical sign used in the diagnosis of knee injuries. The patient lies in a relaxed position with the knee extended and tenses the *quadriceps muscle as the examiner presses the patella into the trochlea. Pain indicates a patellar dysfunction; retropatellar pain indicates chondromalacia patellae, but the sign is not very sensitive.

classical conditioning (Pavlovian conditioning) A form of *learning in which a neutral stimulus becomes a conditional stimulus capable of eliciting a given response after being repeatedly presented with an unconditional (significant) stimulus. For example, in Pavlov's experiment a bell was rung (conditional stimulus) whenever a dog used in the experiment was fed. Eventually the dog would salivate (response)

when it heard the bell ringing, even when the smell of food (unconditional stimulus) was absent. Conditioning is more effective if the conditional stimulus and unconditional stimulus occur simultaneously and are presented in the same location. *Compare* **operant conditioning**; *see also* **principle of contiguity**.

claudication Limping. Intermittent claudication is a cramping pain which limits walking ability. It may be neurogenic or vascular. In neurogenic claudication, pain is due to pressure on a nerve. In vascular claudication, pain is due to ischaemia resulting from a temporary constriction of blood vessels which supply skeletal muscle. Claudication most commonly affects the calf muscle.

clavicle (collar bone) Slender, curved long bone extending horizontally across the upper thorax. The clavicle forms the anterior part of the pectoral girdle. It is attached anteriorly to the sternum and laterally to the acromion of the scapula. Many shoulder and chest muscles attach onto the clavicle which transmits forces from the arms to the axial skeleton. The clavicle resists compression forces poorly and is easily fractured. The thickness of the clavicle depends on the loads that have been placed on it: clavicles are stronger and thicker in those who perform load-bearing exercises involving the shoulder and arm muscles.

clavicle fracture A fracture which commonly occurs when a person falls onto an outstretched arm, for example when falling off a horse. It may also occur from a direct impact with another athlete or obstacle. Fractures in the shoulder area nearly always affect the clavicle. If a clavicle fracture is suspected, the arm is immobilized in a sling in the most comfortable position and secured to the body with an elastic bandage. Ice is applied gently over the area for 20 minutes at a time and medical attention sought so that an X-ray can be taken to confirm diagnosis. Closed treatment (e.g., a clavicle strap or simple sling, depending on the character of the fracture) is often successful. Surgery is required if the bone penetrates the skin. Fractures usually heal in about six weeks (three weeks for children under twelve). However, most athletes should not return to competition until the clavicle is clinically solid and the appropriate muscles rehabilitated. This may take 12 weeks. Rehabilitation includes muscle strengthening exercises that do not involve motion at the fracture site (i.e. they cause no pain).

clavicular Pertaining to the *clavicle.

claw foot *See* cavus foot.

cleated footwear (studded footwear) Athletes of several sports wear cleated or studded footwear (e.g., football, lacrosse, and baseball players). Traditionally, boots have a small number of quite long cleats (studs) to provide good traction, but these tend to increase the risk of injury from twisting motions. Anterior cruciate ligament sprains of the knee often result from the foot being fixed in place by studs stuck in the ground as the upper body is rotated. Wearing footwear with a larger number of shorter cleats can reduce the rates of injury to the lower extremities by more than 40 per cent.

clenbuterol A drug that has stimulatory effects similar to *adrenaline and anabolic effects similar to *steroids. As a stimulant, it is used to treat asthma, but clenbuterol has also been used as an ergogenic aid in sport. Clenbuterol is on the International Olympic Committee list of *banned substances.

clinical examination A medical examination of a person to ascertain the extent to which he or she is suffering from an illness, condition, or injury.

clinical sport and exercise psychologist A medically qualified person with extensive training in psychology who treats athletes and exercisers who have severe emotional disorders (e.g., eating disorders and drug abuse).

clique A small social unit within a group.

clobazam A derivative of benzodiazepine which does not seem to impair psychomotor performance but does retain anti-anxiety properties. This may make it more applicable in a sport context than other *benzodiazepines.

clonic cramp Intermittent contractions and relaxations of muscles. *See also* cramp.

clonidine An alpha$_2$ agonist which inhibits the release of *noradrenaline from postganglionic sympathetic nerves. This drug is used clinically to treat *hypertension and migraine. Clonidine has also been used by athletes to stimulate hGH (human growth hormone) secretion artificially, thus avoiding the direct use of hGH which is a *banned substance.

closed circuit spirometry A method of *indirect calorimetry. The subject inhales via a face mask from a container filled with oxygen. Expired air goes back to the container via soda lime which absorbs carbon dioxide. Changes in the volume of oxygen in the container are recorded as the volume of oxygen consumed. *Compare* open-circuit spirometry.

closed fracture *See* simple fracture.

closed interview Type of interview in which the interviewee is asked questions and picks answers from a limited range of possible responses. *See also* fixed choice questionnaire. *Compare* open-ended question.

closed kinetic chain A movement sequence, starting with a free body segment such as an arm or leg, and finishing at a fixed segment. An example is a dive which starts with movement of the arms and finishes with movement of the feet.

closed loop system (servo; servomechanism) A control system which appears to be self-regulating. Closed-loop systems employ feedback and a reference of correctness (norm or set point). Deviations from the norm are detected and corrections made in order to maintain a desired state in the system. Closed-loop systems provide the homeostatic mechanism of many physiological functions (*see* **negative feedback**) and also control some movement patterns where feedback from proprioceptors and other receptors plays an important part. *Compare* open-loop system.

closed loop theory A cognitive theory of skill acquisition which emphasizes the role played by *feedback. The theory has two key neural components: a memory trace, which selects and initiates an appropriate response; and a perceptual trace, which acts as a record of the movement made over many practices. During and after an attempt of the movement, feedback and *knowledge of results enables the performer to compare the movement with the perceptual trace. The trace acts as a reference of correctness so that appropriate error adjustments can be made for subsequent attempts of the movement.

closed skill A skill performed in a stable or largely predictable environmental setting. The movement patterns for closed skills can be planned in advance. Examples of closed skills are trampolining, golf swing, discus throwing, performing a handstand, diving from a platform or board. *See also* **self-paced tasks**; *compare* **open skill**.

close-packed position The joint position in which the articulating bones have their maximum area of contact with each other. It is in this position that *joint stability is greatest. The close-packed position for the knee, wrist, and interphalangeal joints is at full extension, and for the ankle joint at full dorsiflexion. Any movement away from the close-packed position takes a joint into the loose-packed position in which the area of contact and joint stability is reduced.

closure The formation of a bony union between the diaphysis and epiphysis after the *epiphyseal plate ceases to proliferate and the bone has reached maturity.

clotting *See* **coagulation**.

clo unit Basic measurement for the thermal properties of clothing. One clo unit is the thermal insulation that is comfortable for a resting man at $21\,°C$, where relative humidity is less than 50 per cent and the air movement is 6 metres per minute; it equates to a man wearing a three piece suit and light underclothes. At $-40\,°C$, twelve clo units are required; light activity lowers this to 4 clo units, and a person running at

16 km/hr would be adequately protected by only 1.25 clo units of clothing. The amount of protection required increases when the clothes become wet because water is a poor insulator.

cluster analysis A technique used to differentiate different subgroups within a single collection of information made about a group, people, or objects.

cluster sampling A sample from a representative group where it is not practicable to sample the entire population. For example, if samples of students from universities were required, one university could be selected randomly then a random selection of students made from within the one establishment.

CNS *See* **central nervous system**.

coach Motivator and teacher of athletes. Ideally, a coach is a moulder of theoretical and practical training and translator of technical information. *See also* **coaching**; and **coaching behaviour**.

coach–athlete compatibility Situation in which the coach's behaviour is compatible with the athlete's desires, and vice versa. It is a critical factor in the satisfaction and success of individuals and teams.

coaching The organized provision of assistance to an individual athlete or group of athletes to help them develop and improve the performance of their chosen sport.

coaching behaviour The behaviour of a coach. It is a function of the coach's own characteristics such as personality, ability, and experience, as well as the influences of the situation in which the coach operates. There are many styles of coaching behaviour including training and instruction behaviour, *democratic behaviour, *autocratic behaviour, *social support behaviour, and *rewarding behaviour. A coach may use one type of behaviour exclusively but is more likely to use different styles for different situations and individuals.

coaching behaviour assessment system (CBAS) A system developed to permit the direct observation, analysis, and coding of a coach's behaviour in a natural setting. It consists of twelve behavioural classes divided into eight kinds of reactive behaviour and four kinds of spontaneous behaviour. Reactive behaviour of a coach occurs in response to an athlete's behaviour and level of performance. Spontaneous behaviour is not provoked or directly linked to the observed performance of the athlete, and the behaviour may be either relevant or irrelevant to a game or performance. In one major study, approximately two thirds of all observed behaviours fell into the categories of positive reinforcement, general technical instructions, or general encouragement. The observed behaviour of the coach can be compared with athletes' perception of the coach's behaviour and the coach's self-perception. Coaching behaviour can be modified with training.

coaching competencies *See* managerial competencies.

coaching stereotype The relatively rigid role which has been assigned to coaches and PE teachers by popular belief. A coach is perceived as one who strives for excellence and conditioning, and who otherwise presents a tough and relatively inflexible front to both team and supporters. Some studies have shown that many coaches tend to be rather dominant, able to express aggression easily, and are not interested in the dependency needs of others. However, it is unclear whether this pattern of behaviour is a true reflection of personality or an attempt to act out the role imposed by society, since other studies indicate that coaches do not differ from other members of society in the way and extent to which they exploit situations and people.

coaction 1 A situation in which two or more individuals are engaged in the same activity at the same time. The general affect of coaction is to raise arousal levels. Individuals who are optimally aroused for a sporting event may become over-aroused when joined by other individuals. This may lead competitors to perform less well and spectators to become aggressive. The larger the number of people engaged in an activity and the closer their proximity to one another, the greater the coaction effects will be. **2** The interaction between two or more individuals which produces a motivating effect on performance. *Compare* **audience effect**; and social facilitation. *See also* **dynamogeny**; and **social interactive forces**.

coactive audience An audience of one or more people who are performing the same task as the subject, but independent of the subject.

coactive sports Sports in which athletes perform side by side with little interaction (e.g., archery and sprinting). *Compare* **interactive sports**.

coactor An individual who is performing the same task as the subject, but independent of the subject.

coagulation Precipitation of suspended particles from a dispersed state (e.g., the clotting of blood). Blood coagulation involves the interaction of a number of factors (coagulation factors) which lead to the conversion of soluble fibrinogen into insoluble fibrin fibres, and the formation of a solid mass called a blood clot.

coasting *See* inertial movement.

cobalamin *See* vitamin B12.

cobalt An essential trace element; it is a component of vitamin B_{12}, essential for the production of red blood cells. It is required in very small amounts. Average daily intakes are about 0.3 mg. Very high doses (above 29 mg per day) have proved toxic. Sources include liver, lean meat, poultry, fish, and milk.

cocaine A highly addictive drug that acts as a central nervous system stimulant. Its use is banned by the International Olympic Committee. Cocaine is an alkaloid derived from the leaves of the coca plant, *Erythroxylon coca*, which grows in the Andes. Cocaine abuse has been recorded for American footballers and cyclists. Most take it for recreational use, but some take it as an ergogenic aid. Users report that it increases alertness, and feelings of euphoria and increased mental power. Scientific studies of the effects of cocaine on human performance are rare because of ethical considerations and the results have been contradictory. However, studies of its effects on animals indicate that although cocaine has mood-enhancing properties, it probably has performance-inhibiting effects, at least for endurance activities. Harmful side-effects include serious cardiovascular problems such as arrhythmia, tachycardia, and hypertension. Cocaine abuse can induce coronary occlusion, which was almost certainly the cause of death of at least one basketball player and one US football player in the major leagues.

coccydynia (coccygodynia) Pain in and around the *coccyx.

coccygeal Pertaining to the *coccyx.

coccygodynia *See* coccydynia.

coccyx Vestigial tail-bone consisting of four or, less commonly, three or five fused vertebrae. The coccyx provides some support for the pelvic organs and is the origin of the *gluteus maximus.

cocktail party phenomenon The ability of a person in a crowded, noisy room to selectively attend to a single conversation (often containing personally relevant information), while excluding other inputs. Some individuals lack this ability.

cocktail party problem The problem of being unable to distinguish one voice from another in a crowded room. *Compare* cocktail party phenomenon.

co-contraction The concept that movement usually involves the simultaneous contraction of pairs of antagonistic muscle groups. The contribution which each member of the antagonistic pair makes varies with the type of action. For example, when the external resistance to the agonist is great, the contribution of the antagonist will be minimal. *See also* **reciprocal innervation**.

code A set of rules or guidelines intended to govern or control behaviour.

codeine A drug belonging to the *narcotic analgesics which are on the International Olympic committee list of *banned substances. Codeine is a constituent of a large number of medicines, including many nonprescription preparations to treat colds and coughs when it may be combined with aspirin, a permitted drug. Athletes must therefore take care when choosing a cold cure, especially just before or during competitions.

Codman exercises Flexibility exercises used to rehabilitate a painful shoulder with restricted mobility. For example, the patient bends forwards at the waist with the hand of the uninjured side resting on the knee and performs gentle circumduction movements with the right shoulder. This exercise allows gravity to distract the glenohumeral joint.

coefficient A factor that measures a specific property of a given substance and is constant for that substance under specific conditions.

coefficient of drag A unitless number which indicates a body's ability to generate fluid resistance (*see* **drag**). The coefficient of drag for a human body, and other asymmetrical objects, is usually found experimentally in a wind tunnel. The magnitude of the coefficient depends on the shape of the body and its orientation relative to fluid flow. The coefficient of drag generally decreases as the shape of the body becomes longer and more streamlined.

coefficient of friction A unitless number indicating the mechanical or molecular interaction between two surfaces in contact. Assuming the *normal reaction force is constant, the lower the coefficient of friction, the easier it is for two surfaces to slide over each other. Surfaces with a coefficient of friction of zero, are perfectly smooth and frictionless. Factors affecting the coefficient of friction include the roughness and hardness of the surfaces in contact and the type of molecular interaction between them. The coefficient takes different values depending on whether the bodies with their surfaces in contact are motionless or moving. *See also* **coefficient of limiting friction, coefficient of kinetic friction**.

coefficient of kinetic friction The coefficient of friction for two surfaces in contact with each other. For any two bodies in contact, the coefficient of kinetic friction is always smaller than the coefficient of limiting friction. *See also* **rolling friction**; and **sliding friction**.

coefficient of lift A unitless number which indicates a body's ability to generate *lift as it moves through a fluid. The magnitude of the coefficient depends on the shape of the body and its *angle of attack. For example, the coefficient of lift for a discus in flight is about 1.2 for an angle of attack of 22° and only 0.7 for an angle of attack of 3°.

coefficient of limiting friction (coefficient of static friction) Coefficient of friction which applies to two bodies in contact which have not yet begun to move. Its value equals the maximum *static friction divided by the perpendicular force pressing the two surfaces together (i.e. the normal reaction force). *Compare* **coefficient of kinetic friction**.

coefficient of restitution The ratio of the relative velocity of an object before impact to its relative velocity, in the opposite direction, after impact. The coefficient of restitution is a measure of an object's *elasticity upon striking a given surface. It is a measure of a ball's ability to return to its original shape after being deformed on impact. The coefficient of restitution for a perfectly elastic object is unity (one) and is zero for a perfectly inelastic (plastic) object. The coefficient of restitution is affected by the nature of the surface (using the same ball, a synthetic turf produces a coefficient of restitution twice as great as grass), and speed of impact, composition, temperature, and elasticity of the striking object.

coefficient of rolling friction A measure of how easily a ball will roll on a surface. The coefficient of rolling friction depends on the nature of the ball and the surface, the *normal reaction force, and the diameter of the ball. A heavily grassed, soft, wet surface has a much higher coefficient of rolling friction than one which is bare,

hard, and dry. For any given surface, the coefficient of rolling friction is less than the coefficient of sliding friction. *See also* **coefficient of friction**.

coefficient of sliding friction A measure of how easily two surfaces slide against each other. For any two surfaces, the coefficient of sliding friction is less than the coefficient of limiting friction. Consequently, it is easier to keep a body sliding along a surface than it is to start the body sliding.

coefficient of stability The ratio of the moment tending to maintain a body in equilibrium (M_m), and the moment tending to disrupt the body's equilibrium (M_o). That is, coefficient of stability = M_m/M_o.

coefficient of static friction *See* **coefficient of limiting friction**.

coenzyme An organic, nonprotein cofactor which is needed for the normal functioning of an *enzyme. Many vitamins function as coenzymes.

cofactor A nonprotein substance that is essential for the efficient functioning of an *enzyme, binding with it during a reaction. Tightly bound cofactors are called prosthetic groups. ATP and NAD are cofactors.

coffee *See* **caffeine**.

cognition Mental processes by which knowledge about oneself, others, and the environment is gained and interpreted. It includes thought processes such as perception, problem solving, and creativity.

cognitive-affective stress management A form of *stress management which takes into consideration the aspects of the situation, and the stressed person's cognitive appraisal (feelings and thoughts) of the situation, physiological responses, and overt behaviour. Cognitive-affective stress management can reduce or eliminate negative thoughts or worry.

cognitive anxiety 1 Anxiety as perceived by the individual in terms of how the individual feels about a situation. **2** The anxiety a person is conscious of; actual worrying and anxious feelings (*compare* **physiological arousal**). *See also* **anxiety**.

cognitive appraisal Personal interpretation of a situation (how an individual views a situation). Cognitive appraisal is regarded by some sport psychologists as an important component of *burnout. The perception of a situation can be the cause of a negative psychological reaction, rather than the situation itself. An athlete who loses a string of competitions can view it positively as a challenge and an opportunity to come back from adversity, or view it negatively as evidence that he or she will never be a successful competitor.

cognitive attribution model *See* cognitive model.

cognitive-behavioural orientation An approach to the study of sport psychology which assumes that behaviour is determined by the environment (e.g., rewards and punishments) and cognitions (thoughts and interpretations). *Compare* behavioural orientation; and psychophysiological orientation.

cognitive development Development of the thought processes by which knowledge is acquired including perception, intuition, and reasoning. *Compare* physical development.

cognitive developmental approach A developmental view of how moral reasoning evolves from a low to a high level. It argues that people with a low moral level are unable to conceive acts of aggression as being immoral and are more likely to engage in such acts.

cognitive dissonance The experience of having competing, opposing, or contradictory thoughts, attitudes, or actions leading to a feeling of tension. Dissonance can be removed by making a choice and having positive thoughts about the choice made. *See also* cognitive dissonance theory.

cognitive dissonance theory A theory with the basic premise that people like to be consistent in their thoughts, opinions, attitudes, and behaviours. Therefore, if two cognitive elements conflict, dissonance is created and (according to the theory) people are motivated to reduce dissonance.

Dissonant cognitions exist when belief A implies negation of belief B. For example the belief that drugs can cause illness, is dissonant with the belief that drugs are necessary to win at sport. The dissonance can be reduced by adjusting belief A or B in a number of ways. Belief A could be adjusted by ignoring medical reports which support the belief and studying carefully the reports which state that drugs can be used safely; belief B could be adjusted by taking less drugs and converting to safer drugs. *See also* **cognitive dissonance**.

cognitive evaluation theory A theory dealing with the effect of *extrinsic rewards on *intrinsic motivation. It assumes that intrinsically motivated behaviour is affected by a person's innate need to feel competent and self-determining in dealing with the environment. The theory asserts that there are two main ways extrinsic rewards affect intrinsic motivation. First, the reward may have a controlling affect by being perceived as the primary reason for participating in an activity. Secondly, a reward may have an informational aspect which affects the recipient's opinion of his or her own competence. Most rewards have a controlling aspect and an informational aspect. The combined effects may either increase or decrease an individual's intrinsic motivation. Rewards which have mainly a controlling aspect tend to decrease intrinsic motivation.

cognitive learning A type of *learning which mainly uses cognitive processes, such as perception and reasoning, and in which the contribution of the learner is emphasized. *Compare* observational learning.

cognitive mediational model A model of *anxiety reduction which is aimed at modifying affect-eliciting cognitions. It assumes that emotional arousal is mediated by cognition rather than environmental cues, therefore it is possible to reduce anxiety by modifying thoughts that often elicit and reinforce emotionality.

cognitive model (cognitive attribution model) A model adopted by sport psychologists to study achievement oriented attributions. According to the model, athletes process information about outcomes (e.g., winning or losing) according to whether they perceive the cause as within themselves (*see* **internal locus of control**) or in the environment (*see* **external locus of causality**) and whether the cause is perceived as stable or unstable.

cognitive processes Thought processes include perceiving, remembering, and reasoning.

cognitive psychology The study, by indirect methods, of the nature of unobservable mental processes in human behaviour.

cognitive skills Techniques designed to change levels of *anxiety, *arousal, and *attention using processes such as *imagery.

cognitive somatic anxiety questionnaire A fourteen-item questionnaire designed to assess both somatic and cognitive modes of *trait anxiety, thereby taking into consideration the multidimensional nature of trait anxiety.

cognitive sport involvement Involvement in sport through the process of thinking and knowing about sport indirectly from information supplied by the mass media. Individuals who exhibit strong cognitive sport involvement may accumulate highly detailed information and statistics about their favourite sport. *See also* **affective sport involvement**; **primary behavioural involvement**; and **secondary behavioural involvement**.

cognitive state anxiety (tica, task irrelevant cognitive anxiety) The aspect of *state anxiety which is concerned with worry and anxiety.

cognitive strategy (cognitive therapy) A psychological procedure designed to control *anxiety and improve performance. It is based on the belief that psychological problems, such as anxiety, are the product of faulty ways of thinking about the world. Cognitive strategies are used by sport psychologists to help athletes identify these false ways of thinking so as to avoid them

and to prepare themselves mentally for competition.

cognitive stress management (cognitive affective stress management) Stress management technique used by sport psychologists to reduce or eliminate negative thoughts or worry.

cognitive theory A theory in which the behaviour of individuals is assumed to be directed not only by the occurrence of social events and the individual's own feelings, but also by the individual's thoughts and interpretations of those feelings. It assumes that people think about the results and future consequences of their behaviour and do not react mindlessly to other people, problems, or situations. *See also* **attribution theory**.

cognitive therapy *See* cognitive strategy.

cohesion (group cohesion; team cohesion) The integration of the behaviour of different individuals as a result of social bonds, attractions, or other forces that hold the individuals together as a group or team over a period of time. Cohesion is measured by the degree to which group or team perform efficiently regardless of interpersonal feelings and the emotions prevalent among the individuals, reflecting mutual attraction among members. Research shows that the performance of a team affects cohesion much more than cohesion affects performance. *See also* **life cycle model of cohesion**; **linear model of cohesion**; **pendular model of cohesion**; **sociometric cohesion**; **task cohesion**; and **team cohesion**.

cohort Group of individuals possessing a common characteristic such as being born in the same year, or entering school on the same date.

coincidence–anticipation The ability to produce a response which accurately coincides with the arrival of a moving stimulus. For example, being able to hit a moving ball accurately with a tennis racket.

cold (coryza) The common cold is a virus infection in which blockage and inflammation of the nose (rhinitis) and sinuses are prominent symptoms. Although many athletes train and even compete with a mild cold, it is wise to avoid all strenuous activity during the feverish stage of a cold because there is a danger that the virus will affect the heart (*see* **myocarditis**). Many over-the-counter cold cures contain *stimulants which constrict blood vessels in the upper respiratory tact and nose. Many of these medications contain substances banned by the International Olympic Committee (*see* **codeine**). No product for use in the treatment of colds should be used by a competitor without first checking with a doctor or pharmacist that the product does not contain a drug of the banned stimulants class.

COLD *See* **Chronic Obstructive Lung Disease**.

cold acclimatization Physiological adaptations to repeated, prolonged exposure to low temperatures. Changes in peripheral circulation may keep exposed skin warm and improve cold tolerance, but cold acclimatization has not been thoroughly studied.

cold treatment The treatment of a sports injury by the indirect application of ice or a cold compress. The cold acts reduces pain, inflammation, and bleeding, but only if applied immediately after injury since most bleeding occurs within the first few minutes. The ice is usually applied for 10 to 20 minutes; fatty tissue requires a longer period than lean tissue. Direct application of ice must be avoided because it can cause frostbite. Cold treatment may delay the healing of some conditions. *See also* **RICE**.

colinear force A force which has its *line of action along the same line as another force.

collagen A structural, fibrous protein found in all connective tissues. It is the single most abundant protein in the body. Collagen gives bone its flexibility, helping it to resist tension.

collapse A condition of extreme prostration, associated with sudden loss of consciousness due to faulty circulation such as might occur from a defective heart,

shock, or haemorrhage. Although the collapse of an athlete following strenuous activity may be physiological (for example, a marathon runner who stops suddenly at the end of a race may collapse because of the pooling of blood in the legs), any collapse should be investigated completely to eliminate sinister causes.

collar bone *See* **clavicle**.

collateral circulation Development of alternative routes in the circulatory system. It has been suggested that new blood vessels formed as a response to regular aerobic exercise may take over normal coronary blood circulation after a coronary thrombosis reduces blood flow to heart muscle.

collateral ligament A major ligament that crosses either the medial aspect of a joint (medial collateral ligament) or lateral aspect. Collateral ligaments prevent excessive lateral motion at the knee and elbow. The medial collateral and lateral collateral ligaments of the knee are also known as the tibial and fibular collateral ligaments respectively.

collective aims Aims shared by all members of a group of individuals working together.

collective behaviour Behaviour exhibited by a group of individuals in response to events and by virtue of the fact that the group provides anonymity for, and affects the behaviour of, individuals within the group. Such behaviour is usually unstructured, disorganized, and transitory. *See also* **contagion theory**; **convergence theory**; **crowd behaviour**; and **value-added theory of collective behaviour**.

collective efficacy A group's confident expectation that it will successfully achieve its intended goal. *Compare* **efficacy**; **self-efficacy**.

collectivism Any social doctrine which advocates communal action; in political and economic doctrines collectivism particularly relates to state ownership and control of the means of production and distribution. The term has been applied in sport; for example, to the role of "domestiques" in professional cycling who sacrifice their individual chances of winning for that of the team.

Colles' fracture Fracture of the radius, typically about 1 cm proximal to the wrist. It usually results from a forceful, direct trauma, such as falling on an outstretched hand. It is the most common wrist fracture. Because the ulna plays no part in forming the wrist joint, the radius receives the brunt of the force. Symptoms include local pain, numbness in the fingers, and limited mobility; if the radius is displaced, it produces a classical dinner fork deformity of the wrist. A Colles' fracture often results in a shattering of the ends of the broken bones. Initial treatment consists of splinting the wrist and forearm in the injured position, gently applying ice over the injury, and calling for medical assistance. With mild fractures, a closed reduction (nonsurgical realignment of bones) may be sufficient, but if the injury is more serious, surgical realignment may be required. It is particularly important to maintain the length of the radius. A poorly treated Colles' fracture can result in the radius shortening relative to the ulna, and can give rise to permanent loss of wrist rotation. After reduction, the injured wrist is usually immobilized in a plaster of Paris cast which leaves the fingers and thumbs free so the muscles of the fingers, hand, and forearm can be exercised. Immobilization is often lengthy (4 to 6 weeks). Most sports doctors advocate aggressive rehabilitation which includes an intensive exercise programme to ensure maximum recovery. It may take 3 to 6 months before an athlete can return to full activity. *See also* **carponavicular fracture**.

colloid Small particles (1–100 micrometres) dispersed in a medium. The particles do not dissolve readily, nor do they settle out under gravity. Colloids have a high capacity for binding with water and other substances. They do not pass easily through cell membranes.

colon The main part of the large intestine. It has no digestive function but absorbs large amounts of water and electrolytes from undigested food as it passes through the colon from the small intestine to the rectum.

colour blindness The inability to distinguish certain wavelengths of light. Colour vision is conferred by the light sensitive cells in the retina of the eye, called cones. They belong to three populations with maximum absorption either in the red, blue, or green regions of the spectrum. Colour blind people lack one or more of these pigments. The most common form of colour blindness involves the inability to distinguish between red and green. Even those who are not colour blind respond to some colours more readily than to others. This can be important when considering the colour of team kit, when easy identification of fellow team-members is advantageous.

coma Condition of depressed consciousness in which, unlike sleep, oxygen use is below resting levels and the comatose person is totally unresponsive to sensory stimuli for an extended period of time. A coma can be induced by hypothermia, hyperthermia, and direct trauma. *See also* **Glasgow Coma score**.

combat An activity which involves beating an opponent in a stylized way which has similarities to war or battle. Examples include chess and judo.

comfort index An arbitrary index of the suitability of environmental conditions to physical activity. Comfort Index = (temperature + relative humidity)/4. Since the index was devised in the USA, temperature is measured in degrees Fahrenheit. A comfort index above 95 during low windspeeds may require acclimatization; the presence of wind allows higher values to be tolerated.

comfort zone A range of temperatures and humidity within which people feel comfortable under calm wind conditions. In general, as the temperature increases, tolerance to humidity decreases, and vice versa. In temperate zones, dry-bulb temperatures of 20–25 °C with relative humidity between 25–75 per cent, are regarded as the limits of the comfort zone. In Britain, the optimum conditions for comfort are generally accepted as being 15 °C and 60 per cent relative humidity. The wind chill factor affects this. *See also* **sensible temperature**.

command style A coaching style in which the coach makes all the decisions while the athlete is expected to follow directions.

comminuted fracture Fracture in which the bone shatters into many pieces. It is particularly common in elderly people with brittle bones.

commitment An important psychological attribute, characterized by dedication to completing a particular task. Commitment is one of the most important factors affecting an athlete's success. Athletes who want to achieve their full potential, need high levels of commitment.

communication Any imparting or exchange of information between two or more people. Communication may be verbal, non-verbal, intentional, or unintentional. *See also* **interpersonal communication**; **intrapersonal communication**; **nonverbal communication**.

community 1 Set of social relationships existing within a geographically defined area, or the area itself. **2** Relationships which exist on an abstract ideological or social level; for example, a community of marathon runners.

compact bone (cortical bone) Bone consisting of a central *Haversian canal surrounded by concentric rings of a hard, virtually solid mass of bony tissue intruded by minute canals called canaliculi. Compact bone forms the dense outer shell of bones. It has a smooth and homogeneous appearance.

comparative method A method of testing hypotheses about causal relationships, or establishing social types and classes, by looking at the similarities and differences between phenomena, societies or cultures. It could, for example, be used as a method for studying the role of sport in different countries.

compartment syndrome A painful condition caused by increased pressure within a muscle compartment. An acute compartment syndrome is indicated by an intramuscular compartment pressure above 40 mmHg at rest (normally, it is 0–10 mmHg). It can arise as a result of a direct impact or muscle rupture. If an acute compartment syndrome is not relieved immediately by rest, surgical decompression may be necessary to relieve the pressure against blood vessels, otherwise the blood supply to tissues will be compromised and the tissue may die. Acute compartment syndromes are rare; most cases are associated with fractures or dislocations of the leg, but a few are caused by prolonged increase in exercise intensity (e.g., overambitious marathon training by a novice runner). A chronic compartment syndrome arises as a result of overtraining and is characterized by intermittent excessive pressure. During activity, the muscles within the compartment swell and press nerves and blood vessels against the wall of the compartment. Pain associated with *ischaemia is localized to the muscles. Although the pain is relieved by rest, every time the athlete resumes activity the pain starts again. Although many sportspeople alter their activity patterns until the symptoms settle, usually, the only long-term solution is surgical decompression. The most commonly affected compartment is the anterior tibial compartment of the lower leg (*see* **anterior compartment syndrome**). *See also* **shin splints**.

compartmentalization of muscle The division of a single muscle into anatomical compartments each of which has its own primary nerve branch. Therefore, each anatomical compartment can be recruited independently and may function as a separate entity (*see* **deltoid muscle**).

compensatory movement A reflex movement that maintains a particular body position.

competence Capacity to perform or teach a skill. *See* **technical competency**.

competence motivation *See* **Harter's competence motivation theory**.

competing response theory Theory that explains why *intrinsic motivation is reduced when an external reward is given. According to the theory, the interjection of an external reward acts as a competing response which distracts from and interferes with the responses which facilitate enjoyment of the task (e.g., giving a child a prize for winning a race may detract from the sheer joy of competing).

competition 1 Action in which one person or group vies with another or others to achieve a goal which may be to establish a position of superiority over others, or a goal in which defeating others in a personal sense is of secondary consideration. Competition is a strong motivating force which may be directed against the performance of others, against a person's own standards, or a combination of the two. Generally, competition improves with competition. However, there is some concern about the effects of subjecting young people to frequent competition since, although many situations in life foster competition, many others require cooperation. **2** A contest in which a winner is selected from among two or more participants. In sport, competition is direct, formalized, and socially regulated. *See also* **objective competitive situation**; and **subjective competitive situation**.

competition period A period of training in which competition performance is stabilized as much as possible so that the athlete can produce optimal performances in key competitions. *See also* **peaking**; and **periodization**.

competition training Training in which a competitive environment is simulated over a number of training sessions, usually by gradually introducing more and more aspects of the true competitive environment.

competitive ability The capacity to take part in situations in which a person's performance is judged in relation to that of others.

competitive A-state (competitive anxiety state) A feeling of heightened *anxiety in response to a specific competitive situation which is perceived as threatening.

competitive A-trait (competitive anxiety trait) A relatively enduring *personality disposition to respond with elevated levels of *anxiety before, during, and after any athletic competition.

competitive goal orientation *See* **outcome goal orientation**.

competitive individualism In sociology, the view that achievement and nonachievement should depend on merit. Effort and ability are regarded as prerequisites of success. Competition is seen as an acceptable means of distributing limited resources and rewards. Acceptance of the competitive individualism viewpoint encourages the cult of winning and the belief that competition brings out the best in people.

competitiveness The desire to compete and strive for success in sport.

competitive process A psychological process which sometimes occurs when the objective demands of competition are perceived as threatening, resulting in an increase in *state anxiety.

competitive social situation Situation in which the goals of the separate participants are so linked that there is a negative correlation between their attainments. That is, individuals can only attain goals if other participants do not attain theirs. *Compare* **cooperative social interaction**; and **individualistic social situation**.

competitive state anxiety *See* **competitive A-state**.

competitive state anxiety inventory *See* CSAI.

competitive stress The negative emotional reaction of an athlete when he or she feels that his or her *self-esteem is threatened during a competition. The threat comes from an imbalance between the performance demands of a competition and the athlete's perception of his or her own ability to meet those demands successfully. The degree of stress depends on how important the consequences of failure are perceived by the athlete.

competitive trait anxiety *See* competitive A-trait.

complement system A part of the immune system which includes a group of blood proteins belonging to the globulins involved in removing foreign particles and damaged cells. Complement activation is part of the immune system's response to muscle cell damage after heavy exercise, and it culminates in the release of complement components which cause local inflammatory reactions.

complement The collective term for proteins of the *complement system, known separately as C1, C2, C3 etc. The serum complement tends to be deficient in some endurance athletes. This may contribute to their increased susceptibility to infection.

complete blood count A measure of the composition of blood. It includes haemoglobin concentration and white blood cell count.

completion tendency In the *frustration–aggression hypothesis, the notion that the frustrated individual does not feel satisfied or fulfilled until the urge or drive for *aggression is completed.

complex carbohydrate A carbohydrate that consists mainly of polysaccharides. Complex carbohydrates are common in unrefined foods, such as wholemeal bread. In addition to carbohydrates, these foods are usually a rich source of vitamins, minerals, and fibre.

compliance 1 A form of direct motivation which relies on the use of extrinsic rewards and punishments. For example, compliance is used when a coach offers athletes a day off training if they win a competition; or when the coach threatens extra training if instructions are not listened to and carried out. **2** The elastic resistance of tissue to distension. **3** The volume change in the lungs, measured in litres, produced by a unit change in pressure, measured in centimetres of water. Lung compliance is measured using a balloon placed in the intrathoracic oesophagus so that the pressure can be applied at the end of normal expiration and again after the subject has inhaled a known volume of gas. Compliance is reduced with some diseases and age.

component interaction A feature of some tasks in which adjustments of one component necessitates adjustments of another component.

component vector Two or more vectors the sum of which produces a quantity which may be expressed as a single vector, known as the resultant vector. If a runner on a cross-country course runs two miles east (vector AB), two miles north (vector BC), then two miles west (Vector CD), then the resultant vector is vector AD, two miles due north of where the runner started: $AD = AB + BC + CD$.

compound fracture (open fracture) Fracture in which the broken ends of a bone protrude through soft tissue and skin. It is more serious than a simple fracture because it can more easily lead to severe bone infections that require massive doses of antibiotics.

compress In medicine, a firm bandage that may hold an ice-pad or heat-pad against an injured area.

compressibility A measure of the tendency of a material to change its volume and density when subjected to pressure due to loading.

compression A force squashing, squeezing, or pressing down on an object. The distribution of compression within an object is called compressive stress and is measured as the compression force applied per unit area of the object being squashed. Compression tends to change the shape of an object and reduce its volume. *Compare* **shear force**; and **tension**.

compression bandage *See* bandage.

compression illness An illness that results from an increase in the pressure within gas-containing body spaces (*see* **barotrauma**; and **caisson disease**).

compression modulus *See* modulus of compression.

compression neuropathy Condition in which the fibres of a nerve become compressed, resulting in an inability to transmit impulses. In cycling, the ulnar nerve in the palm of the hand is commonly pressed against the handlebars with a loss of sensation and weakening of the hand. If untreated, it can result in permanent paralysis. However, in its early stages it is easily treated by frequently altering the hand position and protecting the hands with tape or padded gloves.

compression rupture A muscle tear caused by a direct impact pushing the muscle against an underlying bone. Heavy bleeding may result. *See also* **charley horse**. *Compare* **distraction rupture**.

compression syndrome An overuse injury characterized by pain and muscle stiffness in areas where the space available for tissues (e.g., muscles, nerves, and blood vessels) is limited. During exercise, the tissue is pressed against another structure and becomes inflamed or damaged. *See also* **compartment syndrome**; and **compression neuropathy**.

compressive strength The ability to resist compression (a pressing or squeezing force). *Compare* **tensile strength**.

computer assisted tomography *See* **computerized tomography**.

computerized tomography (CAT; computer assisted tomography; CT) An application of computer technology to radiography which involves making X-ray images in layers or 'cuts' through the body. CAT provides excellent visualization of the spatial relationships of body parts in the transverse plane. It is used to diagnose sports injuries (e.g., overuse injuries, such as stress fractures, and the effects of a direct blow to the brain, kidney, and spleen), and in sports science to assess body composition.

conation Mental activities, such as will and drives which lead to purposive action.

conative behaviour Behaviour dependent on effort of mind or willpower. It is the behaviour of a person who is striving for something.

concentration The ability to focus *attention on selected stimuli. Concentration involves the ability to become totally absorbed in the present moment, for example, of a competition or athletic performance, and to focus attention on relevant stimuli and ignore irrelevant stimuli. Concentration is important in all athletic performances. It is a skill which can be improved by specific training (*see* **concentration training**).

concentration grid exercise An exercise used to evaluate and train concentration. Typically, a grid consisting of ten rows and ten columns is drawn up into cells. Each cell has a two-digit number (00–99) randomly assigned to it. The athlete is required to mark in ascending numerical sequence as many numbers as possible in a given time (usually 1 minute). Scores greater than 30 indicate good concentration skills. Once mastered, the exercise can be made more difficult by introducing distractions (e.g., background noises, such as shouts from an audience).

concentration training Training techniques, such as distraction games, used to improve an athlete's *concentration. It also includes mental training which enables an athlete to focus on relevant stimuli and ignore irrelevant stimuli (*see* **attention control training**).

concentric action A form of *isotonic muscle action which occurs when a muscle develops sufficient tension to overcome a resistance, so that the muscle shortens and moves a body part. *Compare* **eccentric action**.

concentric force *See* **direct force**.

concept An abstract idea or conclusion based on a generalization from particular instances.

conceptual competency A managerial competency which refers to a leader's ability to integrate information and make judgements using a number of relevant factors. For example, the successful selection of a team depends on understanding the interactions of a number of factors, such as the interrelationships between players, their level of ability, the environmental conditions of the game, and the characteristics of the opposing team.

conceptual model of team cohesion A model which proposes that individuals are bound and attracted to a group for two basic reasons: group integration and individual attraction.

conceptual schema A mode of thinking. According to Piaget's stage theory, there is a typical conceptual schema for each stage of a child's development.

concomitant variation An empirical relationship in which the magnitude of one variable varies with the magnitude of a second variable. This correlation between variables may be used as a test of causal relationships but there are dangers of false conclusions: two variables may show concomitant variation without any *cause-and-effect relationship.

Conconi heart rate test Test of *aerobic fitness based on the observation that there may be a linear relationship between power and heart rate up to a submaximal rate beyond which the increase in heart rate slows down. In some runners, the deflection point at which the heart increase becomes non-linear is correlated significantly to the *anaerobic threshold, enabling this point to be used as an indicator of fitness. However, the Conconi test has not been generally accepted because many athletes have a linear relationship between heart rate and power output between 50 per cent and 100 per cent maximal oxygen uptake.

concurrent feedback *Feedback which is given at the same time as the action.

concurrent validity In psychology, the extent to which a test involving one task may be used to predict present performance on a different task.

concussion (knock-out) Sudden loss of consciousness due to a blow to the head. It may last a few minutes or a few hours and is often accompanied by pallor, slow movements, feebleness of heart beat, shallow breathing, and loss of normal reflex functions. Athletes suffering from concussion

are usually advised to avoid contact or collision sports for at least three weeks. In some sports, such as Rugby Union football, this lay-off is mandatory. Boxers suffering from concussion after being knocked out in the ring may also be required to avoid boxing. In Britain, amateur boxers are not allowed to box until 28 days after the first knock-out, 84 days after the second knock-out, and 1 year after the third knock-out. *See also* **second impact syndrome**.

conditioned reflex *See* **conditioned response**.

conditioned response (conditioned reflex) A response which is trained or learned. In classical conditioning, a conditioned response is elicited by a stimulus other than that which normally produces the response. In operant conditioning, a conditioned response is one which has become more frequent after being reinforced.

conditioned stimulus A previously neutral stimulus which acquires the property of eliciting a particular response through pairing with an unconditional stimulus. *See also* **classical conditioning**.

conditioning 1 The process of training or changing behaviour by association and reinforcement. There are two main types: *classical conditioning and *operant conditioning. **2** The sum total of all the physiological, anatomical, and psychological changes made by an individual in response to a training program. **3** General training of the whole body to establish aerobic fitness. *See also* **preparation period**.

conditioning exercise An activity which improves cardiovascular endurance as well as muscle strength and muscle endurance. Conditioning exercises increase the energy capacity of the muscle or muscles exercised. They are not primarily concerned with developing skill.

conductance theory Theory that the passage of gases (e.g., oxygen and carbon dioxide), metabolites (e.g., lactate), and heat in a human system is analogous to the passage of electricity along a conductor. Thus, conductance of gases etc. across an individual link in a human system is the reciprocal of resistance, and the overall conductance is given by the reciprocal of the sum of the individual resistances. Conversely, the overall resistance to the passage of a gas etc. is given by the reciprocal of the sum of its individual conductances.

conduction The transfer of heat from one object to another through direct surface contact. When submerged in cold water, much body heat is lost by conduction.

condyle A rounded, knuckle-like projection at the end of a bone which articulates with another bone to form an efficient joint.

condyloid joint (ellipsoid joint) A *synovial joint formed between the convex surface of one bone and the concave surface of another (e.g., the radiocarpal joint of the wrist). It permits free movement in two planes, and slight *circumduction.

confidence A belief and a self-assurance in one's own abilities. In sport, it is essentially a feeling of having an expectation of success. Very often the most successful sportspeople have high aspirations and high levels of confidence. Confidence is situation-specific; for example, a person may be highly confident in tennis but not in swimming.

conflict 1 An overt struggle between individuals or groups. Conflict occurs whenever the action of one person or group prevents, obstructs, or interferes with the goal achievement or action of another person. **2** A group motive where the group functions together to overcome natural obstacles or the opposition. The group motive will be to beat the opposition, or to struggle against opposing forces, whether those forces are from the natural environment or other people. **3** The tension or stress involved when the satisfaction of specific needs is thwarted by equally attractive or unattractive desires.

conflict perspective A view based on the premise that conflict is generated in a society by groups competing for economic and political resources which enable the group to acquire power. Sport is believed by some to replace outright war as a way of one group demonstrating superiority over another group.

conflict perspective on social inequality A point of view which argues that inequality is unjust and that the existing social structure should be changed to eliminate or minimize inequality.

conflict theory Any theory suggesting that change and/or progress in human societies is made by one group mainly at the expense of another. *Compare* **balanced tension theory**.

conformity A tendency of individual members of a group to behave in a manner which agrees with the norms of the group. Groups have norms which members are expected to abide by in order to maintain the integrity of the group. An individual feels the pressure of the group's expectations to conform to these norms. Conformity may involve compliance, in which the member outwardly agrees with the norms but inwardly rejects them; or internalization, in which the member adopts the norms of the group both overtly and internally.

confrontation A face-to-face discussion among two or more people in conflict, for example between team mates or between an athlete and coach. Confrontations, can be negative, exacerbating conflicts, especially if participants are angry and express that anger in hurtful accusations. However, if conducted thoughtfully, with consideration for the feelings and situation of other people, confrontations can be useful in helping to identify and solve problems.

congestive heart failure A clinical condition in which heart muscle becomes too weak to pump blood at a life-sustaining rate. Congestive heart failure may be caused by *hypertension, *atherosclerosis, or heart attack.

conjunctiva *See* **conjunctivitis**.

conjunctivitis Inflammation of the conjunctiva (the thin, protective mucous membrane lining the eyelids and covering the anterior surface of the eye). Conjunctivitis may be due to a viral or bacterial infection, or chemical irritation. Bacterial infections can cause pus formation. Such purulent infections can be exacerbated by exercise. Chlorine in the water of swimming pools commonly acts as a chemical irritant causing conjunctivitis similar to purulent infections. Conjunctivitis in skiers and ice skaters can also be caused by cold injury to the cornea. Wearing goggles offers protection against these conditions.

connective tissue A vascularized tissue composed mainly of extracellular material. It has a number of functions including support, storage, and protection. Connective tissue is found in all parts the body, and includes blood, lymph, bone, cartilage, and adipose (fat) tissue. Joint structures, such as tendons and ligaments, contain connective tissue that is rich in collagen (*see* **dense regular connective tissue**). This enables the tissue to endure high tensile stresses.

conquest activity An activity involving a person or group gaining a victory over another person or group.

conscience A person's sense of right and wrong which constrains behaviour and causes feelings of guilt if its demands are not met. These moral strictures are believed to be learnt through socialization. It is generally agreed that sport can play an important part in the development of a conscience.

conscious experience Experience of which the individual is currently aware as distinguished from past experience. Conscious experiences may be described as those which an individual can describe, such as sensory experience and feelings.

consciousness 1 The condition of a person who is awake rather than asleep so that he or she is able to respond to stimuli. **2** Clinically, different levels of behaviour which can be described on a continuum from a high state of consciousness (alertness and great awareness) to a depressed state of consciousness (coma). **3** The mechanism or process by which humans are aware of sensations, elements in memory, or internal events.

consensus A fundamental agreement within a society, community, or group of basic values.

consensus theory of truth A philosophical viewpoint based on the assumption that truth is a matter of social agreements, including the agreements reached by the scientific community, of reality. *Compare* **correspondence theory of truth**.

consequences 1 The results or effects of an action. **2** In *Cartwright's model of team cohesion, consequences are the outcomes derived from cohesion. These include team success, team performance, and team satisfaction.

conservation of angular momentum The postulate, based on Newton's first law, that a rotating body will continue to turn about its axis of rotation with constant *angular momentum unless an extended *couple or eccentric force is exerted on it. Consequently, given that the angular momentum is constant, the *moment of inertia and angular velocity are inversely proportional. If a spinning person, therefore, changes his or her moment of inertia by changing body shape, the rate of rotation will also change.

conservation of energy (first law of thermodynamics) A law which states that in any system not involving nuclear reactions or velocities approaching the velocity of light, energy cannot be created or destroyed.

conservation of linear momentum The principle which states that in any given system of bodies that exert forces on each other, the total *momentum in any direction remains constant unless some external force acts on the system. Thus the total momentum of two colliding bodies before impact is equal to the sum of their total momentum after impact. In most sports situations the total momentum of bodies is only approximately constant because of the presence of external forces such as friction, but usually the magnitude of these external forces is relatively small.

conservation of mechanical energy A law which states that when gravity is the only external force acting on a body, the mechanical energy of the body remains constant. Therefore, when a trampolinist, for example, is in flight and the effect of air resistance is small enough to be ignored, the sum of the trampolinist's kinetic energy and potential energy remain constant during ascent and descent.

consideration A *leadership behaviour that utilizes friendship, mutual trust, respect, and warmth between coach and athlete. Leadership styles which are at least partly dependent on consideration are those which are democratic, equalitarian, exhibit employee orientation, and use relationship motivation. *See also* **initiating structure**; and **leader behaviour description questionnaire**.

consistency 1 In a naturalistic approach to research, the dependability of the research method. **2** Conformity with previous behaviour, attitudes, performance of a skill, etc.

consolidation theory *See* **continuity theory**.

constant In science, a term or symbol with a constant value.

constant error The average error, with respect to sign, of a set of scores from a target value. It is a measure of a person's accuracy. *See also* **absolute error**; and **variable error**.

constant resistance exercise A form of dynamic resistance exercise in which the load does not vary during the exercise. Constant resistance exercises use simple equipment, such as free weights, which can be moved by concentric and eccentric muscle actions. *See also* **isotonic exercise**.

constipation Infrequent and difficult evacuation of the faeces, usually accompanied by abdominal discomfort. Chronic constipation is generally deemed to occur if there is failure to evacuate the bowels for three days in succession. Intermittent bouts of constipation may occur with changes in environment and diet. Constipation can affect athletic performance adversely. However, it is unwise for athletes to use laxatives to relieve constipation because these often result in the loss of body fluid and dehydration which impairs physical performance. Regular physical activity can play a part in avoiding constipation, especially in the disabled and elderly. Chronic constipation is often linked to low dietary fibre.

constitutional theory A theory based on *somatotyping which posits that each dimension of somatotype is associated with a set of personality characteristics: endomorphy with affection and sociability; ectomorphy with tenseness, introversion, and a preponderance of artistic and intellectual types; and mesomorphy with typical athletic build, aggressiveness, dominance, and risk-taking. The constitutional theory is generally considered to be an oversimplistic view of personality.

constitutive rule An official rule of a sport.

constraint 1 A limiting factor. **2** In biomechanics, a restriction to the performance of free human movement patterns. **3** In sociology, a restraining social influence which leads an individual to conform to social *norms or social expectations.

construct A hypothesized relationship concerning structures or processes underlying observable events. Motives and other theoretical terms such as engrams, subconscious, and insight are constructs. The term is often used in sociology to refer to any theoretical concept.

consumer culture A culture in which the marketing and consumption of goods and services has a dominant influence.

contact force *See* **impact force**.

contact sport A sport in which the impact of one person against another is an inherent part of the sport. Contact sports include boxing, football (especially American football and rugby), ice hockey, lacrosse, martial arts, and wrestling. Contact sports carry a high risk of injury and some people are advised not to take part in them: for example, those with a history of epileptic seizures triggered by collision, and those suffering from contagious skin diseases (e.g., impetigo, herpes, scabies, and boils). It is unwise for an injured person to participate in a contact sport until completely recovered (*see* **concussion**).

contagion theory A theory of collective behaviour which proposes that crowd behaviour depends on emotional interactions which occur when people are in close proximity one with another. Proponents of the contagion theory argue that the anonymity provided by the crowd, combined with high emotional arousal, compels different individuals to act as one body and adopt what has been called herding behaviour. *See also* **collective behaviour**.

content analysis A method of objectively and systematically analyzing communications and written documents by creating categories to classify qualitative information. Content analysis has been used to analyse the behaviour of coaches during a game.

contest A formal game or match in which individuals or teams attempt to demonstrate physical superiority or struggle to gain victory over opponents.

contest mobility A process whereby higher *social status is gained through the personal effort and ability of an individual competing against others in an open contest. *Compare* **sponsored mobility**.

contextural interference The deleterious effect on performance of a skill arising from the environment or context in which the skill is performed.

contextural template matching An analytical technique for exploring and predicting how the characteristics of persons and situations interact to determine certain types of behaviour. Each behavioural pattern of interest is characterized by a number of templates which are based on the *personality descriptions of hypothetical persons most likely to exhibit that behaviour in the situation of interest. An individual's behaviour is predicted by comparing his or her personality description with that of each template. For example, with respect to self-confidence, templates could be constructed for an optimally self-confident person, one who has low self-confidence, and one who is over-confident in the situation of interest.

contingency The relationship between a behaviour and the consequences that are dependent on that behaviour.

contingency principle A coaching principle which states that *reinforcement should occur only after a desired action.

contingency theory Suggestion that the effectiveness of a leader (e.g., coach) and a particular leadership style is dependent on the situation in which the leader is working. *See also* **Fiedler's contingency theory**.

contingent negative variation A slow negative potential recorded in an *electroencephalograph of brain activity that appears to be related to stimulus anticipation and preparation to move.

continuity theory (consolidation theory) A gerontological theory of adjustment to old age which has been applied to the adjustment of athletes to retirement. The continuity theory states that satisfactory adjustment is associated with integration between stages of the life cycle. It stresses the value of continuing activities in old age (or in retirement) which were of value in middle age (or before retirement). It maintains that the best adjusted individuals will replace lost roles with new ones.

continuous skill *See* **continuous task**.

continuous passive motion A physical therapy for treatment of sports injuries which involves the application of an external force to take an injured joint through a predetermined range of motion. Special devices are available to deliver continuous passive motion, but an exercise bike can be used with the noninjured leg creating the required force. Continuous passive motion is sometimes used immediately after surgery to relieve pain, enhance nutrition of the joint, and to discourage the formation of contractures or adhesions in and around the injured joint. It is also used after total joint replacement.

continuous reinforcement A schedule of *reinforcement used in learning, in which every correct response is reinforced.

continuous servo A control mechanism, either behavioural or physiological, consisting of a closed-loop system in which there is a one-to-one relationship between the instruction from the executive level and the state of the controlled system. Therefore, every deviation in output from the controlled system results in a corresponding compensatory response. *Compare* **discontinuous servo.**

continuous task (continuous skill) A task or skill that appears to have no recognizable beginning or end. In theory, a continuous task, such as a gymnastics floor exercise, could be continued as long as the performer wished. The end of one cycle of the skill or task becomes the beginning of the next. *See also* **discrete skill and serial task.**

continuous training Training continuously without rest intervals. It can vary from high-intensity continuous activity of moderate duration to low-intensity activity of long duration. *See also* **fartlek training; high-intensity continuous training;** and **LSD training.**

continuous variable In statistics, a variable, such as time and temperature, whose measurements do not fall into discrete classes but take any value over a defined range.

contraceptive pill (oral contraceptive) A pill containing hormones (or their analogues) which prevent conception. Contraceptive pills containing *steroids are sometimes taken by female athletes to control the menstrual cycle so that menses does not coincide with an important competition. However, these pills are not popular among most endurance athletes because they can cause nausea, weight increases, and lower maximal oxygen consumption. *See also* **menstrual adjustment.**

contract relax, agonist contract technique (hold relax, agonist contract technique; CRAC technique) A form of proprioceptive neuromuscular facilitation. As in the *contract relax technique, the muscles to be stretched are first maximally contracted and passively stretched, but the

subject is asked to assist the stretch with contraction of the agonists.

contract relax (hold relax) technique A form of proprioceptive neuromuscular facilitation. The muscles to be stretched are first maximally contracted and then stretched passively by increasing the stretch torque on the body segments involved either passively by the pull of gravity, by manipulation, or by the application of weights.

contract–relax stretching A method of stretching that incorporates a reflex relaxation of the muscle being stretched. The muscle is contracted against a resistance, usually by pressing against a force exerted by a partner. Then the muscle is relaxed into a static stretch while the partner pushes the muscle into a stretch that extends it further than before. *See also* **proprioceptive neuromuscular facilitation.**

contractile component *See* **contractile element.**

contractile element (contractile component) A part of a muscle which is able to develop tension. The contractile elements comprise the *actin and *myosin filaments in a *sarcomere.

contractile time The time taken for a muscle to reach full tension from a fully relaxed condition.

contractility The ability of a muscle to shorten forcibly when stimulated. This property distinguishes muscle from other types of tissue.

contraction *See* **muscle action.**

contracture A state of prolonged resistance in a muscle which does not involve an *action potential. Contracture may result from mechanical, physical, or chemical agents. It is commonly associated with a *fibrosis which shrinks and shortens muscle tissue.

contra-indicated procedure An inadvisable or undesirable procedure or technique. Contra-indicated exercises include any which pull a body part out of alignment, or force the body beyond its normal limits of tolerance. An exercise may also be contra-indicated because of the poor health or physical condition of an individual.

contrast baths A treatment for sports injuries which uses two baths or basins, one filled with water as hot as the patient can tolerate, and the other filled with water as cold as the patient can tolerate. Alternate immersion of an injured part in the baths stimulates blood flow, accelerates metabolic processes, decreases pain, and helps reduce swelling. The ratio of heating time to cooling time is adjusted according to the likelihood of creating tissue swelling. Short periods in the hot water and longer periods in the cold water are used for acute injuries.

contritely interdependent situation A social situation in which the achievement of a goal by an individual in a team prevents the other team members from reaching their respective goals. For example, the achievement of a 'best player' award. *Compare* **promotively interdependent goals**.

control *See* **social control**.

control dynamics The mechanical characteristics of levers, hand wheels, etc, in systems affected by variables, such as spring tension and inertia, which change the 'feel' of the control.

control group In a trial of a drug or an experimental procedure, a group matched with the experimental group in all respects except the factor under investigation. A control group is an essential part of the scientific research method because it ensures that any changes observed in an experimental group are due solely to the drug or experimental procedure and not to any other factors.

controllability A dimension of *attribution theory which refers to the extent to which the causes for events are perceived by a person to be either within or beyond his or her control. It is sometimes confused with *locus of control.

controlled factors Factors which are varied or held constant according to certain specifications by the investigator of an experiment.

controlled interval method *See* **interval training**.

controlled-variable velocity and resistance testing Measurement of force and velocity change during movements containing both isotonic and isokinetic muscle actions.

controlling aspect The extent to which *extrinsic rewards affect an athlete's perception of what controls his or her behaviour; it is an important component of *cognitive evaluation theory. Rewards which encourage athletes to attribute their participation to external causes can reduce *internal motivation. *Compare* **information aspect**.

control precision A skill-oriented ability underlying the production of a response for which the outcome is rapid and precise, but which is made with movements of a relatively large body segment (e.g., the swing in a golf-drive).

contusion *See* **bruise**.

convection The transfer of heat from one place to another by the motion of a gas or a liquid across the heated surface.

convergence The medial rotation of the eyeballs so that each eye is directed to the object being viewed. Convergence acts with *accommodation and *pupillary constriction to help an athlete retain focus on an approaching projectile, such as a ball.

convergence theory Theory proposing that *collective behaviour is the result of people with similar interests coming together and acting upon those interests. People at a sporting event, for example, often have similar class, racial, or residential backgrounds to which they strongly identify. Consequently, they are likely to respond similarly to precipitating agents.

conversational analysis A method of studying the social interactions within a group by analysing the naturally occurring forms of talk within the group. The group structure (such as dominant personalities and hierarchies) and negotiated meanings within the group may be revealed by how the conversation is managed by the participants.

conversational index A very approximate indicator of *anaerobic threshold given by the activity level at which an exerciser can no longer hold a conversation because the supply of oxygen is only just sufficient to meet the demands of the exercise.

conviction An *attitude dimension which is concerned mainly with how a person is predisposed to think about a situation.

cool-down exercise Light to moderate tapering-off exercises performed after vigorous activity. Cool-down exercises involve a gradual reduction in activity which includes jogging (or slow swimming), and stretching to maintain flexibility and reduce the risk of injury. The low-intensity exercises also prevent blood pooling in the extremities and help to eliminate the waste products of vigorous activity which contribute to muscle stiffness. Cool-down exercises are designed to restore the body as quickly as possible to the pre-exercise condition.

coolant spray See **aerosol administration**.

cooperation Behaviour exhibited by individuals working together towards goals which can be shared. There is much debate concerning the relative merits of co-operation and competition in facilitating learning. Many conditions contain both competitive and cooperative elements and it is not easy to decide which is more beneficial. In team sports, each performer has to learn to play cooperatively as well as to express a desire for defeating opponents. Generally, cooperation requires a greater degree of maturation and intellectual development than competition. See also **social interactive force**; compare **competition**.

cooperative social interaction Situation in which the goals of separate individuals are so linked that there is a positive correlation between their goal attainments. That is, individuals can attain their goals only if other participants can attain theirs. Compare **competitive social situation**; and **individualistic social situation**.

Cooper twelve-minute test A test of *aerobic endurance in which the total distance a subject runs in twelve minutes is recorded. It is a maximal test, that is, the subject must run to exhaustion for the results to be reliable. A variation of the test is based on the time taken for a subject to run 1.5 miles (about 2.4 km).

Cooper points See **aerobic points**.

coordination The ability to integrate the actions of different parts of the body to produce smooth, successful movements. Coordination is very specific (e.g., hand–eye coordination, eye–foot coordination); there is no such thing as all-round coordination.

coordinative structure A group of different muscles which are functionally linked together so that they behave as a single unit.

COPE model A model used as the basis of an instructional programme designed to help athletes cope with acute stress. C represents control of emotions; O, organizing and filtering feedback information; P, planning responses; and E, executing responses.

coping A face-saving mechanism employed to meet perceived threats to prestige and *self-esteem (for example, after losing a competition, or after retirement and desocialization). Coping applies to teams and individuals and is regarded as being positive if it enables threats to be successfully dealt with.

coping skills model Model based on the proposition that cognition (the way we think and feel about things) affects *anxiety. The coping skills model underlies several approaches to reducing anxiety, such as anxiety management training, *stress inoculation training, and *cognitive-affective stress management training. See also **cognitive mediational model of anxiety**.

coplanar forces Two or more forces acting along the same plane.

copper An essential element involved in many processes including red blood cell formation, blood-sugar regulation, and bone formation. Deficiency may cause anaemia and feelings of lassitude. In the UK, the Reference Nutrient Intake for adults is 1.2 mg daily. In the USA, the Recommended Dietary Allowance for adults is 1.5–3.0 mg daily.

coracoacromial ligament A ligament joining the *acromion process to the *coracoid process in the shoulder.

coracobrachialis A small cylindrical muscle which crosses the shoulder joint. The coracobrachialis has its origin on the *coracoid process and its insertion on the inner surface of the humerus. It contributes to adduction, horizontal adduction, and flexion of the humerus, enabling the arm to swing forwards, and it is a *synergist of the *pectoralis minor.

coracoclavicular joint A joint in the shoulder formed between the *coracoid process of the scapula and the inferior surface of the sternum. It is a *syndesmosis, permitting little movement.

coracoclavicular ligament A ligament that binds the lateral end of the clavicle to the *coracoid process. This ligament transmits the weight of the arm to the clavicle and the axial skeleton.

coracoid process (crow's beak projection) A beak-like projection of the shoulder blade which acts as the origin for the *biceps brachii and the *coracobrachialis muscles, and as an insertion for the *pectoralis minor.

core temperature Temperature in the part of the body which contains the vital organs (the brain, heart, lungs, and kidneys). The core temperature is taken internally (e.g., in the rectum or oesophagus) and it normally remains within a narrow range, usually 36.5–37.5 °C. This is the temperature at which the majority of metabolic processes work most efficiently. The temperature of the rest of the body may differ from the core. During exercise, heat is generated and muscle temperature may reach 39–40 °C. Skeletal muscle functions best at 38.5 °C. The thermoregulatory centre for core temperature lies in the hypothalamus.

Cori cycle The cycle of biochemical reactions involving a two-way flow of products between muscles and the liver. During the cycle, muscle glycogen is broken down to lactic acid, transported to the liver and converted to glucose. The glucose can either be passed back to the muscles to serve as an energy source, or be stored in the liver as glycogen.

corn A hard pad of skin which develops on or between the toes as a result of friction or pressure. It is often caused by ill-fitting shoes. The corn has a small fluid sac below the hard pad that allows the pad to slide back and forth without damaging the underlying tissue. Pressure on top of the corn pushes the sac downward causing pain. Corns can be treated with warm water or other softening agents. The pressure on the corn can be relieved by using specially designed pads or plasters. Radical treatment by surgical resectioning of the bone underlying the corn, is generally reserved for very difficult cases that do not respond to other forms of treatment.

corneal abrasion A scratch on the cornea, the transparent epithelium overlying the pupil and iris and through which light is refracted into the eye. Corneal abrasions are very painful, but they usually heal without scarring in a few days. Nevertheless, as with any other eye injury, a corneal abrasion should be evaluated fully by a doctor. If the abrasion is associated with a foreign body on the surface of the eye, this should be removed only by a medical expert. Treatment of an uncomplicated, superficial corneal abrasion is aimed at reducing the pain and preventing secondary infections. It usually consists of applying a firm eye pad over a closed eye and a broad spectrum antibiotic cream.

coronal plane *See* **frontal plane**.

coronary Pertaining to the heart.

coronary artery One of a pair of arteries which branch off the aorta to supply the heart muscle with oxygenated blood.

coronary collateral circulation theory A theory which suggests that regular exercise can improve the blood supply to the heart by *coronary collateral vascularization, and thus reduce the risk of heart attack. It is suggested that when a coronary artery is blocked, additional arteries can form a natural by-pass from one side of the blocked artery to the other.

coronary collateral vascularization Formation of new arteries in the heart. Coronary collateral vascularization has been demonstrated in dogs: the size and number of arteries increases as a result of exercise, but evidence for exercise-induced coronary collateral vascularization in humans is inconclusive.

coronary heart disease A disease of the heart that involves narrowing of the coronary arteries. This may cause a blockage of an artery and a heart attack. Coronary heart disease is one of the major causes of serious illness and death in Western countries.

coronary heart disease risk factor A factor which affects the chances of suffering a coronary heart disease. Risk tends to increase with age, tobacco-smoking, obesity, high blood pressure, high blood cholesterol levels, and high stress. Heredity is probably the single most important factor; those with a family history of heart disease being at a high risk. Males, particularly those who are bald-headed, are at a greater risk than females. Epidemiological studies indicate that physical inactivity doubles the risk of coronary heart disease. However, even low-intensity exercise is sufficient to produce physiological benefits which reduce the risk of coronary heart disease. These benefits include enlargement of the coronary arteries and increased size of the heart muscle and improved pumping capacity.

coronary ligament strain A strain of the coronary ligament (the meniscotibial ligament) which connects knee cartilage (menisci) onto the tibia. The knee joint becomes tender along the top of the tibia, but there is no locking (*compare* **meniscal tear**). It is usually caused by repeated rotational strains of the flexed, weight-bearing knee (e.g., through lateral tackles in rugby or soccer). Chronic ligament strain is common in middle-aged athletes who participate in activities, such as squash, which require frequent knee rotation. It is quite common for the pain to persist for several months, even if the patient rests. The condition usually responds well to ultrasound and *hydrocortisone treatment.

coronary-prone personality A person who exhibits *Type A behaviour, who is aggressive, competitive, and always appears to be short of time. It has been suggested that such a person tends to be prone to *coronary heart disease, though more recent evidence indicates that it might be only particular aspects of the type A constitution that are related to coronary heart disease.

coronary sinus Large vein of the heart which deposits venous blood from coronary veins into the right atrium of the heart.

coronary thrombosis Formation of a clot that blocks a coronary artery.

coronary vein A vein which collects deoxygenated blood from heart muscle and transports the blood to the *coronary sinus.

coronoid fossa Depression above the *trochlea on the anterior surface of the humerus which, with the *olecranon fossa, allows free movement of the ulna during extension and flexion of the elbow.

coronoid process A bony process on the ulna which, with the *olecranon process, forms a stable hinge-joint with the humerus.

corpus Any distinguishable body of tissue.

corpus callossum *See* **cerebrum**.

corpuscle Any small cell or body of tissue. *See also* **red blood cell**.

corrective therapy Therapy, using physical exercises, designed to correct physical abnormalities such as poor posture.

correlation An association between two variables such that when one changes in magnitude the other also changes. A correlation may be positive or negative. If positive, as one variable increases so does the other. If negative, as one variable increases

the other decreases. A statistically significant correlation does not necessarily imply
a *cause-and-effect relationship.

correlation coefficient A statistical measure, referred to as r, of the degree of linear
association between two sets of data; it is a
statistical measure of the association between two variables. *See also* **Spearman
rank correlation coefficient.**

correspondence theory of truth A philosophical viewpoint based on the concept
that truth corresponds to the facts which
exist in a reality external to individual
*cognition. Thus, truth has its own sense
in this independently existing reality and
can be known for what it is. *Compare* **consensus theory of truth.**

cortex The outer part of an organ.

cortical arousal Activation of the *reticular
formation of the brain. Cortical arousal increases wakefulness, vigilance, muscle
tone, *heart rate, and *minute ventilation. *See also* **arousal**; and **inverted U-
hypothesis.**

cortical bone *See* **compact bone.**

cortisol *See* **hydrocortisone.**

coryza *See* **cold.**

cost–benefit analysis A method by which
the benefits of pursuing a particular
action can be weighed against the costs of
pursuing that action. It is suggested that a
cost–benefit analysis could be applied to a
number of sport situations. Coaches, for
example, have been urged to employ the
notion that *anticipation has certain
benefits and costs, and that whether or
not to anticipate in a certain situation
should be determined by weighing the
probable gains against potential losses.

costal cartilage *Cartilage which attaches
the ribs to the sternum.

costal facet An articulating surface on the
centrum (main body) of a thoracic vertebra which receives the head of a rib.

costal In anatomy, pertaining to the ribs.

costochondritis Inflammation of the cartilage connecting the ribs to the sternum.

costoclavicular ligament A short, flat, strong
*ligament attached to the upper part of
the cartilage of the first rib and to the
undersurface of the clavicle.

costovertebral joint Gliding joint consisting
of two sets of points of articulation between the thoracic vertebrae and the ribs.
One set is between the head of the ribs and
the main body of the vertebrae; the other
set is between the tubercles of the ribs and
the transverse processes of the vertebrae.
The joints enable the ribcage to move during inspiration and expiration.

counter conditioning A method of *anxiety
reduction which attempts to break the link
between the stimuli which induce anxiety
and the anxiety-provoked responses. This
is achieved by conditioning pleasant responses, incompatible with anxiety, to the
anxiety-arousing stimuli. *See also* **desensitization.**

countering A *cognitive strategy for improving performance and building confidence by replacing negative, self-defeating
thoughts (e.g., 'No one cares how well I
perform.') with positive, self-enhancing
thoughts (e.g., 'I care, and I will be happier
if I have tried my hardest to perform well').
Countering involves an internal argument that uses facts and reasons to counteract the underlying assumptions that
led to the negative thoughts.

counter-movement jump A jump which utilizes the *stretch-shortening cycle, with
the athlete bobbing down before jumping
upwards.

couple *See* **force couple.**

coupled reactions Two chemical reactions
in which the release of energy and/or the
products of one reaction are used by
the other. In the *ATP–PCr energy system,
the energy released from the breakdown
of phosphocreatine is functionally linked
to the energy needs of resynthesizing
*adenosine triphosphate from adenosine
diphosphate and inorganic phosphate.

covariation principle A principle which suggests that a person's *attributions about a
performance are influenced by the performance of others to whom the subject is

comparing himself or herself. When the performances are similar, attributions tend to be external (*see* **external locus of causality**); when the performances are dissimilar, attributions tend to be internal (*see* **internal locus of control**). *See also* **Big Fish Little Pond Effect**.

covert behaviour Non-observable behaviour.

coxal In anatomy, pertaining to the hip.

coxal bone (hip bone; innominate bone; ossa coxae) One of a pair of large, irregular hip bones which forms the *pelvic girdle. Each bone unites with its partner anteriorly and with the *sacrum posteriorly. In childhood, the coxal bones consist of three separate bones: the ilium, the pubis, and the ischium. In adults, these bones fuse. The point at which the three bones meet is the acetabulum.

coxalgia A pain in the hip.

coxa plana Degeneration and inflammation of the head of the femur.

coxa valga A deformity of the hip-joint in which the angle between the neck and shaft of the femur is greater than normal.

coxa vara A deformity of the hip joint in which the angle between the neck and shaft of the femur is less than normal.

CPI (California Psychological Inventory) A questionnaire-type inventory designed to measure interpersonal behaviour in normal subjects. It has eighteen scales divided into four categories. Class 1 measures poise, ascendancy, self-assurance, and interpersonal adequacy. Class 2 measures socialization, maturity, responsibility, and intrapersonal structuring values. Class 3 measures achievement potential and intellectual efficiency. Class 4 measures intellectual and interest modes.

CP index *See* **cardiopulmonary index**.

CPR *See* **artificial resuscitation**.

C protein *See* **C-stripes**.

CRAC technique *See* **contract relax agonist contract technique**.

cramp A sudden, uncoordinated, prolonged spasm in a muscle, causing it to become taut and excruciatingly painful. Cramps commonly occur in the calf, thigh, and hip muscles after strenuous exercise. As yet, there is no complete explanation for their development. Suggested causes include muscle damage, dehydration, low blood-glucose levels, and restriction of blood supply causing ischaemia. Risk of cramps during exercise is increased by poor condition, wearing low-heel shoes, and not taking sufficient fluid or electrolytes. Cramps are relieved by gentle, static stretching, massage, and rest. *See also* **caecal slap syndrome**; **heat cramps**; and **rigor complex**.

cranial *See* **superior**.

cranium Part of the skull mainly consisting of flat bones enclosing and protecting the fragile brain and organs of hearing and equilibrium.

C reactive protein (CRP) A protein in blood serum involved in inflammatory reactions and general resistance to bacterial infection. Overtraining may reduce serum CRP, increasing susceptibility to infections.

creatine kinase (creatine phosphokinase) An *enzyme which catalyses the interconversion of *phosphocreatine and *adenosine triphosphate. During very intense, short-duration activities, creatine kinase catalyses the reaction in which the phosphate group from phosphocreatine is transferred to ADP to synthesize ATP. Creatine kinase levels increase with isokinetic exercises (*see* **isokinetic action**; and **isokinetic machine**) within *circuit training, but not with heavy resistance training. A high serum creatine kinase concentration is used as a sign of *overreaching because the concentration of the enzyme is often substantially raised in the presence of muscle damage. However, there is such a wide individual variation in serum creatine kinase concentration in response to heavy training that it is not a very reliable indicator of exercise stress and overtraining.

creatine phosphate *See* **phosphocreatine**.

creatine phosphokinase *See* **creatine kinase**.

creative thinking Productive thinking which results in novel rather than routine outcomes.

creativity The aspect of intelligence characterized by originality of thought and problem solving. Creativity involves divergent thinking, that is, thoughts directed widely towards a number of varied solutions.

credulous argument The proposal that athletic performance can be predicted from personality traits. *Compare* **sceptical argument**.

creep effects A process which takes place in the vertebrae when compressive forces exceed the pressure within the intervertebral disc, forcing tissue fluid to be expelled and the disc to narrow and stiffen. Creep effects are caused by excessive and repetitive loading which causes vibrations.

crepitation *See* **crepitus**.

crepitus (crepitation) A crackling sound heard with or without a stethoscope over broken bone, an inflamed lung, or damaged joint. The pressure wave associated with crepitus may be felt as a grating sensation over a joint following inflammation of a tendon sheath.

crest A narrow, usually prominent ridge of bone; a site of muscle attachment.

crestload The highest workload which can be sustained for a long time.

crista Folds of the inner membrane of a *mitochondrion. The folding increases the surface-area-to-volume ratio of the membrane on which enzyme systems facilitate *aerobic metabolism.

crista ampullaris A sensory receptor of dynamic equilibrium in each *semicircular canal of the ear. It consists of a tuft of hair cells which respond to angular or rotary movements in one plane.

criterion-referenced test A test in which an individual's score or performance is compared with some previously established criterion rather than with the performance of others.

criterion variable In studies of prediction, the variable or score that is predicted from predictor variables; the 'best' obtainable measure of the constant that is to be predicted.

critical closing pressure The blood pressure at which a blood vessel closes completely and blood flow is stopped. When the pressure immediately outside a blood vessel exceeds the intravascular pressure, the blood vessel collapses. This happens during a measurement of *blood pressure with a sphygmomanometer.

critical learning period The crucial time in the development of an organism when the ideal intermix of sensory, motor, psychological, and motivational factors is present for learning a specified behaviour. Critical learning periods have been studied mainly on animals other than humans, but many coaches recognize that successful skill attainment is dependent on the timeliness of instruction. In psychology, the critical learning period has special reference to *imprinting, and is the period when imprinting is most likely to occur.

critical mass The minimum number of a group which is needed for the group to be viable and for there to be sufficient exchange of ideas.

critical power The highest exercise intensity which can be maintained without causing exhaustion. *See also* **fatigue threshold**.

critical Reynold's number A critical velocity of fluid in a tube, expressed by a *Reynold's number, above which *laminar flow becomes turbulent.

critical threshold A training guideline proposed by the Finnish physiologist Karvonen. He suggested that, to benefit from aerobic exercise, the training heart rate should be above the critical threshold, calculated as training heart rate = resting heart rate + 60 per cent of (maximum heart rate – resting heart rate).

criticism The analysis of a performance. The term is often used in the pejorative sense of making an unfavourable or severe comment, but criticism of athletes can be a useful motivational strategy if used sensitively, for example when combined with praise and followed with suggestions as to how to improve. It is generally agreed that criticisms consisting only of unspecific exhortations to try harder are not very effective.

critique In sport sociology, a perspective that attempts to problematize the everyday and familiar aspects of sport by questioning how practices in sport are constructed, why they have been constructed in certain ways, and who or what categories of individuals benefit from the way sport is constructed. A critique usually involves an analysis relating individual events to wider social, political, and economic contexts.

cross-adaptation The transfer of an *adaptation acquired from one stressor to another stressor. It has been argued that adaptations to the physical stress of athletic training can be transferred to the emotional stresses experienced in everyday life.

cross bridge (actin–myosin cross bridge) An extension of *myosin which, according to the *sliding-filament theory, attaches onto actin during a muscle action.

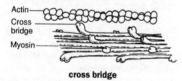

Actin
Cross bridge
Myosin

cross bridge

cross-eyed patellae See **femoral torsion**.

cross frictional massage A form of *massage in which the masseur rubs the body-part using small movements but with a firm pressure across the line of the muscle or tendon growth. Cross-frictional massage is thought to break down scar tissue.

Crossman–Goodeve theory A theory based on the observation that there tends to be a trade off between speed of movements and their accuracy (see **Fitt's law**). The Crossman–Goodeve theory proposes that rapid movements are dependent on intermittent control, with the commands for action being produced alternately with the analysis of *feedback in order to determine movement corrections.

cross-preference The tendency not to prefer organs (eye, hand, or foot) on the same side of the body to perform tasks. The preference is to use a combination such as the right eye, left hand, and right foot.

cross-sectional research design A basic type of research method in which a large cross-section of the population is studied at one specific time and the differences between individual groups within the population compared. It is commonly used by sports scientists to evaluate and compare a given physiological variable or fitness component in individuals already belonging to different groups. *Compare* **longitudinal research design**.

cross-sex effects The effects on an athlete's performance of having members of the opposite sex in the audience (*see* **audience effect**) or performing alongside the athlete. *See also* **coaction**.

cross-training Training that involves more than one type of activity to exercise different muscle groups and provide variety. A cyclist, for example, in addition to cycling may include jogging and swimming in a programme of cross-training. The term is also applied to training multiple fitness components (e.g., strength, flexibility, and endurance) within the same training session. Combining strength training and endurance training does not appear to diminish improvements in aerobic fitness. However, gains in strength are greater when strength training is performed on its own.

crow's beak projection See **coracoid process**.

crowd A relatively unstructured mass of people who group together in a given area in a more or less spontaneous way for a short time in response to an attraction, such as a sports event.

crowd behaviour The behaviour of people in large groups or a crowd. The close physical proximity of large numbers of people provides relative anonymity and protection for individuals whose behaviour often departs from what would be expected when they are alone. The unruly behaviour of a few individuals may quickly spread and crowd behaviour may be more than usually explosive and unpredictable. In a number of sociological studies crowd behaviour is seen as a potential threat to normal social order. *See also* **collective behaviour, hooliganism**.

CRP *See* **C-reactive protein**.

cruciate ligaments Ligaments which cross each other to form an X-shaped configuration within the notch between the femoral condyles of the knee capsule. The anterior cruciate ligament attaches the femur to the anterior tibia. It prevents backward sliding of the femur and overextension at the knee. It is lax when the knee is flexed and taut when the knee is extended. The posterior cruciate ligament attaches the femur to the posterior tibia. It prevents the femur from sliding forwards and the tibia from being displaced backwards.

cryokinetic A form of *cryotherapy which combines ice and exercise. It is used to treat a sports injury during rehabilitation. Ice is applied to numb the injured part which the patient can then move actively. The procedure is repeated three or four times. The ice reduces but does not remove sensation. Thus the ice increases the pain-free range of motion while ensuring that the patient moves the injured part within tolerance levels.

crural Pertaining to the leg.

crural index The ratio of thigh length to leg length. A high crural index is advantageous to long-jumpers since it enables the jumper to apply a force against the ground for a longer time than someone with a low crural index.

crutch walking Walking with the assistance of elbow or axillary crutches to support an injured leg and avoid putting weight on the leg. Crutches should be carefully measured to suit the patient. There should be sufficient space between the top of the crutch and the axilla (arm pit) to prevent damaging the nerves. The hand rest should be level with the crease of the wrist or the styloid process. The patient should use two-point walking, with both crutches being moved forwards together, then the patient pushes down on the hand rests, straightens the elbow, and hops forwards.

cryogenic Pertaining to the production of low temperatures.

cryotherapy The use of low temperatures to treat an injury or disorder. *See also* **cold treatment**.

CSAI (Competitive State Anxiety Inventory) A ten item test of *competitive state anxiety; it is a shortened, situation specific version of the *SAI.

CSAI-2 (Competitive State Anxiety Inventory-2) A multi-dimensional test of *competitive A state which is situation specific and accurately assesses three different dimensions or manifestations of state anxiety: cognitive state anxiety, somatic state anxiety, and self-confidence state anxiety. It has been adopted by many sport psychologists as an appropriate tool for measuring sport competition state anxiety.

CSAQ *See* **cognitive somatic anxiety questionnaire**.

C stripes Fibrous protein (C-protein, X-protein, and H-protein) that appear as thin lines running at right angles to thick filaments in electron micrographs of muscle fibres. C-protein is thought to hold adjacent thick filaments at an even distance during force generation, and it may also control the number of myosin molecules in a thick filament.

CT *See* **computerized tomography**.

cubital Pertaining to the elbow or forearm.

cubital tunnel syndrome *See* **ulnar compression syndrome**.

cubital vein A vein in the forearm which crosses the elbow joint.

cubitus recurvatus *Hyperextension of the elbow joint which may occur in isolation or as part of *hypermobile joint disease.

cuboid In anatomy, the *tarsal bone articulating with the fourth and fifth digits in the foot.

cue A signal for some particular action. The term is used in performance models of behaviour to describe that to which a person reacts or that which precipitates behaviour in a particular situation. Cues may be verbal, visual, or kinaesthetic. *See also* **stimulus**.

cue utilization theory A theory which predicts that as an athlete's *arousal increases, his or her attention focus narrows and the narrowing process tends to gate out irrelevant environmental cues first and then, if arousal is high enough, the relevant ones. This results in reducing the availability of important information to an over-aroused performer, and the overwhelming influx of irrelevant information in an underaroused performer.

cue words Words which have developed a special meaning through training and which are used to evoke a particular behaviour. A coach may, for example, use special cue words to remind a competitor to concentrate.

cult-of-personality An intense interest in or devotion to a person, idea, or activity. The phrase was originally used to describe the practice of totalitarian regimes in which a leader (e.g., Hitler) was elevated to a position of pre-eminence and presented as a source of all political wisdom and the architect of all worthwhile political and social actions. The phrase has been applied to pre-eminent, famous sports personalities who have acquired a similar following.

cult of slenderness An intense interest in and devotion to the development of a body that is not obese but that is shapely and slender. The cult of slenderness is a manifestation of the wider ideology of shapism in which definitions of the desirable body image are constructed by groups who have a vested interest in promoting the ideal shape of women as slim, and that for men as slim muscularity. *See also* **mesomorphism**.

cultural assimilation The incorporation of a *culture into the general host society (*see* **melting pot theory**). The acceptance of the host culture may result in the loss of cultural identity of an ethnic group. In reality, cultural assimilation can range along a continuum from complete isolation, or segregation (*see* **apartheid**) to complete assimilation. *Compare* **structural assimilation**.

cultural diffusion A social process resulting in the transfer of beliefs, values, and social activities (e.g., games or sports) from one society to another.

cultural mosaic theory A theory which suggests that society should encourage ethnic groups to maintain their ethnic diversity and identity. Participation in sports may strengthen ethnic identity, for example, when a team comprised of members from one ethnic background compete against another team with members from a different ethnic background. *Compare* **melting pot theory**.

cultural norm The norms of a culture.

cultural norms theory A theory of mass communication which suggests that the *mass media selectively presents and emphasizes certain contemporary ideas or values. According to this theory, the mass media influences norms by reinforcing or changing them. For example, the cultural norm theorists argue that television programmes presenting an active lifestyle for older people can change the attitudes of viewers in that direction.

culture The ways of behaving and the ultimate goals of society; the norms and values of a society. Culture has been taken as constituting the way of life of an entire society, including the codes of manners, language, rituals, norms of behaviour, and systems of belief. Sociologists stress the importance of culture in determining human behaviour; thus the attitude of individuals to sport may be greatly influenced by the culture; for example in North America there is a very strong cultural influence to win at all costs. But sport has also been seen as an important means of encouraging people to conform to a particular culture. *See also* **acculturation; high culture, idioculture, mass culture.**

Cumming test A cycle ergometer test of alactacid *anaerobic power. The subject pedals from a standing position on a cycle ergometer with known resistance for 30 seconds at maximum effort. The highest power is determined by the highest number of pushes in any 5 second period. The force which the subject overcomes is usually proportional to body weight, and the distance the force moves is the product of the number of pedal pushes and the flywheel circumference.

cumulation The process by which blood levels of a drug build-up, thereby increasing its therapeutic and toxic effects. If drug dosage exceeds the elimination rate, the drug will cumulate. Cumulation may result from poor elimination due to slow metabolism, binding the drug to plasma proteins, or inhibition of excretion as occurs in sufferers of a kidney disease. *Compare* **drug tolerance**.

cuneiform bones Three bones in the tarsus which articulate with the navicular bone posteriorly, and the first, second, and third metatarsals anteriorly.

Cunningham and Faulkner treadmill test A *long-term anaerobic test in which the subject runs maximally on a treadmill with a 20 per cent gradient, at 8 miles per hour. The time to exhaustion in seconds is recorded.

Cureton's tables A set of tables based on over one hundred parameters which indicate *aerobic endurance. The parameters include pulmonary gas and blood examinations, ECGs, heart rate, and blood pressure.

Cureton's test of minimal flexibility A series of indirect tests of flexibility which includes the standing toe-touch.

curl-up 1 A weight-training exercise which strengthens the anterior muscles of the arm. The subject stands with feet shoulder-width apart and holds a barbell or dumbbells with an underhand grip at thigh level, then brings the weight up to the chest and lowers it back to the thigh. **2** Form of abdominal exercise similar to a sit-up but which involves curling the chin onto the chest while the lower back retains contact with the ground.

curvilinear motion Motion along a curved line or path in which all parts of the system move in the same direction at the same speed. *Compare* **rectilinear motion**.

custom Any established pattern of behaviour within a community or society. A custom is an accepted rule of behaviour which is informally regulated. Shaking hands with the umpire is the custom after a tennis match.

cutaneous Pertaining to the skin.

cyanocobalamin *See* **vitamin B$_{12}$**.

cyanosis Bluish discoloration of the skin and mucous membranes caused by lack of oxygen.

cybernetics *See* **negative feedback**.

cycle ergometer (bicycle ergometer) A stationary one-wheeled cycle used as an *ergometer to measure a person's work output under controlled conditions. The resistance (and therefore work output) is controlled usually by one of four main methods: varying mechanical resistance (by tightening or loosening a flywheel), electrical resistance (by changing the strength of the magnetic field through which an electrical conductor moves), air resistance (produced by fan blades displacing air as the wheel turns), or hydraulic fluid resistance. A cycle ergometer supports the upper body, keeping it relatively immobile. This makes it relatively easy to measure blood pressure and take blood samples. It also makes the cycle ergometer a good device for measuring physiological responses to a standard rate of work output (power output) in people whose weights have changed. Because much of the body weight is supported by the cycle, resistance is relatively independent of body weight (*compare* **treadmill**). Cycle ergometers are not very good at measuring peak performances in people not used to cycling because the leg muscles usually fatigue before the rest of the body.

cyclic activity An activity, such as rowing, in which body movements are regularly repeated.

cyclical involvement A sporadic involvement in sport, for example, of an individual who plays golf only during his or her holiday.

cyclic AMP An important intracellular chemical that mediates intracellular responses to some nonsteroid hormones; it acts as a second messenger. Cyclic AMP is formed from ATP by the action of adenylate cyclase, an enzyme on the cell surface membrane.

cycling of training *See* periodization.

cyclist's melanoma A melanoma (malignant tumour of cancer-producing cells) on the exposed part of the lower limb. The development of this type of melanoma has been linked with cycling because the skin of the calf and thigh are intermittently exposed to high levels of UV light when in the flexed cycling position. To reduce risks, cyclists should wear protective clothing and high protective factor sunscreen on skin areas exposed to the sun.

cyproheptadine hydrochloride A drug used to increase appetite and weight, possibly through its actions on the *appetite centre in the *hypothalamus. Drowsiness is a common side-effect.

cyst A cavity lined with epithelium and filled with fluid or a semi-solid substance, usually formed as a result of a pathological process in a tissue or organ. Cysts or cyst-like structures can form as a result of soft tissue sports injuries (for example, a *meniscal tear). A swelling similar to a cyst can develop when a large muscle haematoma fails to reabsorb. Treatment may involve surgical removal of the cyst or drainage of the excess fluid under sterile conditions.

cytochrome A protein pigment containing a metal involved in redox reactions in the *electron transport chain in *mitochondria.

cytochrome oxidase Enzyme which catalyses the final stage of *aerobic metabolism when oxygen combines with hydrogen ions to form water. The amount of cytochrome oxidase is commonly used in exercise physiology as a measure of the capacity of the respiratory chain to generate energy.

cytology The study of the structure and function of cells.

cytoplasm The part of a cell inside the cell surface membrane but outside the nucleus. It consists of a watery fluid, the cytosol, in which cell organelles are suspended.

cytosol *See* cytoplasm.

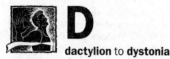

D

dactylion to **dystonia**

dactylion An anatomical landmark located at the tip of the middle (third finger), or the most distal point of the middle finger when the arm is hanging down at the side and the fingers are stretched downward.

dactylion height A body height measured from *dactylion to base.

Dal Monte five sprint test A test of an athlete's ability to perform alternate aerobic and anaerobic activities. The athlete performs 5 sprints at maximal effort from standing starts over distances of 50 m for men and 40 m for women, at intervals of 1 min. The athlete's time for each sprint is recorded to indicate the ability to repeat an anaerobic activity. Heart rate is taken between the 40th and 55th second after each sprint, and between the 60th and 90th second after the fifth sprint, and finally at the end of the third minute to evaluate recovery capacity.

Dal Monte test A test of anaerobic power which estimates the heaviest thrust applied by a subject against a dynametric bar set at the level of the centre of gravity, whilst running for 5 s up a 10 per cent gradient on a treadmill. The test is performed at three different speeds.

Dalton's Law A law which states that the total pressure of a mixture of two or more gases or vapours is equal to the sum of the pressures that each gas would exert if it was present alone and occupied the same volume as the whole mixture.

dark adaptation An increase in the sensitivity of the eye to light when a person remains in darkness or in low illumination.

dart thrower's elbow A tender swelling around the tip of an elbow due to a *bursitis. It is caused by repeated physical flexing of the elbow or rubbing the elbow.

data set In sociology, a collection of information or observations made on a group of individuals relating to certain variables of interest to the investigator. The data may be gathered in a number of ways, for example, from interviews, surveys, and experiments.

datum (pl. data) A single piece of information.

dead arm syndrome A condition characterized by sudden pain and a complete lack of strength in the upper arm when it is abducted and externally rotated. It is usually associated with a shoulder instability, such as a dislocation or recurrent subluxation of the glenohumeral joint, caused by repeated throwing.

dead leg *See* **charley horse**.

dead space The volume of gas taken into the lungs which does not contribute to gaseous exchange. It consists of the *anatomical dead space, the volume of the alveoli which are not perfused with blood, and the volume of underperfused alveoli.

dead space to tidal volume ratio The proportion of *tidal volume taken up by the *dead space; the ratio gives a measure of the efficiency of pulmonary gas exchange.

deamination Removal of an amino ($-NH_2$) from an organic compound by hydrolysis or oxidation. Deamination occurs in the liver where amino acids are converted into ammonia which is ultimately converted into urea and excreted.

de Bruyn–Prevost constant load test A *short-term anaerobic test performed to exhaustion on a bicycle ergometer at a constant workload of 400 W and pedal speed of 124–128 rpm for males, and at a work load of 350 W and pedal speed of 104–108 rpm for females. The time taken to reach the required pedal speed (known as the delay time) and the total time the subject can maintain the required speed (known as total time) are used to compute an index of total time divided by delay time which is used to evaluate anaerobic tolerance and performance.

decalcification Loss of calcium or calcium salts from bone.

decarboxylation Removal of carbon dioxide from a molecule. Decarboxylation takes place in the *Krebs cycle during *aerobic metabolism. The carbon dioxide is eventually exhaled.

decay theory A theory of loss of *learning of motor skills based on the premise that *engrams storing the motor patterns required for the performance of a motor skill deteriorate when they are not activated.

deceleration A reduction in the acceleration of a body; the non technical term for negative acceleration.

deceleration injury An injury incurred when a moving person stops suddenly (e.g., when a polevaulter lands, a ice hockey player collides with a sidewall, and when a concussed boxer falls onto the boxing ring floor). These injuries can be very traumatic because even in an unrestrained fall from standing height, the head can strike the floor with a force exceeding 300 G.

decision-making The important cognitive process of selecting one action or policy from two or more choices to achieve a desired goal. A decision is made by using perceptual information about a current situation and integrating this with information held in the memory to determine the best course of action. Sport sociologists and sport psychologists are particularly interested in decision-making strategies of individuals and teams in competitive situations (see **game theory**). The time taken to make a decision is a component of *reaction time and varies according to the activity. In some activities, decision-making is similar to a reflex action and is quick and simple; in others it is very complex and is the longest component of reaction time. Decision-making is prolonged by anxiety, causing reaction times to become slower. See also **response-selection stage**.

decompensation Inability of the heart to maintain an adequate circulation, for example, when confronted with increased workloads.

decompression 1 Any medical procedure for relieving pressure or the effects of pressure. **2** The reduction of gas pressure within a body space (for example, during ascent to high altitudes or from deep water to shallow water).

decompression sickness See **caisson disease**.

deconditioning Loss of fitness due to inactivity or inadequate training. A decrease in the cardiovascular system's ability to transport oxygen and nutrients to muscles (cardiovascular deconditioning) for example, results from insufficient endurance training. See also **detraining effects**.

decongestant A medication that reduces or relieves a blocked up nose. Many nasal decongestants are sympathomimetic drugs, most of which are on the International Olympic Committee's list of *banned substances. Xylometazoline and oxymetazoline are permitted decongestants.

dedication A strongly positive attitude that leads to intensive activity; it is often associated with self-sacrifice.

deduction A logical method of reasoning from generalizations to specific relations or facts. Compare **induction**.

deductive explanation An explanation in which a specific phenomenon is deduced from an established general law. Compare **induction**.

deep In anatomy, away from the body surface, more internal, as in deep muscle.

deep-body temperature See **core temperature**.

deep friction massage Massage in which a firm pressure is applied to treat deep muscle injuries.

deep peroneal nerve compression A compression injury of the peroneal nerve, deep in the anterior compartment of the lower leg. It occasionally occurs in a normally sedentary person who performs a very intensive burst of activity. It may also occur after serious bruising of the shin or after a fracture. Symptoms include throbbing and paraesthesia (e.g., an abnormal tingling sensation) followed by anaesthesia (lack of sensation) in the web between the first and second toes. Treatment includes ice and elevation. Surgical decompression may be required if motor weakness develops, or if the tissues within the compartment are compromised (see **compression syndrome**).

deep spinal muscles Muscles with their proximal attachments on the posterior processes of all vertebrae and the posterior of the sacrum, and with their distal attachments on the neural spines, transverse processes, and laminae of all the vertebrae below their proximal attachments. The deep spinal muscles include the multifidus, rotatores, interspinales, intertransversii, and levatores costarum. Their primary actions are extension, lateral flexion, and rotation (to the opposite side) of the spine.

deep stroking A form of *massage performed by moving the pads of the thumbs along the length of muscle, starting from the point farthest from the heart and moving towards it. Deep stroking moves much blood and lymph through the muscle, removing fluid which might have accumulated during exercise. This form of massage is quite aggressive and can be painful, causing the subject to tense the muscles; this tension can be relieved by *jostling.

defence mechanism A behaviour pattern primarily concerned with protecting the ego. See also **ego defence mechanism, rationalization, repression**.

deferred gratification Behaviour in which sacrifices are made in the present in the hope of future rewards.

deficiency disease A disease caused by lack of an essential nutrient. See also **vitamin-deficiency disease**.

definition of situation Concerns the importance of subjective perspectives of *actors for the objective consequences of social interactions. Therefore, if a situation is defined as real, its consequences are real. For example, if an athlete assumes that a coach does not like him or her and acts accordingly, the assumption (whether true or not) will have real consequences.

deformation A change in the shape of a structure.

degeneration Deterioration and loss of function in body structures. Degeneration is usually associated with ageing, but it can also result from disease and inactivity. See also **atrophy**.

degree 1 A unit of angular distance. One degree equals 1/360 revolutions of a circle. **2** The loft of a golf-club which is usually given as the number of degrees the club-face is set back from the vertical. **3** Unit of temperature.

dehydration A depletion of fluids from the body which can hinder *thermoregulation and cause an increase in core temperature. A reduction of the body's fluid volume may result in a lowering of blood pressure and cardiac output. Dehydration occurs during exercise if the fluid lost through perspiration and urine exceeds fluid replacement. Mild dehydration may cause a general malaise and insomnia,

and it leads to poor performances even in temperate climates. A two per cent loss of body-weight due to water loss can lead to a 20 per cent drop in the working capacity of muscles. Training may increase tolerance to dehydration. See also **heat stroke**; and **water replacement**.

dehydroepiandrosterone (DHEA) A *steroid produced from cholesterol in the adrenal glands. It is found naturally in the blood and tissues. Its physiological functions are unclear, but it may be used to manufacture either *testosterone or *oestrogen. It could, therefore, play a role in any of the actions associated with these hormones (e.g., growth and repair of muscles). Levels of DHEA decline with age and it has been suggested that some age-related diseases (e.g., atherosclerosis) are associated with this decline. DHEA supplements have been promoted by some health food shops as a 'miracle drug', increasing muscle mass, lowering body fat, and reducing the risk of heart disease. The supplements are used as an ergogenic aid by athletes who believe the claims that DHEA promotes faster recovery from physical stress and that it can reduce excess body fat. However, there is little scientific evidence to support these claims. Excess DHEA may be harmful. Preliminary studies suggest that it may increase the risk of certain cancers, and high levels may have a masculinizing effect on women.

deinhibition training A potentially dangerous form of training performed by some weight-lifters and body-builders. Usually, when the mechanical strain on muscles exceeds a threshold level, responses initiated by the *Golgi tendon organs cause the central nervous system to inhibit further muscle activity. This is an important safety mechanism designed to prevent muscles from being overstretched, but it tends to stop them from working to their full capacity. Deinhibition training aims to remove the inhibition, enabling muscles to work with greater loads, thus accelerating strength development. It requires high amplitude or explosive movements that stretch muscles and tendons fully.

However, with the natural safety mechanism removed, the risk of overstretching and damaging nerves, muscles, and tendons is high.

delayed feedback Situation in which there is a time-lag between a performance of a skill and the *feedback which is given to a subject about the performance.

delayed-onset muscle soreness (DOMS) Muscular discomfort which develops one or two days after exercise has stopped. DOMS may be caused by structural damage to the muscle cells or inflammatory reactions in and around the muscles. DOMS typically affects those who only exercise occasionally or who perform strenuos exercises to which they are unaccustomed. It is greatest following *eccentric training. For example, muscle soreness is far less after running on a flat track than after an equivalent bout of downhill running. Treatment of DOMS consists of rest and use of nonsteroidal anti-inflammatory drugs (NSAIDS), such as aspirin, to relieve the pain. Muscle soreness can be minimized by reducing eccentric actions during early training periods; by training at low intensity during early training and gradually increasing intensity; or by beginning a training programme with an exhaustive bout of high-intensity exercise. The exhaustive, high intensity exercise causes great soreness for the first few days, but seems to offer some protection against further muscle soreness. *Compare* **acute muscle soreness**.

delegated performance Group performance in which various individual members are assigned specific functions. Delegated performance affects social interaction and social facilitation. Types of delegated performance are sequentially independent tasks and sequentially dependent tasks. *Compare* **interdependent performance**.

deliberation The initial phase of *decision-making during which the subject considers perceptual information about the situation and information held in the memory before deciding on a choice of action.

delinquency Antisocial or illegal acts, commonly performed by young males. *See also* **football hooliganism**.

delinquency deterrence hypothesis A proposition that participation in sports reduces the tendency towards anti-social behaviour in young people.

delinquent subculture A social group committed to values considered within the general society to be criminal or antisocial.

deltoideus *See* **deltoid muscle**.

deltoid ligament *Ligament connecting the *tibia to the *calcaneus in the ankle.

deltoid muscle (deltoideus) A thick pennate muscle responsible for the roundness of the shoulder. The anterior deltoid originates from the outer third of the *clavicle; the middle deltoid originates from the top of the *acromion process, and the posterior deltoid originates from the scapular spine. All parts of the deltoid insert onto the deltoid tuberosity of the humerus. The deltoids take part in all movements of the upper arm. They are prime movers of arm abduction and also act as antagonists of the *pectoralis major and *latissimus dorsi which adduct the arm. The primary actions about the shoulder of the anterior fibres of the deltoids are flexion and horizontal adduction; those of the middle fibres are abduction and horizontal abduction; and those of the posterior fibres are extension and horizontal abduction.

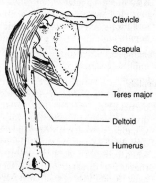

Clavicle

Scapula

Teres major

Deltoid

Humerus

deltoid muscle

The deltoids are particularly active during rhythmic swinging movements of the arms during walking.

deltoid tuberosity An attachment site of the fleshy deltoid muscle onto the shaft of the humerus.

deltoideus See **deltoid muscle**.

delusion A false judgement or conclusion; usually used in reference to a mentally ill person, but it has also been applied to sports people, particularly when they act irrationally under the pressure of competition.

dementia pugilistica See **encephalopathy, traumatic**.

democratic behaviour Coaching behaviour which allows high levels of participation by the athletes in decisions pertaining to group goals, practice methods, game tactics, and strategies.

democratic leadership A relationship-oriented form of leadership that encourages coach–athlete interaction. It is a leadership style which can best be explained in terms of *consideration.

democratization A process whereby a social activity such as sport becomes more accessible to, and popular among, different segments of society, such as across different groups of age, gender, race, and social class.

demography The scientific study of populations, their age-structure, migrations, mortality rate, occupations, and other factors affecting the quality of life within the populations.

dendron Part of a neurone carrying a *nerve impulse towards a cell body. *Compare* **axon**.

denial A mechanism of *ego defence in which an individual under threat may, particularly if immature or emotionally disturbed, deny the existence of an object, situation, person, or threat. Mild forms of denial can be seen in young athletes who, when facing formidable opponents, reject the obvious threat to their self-esteem and deny the abilities of their adversaries. As people mature and form more accurate perceptions of reality, this form of ego defence is less likely to occur.

dense fibrous connective tissue See **dense regular connective tissue**.

dense irregular connective tissue Connective tissue consisting mainly of *collagen fibres interwoven and arranged irregularly in more than one plane to form sheets. It occurs particularly in areas where tension is exerted in many different directions (e.g., in the *fascia surrounding muscle). *Compare* **dense regular connective tissue**.

dense regular connective tissue (dense fibrous connective tissue) A white, flexible connective tissue comprised mainly of collagen fibres running in the same direction. It provides great tensile strength to tissue which tends to be pulled in one plane. It occurs in tendons, aponeuroses, and ligaments. *Compare* **dense irregular connective tissue**.

densitometry Measurements of body density, defined as body mass (scale weight) divided by volume. Body volume can be obtained in a number of ways (see **hydrostatic weighing**). Densitometry is used to estimate the percentage body fat, since fatty tissue is less dense than lean tissue. The standard equation used is that of Siri: % body fat = (495/body density) −450. The equation assumes that the densities of fatty tissue and lean tissue are relatively constant in all people. Unfortunately, the densities of lean tissues varies considerably between people.

density The mass per unit volume of an object: density = mass/volume. A common unit of density is the kilogram per cubic metre.

deoxyribonucleic acid (DNA) An organic chemical which carries genetic information found in the nucleus of all cells, and which is inherited from parents to offspring. The genetic information determines which proteins can be synthesized by each cell. These proteins include enzymes which determine the inherited characteristics of an individual. It is possible that as we age, DNA becomes damaged by intrinsic or extrinsic factors. This may lead to errors in the synthesis of various proteins, contributing to age-related degeneration in physical performance.

dependent variable A variable which is acted on or influenced by another variable. For example, in an investigation of the affects of age on running speed, the independent variable (e.g., the age of the athlete) is manipulated, selected, or otherwise controlled, and the affect of this manipulation can be seen in the change in the dependent variable (running speed). It is, therefore, an aspect of behaviour or experience which goes with or depends on the changes in the independent variable.

depolarization A decrease in the electrical potential across a cell membrane. Depolarization occurs during an *action potential when the potential difference across a cell membrane (especially that of a muscle fibre or neurone) becomes reversed. The inside of the cell loses its negative charge and becomes positive relative to the outside due to an influx of sodium ions. *Compare* resting membrane potential. *See also* **hyperpolarization**.

depot preparation A preparation of a medicine in which the active ingredients are released slowly into tissue.

depressed fracture A fracture that results in the depression of bone fragments into underlying structures.

depression 1 Movement of the shoulder girdle or another body part downwards (i.e. in an inferior direction). *Compare* **elevation**. **2** A melancholy mood; a feeling of hopelessness, or an attitude of dejection. Depression can adversely affect the motivation to train and compete. In serious cases, depression is a symptom of mental illness. Exercise is often used in the treatment of mild depression and anxiety. Research has shown that aerobic exercise sustained for at least 30 minutes, five times a week can have anti-depressant effects, and the exercise produces physiological benefits which extend the range of activities that the patient can undertake with ease. Some of the psychological

benefits are probably linked to an improved general feeling of wellbeing.

deprivation–satiation proposition A proposition that the more often in the recent past a person has received a particular reward, the less valuable any further unit of that reward becomes.

deprofessionalization The process by which members of a high-status occupation loses the facility to have autonomous control over its internal affairs and the behaviour of its membership. Deprofessionalization also results in a loss of the monopoly of the members of the profession to have exclusive rights to do certain kinds of work and a loss of control over the expert knowledge which, before deprofessionalization, was not available to the general public. It could be claimed that aerobic fitness clubs and diet clubs act to deprofessionalize sport scientists, qualified athletic coaches, and health physiologists who are now not seen as having a monopoly of knowledge in these areas.

depth of processing The level to which information is processed after being introduced into the memory. The concept is based on the rejection of the idea that information is stored in discrete memory stores. It adopts the view that an item enters the information-processing system and undergoes an increasing amount of processing thereby moving deeper into the system. It is postulated that the retention characteristics of information are determined by the depth of processing, with deeper levels being associated with more abstract coding and greater retention.

depth perception Three-dimensional perception which is essential for the ability of a person to judge quickly and accurately the speed and distance relationships between an object and the individual.

de Quervain's disease Tendinitis of the extensor pollicis brevis and the abductor pollicis longus tendons at the base of the thumb; an overuse injury of the wrist common among racket players and golfers, especially those golfers who use a larger than average range of motion during the swing. Right handed golfers tend to injure the left wrist. This injury is characterized by local swelling and tenderness on the thumb side of the wrist, and difficulty in moving the thumb into a 90 degree, 'thumbs up', angle. Initial treatment consists of RICE and anti-inflammatories. If symptoms persist, medical advice should be sought. Nonsurgical treatment, which may include splinting and cortisone injections, usually resolves the condition, but sometimes surgery may be necessary to release the tendon or remove calcium deposits that might have accumulated. Recovery from nonsurgical treatment usually takes about 1 to 2 weeks; recovery after surgery includes a period of immobilization in a cast (about 2 weeks), followed by a few weeks of rehabilitation.

dermatitis Inflammation of the skin, often accompanied by a rash. *See also* **allergic contact dermatitis**.

dermatome An area of skin innervated by the branches of a single spinal nerve. Dermatomes are represented as distinct areas on a dermatome map, but in reality their distribution is much more complex as there is considerable overlap between dermatomes (about 50 per cent). *See also* **Transcutaneous Nerve Stimulation**.

dermis Deep layer of the skin, beneath the epidermis, containing blood vessels, muscles, nerve endings, and dense irregular connective tissue.

descriptive statistics Statistics which summarize the characteristics of a particular sample such as the attitude of a group towards aggression. *Compare* **inferential statistics**.

desensitization A *stress-management technique, more accurately called systematic desensitization, which uses relaxation techniques to cope with anxiety-inducing situations. The subject compiles a hierarchical list of anxiety-inducing situations (such as those associated with competition) with the one inducing the most anxiety at the top, and so on. The subject then undergoes *progressive muscle relaxation. Once relaxation is achieved, each anxiety-inducing situation is visualized, starting with the least stressful. At the same time, the subject visualizes himself or herself performing very well in the competition. Desensitization is a form of *counter-conditioning.

designer drug A synthetic drug designed to produce a specific effect on athletic performance and to escape detection in dope tests, either because it can be used in concentrations too low to be detected, or because the test cannot detect the drug at all. The International Olympic committee lists classes of banned substances rather than specific drugs in order to minimize the risk of non-listed designer drugs being used to circumvent the rules.

desire for group failure A group-member's expectations and hopes that the group will fail to achieve a goal. A substitute, for example, may sit on the bench secretly willing his or her team to lose. Those with a desire for group failure have a sense of satisfaction when failure has been realized.

desire for group success A group-member's expectations and hopes that the group will succeed. Desire for group success is a key, situation-specific element in group motivation which spurs group members to set and strive for challenging goals. Those with a desire for group success generally have a sense of pride and satisfaction when a goal has been achieved.

desmin A muscle protein associated with the *Z-line of sarcomeres. Desmin forms the connection between adjacent Z-lines from different myofibrils, keeping sarcomeres in register. It is responsible for the regular striated appearance of muscle fibres.

desocialization The process by which an individual experiences role loss and an accompanying loss of associated power or prestige (for example, following retirement from a sport). The individual may experience a loss of social identity resulting in an identity crisis, loss of peer status, loss of self image and self-esteem, and have difficulty finding a substitute activity or another peer group. *See also* **resocialization**.

detached retina Separation of the whole or part of the retina from the choroid coat, the vascularized intermediate layer of the eye. The actual separation may be due to a blow to the head or extreme physical exertion, such as lifting a heavy weight, but the underlying cause may be a hole or tear in the retina associated with degenerative changes. The actual detachment may be painless, but the athlete may complain of seeing specks floating in the eye, flashes of light, or blurred vision. Treatment is by fixation of the retina. Those who have had a detached retina are advised to avoid contact sports or very strenuous activity. Medical attention should be sought in all cases of eye injury.

detachment training Psychological training which enables athletes to create an inner, mental state of calm despite distractions and disturbances, such as other people watching, loud sounds, and bright lights. Detachment training includes practising mental relaxation techniques in unprotected environments in which distractions can occur.

detection *See* **stimulus identification**.

determinant Any factor which causes a particular phenomenon. For example, in *Cartwright's model of team cohesion, determinants are factors that lead to the development of *team cohesion and include cooperation, team stability, team homogeneity, and the size of the group.

determinism 1 The assumption that nothing occurs without it having a cause, implying that if the cause of a phenomenon can be identified, the occurrence of the phenomenon can be predicted. **2** In psychology, the view that every aspect of behaviour or experience is related to an antecedent event, external or internal to the individual.

deterministic model A model which proposes that behaviour is determined *for* an individual rather than *by* an individual. Proponents place much weight on the

regulation of behaviour by subconscious processes.

detoxify To remove poisonous substances.

detraining effects The changes the body undergoes when a person reduces or stops physical training. If a person stops exercising completely, most training effects are lost within eight weeks; detraining losses in speed and agility are relatively slow, but flexibility is lost quickly. If exercise is continued at a moderate level, many of the beneficial effects are retained. Endurance levels, for example, can be maintained for several months by continuing a light exercise programme for one or two days a week. In addition, detraining is affected by the way people have acquired their training benefits. Those who have trained at gradually increased intensities over a number of years, tend to lose the training effects much more slowly than those who have trained intensively for only short periods.

Deutschlander's fracture A *stress fracture in the metatarsal bones associated with long distance walking or running; the first type of stress fracture to be confirmed by radiography.

development The process of continuous change that occurs in the body, starting at conception and continuing through adulthood. Physical development usually results in greater complexity and specialization of body structures. Intellectual development results from learning and leads to more complex behaviour.

deviance Any social behaviour which departs from that regarded as 'normal' or socially accepted within a society or social context.

deviance amplification Process, often performed by the *mass media, in which the extent and seriousness of deviant behaviour, such as football hooliganism, is exaggerated. The effect is to create a greater awareness and interest in deviance which results in more deviance being uncovered, giving the impression that the initial exaggeration was actually a true representation.

deviant behaviour The conduct of individuals whose behaviour is contrary to the generally accepted norms or values of a society. *See also* **deviant sport acts**.

deviant sport acts Actions, on or off the field of play, which involve violating the rules of the sport or contravening the commonly accepted definitions of fair play or sportsmanship.

deviant sport subculture A sport group whose members' behaviour is contrary to some of the norms or values of the wider society. For example, some regard boxing as a deviant sport subculture because of the intent to inflict physical harm on the opponent. *Compare* **avocational sport subculture**; **occupational sport culture**.

deviation In statistics, the difference between one value and the mean of the set of values. Mean deviation is the mean of all the individual deviations of a set.

Dewey's theory of experiential continuum A theory maintaining that every experience takes up something from those experiences which have gone before and modifies in some way the quality of those experiences which occur later. Dewey argued that education should at each stage build on what has been learnt in the previous stage.

dexterity Ability to manipulate fine objects with the hands.

DHEA *See* **dehydroepiandrosterone**.

dhobie itch (groin itch) Infection, particularly of the groin, caused by fungi belonging to the genus *Tricophyton* or *Epidermophyton*.

diabetes mellitus A disorder of carbohydrate metabolism characterized by an increased blood glucose level (hyperglycaemia) and the presence of glucose in the urine (glycosuria). There are two main types of diabetes mellitus: Type I diabetes (also known as juvenile-onset diabetes and insulin-dependent diabetes) generally has a sudden onset in young people who develop almost total insulin deficiency that usually requires daily insulin injections; Type II diabetes (also known as adult-onset diabetes and noninsulin-dependent diabetes) usually develops gradually in adulthood and is caused by delayed or impaired insulin secretion, impaired insulin action (*see* **insulin resistance**), or excessive glucose output by the liver. Exercise is often an important part of the management of diabetes. It can be effective in modifying the course of the disease, helping to reduce the risk of vascular complications (e.g., coronary artery disease). Regular aerobic exercise might also reduce the risk of developing Type II diabetes, and it improves the control of blood glucose levels in those who already have the disease. However, it is important that the diabetic, coach, and friends are well acquainted with potential problems during exercise, such as *hypoglycaemia. A glucose drink or some other simple and quick source of glucose should be available if needed to prevent insulin shock. Physical activity reduces the concentration of insulin in the blood, and acute bouts of exercise increases the sensitivity of target cells to insulin, reducing the dosages required by a diabetic. Diabetics often suffer complications such as peripheral neuropathy which can reduce sensation in the feet and peripheral vascular disease which may impair blood circulation in the feet. They therefore need to pay particular attention to their feet, taking care to select proper footwear, especially if they perform weight-bearing exercises (e.g., road running).

dialectics The process of assessing the truth of a theory by logical reasoning and argument.

dialysis Separation of small molecules from larger ones through a differentially permeable membrane.

diapedesis Passage of cells through intact vessel walls into tissue spaces. It is a feature of inflammation.

diaphragm 1 A sheet of muscle and tendon between the abdominal cavity and the thoracic cavity. The diaphragm is attached on each side to the inferior border of the ribcage, in front to the sternum, and at the back to the vertebrae. Its insertion consists of a boomerang-shaped central tendon. The diaphragm plays an important role in breathing: contraction of the diaphragm increases the volume of the thoracic cavity, drawing air into the lungs; relaxation and elastic recoil of the diaphragm decreases the volume of the thoracic cavity, pumping air out. When the diaphragm contracts strongly, it increases the intrabdominal pressure. This may help to support the backbone and reduce flexion of the spine when lifting heavy weights. **2** Any partition or wall separating one body area from another.

diaphysis The central shaft of a long bone consisting mainly of compact bone surrounding a cavity (*see* **medullary cavity**).

diarrhoea Frequent evacuation of the bowels or the passage of soft, watery faeces. Diarrhoea may be associated with an intestinal infection, change of diet, exhaustion, nervous tension, or extreme physical exertion. The loss of fluid during diarrhoea impairs physical performances and increases the risk of muscle cramps. *See also* **runner's diarrhoea**; **traveller's diarrhoea**.

diarthrosis *See* **synovial joint**.

diastole Resting phase of the *cardiac cycle when all parts of the heart are relaxed. It occurs immediately after *systole and lasts about 0.5 s, assuming one complete cardiac cycle takes 0.8 s.

diastolic blood pressure The lowest arterial blood pressure associated with the resting phase (diastole) of the cardiac cycle during which the heart is filling up with blood.

diastolic volume The volume of blood which fills the ventricles during diastole.

diathermy Form of heat treatment of which there are two main types: short wave diathermy and microwave diathermy. Short wave diathermy (SWD) uses a high frequency alternating electric current to produce wireless waves 11 m in length. These can penetrate deep structures in which they generate heat. SWD is used to relieve pain and accelerate healing of deepseated sports injuries, such as chronic lesions in the hip joint. Microwave diathermy uses shorter wireless waves (in

physiotherapy, 12.25 cm or 69 cm in length). Its depth of penetration is only about 3 cm so it can be used only on superficial structures. However, microwave diathermy has a greater heating affect on muscles than SWD, so it is particularly useful for treating small, subcutaneous muscle lesions. Like other forms of heat treatment, diathermy should not be used immediately after an injury when there is a haemorrhage. Protective goggles should be worn, and microwaves should not be applied to the genitalia.

diencephalon The central core of the forebrain, between the cerebral hemispheres. It is mostly composed of the *thalamus and *hypothalamus.

diet Pattern of eating. The quality, quantity, and times of the day a person eats. *See also* **balanced diet**.

dietary fibre *See* **fibre**.

diet induced thermogenesis *See* **thermic effect of a meal**.

differential approach Approach to study of behaviour that focuses on individual differences, abilities, and predictions.

differential diagnosis The recognition of one disorder from another or others which have similar signs and symptoms. Some relatively innocuous sport-related disorders can be difficult to diagnose because they mimic other more serious complaints (*see* **athletic pseudonephritis**).

differential relaxation A relaxation technique which involves producing just the right degree of tension in different muscles to perform a particular movement. Muscles not involved in the required movement are relaxed so that energy is not wasted. Differential relaxation avoids the production of unwanted tension which can interfere with the performance of skilled movements. Elite athletes appear to be able to achieve a state of differential relaxation more easily than lower ability athletes.

differential threshold 1 The smallest perceptible difference between two stimuli. **2** The least amount of change in a stimulus in order for it to be recognized.

difficulty The state or quality of being not easy to perform. In some models of movement-behaviour, difficulty depends on both the distance a limb has to move and the narrowness of the target. As the movement becomes more difficult, the time to complete the movement accurately increases (*see* **Fitt's law**).

diffidence Lack of *self-confidence. Diffident individuals typically respond to competitive situations with fear of failure, are easily intimidated, and act with trepidation.

diffusing capacity of lung *See* pulmonary diffusion capacity.

diffusion 1 The net movement of molecules of a fluid from a high concentration to a low concentration. Diffusion is a passive process resulting from the random movement of molecules as a result of their kinetic energy. Gaseous exchange in the lungs and tissues takes place by diffusion through biological membranes. The rate of diffusion depends on the concentration gradient, diffusion distance, and the surface area and properties of the membrane. **2** The spread of cultural traits, such as language, technological ideas, or social practices from one society to another.

digestion The process which breaks down large food molecules in the alimentary canal, into smaller substances which can be absorbed from the gut into the blood stream. Digestion involves mechanical processes, such as chewing, and chemical processes involving enzymes.

digit One of the five fingers on each hand or five toes on each foot.

digital In anatomy, pertaining to the toes or fingers.

diphosphoglycerate (2,3-DPG) An organic phosphate bound to haemoglobin in red blood cells. 2,3-DPG is a by-product of the breakdown of glycogen to glucose. It reduces the affinity of *haemoglobin for oxygen, shifting the oxygen dissociation curve to the right and thereby assisting the unloading of oxygen to respiring tissues. Regular aerobic training increases the 2,3-DPG concentration in red blood cells. *See also* **altitude acclimatization**.

diploe Layer of spongy bone sandwiched between the inner and outer layer of compact tissue in the skull.

diplopia Double vision; seeing two images of the same object. It is one of the signs of a potentially serious eye injury.

direct calorimetry A method of determining a person's energy expenditure by direct measurement of the body's heat production in a *calorimeter.

direct competition Competition involving persons in a clearly personal contest against each other. Opponents may confront one another as teams or as individuals.

direct descriptive feedback *Feedback, usually given to athletes by their coaches, consisting of a description of a performance followed by a description of how the coach reacted to it.

direct evaluative feedback Feedback given to an athlete by coach (or other observer) in which the coach directly evaluates the athlete's behaviour without describing what led to that evaluation. Direct evaluative feedback may consist of a statement such as 'You were terrible', or 'You were great'. *Compare* **direct descriptive feedback**.

direct force (centric force: concentric force) A force which has its *line of action passing through the *centre of gravity of the body on which it acts. *Compare* **eccentric force**.

direct gene activation The method by which steroid hormones affect the activity of their target cells. The hormones attach onto specific receptors on the cell surface membrane to form a hormone–receptor complex which enters into the nucleus and activates certain genes.

direct impact The collision between two bodies moving along the same straight line before impact, or the collision of a stationary body with another body travelling at right angles to the surface against

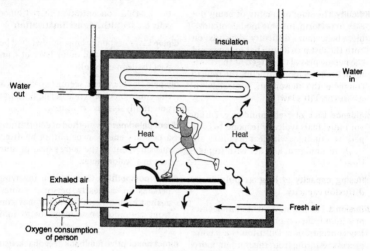

direct calorimetry

which the impact occurs. *Compare* **oblique impact**.

directional terms Terms used by physiologists, medical personnel, and biomechanics to describe the relative position of body parts or the location of an external object with respect to the body (*see* **anterior, deep, distal, inferior, lateral, medial, posterior, proximal, superficial,** and **superior**).

direct measure In sports psychology, a measurement in which individuals are asked direct questions. In the assessment of *team cohesion, for example, team members might be asked direct questions about how well they work together in the pursuit of team goals.

direct motivation *Motivation which is clear and unambiguous, such as when a coach makes a direct appeal to an athlete to try harder for the sake of the team. There are three main forms of direct motivation: *compliance, *identification, and *internalization. *Compare* **indirect motivation**.

direct trauma An injury caused by a *direct impact.

DIRT Mnemonic used to remember the components of interval training. 'D' represents the distance to be covered in each bout of activity (run, swim, cycle–ride etc.); 'I' is the interval of rest between each bout of activity; 'R' is the number of times the activity is repeated (i.e. the repetitions); and 'T' is the target time for each activity.

disability Any partial or total, mental or physical inability to perform any activity (sporting, social, or occupational) the affected person wishes to perform.

disaccharide (double sugar) A sugar formed when two monosaccharides join together by a reaction in which water is removed (condensation). For example, glucose and fructose combine to form sucrose. Other common disaccharides are lactose (formed from glucose and galactose) and maltose (formed from two molecules of glucose).

disc *See* **intervertebral disc**.

disc displacement Displacement of an intervertebral disc from its normal position, without the disc being herniated (*see* **prolapsed intervertebral disc**). Some of the cushioning effects of the disc are lost as a result of displacement. Disc displacement is a common cause of low back pain.

discontinuous servo A closed-loop control system in which the control actions of the effector are not continuously related to the state of the system being controlled. A simple home thermostat controlling room temperature is an example of a discontinuous servo: the room temperature continuously fluctuates but the heater (which acts as the effector) does not behave in the same way: it is either on or off with no one-to-one relationship between the changes in room temperature and the state of the heater. *Compare* continuous servo.

discounting principle A principle concerning the effect of rewards on the motivation of athletes. According to the principle, if an extrinsic reward is perceived by an athlete to be more important than the intrinsic motivation to participate in an activity, the value of the intrinsic motivation is discounted. For example, if an athlete who started playing a sport for its own sake is given money to play, the athlete comes to perceive that he or she is playing only for money rather than for any intrinsic reason. Consequently, the athlete is likely to stop playing in the absence of a monetary reward.

discovery learning Type of learning in which the learner discovers for himself or herself the chief contents or principles of the phenomenon to be learnt, and then incorporates them into his or her behaviour and thinking.

discrete skill (discrete task) A skill containing a single unit of activity with a definite beginning and end. A tennis serve and golf swing are examples of discrete skills. *Compare* continuous task.

discrete task *See* discrete skill.

discrimination 1 Prejudicial and therefore unequal treatment of a group of persons. Discrimination can apply to race or ethnic group (*see* racial discrimination), gender (*see* sexism), or age (*see* ageism). **2** The ability to distinguish between different levels or types of stimulation when they are presented simultaneously. **3** The ability to make precise distinctions between different stimulus-response conditions, as when a person distinguishes between a reinforced stimulus, to which a response is given, and an unreinforced stimulus, to which no response or a different response is given.

discrimination reaction time The *reaction time for a task in which different combinations of different stimuli are presented, with a response being made only if the combination includes a given stimulus.

disease Any disorder with a characteristic set of signs and symptoms, except that resulting from physical trauma.

disengagement The withdrawal from participation in an activity. In sport, disengagement tends to increase with age, and it is common during certain critical periods of the life course, for example during adolescence.

disengagement theory A theory which proposes that society and the ageing individual mutually withdraw from one another for the benefit and satisfaction of both. Thus, as a person ages he or she should withdraw from their roles of middle age thereby allowing these roles to be filled by younger people, and releasing the aged person to pursue new leisure pursuits. The theory is not supported by many gerontologists.

disinhibition The suppression of *inhibition, such as might occur through the inhibitory action of one neurone on another inhibitory neurone.

dislocating component When a joint is at certain angles, a component of muscle force directed away from the joint centre and which tends to pull the articulating ends of bones away from each other. *Compare* stabilizing component.

dislocation Complete separation (displacement) of articulating bones as a result of a joint being forced beyond its *maximum passive range. The joint becomes immobile and unstable, but there is little pain unless a displaced bone presses on a nerve. Considerable care is required when putting a dislocated bone back in its correct place as great damage can be done to surrounding blood vessels and nerves by an unskilled person. It is usually quite easy for a skilled person to reposition a dislocated bone (it may even realign automatically) within a few hours of injury. If, however, treatment is delayed, the condition is usually difficult to correct because the ligaments damaged during the injury tend to stick together. *Compare* **subluxation**.

disordered eating *See* **eating disorder**.

disorientation A mental state characterized by loss of awareness of space, time, or personality. In sport, disorientation can result from *dehydration, *heat exhaustion, and *hypothermia. Individuals who become disoriented during a physical activity often have problems of thermoregulation and they should not continue with the activity. Athletes, especially those who are not well conditioned, commonly become disorientated at the end of endurance events. Most respond well to a supervised warm-down of slow walking and the administration of oral fluids.

displaced aggression Hostility directed against an inanimate object or a person, other than the source of the hostility, from which retaliation is unlikely. The person to whom the *aggression is displaced is usually weaker than the aggressor.

displacement 1 A vector quantity which refers to the distance which an object has moved in a given direction. It is measured as the length of a straight line between the initial and final positions of a body. For example, in a race around one complete circuit of a 400 metre track, the displacement is 0 metres. *Compare* **distance**. **2** Volume of fluid displaced by a body completely or partially submerged in a fluid. **3** In psychology, applied to behaviours and emotions which are transferred from their original object onto a more acceptable substitute. For example, a tennis player who feels aggrieved about an umpiring decision may throw his or her tennis racket at the ground rather than at the umpire.

display A specific learning situation or task which confronts an individual. In sport, the display includes the equipment, cues, and environment in which an athlete acquires skills. One of the challenges of a coach is to be able to modify displays to make it easier for athletes to achieve desired learning outcomes.

dispositional theory *See* **trait theory**.

dissociation An attentional style characterized by distraction. Dissociation is exhibited by athletes who are unaware of their surroundings because they are mentally absorbed thinking about other things while participating in their sport. *Compare* **association**.

dissociators Individuals who externalize or adopt an external attentional focus. Those participating in contact sports are often dissociators because they attempt to focus on things unrelated to body sensations. *Compare* **associators**.

dissonance *See* **cognitive dissonance**.

distal Away from the midline of the trunk (e.g., the ankle is distal to the knee). *Compare* **proximal**; *see also* **directional terms**.

distance A scalar measurement of the extent of a body's motion, irrespective of the direction in which it has travelled. Thus, when a body moves from one location to another, the distance through which it moves is the length of path it follows. In a race around a 400 m track, the distance travelled is 400 m. *Compare* **displacement**.

distance acuity The ability to focus on and distinguish fine detail at 6 metres or more with either eye separately and together under a variety of lighting conditions.

distance–time curve A smooth line or curve which best fits the points on a graph in which distance is plotted on the y-axis and time on the x-axis. The distance–time curve enables changes in speed (e.g., during a 100 m race) to be identified since the slope (gradient) at any point of time gives the speed of the body at that time. *See also* **instantaneous speed**.

distensibility The capacity to expand or stretch under pressure.

distorting force A force which changes the dimensions of a body. *Compare* **rotary force**.

distractibility The ease with which irrelevant thoughts and external stimuli interfere with concentration on the task in hand. Distractibility is affected by levels of arousal: as arousal increases up to the optimum, the athlete's attention narrows and distractability decreases, but with levels of arousal above an optimum, the athlete's attention shifts sporadically from one cue to another, increasing distractibility and increasing the chances of a poor performance.

distraction conflict theory The suggestion that when a person is performing a task the *mere presence of others creates a conflict between concentrating on the task and concentrating on the other people. This conflict increases *arousal which leads to *social facilitation. *See also* **Zajonc's model**.

distraction game A form of *concentration training in which attempts are made to distract the players without physically impeding them.

distraction hypothesis A hypothesis which maintains that exercise enhances psychological well-being by acting as a distraction from stressful life events, and it is this distraction rather than the physical exercise itself that reduces anxiety. *Compare* **endorphin hypothesis**.

distraction rupture An injury resulting in a muscle-tear caused by overstretching or overloading. Distraction ruptures commonly occur in biarticulate muscles (muscles, such as the hamstrings, which span two joints) in performers of explosive events when demands on muscles exceed their strength. *See also* **distraction strain**.

distraction strain A muscle strain which occurs when a muscle accidentally contracts when it is being stretched. Distraction strains often occur among athletes who do not warm up properly or who are suffering from fatigue and are not able to respond adequately to neuromuscular reflexes. There are three degrees of distraction strain: first degree strain, where there is some swelling, inflammation, and discomfort, but no appreciable tear; second degree strain, in which there is considerable pain, more damage to the muscle, but there is no complete tear; and a third degree strain, in which there is a complete tear of the muscle (*see* **distraction rupture**).

distress The negative, harmful aspects of stress. *Compare* **eustress**.

distributed practice A procedure for learning a skill in which small units of practice are alternated with rest periods; usually the practice time is less than the rest time. *Compare* **massed practice**.

distributive justice proposition The proposition that the perceived adequacy of a reward depends not so much on a person's needs but on what rewards are available and how they are shared. Individuals may compare their own reward with those of other team mates.

disuse atrophy A degeneration or loss of muscle mass resulting from inactivity. It can lead to paralysis if muscles are reduced less than one quarter of their original size. Connective tissue consisting mainly of dense collagen fibres replaces the muscle making complete rehabilitation impossible. *See also* **principle of disuse**.

diuresis Excretion of large volumes of urine. An increase in urine output may be induced by disease or drugs. *See also* **diuretic drugs**.

diuretic drugs 1 A class of pharmacological agents banned by the International Olympic Committee (IOC). Diuretics increase urine flow which helps to eliminate tissue fluid. This is important for the treatment of certain pathological conditions such as oedema (excess water retention), but diuretics have been misused to reduce quickly the weight of participants in sports with strict weight-controls. They have also been misused to flush out drugs and reduce the concentration of banned substances in a urine sample. Diuretics can be harmful: they may accelerate the removal of valuable water-soluble minerals and vitamins and hinder thermoregulation. Electrolyte imbalances caused by diuretics may lead to exhaustion, heart abnormalities, and even death. **2** Any substance that increases the elimination of fluid from the body through urination. In addition to the pharmacological agents banned by the IOC, diuretics include alcohol and caffeine.

diurnal cycles Fluctuations in physiological processes (e.g., heart rate and body core temperature) that occur during a normal 24-hour day. *See also* **circadian rhythms**.

divergent involvement Sport involvement which almost amounts to an obsession, with a disproportionate amount of time being devoted to sport, often to the detriment of family and career. Primary divergent involvement in sport is exhibited by individuals who play sports to the exclusion of most other things; secondary divergent involvement refers to individuals who consume sport to excess and become sports addicts.

divergent sport involvement *See* **divergent involvement**.

divergent thinking A form of thinking in which a single idea or problem generates many other ideas or solutions.

diverting activity In sports training, a physical or mental activity performed during rest periods which is distinctly different from that performed during work bouts. Diverting activities can enhance recovery.

divided-target-type-test A test of accuracy in which the target is divided up into several parts each of which receives a different score.

divisible task A group task which can be divided into different components each of which is performed by different members of the group.

division of labour The process by which tasks are separated and become more specialized. American football teams with their highly specialized teams of offence and defence, their specialized kickers and punters, provide an example of division of labour in sport.

DNA *See* **deoxyribonucleic acid**.

dominant response *See* **reaction potential**.

domination In general usage, the influence exerted by one person or group over another person or groups. In sociology, domination is indicated by the likelihood that a command will be obeyed, and is distinguished from power which may be imposed despite resistance.

DOMS *See* **delayed-onset muscle soreness**.

Donnagio test A qualitative test of mucoproteins used as an indicator of *stress. An increase in mucoproteins is associated with a stress reaction induced in the adrenal cortex as a result of metabolic fatigue. The test consists of taking a 2 ml sample of urine and adding to it 1 ml of 1 per cent thionin and 2 mls of a 4 per cent solution of ammonium molybdate. A positive reaction is indicated by the urine turning violet. The degree of coloration indicates the degree of positive reaction which may be represented as +, ++, or +++.

Donnan equilibrium An electrochemical equilibrium established when two solutions are separated by a membrane that is impermeable to some of the ions in the solution.

Donway traction splint A traction splint specially designed for a fractured femur shaft and supplied for the use of UK racecourse medical officers. The splint applies gentle traction to align the injured leg.

dopamine A metabolic neurotransmitter belonging to the *biogenic amines. It is an intermediate in the synthesis of *noradrenaline. Dopamine is regarded as a stimulant; as such, it is on the International Olympic Committee list of *banned substances. It is secreted by some sympathetic ganglia in the *hypothalamus and by some neurones in the midbrain. It is the main neurotransmitter in *extrapyramidal tracts. Its release is enhanced by *amphetamines. High dopamine levels

dopamine

have been linked to *aggression. Antipsychotic drugs such as thorazine, have been used to block dopamine receptors and reduce aggression. However, overuse of these antipsychotics may cause motor problems because dopamine levels may be reduced in parts of the brain controlling skeletal muscle.

dopaminergic system Part of the nervous system which uses *dopamine as a neurotransmitter.

doping A term derived from the African Kaffirs who used a local brew called 'dop' as a stimulant. Doping is generally regarded as the administering or use of substances which are alien to the body, the use of physiological substances in abnormal quantities, or the use of abnormal procedures by persons with the intention of gaining an artificial and unfair improvement of performance in competitions. Doping includes the use of medicines if these raise the physical capacity above the normal level. Defining which drugs and methods constitute doping is a major problem and there is no universally agreed definition for all sports. The International Olympic Committee (IOC) has a list of *banned substances which must be avoided by athletes competing in the Olympic Games, but governing bodies of individual sports have their own lists which may differ from that of the IOC.

doping classes A classification of substances banned by the IOC, based on pharmacological classes of agents (*see* **banned substances**).

doping methods Pharmacological, chemical, and physical manipulations which are banned by the International Olympic Committee. They include the use of substances and methods which alter the integrity of urine samples taken for dope testing (e.g., urine substitution by catheterization). *See also* **blood doping**.

dorsal Towards the upper surface or back.

dorsal interossei Four muscles at the back of the hand. They originate at the sides of the metacarpals of all digits and insert onto the base of the proximal phalanx of all dig-

its. Their primary actions are abduction of the second and fourth metacarpophalangeal joints, radial and ulnar deviation of the third metacarpophalangeal joint, and flexion of the second, third, and fourth metacarpophalangeal joints.

dorsal root The collection of nerve fibres from the peripheral nervous system which occurs as a bundle near the upper surface of the spinal cord at each spinal level; the major sensory input to the cord.

dorsiflexion Movement that brings the top of the foot towards the lower leg. Dorsiflexion involves the combined action of the tibialis anterior, peroneus tertius, extensor hallucis longus, and extensor digitorum longus muscles. It is not a powerful movement, but it helps prevent the toes from dragging during walking.

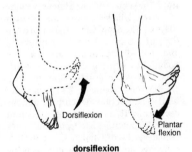

Dorsiflexion

Plantar flexion

dorsiflexion

dorsum In anatomy, pertaining to the back.

dose The precise amount of a drug prescribed by a doctor to be given to a patient at any one time.

dose regime The amount of drug taken, expressed in terms of the quantity of the drug and the frequency at which it is taken.

double-blind situation A situation in which contradictory demands or meanings are communicated in the same message or environment. A coach, for example, may encourage an athlete to be competitive and follow the 'law of the jungle', while family and teachers urge the athlete to cooperate with others or to turn the other cheek. The athlete is then in a double-blind situation.

double-blind study An experimental protocol used when studying the effects of an experimental treatment in which one group is given the experimental treatment (e.g., a certain drug) while the other group receives a control treatment (e.g., a placebo). In a double-blind study neither the investigator nor the subjects know who is receiving the experimental or control treatments.

double circulation Circulation in which blood goes through the heart twice for each complete circuit of the body. It consists of a systemic circulation and a pulmonary circulation.

double jointed *See* **hypermobile joint disease.**

double labelled water technique A method of indirectly estimating energy expenditure. The subject ingests a known volume of water labelled with two isotopes ($^2H_2$$^{18}O$). The deuterium ($^2H_2$) and oxygen ($^{18}O$) diffuse throughout the body's water, and their disappearance rate from the body fluid (e.g., in blood, urine, or saliva) is measured. When a subject is loaded with $^2H_2$$^{18}O$, the decrease in ^{18}O is a measure for H_2O output plus CO_2 outputs, and the decrease in $^2H_2$ is a measure of H_2O output alone. Therefore CO_2 output can be obtained by the difference. CO_2 output is converted to energy expenditure using the energy equivalent of CO_2, calculated using additional information on the substrate mixture respired.

double pendulum Two rigid bodies joined together with one of the bodies supported at a fixed point in such a way that the whole assembly can swing smoothly about that point. In biomechanics, the arm and the golf club can be regarded as a double pendulum during a golf swing.

double product The product of heart rate and systolic blood pressure. Double product is used as an estimate of myocardial (heart muscle) work and is proportional to myocardial oxygen consumption. Strength training reduces the resting double product, indicating a decrease in myocardial oxygen consumption at rest.

double progressive system A system of strength training in which both the resistance and the number of repetitions are adjusted.

double pull The simultaneous production of tension in an antagonistic pair of muscles. The double pull is essential for normal movement of a body segment: when one muscle shortens, its opposite partner produces a counter tension to hold the body segment in place. However, the production of excessive counter tension can interfere with the performance of a skilled movement; this can be avoided by differential relaxation.

double sugar *See* **disaccharide.**

Douglas bag A rubber-lined canvas bag used for the collection of gas exhaled by a person. A Douglas bag can be used to measure oxygen uptake during exercise.

down-regulation A decreased sensitivity of cells to a particular hormone, probably caused by a reduction in the number of receptors on cell surface membranes that bind to that hormone. Down-regulation occurs, for example, in response to obesity when cells become less sensitive to insulin. *Compare* **up-regulation.**

downward social mobility A form of *social mobility which results in a person moving from a higher social class or socioeconomic status to a lower social class or socioeconomic status. The term is also applied to sportspersons moving from high levels of sport to a lower levels. Downward social mobility results in a decrease in social status. *Compare* **upward social mobility.**

drafting *See* **form drag.**

drag A force that resists the motion of a body moving through a fluid. As applied to a projectile in flight or any other body moving through a fluid (e.g., a swimmer), drag is the component of the resultant force due to relative fluid flow measured parallel to the direction of freestream fluid flow. *See also* form drag; surface drag; and wave drag.

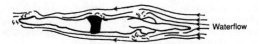

Small drag in streamlined position

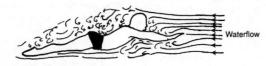

Large drag in unstreamlined position

drag force

drain A medical procedure which allows the outflow of fluid from, for example, a sports injury.

drawer sign *See* **anterior drawer sign**.

dressing Material applied to an injured body-part to protect it and assist healing. The material may also act as a means of carrying or enclosing medicines.

drill 1 A precise, well-defined motor skill practised repeatedly. **2** A pre-determined series of actions.

drive 1 A physiological condition involving sensitivity to certain types of stimulation which activates behaviour. Drives are distinguished from motives in being initially indiscriminate and without any appropriate direction. Drives may be grouped into two main categories: primary, innate drives which include hunger, pain, thirst, and sex; and secondary drives including socially learned rewards not directly dependent on biological needs, and other rewards including verbal and monetary reinforcements. **2** In sport psychology, a term often equated with arousal.

drive theory Theory of learning that predicts a linear relationship between drive (arousal) and learning. According to the theory, as an athlete's arousal or state anxiety increases, so too does his or her performance. Few sport psychologists support drive theory because they recognize that overarousal can diminish the quality of performance. *See also* **inverted-U hypothesis**.

drop jump A jump in which the performer drops down from a specified height and then jumps upwards. A drop jump uses the *stretch-shortening cycle.

drop out An individual who has stopped taking part in sport or an exercise programme. Lack of time, loss of interest, and, especially, failure to achieve performance goals seem to be critical factors.

drug Any substance which alters the body's actions and natural chemical environment. In sport, drugs are often misused to enhance physical or mental performance. Drugs taken to prevent or cure a disease or other body disorder are often called medicines to distinguish them from addictive substances, such as *narcotic analgesics, taken illegally for some other purpose. *See also* **doping**.

drug addiction Chronic physical craving or compulsion to continue to take a drug to avoid the unpleasant physical effects

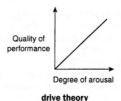

drive theory

resulting from withdrawal of the drug. Many drugs are associated with addiction including barbiturates, opiates (e.g., heroin), morphine, and alcohol. Use of the term often includes psychological dependence.

drug allergy An antigen–antibody reaction induced by a drug. The drug or one of its products sensitizes its user by combining with a protein in the body to produce an antigen which, in its turn, leads to the formation of antibodies. Subsequent exposure to the drug initiates an antigen–antibody reaction which may manifest itself as anything from a mild skin irritation to a potentially fatal *anaphylaxis.

drug control policy A policy to control the procedures and drugs used to gain an unfair advantage in sports. A good drugs control policy not only lists banned substances and procedures, but has a fair and effective testing programme (including good collection and testing procedures), and takes strong action against any well-proven contraventions of the policy. The most influential drug control policy is that of the International Olympic Committee. Its policy is based on a list of *banned substances and procedures compiled by its Medical Commission. An effective drug control policy incorporates out-of-competition testing as well as in-competition testing for drugs. Many sports governing bodies conduct such tests, but they are likely to take action only if an *anabolic steroid or one of its masking agents is found. A doctor may prescribe a banned drug or a coach may encourage an athlete to take drugs, but in the eyes of sporting authorities administering drug control policies, the responsibility for adhering to the policy rests solely with the athlete.

drug dependence A compulsion to take drugs because of the physical and/or the psychological effects produced by the habitual taking of the drug. Many drugs, such as cannabis, are associated with psychological dependence only when repeated use induces reliance on it for a state of well-being. Other drugs, such as mor-

phine, are associated with both a psychological and a physical need to take the drug to avoid unpleasant withdrawal symptoms.

drug detection *See* drug screening.

drug idiosyncrasy A genetically determined, abnormal reaction to a drug.

drug screening Methods carried out on a group of athletes to distinguish between those who have used a banned substance and those who have not. Screening is essentially a procedure to clear athletes of any possibility of having used drugs. If a test is positive, then specific identification is needed. Techniques used in drug detection include chromatography, mass spectrometry, and radioimmunoassay. *See also* **drug control policy**.

drug tolerance An acquired resistance to the effects of a repeatedly administered drug. When tolerance occurs, more drug is needed to produce the same pharmacological effects.

dry bulb thermometer The usual type of thermometer used to record the temperature of air.

duct A canal or passageway, especially one for carrying secretions from an *exocrine gland.

dumb-bells A short bar with weights, sometimes adjustable, at each end. They are usually used in pairs during weight training, one for each hand.

duodenum The first part of the small intestine connecting the stomach to the ileum. In addition to secreting its own enzymes and mucus, the duodenum also receives bile from the gall bladder and juices from the pancreas to aid digestion of food. The walls of the duodenum are highly folded to absorb digested substances.

duration *See* **training duration**.

Dutoit procedure A surgical procedure for treating recurrent anterior dislocation of the shoulder. During the procedure, large metal staples are placed through a longitudinal splint in the subscapularis to reattach the capsule to the anterior glenoid neck. Because of the risk of arthrosis if the staples are not inserted properly, most surgeons avoid this procedure.

dynamic Pertaining to forces which produce motion.

dynamic action A muscle action in which the muscle changes length, producing forces that result in movement and a change in joint angle.

dynamic balance Balance maintained either on a moving surface or while the body is moving.

dynamic balance movements Movements made in order to maintain a balanced position. Such movements often take the form of irregular oscillations. *See also* **balance**.

dynamic contraction *See* **dynamic action**.

dynamic endurance The ability of a muscle to contract and relax repeatedly. Dynamic endurance can be tested, for example, during an isotonic exercise such as raising and lowering the arm. *Compare* **static endurance**.

dynamic equilibrium State of an object which is moving with constant (uniform) linear velocity and angular velocity; that is, it is moving with zero acceleration. Dynamic equilibrium exists if there is a balance between the applied forces and inertial forces for a body in motion, with all the applied forces resulting in equal and oppositely directed inertial forces.

dynamic flexibility The range of motion that can be achieved by actively moving a body segment using muscle actions. Dynamic flexibility also refers to the relative ease of making rapid or repeated movements over any range, rather than the range itself (*compare* **extent flexibility**). It is determined by the forces which oppose or resist the movements, and is affected by the ability of muscles to recover quickly. Dynamic flexibility is an important ability underlying many gross motor skills and is important for developing speed and power.

dynamic friction *See* **sliding friction**.

dynamics A branch of mechanics concerned with the study of the mathematical and physical properties of bodies in motion,

and the forces that produce or change the motion. *Compare* **statics**.

dynamic strength (ballistic strength) The ability to exert muscular force repeatedly or over a period of time. It is especially concerned with forces which produce or change the motion of a mechanical system.

dynamic stretching *See* **ballistic stretching**.

dynamic visual acuity Ability of an observer to detect details of an object when either the object and/or the person is moving.

dynamogeny The concept that the presence of others moving alongside or faster than an athlete (e.g., runner, swimmer, or cyclist) stimulates the production of nervous energy which increases the kinetic energy of the athlete. Dynamogeny has been proposed to explain the improved performances of athletes in competition or when using a pace maker.

dynamography The measurement and recording of forces and pressure. Force platforms and pressure platforms have been used in gait research and to study starts, take-offs, and landings in running and jumping events; swings in baseball and golf; and balance in gymnastics.

dynamometer An instrument designed to measure the *torque or force exerted by a muscle or muscle group.

dyne Unit of *force; one dyne is required to give a mass of 1 g an acceleration of 1 cms^{-2}.

dysfunctional activity Any social activity that has a negative effect on the maintenance and efficient functioning of a social system.

dysfunctional aggressive behaviour Aggressive or assertive behaviour that interferes with attaining a goal. A footballer who intentionally fouls an opponent rather than intercept the ball is guilty of dysfunctional aggressive behaviour. *Compare* **functional aggressive behaviour**.

dysmenorrhoea Severe pain during menstruation. This often interferes with training and competition, but it is sometimes possible to change the timing of the menstrual cycle by using contraceptive pills or other substances. It is important that athletes taking medication to treat dysmenorrhoea check that the medication does not include any *banned substances. There is some evidence that regular aerobic exercise reduces the incidence of dysmenorrhoea.

dyspnoea Laboured breathing which usually causes some distress because it seems inappropriate for the demands being placed on the body. Shortness of breath at the end of a race is not dyspnoea because

the effort of breathing is appropriate, passes quite quickly, and causes no real distress. Dyspnoea occurs when there is a malfunction in the air supply to the lungs, as in bronchitis and asthma; when circulation to the lungs is impaired, as in heart failure; or if the blood cannot carry sufficient oxygen, as in anaemia.

dystonia 1 An impairment of tone in tissue, particularly muscle (*see* **muscle tone**). **2** A postural disorder affecting muscles of the head, neck, and trunk due to disease of *basal ganglia.

 E

ear drum rupture to **Eysenck personality inventory**

ear drum rupture A perforation in the eardrum (tympanic membrane). It occurs most often when an underwater diver fails to equalize the pressure in the middle ear. A rupture underwater usually causes an immediate and debilitating vertigo as cold water enters the middle ear. This carries with it the risk of infection so a prophylactic antibiotic should be given. No one with an eardrum rupture should dive underwater until the eardrum has completely healed and its mobility is restored (this usually takes about 6 weeks). An eardrum rupture may also result from a blow to the side of the head, or from the pressure wave produced from a gun shot.

ear drum temperature The temperature of the outer ear taken with a thermocouple next to the eardrum. Eardrum temperature is used as an approximation of body core temperature, but it varies more than *core temperature.

ear guards Headgear which protects the ears. They are commonly used by wrestlers and rugby players to minimize the risk of auricular haematomas (cauliflower ears).

Ear guards may also reduce concussive forces to the head.

ear injuries Damage to either the outer, middle, or inner ear. In sport, if the outer ear is repeatedly damaged by blows there is a risk of bleeding and inflammation of the ear lobe which can lead to a permanent deformity commonly called a cauliflower ear (*see* **auricular haematoma**). Sports linked with this type of injury are boxing, rugby football, and wrestling. Sometimes a blow to the side of the head can increase the pressure in the middle ear, rupturing the eardrum (*see* **eardrum rupture**). An eardrum rupture may also occur as a result of barotrauma, for example, during a scuba underwater dive when changes in air pressure in the middle ear are not equalized.

early recall Recall of information within two hours or so of its being stored. In most sports, this is the approximate time interval during which an athlete must be able to retain information about opponents' strengths and weaknesses. *See* **short-term memory**.

early responding Anticipation of a stimulus so that a movement can occur at or before the stimulus is given. During a 100 metre sprint, for example, early responding may result in a false start when an athlete anticipates the starting gun. Early responding must be taken into consideration when designing tests of *reaction times.

eating disorder A group of clinical disorders involving disturbed eating patterns. Eating disorders are usually classified into two main groups (*see* **anorexia nervosa, and bulimia nervosa**) but in reality there is a spectrum of disorders. Eating disorders are much more prevalent among women (especially adolescents) than men. Many sociologists blame the disorders on the preoccupation of Western culture with slimness. Eating disorders are of major concern in female athletes. Some estimates suggest that as many as 50 per cent of elite athletes in certain sports may have an eating disorder. High-risk sports include appearance sports (e.g., diving, figure skating, and gymnastics), endurance sports (e.g., distance running and swimming), and weight-classification sports (e.g., judo). A mild eating disorder (loss of appetite and weight) is one of the symptoms of overtraining.

eburnation The wearing away of *articular cartilage exposing underlying bone. Eburnation is the end-result of *osteoarthritis.

eccentric action A muscle action in which a muscle exerts a force while lengthening. Such actions are used to resist external forces, such as gravity. They also occur during the deceleration phases of locomotion. For example, the *quadriceps produces an eccentric action when a person walks down a hill. During eccentric actions, muscle fibres move in the opposite direction to the change in joint angle and the mechanical work done is negative: $W = F - D$; where W = work; F = force; and D = distance. *Compare* **concentric action**.

eccentric force A force which does not pass through the *centre of gravity of the body on which it acts, or through a point at

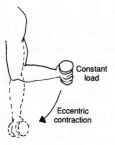

eccentric action

which the body is fixed. Such a force produces translation and rotation. Its rotatory effect is known as *torque.

eccentric training Training that focuses on *eccentric actions of muscles. There appears to be no clear advantage of eccentric training over other types of concentric or static action training, but in resistance training (e.g., weight-lifting) it is important to include the eccentric phase with the concentric phase to maximize strength gains.

ecchymosis A bruise caused by an injury or spontaneous diffusion of blood from blood vessels, characterized by a red or bluish-black discoloration just under the skin. An ecchymosis under the conjunctiva in the eye (a 'bloodshot' eye) may result from chemical or physical irritation.

Eccles' expectancy model A model of sporting achievement and activity choice in which key components are expectations (i.e., how well individuals are expected by others and themselves to do), social environment, gender roles, and individual differences. The model has been used to explain male/female differences in sport participation and success. If parents, for example, rate a daughter's potential for success in a sport lower than a son's, the daughter is less likely to take part in the sport. *See also* **self-fulfilling prophecy**.

eccrine gland Applied to a *sweat gland which releases its secretion directly onto the skin surface. Eccrine glands are distributed over most of the body, but occur in greatest density on the palms of the hands, soles of the feet, in the axillae (armpits), and on the forehead. Eccrine sweat glands are involved in thermoregulation.

ECG *See* **electrocardiogram**.

echocardiography A non-invasive technique which uses ultrasound waves to produce a real-time image of the internal structure of an active heart. Echocardiography enables the cavity size and wall thickness of the heart chambers to be measured. In addition, structural abnormalities (such as defective heart valves) can be detected. Because of its non-invasive nature, electrocardiography is an ideal technique for studying heart function in athletes.

eclectism A method of study which selects theories and ideas from a variety of disparate sources.

ecological viewpoint A point of view emphasizing the study of movement in the natural environment, and the evolutionary, physical, and biological constraints of movement. *Compare* **SR approach**.

ectomorph A dimension of somatotype (body build) characterized by a tall, thin, and linearly constructed body. *See also* **somatotype**.

ectopic bone Bone which forms outside the area in which it is normally expected to occur. *See also* **myositis ossificans**.

ectopic heartbeat A heartbeat which momentarily loses its rhythm. The heart may miss a beat which is then followed by a heavy jolt. This is not sinister as long as the heart is otherwise normal, and as long as the ectopic heartbeat occurs at rest. If it occurs during exercise, or increases with intensity of exercise, or if it combines with other abnormalities, medical advice should be sought.

eczema A non-infectious skin complaint characterized by itching and often accompanied by small blisters. One form may be induced by cold, windy conditions, or chemical irritants dissolved in water. Another form is caused by an allergy to one of a wide range of substances. Flexural or atopic eczema primarily affects children at sites which are frequently flexed, such

as the back of the knee. Although swimming is not generally suitable for eczema sufferers, irritant eczema has little effect on sports participation. Contact sports are generally not suitable for sufferers of flexural eczema because of the risk of bacterial infection of eczematous blisters.

eddy currents Whirling currents of fluid (e.g., air or water) formed during turbulent flow. Eddy currents turn back on themselves and eventually become detached from the main body of fluid, thereby opposing the main current flow.

eddy resistance (tail suction) A *drag force caused by eddy currents. Eddy resistance is reduced by *streamlining and increased by certain positions and movements of a body in the fluid. For example, lateral movements of a swimmer such as wriggling the hips and legs, increase eddy resistance. *See also* **form drag**.

edema See oedema.

EDV *See* **end-diastolic volume**.

EEG *See* **electroencephalograph**.

effective anticipation An ability to predict the duration of internal processes and planned movement so that a response can be made coincident with an anticipated external event. Effective anticipation is needed when swinging a bat or racket to hit a moving ball.

effective behaviour Behaviour resulting in desirable outcomes.

effective force A force producing a desired outcome. An effective force is produced by a limb when it accelerates sufficiently to overcome a resistance which a subject wishes to overcome.

effectiveness The degree to which a purpose is achieved. In biomechanics effectiveness refers, for example, to how well a particular running technique helps a sprinter complete the 100 m as quickly as possible. A technique may be effective in enabling the sprinter to run fast, but inefficient in terms of energy expenditure.

effective synergy *See* **synergy**.

effector Any body structure, such as a muscle, gland, or organ, that brings about an action (e.g., a muscle action or glandular secretion) as a result of a stimulus it receives. The stimulus may be neuronal or hormonal.

effeminacy The presence of or manifestation of feminine characteristics, either physical or behavioural, in a male.

efficacy The ability to successfully achieve an intended result. *See* **collective efficacy**; and **self-efficacy**.

efficiency In human movements, the relationship between the amount of work done and the energy expended in doing the work. It is usually expressed as a percentage of the ratio of work accomplished to energy expended: efficiency = (work done/energy expended) × 100. Efficiency is always less than 100 per cent because some useful energy is always dissipated as heat. Until recently, it was assumed that the efficiency of human movements was only about 20–25 per cent. However, it is now believed that the elastic components in the limbs can store energy after impact enabling greater efficiencies to be achieved.

effleurage A form of *massage consisting of superficial or deep stroking movements towards the heart. It is administered with the flat of the hand and fingers. Effleurage helps stimulate circulation of blood and lymph, relieving congestion and swelling around joint injuries.

effluage *See* **effleurage**.

effort The force applied to a lever which is used to move a load or overcome a resistance. In human locomotion, an effort is produced by a muscle action at its attachment point on the skeleton.

effort headache A headache commonly experienced at the completion of sporting activities, such as the marathon and triathlon, in which participants are exposed to extremes of heat, humidity, and inadequate hydration. The headache usually lasts for about 1 hour and has symptoms similar to a migraine, such as affecting one side, visual aura, and vomiting. An effort headache can be prevented by proper conditioning and maintaining adequate hydration during the activity. *See also* **headache**.

effusion A form of *oedema in which there is an accumulation of fluid in a potential space, such as a joint capsule.

ego An individual's concept of himself or herself. Ego is a part of the mind which develops from the individual's experience of the outside world. It operates in direct contact with reality and is concerned with processing and evaluating information about the importance of, and relationships between, specific actions and behaviours of the individual. It is one of the three elements of Freudian theory. The ego, which is thought to have developed from the *id, attempts to reconcile the unconscious primitive demands of the id with the constraints imposed by the *superego and with the individual's awareness of the real world.

ego defence mechanism A mechanism whereby the *ego reconciles basic instincts of the id with the more sedate cultural values of the superego to make them acceptable to reality. Ego defences include projection, reaction formation, denial, and sublimation. *See also* **intellectualization**; and **repression**.

ego enhancing strategy A psychological device by which a person attributes all success to internal causes.

ego protecting strategy A psychological device by which a person attributes all failures to external causes.

ego threat Any factor which tends to diminish a person's opinion of himself or herself.

eight-state questionnaire A questionnaire designed to measure eight *affective characteristics which are believed to be important in athletic performance. The questionnaire has been used successfully in measuring the psychological states of élite, world-class runners.

ejection fraction The proportion of blood ejected out of the left ventricles during each heartbeat. It is equal to the *stroke volume divided by the *end diastolic volume. The ejection fraction, is usually expressed as a percentage. It averages about 60 per cent at rest.

elastic Applied to a material which regains its original shape on removal of a distorting force. *Compare* **plastic**.

elastic cartilage *Cartilage with an amorphous, unstructured matrix containing elastic fibres in addition to *chondrocytes. Elastic cartilage supports the pinna (outer ear) maintaining its structure while allowing it to be flexible.

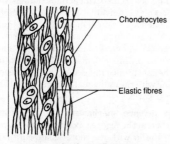

Chondrocytes

Elastic fibres

elastic cartilage

elastic components The viscoelastic structures associated with the contractile elements of muscle. *See also* **parallel elastic components**; and **series elastic components**.

elastic energy *See* **strain energy**.

elastic filament A protein filament in a *sarcomere which stretches from the M-line to the Z-line. It is thought to consist of one molecule of the protein titin. Elastic filaments keep thick filaments exactly in the middle between the two Z-lines of a sarcomere during a muscle action.

elasticity (restitution) **1** Property of a body that causes it to tend to regain its original shape after being compressed or deformed. **2** The ability of a tissue to resume its resting length after it has contracted or been stretched.

elastic limit The limit of *stress within which the *strain in a material completely disappears when the stress is removed. If a solid material is stretched beyond its elastic limit, it becomes permanently deformed.

elastic modulus Ratio of *stress to *strain in a given material. Strain may be a change in length, a twist, or a change in volume. *See also* **flexural rigidity**; **modulus of compression**; **modulus of rigidity**; **torsional modulus**; and **Young's modulus**.

elastic strength The ability of muscles to exert forces quickly and to overcome resistance with a high speed of muscle action. High levels of elastic strength requires good coordination and a combination of speed and strength of muscle action. It is important in explosive activities such as jumping and sprinting. In old textbooks, elastic strength was used synonymously with power. *Plyometric exercises are used to improve elastic strength.

elastin Elastic fibrous protein found in connective tissue.

elbow The structures in and around the joint formed between the humerus of the upper arm and the ulna and radius of the forearm (*see* **elbow joint**).

elbow dislocation Forceful displacement anteriorly, laterally, or posteriorly of the ulna or radius on the humerus. Posterior dislocation which pushes the forearm backwards on the upper arm can be very serious: it is often associated with disruption of the blood supply which requires urgent surgical treatment.

elbow extension Movement of the forearm about the elbow which straightens the arm.

elbow extensor A muscle which effects *elbow extension. The major elbow extensors are the *triceps brachii (long head and lateral head). The anconeus is an assister, pulling the joint capsule of the elbow out of the way of the advancing *olecranon process during extension.

elbow flexion Movement of the forearm about the elbow joint which bends the arm.

elbow flexor A muscle that effects *elbow flexion. The main elbow flexors are the *biceps brachii, *brachialis, and *brachioradialis.

elbow injury Damage to structures in and around the elbow. Elbow injuries require skilled help, particularly in children, because they can be permanently disabling. In sport, acute elbow injuries usually result from a fall onto an outstretched hand with the elbow locked into extension (*see* **elbow dislocation**). Contusions resulting from a blow to the elbow are common, but X-ray diagnosis should be made to exclude a fracture. Elbow fractures should always be dealt with by an orthopaedic surgeon, as fixation may be required and it is important that the blood supply has not been impaired. Even partial damage to the blood supply can be very serious, causing a *compartment syndrome. Anyone who experiences tingling in the fingers or loss of sensation in the arm and hands following an acute elbow injury should receive immediate medical attention. Chronic, overuse injuries are especially common in golfers, throwers, racket players, and young gymnasts (*see* **golfer's elbow**; **thrower's elbow**; and **tennis elbow**). Common overuse elbow injuries in young gymnasts are *Panner's disease, *osteochondrosis of the capitellum, *osteochondritis dissecans of the radial head, and a *stress fracture of the olecranon epiphysis. Repeated forceful elbow extension in throwers may stimulate hypertrophy (growth) of the olecranon process and an *impingement syndrome.

elbow joint A complex of three synovial joints enclosed in a common joint capsule. The humeroulnar joint (considered *the* elbow joint) is a hinge joint between the trochlear fossa of the humerus and the trochlear notch of the ulna, permitting extension and flexion. The humeroradial joint is a gliding joint between the capitellum of the humerus and the radius. The radioulnar joint is a pivot joint between the radius and ulna, around which *pronation and *supination occur. The articular surfaces of the bones in the elbow are highly complementary and is the main reason why this joint is very stable.

elbow pronation Inward rotation of the radius around the ulna so that the hand moves from a palm-up to a palm-down position.

elbow pronator A muscle which effects *elbow pronation. The main elbow pronator is the *pronator quadratus.

elbow supination Outward rotation of the radius around the ulna so that the hand moves from a palm-down to a palm-up position (the anatomical position).

elbow supinator A muscle that effects *elbow supination. The chief elbow supinator is the supinator muscle, deep in the forearm, assisted by the *biceps brachii.

electrical stimulation training Training achieved passively by stimulating muscle with an electrical current. The device used for this type of stimulation is called an electrical muscle stimulator. It is used to treat muscle injuries and muscle atrophy when a limb has been immobilized. Some coaches believe that electrical stimulation training accelerates muscle growth and they have used the technique to train élite athletes. Most exercise scientists believe that this form of training is a valuable aid to rehabilitation, but that its use for muscle building purposes is unproven. Improper use of EMS or poorly designed devices can be dangerous. In 1970, a home EMS device was banned by the Food and Drug Administration after users testified that they suffered varying degrees of injury, including severe burns.

electrical synapse A synapse which allows ions to flow directly through protein channels from one neurone to another. Electrical synapses provide low-resistance electrical pathways for rapid unidirectional or bidirectional transmission of information from one neurone to another. They are found in regions of the brain responsible for the normal jerky movements of the eye.

electric muscle stimulation The use of electricity (direct current, alternating current, or both) to treat muscle injuries. Electric muscle stimulation has been used to treat muscle atrophy which occurs when a limb is immobilized. *See also* **electrical stimulation training**; and **Faradism**.

electrocardiogram (ECG) A graphical record of the electrical changes occurring during a heartbeat. A typical ECG is composed of a P wave, representing depolarization of the atria; the P–R interval, indicating the delay in conduction at the atrioventricular node; the QRS complex, produced during ventricular depolarization and contraction; and the T wave and ST segment, corresponding to ventricular repolarization. When read and interpreted by a highly skilled and experienced physician, an ECG is probably the most useful record of heart function. It can reveal the cause of irregular heart beats and damage to the heart muscle. It can also show enlargement of heart chambers, mineral imbalances in the blood, and whether someone has had or is having a heart attack. ECGs are recorded while the subject is resting or exercising. An exercise ECG, also called a stress test, can provide information on cardiorespiratory fitness and how the heart responds to strenuous exercise; it often forms part of the medical screening process of potential exercisers.

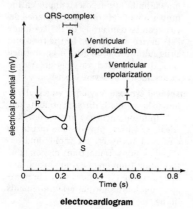

electrocardiogram

electroencephalogram (EEG) A graphical recording of the electrical activity of the brain made during *electroencephalography.

electroencephalography Measurement of the electrical activity of the cortex of the brain. Different types of brainwaves are associated with at least three different arousal states: sleep, wakefulness, and excitement. There is a strong correlation between the type of electroencephalograms and fatigue and overtraining. EEGs are used to assess brain injuries resulting from blows to the head in contact sports, such as boxing.

electrogoniometer (elgon) An electrical device for measuring *flexibility. The protractor used in a traditional goniometer is replaced by a potentiometer positioned over the centre of rotation of the joint being monitored. When motion occurs at the joint, an electrical output from the potentiometer provides a continuous record of the angle present at the joint. Goniometers measure angles of joints in stationary positions only.

electrolyte A substance (acid, base, or salt) that can be dissolved in water and which conducts an electric current. *See also* **electrolyte drink**.

electrolyte drink A drink containing electrolytes, such as sodium and potassium salts, usually taken to replace mineral salts lost during sweating and to avoid *heat cramps. Sodium salts are the most important electrolytes in these salt-replacement drinks. As exercise progresses, the salt content of sweat tends to decrease, proportionately more water is lost, increasing the salt concentration in the body. Therefore, electrolyte replacement without adequate water replenishment will increase the state of *dehydration and may adversely affect performance. *See also* **energy drink**.

electromechanical delay The delay between neural stimulation of a muscle and the development of muscle tension. The delay is partly due to the time required for the *contractile elements of muscles to stretch the *series elastic components. *See also* **reaction time**.

electromyogram (EMG) A record of the electrical activity of muscle made by electromyography.

electromyography The measurement and recording of electrical activity produced by muscle. Electromyography is used as a diagnostic tool to assess nerve conduction and muscle response in injured tissue, and to identify and measure muscle activity during a movement.

electron transport chain (electron transport system) A series of biochemical reactions by which free energy contained within hydrogen (derived from the *Krebs cycle) is released so that it can be used to synthesize ATP during aerobic metabolism. Electron transport chains occur in mitochondria. Each reaction involves a specific electron-carrier molecule which has a particular affinity for hydrogen or an electron derived from hydrogen. The carriers are organized in a sequence of increasing affinity. The final link in the electron transport chain is oxygen which combines with the hydrogen and electrons to form water.

electron transport system *See* **electron transport chain**.

electrophysiology The study of the electrical activity of the human body.

elevation 1 Movement of the shoulder girdle or another body part upwards (i.e. in a superior direction), as when shrugging the shoulders. *Compare* **depression**. **2** The process of raising a limb after an acute injury. Damage to the limb usually reduces mobility and causes swelling. Blood is not pumped back to the heart by muscles (*see* **muscle pump**), resulting in pooling of blood in the extremities. Elevation enables gravity to help the blood return to heart. Whenever possible, the injured limb should be raised above the heart. *See also* **RICE**.

elgon *See* **electrogoniometer**.

eliasian An approach to sociological analysis which follows that of Norbert Elias (1897–1990). He promoted a figurational developmental viewpoint to sociological analyses in which social configurations rather than individuals or societies are analysed.

élite athlete An athlete who has reached the highest level of a particular sport.

élitism The restriction of an activity to a privileged group. Some sports clubs restrict access on the basis of social characteristics and not athletic ability. Such élitism has resulted in the sports being associated with certain social classes and social statuses.

elliposid joint *See* **condyloid joint**.

emancipation A term applied specifically to the freeing of slaves from bondage, but which is used more generally in relation to the liberation of any person or group from social or legal restraint.

Embden–Meyerhoff pathway Sequence of chemical reactions which make up anaerobic glycolysis, discovered in the 1930s by the Germans, Otto Embden and Gustav Meyerhoff.

embolism Obstruction of a blood vessel with an embolus, such as fat, a blood clot, or an air bubble.

embrocation A liquid rubbed onto the skin to treat sprains and strains.

emergency muscle An assistant mover brought into action only when an exceptional amount of total force is needed. The long head of the biceps brachii, for example, contributes to abduction of the shoulder joint only in times of great need.

emergent leader A leader who arises from within a group. *Compare* **prescribed leader**.

EMG *See* **electromyogram**.

emic perspective Applied to linguistic analyses and sociological accounts made from a perspective internal to a language or social situation. In sport, an emic perspective involves gaining an understanding of the sport situation from an athlete's point of view. *Compare* **etic perspective**.

eminence A projection, usually rounded, on the surface of an organ or tissue, particularly bone.

emotion A complex state of arousal which occurs as a reaction to a perceived situation. In its most obvious manifestation, an emotion is an acute condition characterized by disruption of routine experience and activities; as such, emotions may provoke subjective feelings of pleasure or displeasure, physiological responses (such as changes in heart rate), and behavioural responses. There is much disagreement as to the exact nature of emotions and how they differ from motives and distractions, but there is no doubt that emotions may have an organizing or disorganizing effect on performance in sport.

empathy The ability to project oneself into the situation of another person and thereby understand the feelings and thoughts of that person. Empathy is an important characteristic of an effective coach–athlete relationship, since an athlete's problems can only be understood if the coach experiences the athlete's subjective perception of the problems. *Compare* **sympathy**.

emphysema A degenerative disease, fairly common in the elderly, in which living tissue in the airway loses its elasticity so that air tends to remain trapped in the lungs. This effectively reduces breathing capacity and the ability to perform physical work. A sensibly prescribed programme of aerobic exercise can improve the work capacity of those with emphysema, but it will not cure the condition.

empirical Pertaining to *empiricism.

empirical method A method of scientific investigation which involves systematic observation or experiments rather than speculation or mere theorizing. Observations are made, experiments performed, and facts gathered primarily for their own sake without regard to theories.

empiricism Philosophy of science that regards experience as the only source of knowledge. Empiricists seek evidence through direct experience rather than through reasoning or intuition. Their standard method of investigation consists of observations made via the senses, although the observations may be mediated by scientific instruments.

employee enrichment model A model, adopted by some sport psychologists and coaches, which proposes that task enrichment increases the employees' (or athletes') capacity for increased motivation, success, and satisfaction.

employee orientation A leadership style used by coaches which may be considered as equivalent to *consideration.

empty calories Foods which are highly refined, such as sweets and soft drinks, which provide a quick source of energy but are very low in nutrients such as vitamins and minerals.

emulsification Process in which a liquid, known as the emulsion, containing very small droplets of another immiscible liquid is formed. Fats are made into an emulsion in the duodenum by the action of bile. The process increases the surface area of the fat making it easier to digest. Unemulsified fats usually pass down the intestine and are egested in the faeces.

enarthrosis A ball-and-socket joint in which a long bone is able to move freely in all planes.

encephalin *See* **enkephalin**.

encephalopathy, traumatic (chronic cerebral injury; dementia pugilistica; punch drunk syndrome; traumatic encephalopathy) A neurological disorder induced by repeated blows to the head which are thought to cause microhaemorrhages of the brain stem and permanent neuronal damage. Typically, the victim is unsteady when standing; fatuous, euphoric, and voluble when speaking; and even aggressive. Memory and intellect may become impaired and, in advanced cases, encephalopathy causes chronic tremors, rigidity, and shaky movements (ataxia). Several studies have linked boxing (particularly professional boxing) with chronic brain dysfunction. Traditionally, the medical profession has based its opposition to boxing on this link. *See also* **second impact syndrome**.

encoding In psychology, the ability to perceive and understand the meaning of the important features of a situation, and to change this information into a form which can be stored in the memory.

encounter Any meeting between two or more people in face-to-face interactions. Sporting competitions are made up of many such interactions.

enculturation The process of formally and informally learning and internalizing the prevailing values and accepted behavioural patterns of a *culture. The term is sometimes used synonymously with socialization. Sport can play a major role in enculturation.

end-diastolic volume (EDV) The volume of blood in the left ventricle at the end of *diastole, just before systole (contraction). Endurance training increases blood plasma volume, which means more blood is available to fill the heart, causing an increase in end-diastolic volume. With more blood in the ventricles, the heart is able to contract more forcefully (see **Starling's law**).

endergonic reaction (endothermic reaction) Reaction requiring an external source of free energy (usually heat).

endocarditis Inflammation and infection of the inner lining of the heart, usually including the valves. It may be due to a bacterial infection (frequently originating from a dental infection) or rheumatic fever. Endocarditis is characterized by fever, abnormal changes in the rhythm of the heartbeat, and heart murmurs. Strenuous exercise should be avoided during endocarditis and not be resumed until after full recovery and consultation with the treating physician.

endocardium The inner lining of the heart, consisting of endothelium (a simple sheet of tissue).

endochondral ossification A form of *indirect ossification in which bone is formed by replacing *hyaline cartilage in the fetus.

endocrine gland A ductless gland producing hormones which are secreted directly into the blood stream.

endocrine system The body system consisting of organs and tissues which secrete *hormones.

endogenous opiate A chemical produced inside the body that binds to opiate receptors in the brain, mimicking the analgesic effects of morphine. Endogenous opiates include the enkephalins and *endorphins.

endogenous substance A substance such as a hormone or neurotransmitter produced naturally in the body.

endomorph Dimension of somatotype (body build) characterized by a rounded body shape and predominance of fat, especially in the abdominal and lower body region.

endomysium The connective tissue surrounding each individual muscle fibre.

endorphin A peptide found in the gut, brain, and pituitary gland which acts as *neurotransmitter. Endorphins, like enkephalins, are endogenous opiates. They can bind onto opiate receptors in the brain and mimic the analgesic effect of morphine. The release of endorphins is believed to increase when an athlete gets his or her second wind. Endorphins may be responsible for some of the pleasant feelings associated with exercise, such as runner's high.

endorphin hypothesis The hypothesis that exercise promotes psychological well-being by increasing the secretion of endorphins which reduce the sensation of pain and produce a state of euphoria.

endosteum The membrane lining the medullary cavity of bones; it contains osteoblasts and *osteoclasts.

endothelium Simple sheet of tissue composed of a single layer of cells which provide a friction-reducing lining in lymph vessels, blood vessels, and the heart.

endothermic reaction See **endergonic reaction**.

endothermy The process of generating metabolic heat to maintain body *core temperature.

endplate A modified muscle fibre membrane occurring at the junction between muscles and nerves. In stimulatory nerve fibres, *acetylcholine acts as the neurotransmitter released by the nerve-ending and attaches to receptor sites on the endplate, depolarizing the muscle membrane. If depolarization exceeds the threshold level, an *action potential occurs in the muscle fibre.

end-position Limit of the *range of motion of a joint that can be attained unaided. It is generally believed that mobility can be improved only if a joint is taken to this position during stretching and flexibility exercises.

end-systolic volume (ESV) The volume of blood remaining in the ventricles just after ventricular systole (heart contraction). The difference between the end-systolic volume and *end-diastolic volume equals the *stroke volume.

end-tidal carbon dioxide partial pressure Partial pressure of carbon dioxide at the end of exhalation.

end-tidal oxygen partial pressure Partial pressure of oxygen at the end of exhalation.

endurance (staying power) Ability to sustain a specific activity for a long period of time. Endurance has two main components which differ in the contribution they make to different types of activity. Cardiorespiratory endurance is of greatest importance in whole body activities, and muscular endurance is of greatest importance in activities involving individual muscles. Sports scientists investigating functional systems have found it useful to divide endurance into short-term endurance (35 s–2 min), medium-term endurance (2–10 min), and long-term endurance (longer than 10 min). Success in endurance activities is generally associated with high VO2 max; high lactate threshold; high economy of effort; and a high percentage of slow twitch fibres.

endurance capacity In physiological investigations, for example, on the effects of diet, endurance capacity is the time to exhaustion during exercise of constant intensity (*compare* **endurance performance**).

endurance force A force identified on the basis of the formula: force = mass × acceleration, where neither the mass or acceleration component prevails.

endurance performance The time taken to complete a prescribed exercise, such as swimming a certain distance.

endurance sport A sport that involves continuous high intensity exercise; for example, cross-country skiing, and long-distance running, swimming, cycling, and walking.

endurance training Training of relatively long duration and moderate intensity which enhances *maximal oxygen uptake. Endurance training is often regarded as the prerogative of endurance athletes, but it also benefits athletes who take part in burst-type sports (e.g., football and basketball) and moderate intensity sports requiring skill.

energizing technique A technique for increasing *arousal. Energizing techniques are used by athletes when they are not psyched-up enough for their activity and competition. They may also be used to overcome fatigue during competition. Energizing techniques include combining controlled breathing with positive self-talk, positive verbal cues (e.g., 'explode' and 'psyche up'), and imagery. *See also* **psyching-up**.

energy The capacity for doing work. The SI unit for energy is the *joule, although the calorie is still commonly used in nutritional studies. There are many different interconvertible forms of energy, including chemical energy, mechanical energy, electrical energy, heat energy, nuclear energy, and radiant energy.

energy balance The relationship between energy input (caloric intake) and energy output (caloric expenditure). A balance occurs when the energy input equals energy expenditure. *See also* **set point theory**.

energy continuum A concept used to describe the type of metabolism demanded by different physical activities. Those

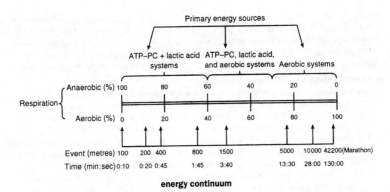

energy continuum

activities requiring 100 per cent *aerobic metabolism are at one end of the continuum, those requiring 100 per cent *anaerobic metabolism are at the other end. In between these two extremes are activities which require various proportions of aerobic and anaerobic metabolism.

energy coupling *See* **coupled reactions**.

energy drink A drink, usually containing glucose, especially designed to replace or supplement energy expended during exercise. Consumption of low concentrations of liquid glucose (less than 2.5 g per 100 ml) may prevent *hypoglycaemia and *dehydration, and delay fatigue. An intake of large doses of energy drink can cause dehydration and *insulin rebound. *See also* **electrolyte drink**.

energy expenditure The amount of energy used, for example in an activity. The most common unit of energy expenditure is the kilocalorie, but in scientific work the joule is preferred. The daily energy expenditure of an individual is dependent on sex, *basal metabolic rate, body mass, body composition and activity level. The approximate expenditure of an adult male lying in bed is 1.0 kcal/h/kg body-mass; for slow walking at 25 min per mile (1.6 km), 3.0 kcal/h/kg; and for fast steady running at 6 min per mile, 16.3 kcal/h/kg. Females have an energy expenditure 10 per cent lower than males doing a comparable activity. *See also* **metabolic equivalent**.

energy nutrient A food which is a major source of energy. Fats, carbohydrates, and (to a lesser extent) proteins are the main sources of energy.

energy of rotation The kinetic energy associated with rotation of a mass about an axis. It is expressed by $E=Iw^2$, where E is the kinetic energy of the mass, I is the mass's *moment of inertia, and w is the *angular velocity of the mass.

energy potential The maximum capability of an energy system to supply ATP. Tests of energy potential are designed to create a situation in which ATP is supplied predominantly by a single energy system and either capacity (total amount of ATP generated, irrespective of time) or power (amount of ATP generated per unit time) is measured.

energy-rich bond A concept which suggests that certain chemical bonds, such as the terminal bond in *adenosine triphosphate, contain large amounts of energy which, when the bond is broken during hydrolysis, yield large amounts of energy. In reality, the energy generated by the hydrolysis of ATP does not derive from the bond, but comes from the whole reaction which includes bond formation and bond breakage.

engram An altered state of living tissue which is believed to underlie memory. An engram may occur as a permanent trace left by a stimulus in nervous tissue. An example of an engram is a specific, learned, and memorized motor pattern stored in both the sensory and motor portions of the brain, that can be replayed on request.

enjoyment rating A scale in arbitrary units that reflects the enjoyment of an exercise or training session. On the scale, a score of 1 indicates a very unpleasant session; a score of 3, a neutral session; and a score of 5, a very enjoyable session. Consistent low scores demand urgent action and the exerciser should analyse the cause. For example, the sessions may be too exhausting, increasing the risk of *overtraining. Unpleasant sessions are the main reason for people dropping out of an exercise programme. Enjoyment ratings have been used by health experts as a behavioural management strategy for improving health and fitness. They recommend that an exerciser's motivation can be improved by recording the rating in a daily training logbook.

enkephalin (encephalin) A pentapeptide found in the brain, gut, and adrenal glands. In the brain, enkephalins bind onto opiate receptors, mimicking the analgesic effects of *morphine. *See also* **endorphin.**

ensemble In psychology, the combination of various sources of sensory information that enable the accurate perception of movement and position.

enthesis The junction between a tendon and a bone.

enthesitis A lesion at an *enthesis.

enthesopathy Any pathological condition of the enthesis (teno-osseous junction), for example *tennis elbow, and *jumper's knee.

entramine *See* **serotonin.**

entrapment The trapping of a nerve between two other structures with subsequent mechanical irritation and usually some loss of function.

entropy The amount of disorder or degree of randomness in a system. Heat has a higher level of disorder than other forms of energy. Therefore, since heat is always produced during energy transformations (e.g., during the transformation of chemical energy from food to the kinetic energy of a runner), entropy increases during these changes.

environment In a sporting context, the surroundings in which the sport takes place. It is the sum of the outside influences on the athletes, including all the physical conditions, the surrounding buildings, weather, and the audience. This external environment may also include the social or cultural conditions. Other types of environment include the intracellular environment, consisting of the conditions within a cell; the intercellular environment, composed of tissue fluid between cells; and the prenatal environment, which is the immediate surroundings of an embryo or fetus.

enzyme A protein that acts as a biological catalyst, accelerating the rate of specific biochemical reactions. An enzyme is not used up or changed in the reaction, and the enzyme cannot force a reaction to occur between molecules that would not otherwise react. Enzymes are denatured with time, and by changes in pH and temperature. The concentration of specific enzymes involved in energy systems, is an important determinant of athletic ability.

ephedrine A *sympathomimetic drug used in the treatment of asthma and respiratory ailments. Ephedrine belongs to the stimulants which are on the International Olympic committee list of banned substances. *See also* **beta$_2$ agonists.**

epicardium The outermost layer of the heart wall. It forms the inner wall of the pericardium.

epicondyle Protuberance of bone on or above a *condyle, which forms part of a joint. Epicondyles act as attachment points for muscles.

epicondylitis Inflammation of muscles and tendons attached to an *epicondyle. Epicondylitis on the lateral side of the distal humerus is commonly referred to as tennis elbow; epicondylitis on the medial side of the distal humerus is sometimes called little leaguer's elbow. Both medial and lateral epicondylitis are common injuries of golfers.

epidermis Outer layer of skin made of stratified epithelium and covered by dead cells impregnated with the fibrous protein, keratin.

Epidermophyton A genus of fungi which grows on the epidermis and is responsible for *athlete's foot and *dhobie itch.

epidural haematoma (extradural haematoma) A clot between the outermost membrane of the brain and the skull. This can occur as a result of a blow to the head, for example from a boxing punch or a fall from a bicycle. The blood and fluid can accumulate in and around the clot, pressing on the soft structures of the brain causing brain injury that can rapidly lead to death. If such an injury occurs, surgical relief of intracranial pressure is required urgently. The amount of energy required to produce an extradural haematoma is less than that required to produce unconsciousness. Therefore, any sportsperson who has suffered a head injury should be observed carefully, especially if consciousness is lost, and must be considered at risk until proved otherwise.

epigastrale An anatomical landmark located on the anterior surface of the trunk at the intersection of the midsaggital plane and the transverse plane through the most inferior point on the tenth rib.

epiglottis Flexible cartilage guarding the entrance to the larynx. The epiglottis prevents food from entering the trachea.

epilepsy An established tendency to recurrent seizures of varying degrees of seriousness, brought about by sudden abnormal discharges from brain cells. Epileptics can participate in many sports. The British Epilepsy Association advises only against those sports in which a blow to the head is likely, and underwater sports or climbing where an epileptic seizure could be fatal. Regular exercise may be helpful in controlling epilepsy (endorphins secreted by

the brain during exercise tend to inhibit seizures).

epimysium A layer of connective tissue, mainly *collagen, surrounding an entire muscle. The epimysium provides a smooth surface against which other muscles can slide.

epinephrine *See* **adrenaline**.

epiphyseal avulsion A dramatic injury resulting in partial or complete detachment of the *epiphysis from the rest of the bone. A complete avulsion is most common in boys 12–14 years old. It may occur during rapid deceleration, such as when a basketball player comes to a sudden stop or a long-jumper lands, causing the epiphysis to be pulled upward by the contracting quadriceps muscle. The resulting fracture may extend right through the knee joint.

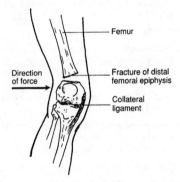

epiphyseal avulsion

epiphyseal plate (growth plate) A plate or disc of cartilage between the *epihysis and *diaphysis of a bone. It is the only region in a long bone which can generate new cells. Elongation of a bone stops when the cartilage in the plate ossifies (*see* **ossification**).

epiphyseal line An elevated ridge on the surface of a mature bone which marks the point of fusion between the *epiphysis and *diaphysis.

epiphysiolysis (slipped epiphyseal plate) An injury to the growth centre of a bone in which the growth zones or epiphyses are displaced in relation to the bone.

epiphysis The end portion of a long bone. It consists of a thin outer layer of compact bone enclosing spongy bone. The epiphysis ossifies separately from the diaphysis to which it fuses when growth is complete (*see* **ossification**).

epiphysitis Inflammation of the *epiphysis. Epiphysitis is a common overuse injury of young athletes. One form is 'Little Leaguer's elbow'. This is a repetitive strain injury of the medial epiocondylar epiphysis of the humerus on the inner aspect of the elbow. It is caused by repeated throwing. Boys as young as twelve years old can pitch baseballs at speeds exceeding 80 mph (129 kmh), imposing tremendous forces on the elbow. The injury can be extremely uncomfortable and may lead to retarded growth of the bone and disability.

epistaxis *See* **nosebleed**.

epistemology A branch of philosophy which deals with the nature and validity of knowledge. Epistemology is concerned with establishing the kinds of things which exist and to establish how we can know about the world.

epitestosterone An *anabolic steroid on the International Olympic Committee list of banned substances. *See also* **testosterone**.

epithelial Pertaining to the *epithelium.

epithelium A sheet of tissue consisting of tightly bound cells lining the external surface (e.g., epidermis) or internal surface of a body cavity.

EPO *See* **erythropoietin**.

EPOC *See* **excess post-exercise oxygen consumption**.

epoietin A drug which is an analogue of *erythropoietin. It is on the International Olympic Committee list of banned substances.

EPSP *See* **excitatory postsynaptic potential**.

equalitarian Leadership style which may be regarded as equivalent to *consideration.

equality The state of being equal. In sociology, equality is viewed mainly in a social context and the lack of equality is regarded as being profoundly shaped by social structures.

equality of access The concept that all persons should have equal rights of access, for example, to sporting facilities. Equality of access does not necessarily lead to *equality of opportunity.

equality of opportunity The concept that all persons regardless of social class, age, race, or gender should have equal rights to compete for and attain sought-after positions in society.

equilibrium The state of an object when the resultant forces acting on it are zero; that is, when the object is at rest or moving with uniform velocity and zero acceleration. The stability of a person depends on whether he or she is in a state of *stable equilibrium, *neutral equilibrium, or *unstable equilibrium. *See also* **dynamic equilibrium and static equilibrium**.

equilibrium point For a given level of neuronal stimulation, the hypothetical joint angle at which the *torque from each of the opposing muscle groups in an antagonistic pair of muscles is equal and opposite.

equilibrium principle A principle which states that the *line of gravity of a body must be located within its supporting base if the body is to be in a state of equilibrium at rest.

equilibrium sense An ability to use sensory information from the eyes, balance organs in the ear, and *proprioceptors in the muscles, to maintain *balance and be aware of body position relative to gravity.

erector pili Muscle in the dermis which raises hair, improving heat retention in the body by trapping a layer of air on the skin surface. *See also* **thermoregulation**.

erector spinae A massive group of back muscles that are prime movers of extension, lateral flexion, and rotation of the spine. The erector spinae consist of three columns: the iliocostalis, longissimus, and spinalis muscles. These muscles resist forward bending at the waist, and act as powerful extensors to raise the trunk from a flexed position to an upright position; they also help a person to maintain an upright stance.

erg A unit of *work or *energy; the work done by a force of one dyne acting through a distance of 1 cm.

ergocalciferol *See* **vitamin D**.

ergogenic aid Any factor which enhances physical performance. Ergogenic aids are frequently thought of as artificial drugs only, but they may also include psychological techniques, such as hypnosis and mental practice, music, and nutritional substances.

ergo jump test *See* **Bosco jump test**.

ergolytic Applied to a substance or factor which has a detrimental effect on physical performance.

ergometer An exercise device that enables the amount and rate of a person's physical work to be measured under controlled conditions. There are several different types of ergometer, each with its own particular advantages and disadvantages. The best ergometer for athletes is one which closely matches their training or competition. Rowing ergometers simulate the action of pulling on oars and have been designed to measure work output of competitive oarsmen under controlled conditions. Arm ergometers consist of a flywheel moved by a pedalling action of the arms. They are especially suitable for people who primarily use their arms and shoulders in physical activity. *See also* **cycle ergometer, swimming flume, treadmill, and tethered swimming**.

ergonomics The study of relationship between workers and their environment with particular emphasis on engineering aspects. In sport, ergonomics includes the study of designs which produce the most efficient racing cycles, canoes, and other sports equipment.

error A deviation from accuracy or correctness. *See also* **absolute error; constant**

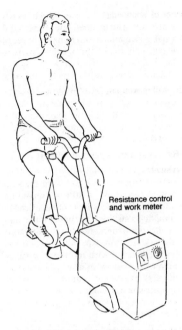

Resistance control and work meter

Electrically braked bicycle ergometer

ergometer

error; error of movement; and **variable error**.

error in execution A movement error in which the planned movement, with respect to its timing and direction, is appropriate, but in which the movement deviates from the desired path because some unexpected event occurs that disrupts the movement. A gust of wind, for example, could slow an otherwise well-timed swing of the racket during tennis, resulting in an error of execution.

error in selection A movement error in which the planned direction and/or timing of the movement is inappropriate. For example, a goalkeeper facing a penalty may move to the right when a movement to the left was appropriate; or the goalkeeper may move in the correct direction, but the move is made slightly late. *Compare* **error in execution**.

error of knowledge An error which occurs when an athlete does not understand what is demanded, or is unable to recall what is expected of him or her in a particular situation. The athlete may be capable of doing something but forgets what to do.

error of movement Error in retrieval and/or execution of a motor program. Errors which occur during the execution of a movement include two main types: *error of execution and *error in selection.

ERV *See* **expiratory reserve volume**.

erysipelas A severe, contagious bacterial infection (*Streptococcus pyogenes*) of the skin which can cause a diffuse spreading inflammation, high fever, and may lead to complications such as pneumonia and nephritis (inflammation of the kidneys). It is a risk after any skin injury (e.g., it has been associated with scrumpox in rugby players and elbow injuries in basketball players). Treatment requires the use of appropriate antibiotics. Physical activity should not be resumed until after complete recovery.

erythema Abnormal reddening of the skin due to dilation of capillaries. Erythema may be due to a number of conditions, but it is often a sign of inflammation and infection.

erythrocyte *See* **red blood cell**.

erythrocythaemia An abnormally high concentration of erythrocytes (red blood cells) in the blood. Erythrocythaemia is induced by blood doping and the administration of erythropoietin.

erythrogenin An enzyme released by the kidney when exposed to low partial pressures of oxygen. Erythrogenin transforms a plasma globulin into *erythropoietin which stimulates the production of red blood cells.

erythropoiesis The production of red blood cells. It occurs in the bone marrow and is stimulated by erythropoietin.

erythropoietin (EPO) A hormone which stimulates the production of red blood cells in bone marrow. Erythropoietin is a blood protein produced primarily in the kidneys by the action of an enzyme released in response to hypoxia: a reduction in tissue oxygen pressure can increase red cell production by as much as 6–9 times. Altitude training, because of exposure to low oxygen partial pressures, increases EPO secretion and boosts the red blood cell count. Eythropoietin (especially rEPO, recombinant human erythropoietin synthesized by genetic engineering) has been used by athletes to artificially raise the blood cell count and increase the oxygen-carrying capacity of blood. In addition to giving athletes an unfair advantage, blood boosting with rEPO is potentially dangerous. The red blood cell count may be raised to dangerously high levels, increasing the viscosity of the blood and elevating blood pressure; this can lead to heart failure and increase the risk of stroke and thrombosis. Erythropoietin and rEPO are on the International Olympic Committee list of *banned substances. Unfortunately, artificial blood boosting is difficult to detect with confidence. *See also* **erythrogenin**.

escape training Training which enables a person to behave in such a way as to extricate himself or herself from an unpleasant situation.

essential amino acids An amino acid, essential for the synthesis of body proteins, that can only be obtained from the diet. The essential amino acids are arginine, histidine, isoleucine, leucine, lysine, methionine, phenylalanine, threonine, tryptophan, and valine. (Histidine is required by infants, but it has not been fully established that it is essential for adults.) They must be available simultaneously in the correct proportion for protein synthesis to take place efficiently.

essential fat Storage fat which forms an essential part of the body. Fats needed for normal functioning of the body occur in bone marrow, heart, lungs, spleen, kidney, muscles, and CNS, and, in women, the breasts.

essential fatty acid An unsaturated fatty acid, such as linoleic acid, needed for normal, healthy functioning of the body, but which cannot be synthesized by the body. Lack of essential fatty acid may result in hyperactivity, reduced growth, and even death.

essential nutrient A substance that is essential for health, but which can be obtained only from the diet.

ESV *See* end-systolic volume.

ethic A belief or attitude which contributes to the moral values of a society, culture, or organization.

ethics 1 The study of how people ought to act in order to be moral. **2** A moral code that guides the conduct of a group of professionals such as medical doctors. Medical ethics is particularly relevant to the application of drugs and ergogenic aids in sport.

ethmoid bone A plate-like bone found behind the nose.

ethnic group A group of individuals with a shared sense of belonging based on a common heritage and sociocultural background. The individuals within an ethnic group are often visibly different from other individuals by virtue of unique lifestyle or appearance, and they usually share a common culture, customs, and norms.

ethnic resistance Opposition of an ethnic group to the dominant culture. For example, an ethnic group may resist attempts to eliminate or discourage their traditional sporting activities.

ethnicity A social stratification system based on the ethnic group to which individuals belong.

ethnocentrism The tendency of members of one social group to mistrust individuals belonging to another social group. It involves the belief that one's own social group is culturally superior to another group. It also involves the inability to understand that cultural differences do not imply the inferiority of those groups which are distinct from one's own.

ethnography A written description of an organization or small group based on direct observation. The researcher usually gathers data by living and working in the social setting being researched.

ethnomethodology An approach to sociology which attempts to reveal the methods and social competencies used by members of social groups to establish their sense of social reality. It emphasizes the role of individuals in creating social reality.

etic perspective Applied to linguistic analyses and sociological accounts made from a perspective external to a language or social situation. *Compare* **emic perspective**.

eumenorrhoea Normal menstrual function. *Compare* **amenorrhoea**.

Eustachian tube The tube, sometimes called the auditory canal, which connects the middle ear to the pharynx. It allows pressure to be equalized on either side of the eardrum.

eustress The positive or pleasant aspect of *stress; for example the demands of competition which produce positive responses of excitement and happiness. *Compare* **distress**.

evaluation apprehension The idea that an audience heightens the *arousal level of performers only if the audience is perceived as evaluating the performance. *See also* **Zajonc's model**.

evaporation The conversion of liquid into vapour. Evaporation of sweat is the primary route for heat dissipation during exercise, accounting for up to 80 per cent of heat lost from the body.

event importance A situational source of stress. The more important an athlete perceives an event, the more stress-provoking it will be.

eversion (plantar eversion) Outward rotation (a sideways movement) of the foot so that the sole faces laterally. *Compare* **inversion of foot**.

excessive lateral pressure syndrome Abnormalities of the patellofemoral articulation in the knee associated with excessive lateral pressure on the patella. The syndrome is characterized by anterior knee pain, hypoplasia (deficient growth) of the lateral femoral condyle and patella, and

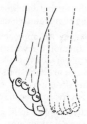

eversion

abnormalities of the supporting structures about the knee, including weakness and/or atrophy of the *vastus medialis muscle.

excessive training Training in which the frequency, duration, or intensity (or any combination of the preceding) is too great or is increased too rapidly without suitable progression. *See also* **overtraining syndrome**.

excess post-exercise oxygen consumption (EPOC) The amount of oxygen consumed during recovery from exercise above that which would be consumed at rest in the same period. The extra oxygen consumption helps restore the body to its pre-exercise condition. EPOC was once referred to as oxygen debt or oxygen recovery because the extra oxygen consumed after exercise was thought to compensate for *anaerobic metabolism during the exercise (*see* **oxygen deficit**). However, it is now thought that the physiological mechanisms responsible for EPOC are complex, involving the combination of several factors. In trained athletes, EPOC may be as high as 18 litres.

exchange theory (social exchange theory) A theoretical viewpoint of human social relationships based on the idea that individuals always seek to maximize the rewards they obtain from their interactions with others.

excitability The ability to receive and respond to a stimulus.

excitation The act of stimulating a neurone or muscle fibre to conduct an impulse.

excitation–contraction coupling The events occurring between the excitation of a muscle fibre and the resulting contraction. They include spread of depolarization over the muscle fibre via the transverse tubular system (*see* **transverse tubules**), the release of calcium into the sarcoplasm, and the sliding of actin and myosin myofilaments which causes the muscle action (*see* **sliding filament theory**).

excitatory postsynaptic potential (EPSP) A transient, graded reduction in resting potential of a postsynaptic membrane of a neurone or muscle fibre due to the release of a neurotransmitter from a presynaptic neurone. If the EPSP exceeds a critical level an action potential will form (*see* **threshold**).

excretion the elimination of metabolic wastes (including carbon dioxide and urea) from the body.

excretory system The body system concerned with elimination of metabolic wastes, mainly through the action of the kidneys.

executive program A *motor program for a skill consisting of several movements. Movements performed during a tennis serve, for example, include taking a stance, throwing the ball in the air, swinging the racket, transferring the weight from one foot to the other, and striking the ball. The executive program for the whole action consists of subroutines for each component movement.

executive level In *cybernetics, part of a control system which compares deviations of output from the norm and decides how to reduce the error towards zero.

exercise 1 Human movements and physical activities involving large muscle groups rather than highly specific, relatively non-taxing movements of small muscle groups. Exercise includes dance, callisthenics, games, and more formal activities such as jogging, swimming, and running. **2** Any set of movements designed to train or improve a skill. **3** The voluntary component of physical activity. Exercise may be spontaneous and playful, but it is usually performed with a specific objective (e.g., to become healthier, or to prepare for a competition).

exercise addiction An unhealthy reliance on exercise for daily functioning. The exercise often becomes the main mechanism for coping with everyday stresses. Exercise addiction is characterized by dependence (a belief that exercise is essential for feeling good), tolerance (the need to progressively increase the level of exercise in order to achieve the same level of feeling good), and withdrawal (unpleasant feelings, such as tiredness and irritability, associated with stopping or reducing exercise levels). The cause of exercise addiction is not known, although tentative links have been made with release of endorphins during exercise. In many cases exercise addiction is associated with an underlying problem, such as career or family stress. Treatment is notoriously difficult (some exercise addicts will not stop no matter what enticements or warnings you offer them), but it may be successful if the underlying problem causing it is identified and remedied. Continued exercise addiction can lead to overuse injuries, and social, family, and career problems. Running is the most common sport associated with exercise addiction.

exercise adherence Maintenance of an active involvement in physical exercise. Those with strong exercise adherence continue participating in physical activity despite opportunities and pressures to withdraw.

exercise-induced anaphylaxis A life-threatening exercise-associated syndrome similar to *anaphylaxis. Exercise-induced anaphylaxis is characterized by the onset during exercise (usually the first 5 minutes) of severe redness and blistering of the skin (*see also* **urticaria**). It may be associated with cardiovascular collapse, severe respiratory distress, nausea, gastrointestinal disturbances, and headaches which persist for up to three days after the initial attack. Exercise-induced anaphylaxis appears to occur when exercise follows exposure to specific substances (allergens)

to which the exerciser is sensitive. Sources of allergens that have acted as co-precipitators of exercise-induced anaphylaxis include raw celery, alcohol, cabbage, wheat, shellfish, caffeine, aspirin, and alcohol. Attacks are unpredictable; they do not occur with every exercise session. Reported frequencies range from once a month to once every decade. Treatment must be given immediately if there is any evidence of shock or serious respiratory distress. It includes the subcutaneous injection of adrenaline and intravenous injection of antihistamine drugs. Prevention depends on the identification and avoidance of the allergen for about 6 hours before exercise. Individuals with exercise-induced anaphylaxis should never exercise alone and should always carry epinephrine (adrenaline) during exercise.

exercise-induced asthma A form of asthma induced by physical activity. All asthmatics have their symptoms exaggerated by exercise, but exercise appears to actually precipitate an asthmatic attack in some people. It is believed that exercise and hyperventilation with dry air, dries the mucous membrane lining the airway, leading to the release of chemicals which cause the bronchioles to constrict (exercise-induced bronchospasm). Normally, bronchioles in the airways are dilated during exercise, but in exercise-induced asthma they constrict either during or a few minutes after cessation of the activity, making breathing difficult. The same level of exertion may produce different degrees of asthmatic attack depending on the nature of the activity. Running tends to provoke worse attacks than cycling, and both running and cycling provoke worse attacks than swimming, which is among the best sports for asthmatics. Factors which increase the risk of an asthmatic attack include activity performed in cold weather or a smoky environment; continuous exercise running; high intensity exercise; poor physical fitness; cold, dry air; air pollutants; pollens and grass; recent respiratory infection; and taking *beta blockers. Those which tend to decrease the risk include intermittent exercise; swimming; low exercise intensity; good physical fitness; and warm, moist air. Sodium cromoglycate and certain beta-agonists (e.g., salbutamol) help to relieve exercise-induced asthma. Use of these by athletes is permitted by the International Olympic Committee (IOC), but by inhalation only, and their use must be declared to the relevant medical authority. (Note, a compound of sodium cromoglycate and isoprenaline is banned under IOC rules.) Use of approved medication *before* exercise can be highly effective. *See also* **exercise test**.

exercise-induced bronchospasm *See* exercise-induced asthma.

exercise-induced urticaria *See* urticaria.

exercise intensity A specific level of muscular activity that can be quantified, for example, in terms of power output (work done or energy expended per unit time), forces resisted (e.g., free weights lifted) per unit time, the amount and duration an isometric force is sustained, or the velocity of progression. *See also* **intensity of training**.

exercise machine A machine used in strength and general fitness training. Exercise machines may be multi-units or single units. Machines differ with respect to the type of resistance they provide and the way that the resistance is applied.

exercise myoglobinuria *See* myoglobinuria.

exercise physiology A branch of *physiology concerned with how the body adapts physiologically to the acute (short-term) stress of exercise or physical activity, and the chronic (long-term) stress of physical training. Exercise physiologists, for example, study how our bodies obtain energy from the food we eat and use the energy to initiate and sustain muscle activity. A sound knowledge of exercise physiology enables coaches and athletes to optimize the amount and type of *training.

exercise prescription An individualized programme of exercise which prescribes the exercise frequency, duration, intensity, and mode according to an individual's level of health, fitness, and aspirations.

exercise psychology 1 The study of the psychological factors which affect participation in physical activity and the application of psychological principles to explain and improve the participation in physical activity. **2** The study of the psychological outcomes (or mental health aspects) of exercise.

exercise psychologist A professionally trained practitioner of *exercise psychology. Exercise psychologists develop strategies to encourage sedentary people to exercise, and assess the effectiveness of exercise as a treatment for mental disorders such as *depression. *See also* **sport psychologist**.

exercise recovery (active recovery) Performance of light exercise during the recovery phase of training. Exercise recovery often forms a part of interval training to enhance the removal of lactic acid.

exercise science The study of the natural phenomena associated with physical activity and sport. *See also* **sports science**.

exercise stress *Stress associated with *exercise.

exercise stress test (exercise tolerance test; graded exercise test) A test that evaluates an individual's physiological response to exercise, the intensity of which is increased in stages. Functions such as heart rate and blood pressure are usually monitored during the test. An exercise stress test is used to evaluate a person's health and fitness status before commencing an exercise program, but it is not very reliable. Most people who die a sudden death during exercise have negative test results, and most people who test 'positive' (i.e., appear to have cardiovascular problems according to the test results) do not actually have significant coronary artery disease. However, the test has great value as a means of quantifying fitness levels, and for determining a true maximum heart rate for an exercise prescription.

exercise test A simple and inherently safe test of pulmonary function following exercise. Formal testing consists of measuring pulmonary function before and after 5–8 minutes of vigorous exercise on a treadmill at 90 per cent of predicted maximum heart rate. Informal tests are often conducted outdoors where the subject runs as hard as possible, or at a pace which usually precipitates an asthmatic attack, for about 3 to 4 minutes. Measurements are made of the peak expiratory flow or *forced expiratory volume for 1 minute (PEF_1 or FEV_1) at 5, 10, and 15 minute intervals after exercise. A significant fall in values at any time is abnormal, and a fall of 15 per cent or more indicates a diagnosis of exercise-induced asthma. As all asthmatics develop bronchospasm after exercise, the test can also be valuable where there is doubt about the diagnosis of mild asthma.

exercise therapy Use of exercise as a mode of therapy for promoting psychological or physical well-being. Running is often used as an effective psychotherapeutic tool. In rehabilitation from illness and injury, controlled exercise is a key factor in returning a sportsperson to normal activity.

exercise tolerance test See **exercise stress test**.

exergonic reaction A chemical reaction that releases energy.

exertion Effort expended in performing a physical activity. See also **rating of perceived exertion**.

exertional sudden death See **sudden death**.

exertional haemolysis See **haemolysis**.

exhalation See **expiration**.

exhaustion A condition of extreme *fatigue when a person can no longer continue physical activity. See also **heat exhaustion**.

exocrine gland A gland with ducts through which secretions are carried to a particular site.

exogenous Developing or originating outside an organ or body-part.

exostosis A benign growth of cartilage or bony material which may occur spontaneously or as a result of the margins of a joint knocking against each other. See also **blocker's exostosis**.

expectancy The expectation that a particular *reinforcement will be given to an individual who behaves in a specific manner in a particular situation. During training, for example, an athlete who is performing well might expect praise from the coach.

expedition-type endurance A special type of *endurance which enables participants to successfully complete demanding expedition-type events (long duration, ultra-long distance activities). In addition to aerobic fitness, expedition-type endurance may require *acclimatization to high altitudes or high environmental temperatures, the ability to judge the degree of exhaustion in a team, and the conscious marshalling of physical, psychological, and spiritual resources for a supreme effort.

experiential continuum See **Dewey's theory of experiential continuum**.

experiential learning Learning from experience.

experiment An observation made or procedure carried out for scientific purposes under conditions which are controlled as far as possible by the experimenter. Experiments are conducted to formulate and test hypotheses. In a classical experiment (sometimes called a single factor experiment) only one condition, called the independent variable, is manipulated at any given time to determine its influence on a dependent variable (compare **multifactorial study**). Most experiments in sports science are conducted on human subjects whose behaviour and physiological functions are affected by many factors, therefore it is imperative that a strict protocol is adopted for the experiment.

experimental error A source of variation in experimental results due to the way in which a test has been conducted. Experimental error can be minimized by following a protocol which incorporates strict standardization.

experimental group A group of subjects exposed to the *independent variable of an experiment (*compare* **control group**). Typically, the experimental group is treated with the independent variable to test an *experimental hypothesis. The resultant effect, measured by a dependent variable, is compared with the control group. If a statistically significant difference (*see* **statistical significance**) is found between measurements of the dependent variable in the experimental and control groups, then the experimental hypothesis is supported. If there is no significant difference, the *null hypothesis is supported.

experimental hypothesis The hypothesis that in an experiment, the results of the experimental group will differ significantly from those of a control group, and that the difference will be caused by the *independent variable (or variables) under investigation. *Compare* **null hypothesis**.

experimental method Scientific method that involves a sequence of procedures: observation, identification of a problem, hypothesis formulation, experimentation, analysis of data, and interpretation that involves acceptance, rejection, or modification of a *hypothesis. In sports science and medicine, the effects of a variable on an experimental group is often compared with its effects on a control group of subjects.

experimenter effects The influence of an experimenter's behaviour, personality traits, or expectations on the outcome of an experiment. These effects can be significant when, for example, a scientist studying the action of a drug on athletic performance knows which group is given a placebo and which group is given the drug: the effect can be nullified by conducting a *double-blind study.

expiration (exhalation) Breathing out or exhalation. Normally, expiration is a passive process involving the relaxation of the diaphragm and the external intercostal muscles. During strenuous activity, it is an active process in which internal intercostals pull the ribcage downwards and inwards to reduce the volume and increase the pressure within the thoracic cavity.

expiratory reserve volume Maximal volume of air expired from end-expiration (i.e., the volume of air in the deepest exhalation possible at the end of normal expiration). The expiratory reserve volume (ERV) is about 1.5 litres.

expiratory mechanism Mechanism by which air is forced out of the lungs. During forced expiration, the diaphragm muscles relax, and the ribcage moves downwards and inwards (a movement brought about by contraction of the internal intercostal muscles). These actions combine to increase the intrapulmonary and intrapleural pressures, forcing air out of the lungs. *See also* **inspiratory mechanism**.

explanation An account which attempts to identify the cause, nature, and interrelationships of a phenomenon. Scientific explanations, especially those of the physical sciences, often involve the use of scientific laws and theories. In the social sciences, explanations may also involve the reasons and meanings provided by actors.

explosive power *See* **explosive strength**.

explosive strength (explosive power) The ability to expend energy in one explosive act or in a series of strong sudden movements as in jumping, or projecting some object (e.g., a javelin) as far as possible.

extensibility The ability to stretch a material beyond its resting length.

extension Straightening of a joint; a movement which returns a body segment to the *anatomical position from a flexed position. *Compare* **flexion**.

extensive interval work Interval training over a long distance (typically 800–3000 m in running) or long duration (typically 1–5 minutes) with short recovery periods. Extensive interval work helps develop endurance and tolerance of pH changes.

extensor A muscle that straightens a joint. *Compare* **flexor**.

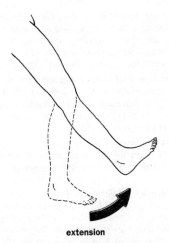

extension

wrist extension and is an extensor of the fifth metacarpophalangeal joint.

extensor digitorum A slender muscle that runs along the posterior fascial compartment of the forearm. It has its origin on the lateral epicondyle of the humerus and its insertion consists of four tendons attached to distal phalanges 2 to 5. It acts as a wrist extensor, and extensor of the finger joints 2–5.

extensor digitorum longus A slender muscle in the anterior compartment of the lower leg. It has its origin on the upper, anterior surface of the fibula, and its insertion on the second and third phalanges of the four lesser toes. Its primary actions are *dorsiflexion and *eversion of the foot, and extension of the toes.

extensor hallucis longus A muscle in the anterior compartment of the lower leg. It has its origins on the anteromedial surface of the fibula and its insertion on the distal phalanx of the great toe. Its primary actions are *dorsiflexion and *inversion of the foot, and extension of the great toe.

extensor indicis A small deep muscle with its origin on the posterior dorsal surface of the ulna and its insertion on the extensor expansion of the index finger where it joins with the tendon of the extensor digitorum. It primary action is extension of the metacarpophalangeal joint of the index finger (digit 2).

extensor pollicis brevis A deep muscle in the posterior compartment of the forearm which bends the thumb by causing flexion of the interphalangeal and metacarpophalangeal joints. Its origin is on the dorsal shaft of the radius and its insertion is on the dorsal proximal phalanx of the thumb.

extensor pollicis longus A muscle with its origin on the middle dorsal surface of the ulna, and its insertion on the dorsal distal phalanx of the thumb. Its primary actions are extension at the metacarpophalangeal and interphalangeal joints, and abduction of the hand.

extensor tenosynovitis 1 In the wrist, inflammation of the tissue around the

extensor carpi radialis brevis One of a group of superficial muscles lying in the posterior fascial compartment of the forearm acting on the wrists and fingers. It lies a little deeper than the extensor carpi radialis longus. It has its origin on the lateral condyle of the humerus and insertion on the base of the third metacarpal. It is a major wrist extensor muscle, also contributing to abduction and steadies the wrist during finger flexion.

extensor carpi radialis longus One of a group of superficial muscles lying in the posterior fascial compartment of the forearm acting on the wrists and fingers. It has its origin on the lateral supracondylar ridge of the humerus and insertion on the second metacarpal. It is a major wrist extensor, contributes to wrist abduction, and steadies the wrist during finger flexion.

extensor carpi ulnaris A superficial muscle in the posterior fascial compartment of the forearm which acts as a major wrist extensor and wrist adductor. It has its origin on the lateral condyle of the humerus and insertion on the fifth metacarpal.

extensor digiti minimi A slender muscle in the forearm which lies medial to the extensor digitorum. It has its origin on the proximal tendon of the *extensor digitorum and its insertion on digit 5. It assists tendons that extend or straighten the wrist and fingers. In the past, the condition was treated with injections, ointments, and splints. A newer treatment uses a small operation which relieves symptoms and allows resumption of activity within days. **2** In the foot, localized swelling of the extensor tendons at the front (anterior) of the ankle. It is usually caused by unaccustomed, intensive distance running or from overtight lacing of running shoes. It is characterized by pain when the foot or toes are passively pointed downwards away from the shin, or when they move towards the shin against a resistance. Treatment includes application of anti-inflammatories and reduction of mechanical stress. In chronic cases, it may be necessary to release the tendons surgically.

extent flexibility The maximum range of motion possible at a particular joint or series of joints working together. Extent flexibility is largely joint-specific; good flexibility at one joint does not guarantee good flexibility elsewhere. Use of the term is sometimes restricted to the ability to flex and stretch the trunk and back muscles as far as possible in any direction. *See also* **flexibility**.

external axis An axis which is outside the body. For example, the high bar in gymnastics is the external axis around which the gymnast rotates.

external cardiac massage Rhythmic pressure exerted by the heel of the hand on the lower half of the sternum in order to stimulate the heart to beat after a cardiac arrest.

external control An individual's perception that external factors determine performance outcomes. *See also* **externals**. *Compare* **internal controls**.

external controls *See* **externals**.

external force A force outside the system under consideration. The classification of forces as external or internal is largely a matter of convenience and depends on how the system is defined. In biomechanics, the human body is generally regarded as the system and any force acting on it from the outside environment, such as *air resistance or the impact force of an external object, is regarded as an external force. *Compare* **internal force**.

external heel-counter support Part of a training shoe which usually consists of a nylon collar supporting the heel counter and helping to prevent excessive sideways movement of the foot inside the shoe.

external imagery A form of mental practice in which individuals imagine they are external observers watching themselves perform.

external intercostals Eleven pairs of muscles which lie between the ribs. The fibres run downwards and forwards from each rib onto the rib below. The external intercostals take part in inspiration, elevating the ribcage, and act as *synergists to the *diaphragm.

external locus of causality A cause of an outcome perceived by the individual as being in the environment and beyond his or her control.

externally paced skill A skill in which the timing and form are determined by factors outside the control of the performer; for example a sailor adjusts the sails according to the wind direction and speed. *Compare* **self-paced task**.

external obliques The largest and most superficial of the three pairs of muscles which form the lateral abdominal wall. The external obliques have their origin on the outer surface of the lower ribs and most fibres insert via a broad *aponeurosis onto the *linea alba with their fibres inserting onto the pubic tubercle or the iliac crest. When the pair of external obliques contract simultaneously they cause flexion of the spinal column, compress the abdominal wall, and increase abdominal pressure. When acting individually on one side of the body, they contribute to spinal rotation and lateral flexion.

external overload An *attentional style in which an individual has the tendency to become confused and overloaded with external stimuli. *Compare* **broad external**.

external reinforcement *Reinforcement provided by another person (for example, through praise) or an object (for example, a trophy).

external respiration Ventilation and gaseous exchange; the process of drawing air into the lungs and the exchange of gases between the alveoli and the blood capillaries. *Compare* **cellular respiration**.

external rotation Movement of the limbs around their long axis, away from the midline of the body. *Compare* **internal rotation**.

externals (external controls) Individuals who tend to believe that events in their lives result from external factors beyond their control, such as luck and referee's decisions. Whether players are external controls or internal controls may influence their performance and the method most appropriate to motivate them. External controls tend to fear failure and are chance-oriented.

external validity 1 The applicability of experimental results to real situations. **2** In statistics, the extent to which the results of an investigation may be generalized to the population as a whole, and to other populations, settings, measurement devices, etc. External validity depends, among other things, on the adequacy of the sample.

exteroceptor A sensory receptor that responds to stimuli from outside the body. Exteroceptors include touch, pressure, pain, and skin-temperature receptors, as well as special receptors in the eye and ear concerned with sight and hearing. *Compare* **interoceptor**.

extinction The gradual elimination of a learned response due to lack of *reinforcement. In *classical conditioning, extinction of the conditioned response occurs when the conditioned stimulus is repeatedly presented in the absence of the unconditioned stimulus.

extinction model A model of anxiety reduction which conceives *anxiety as an emotional response. The extinction model is based on the idea that anxiety is elicited through a process of *classical conditioning by stimuli which were originally neutral. Because of pairing with painful or aversive stimuli (which thereby act as unconditioned stimuli), the neutral stimulus becomes a conditioned stimulus capable of eliciting a conditioned reflex. For example, a horse rider thrown during a race who suffers painful fractures may later find that riding a horse elicits intense anxiety. The anxiety is reduced by exposing the sufferer to anxiety-arousing stimuli in the absence of the primary aversive stimuli in the expectation that the anxiety will be eliminated by extinction.

extracellular Outside the cell.

extracellular fluid A body fluid outside cells. It makes up about 35 to 45 per cent of the body water and includes blood plasma, interstitial fluid, lymph, and cerebrospinal fluid.

extradural haematoma *See* **epidural haematoma**.

extrafusal fibre A typical contractile muscle cell or *muscle fibre that lies outside muscle spindles.

extrapolation The process of extending the values or terms of a series on either side of the known values, thus increasing the range of values, for example on a graph.

extrapyramidal system *See* **extrapyramidal tracts**.

extrapyramidal tracts (extrapyramidal system) A system of nerve pathways in the brain between the *cerebral cortex, *basal ganglia, *thalamus, *cerebellum, *reticular formation, and the spinal motor neurones. The tracts are mainly concerned with *coordination of stereotype reflex movements.

extrasensory perception *Perception which allegedly occurs without sensory awareness; for example, communication between two individuals when there appears to be no channels of information exchange.

extrasystole An extra heartbeat. *See also* **ectopic heartbeat**.

extremity The distal part of the body or of a limb.

extrinsic Outside an organ or body-part.

extrinsic factor A factor external to the human body, such as equipment and playing surfaces.

extrinsic injury An injury resulting from forces outside the body. The external force may be produced by another person, a piece of equipment, or some other environmental factor. Dramatic, acute injuries such as *fractures, tend to belong to this group. Compare **intrinsic injury**.

extrinsic motivation Motivation derived from external rewards, such as praise, money, and trophies. Extrinsic motivation may encourage a person with a low motivation for success, or one with a high motivation to avoid failure, to take part in an *achievement situation, contrary to what is expected from the *McClelland–Atkinson model. Compare **cognitive evaluation theory**.

extrinsic muscle A muscle which has at least one point of attachment inside the body-part upon which it acts, and at least one attachment point outside. In the hand, nine extrinsic muscles cross the wrist so that their origins are proximal to the wrist and their insertions are distal to the wrist. Compare **intrinsic muscle**.

extrinsic neural-control Modification of heart rate by nervous stimulation, and the regulation of the redistribution of blood by nervous stimulation. The lowering of heart rate associated with endurance training, for example, is thought to be due mainly to an increase in stimulation from the vagus nerve (an inhibitory nerve). Most blood vessels are supplied with nerves from the sympathetic nervous system. During exercise, sympathetic stimulation increased. This causes blood vessels in the gut to constrict and those in the heart and skeletal muscle to dilate, enabling blood to be shunted from the gut to the heart and skeletal muscles (see **shunting**).

extrinsic reward An external *reinforcement which takes the form of a tangible item such as a trophy or money, or something intangible such as praise and public recognition. See **motivation**.

extrinsic risk factor In sports science, an extrinsic factor that increases the risk of sustaining a sports injuries. Extrinsic risk factors include inappropriate training (e.g., too frequent or too intense), improper equipment, inappropriate clothing or protective gear, and poor technique. Compare **intrinsic risk factor**.

extropunitive behaviour See **aggression**.

extroversion A *personality dimension characterized by orientation towards the outside world, sociability, and impulsiveness.

extrovert A *personality type characterized by individuals being socially cooperative and liking others. Extroverts are generally outwardly expressive, active, and readily engage in social activities. Compare **introvert**.

exudate Material including pus, fluid, and cells that has slowly escaped from intact blood vessels and has been deposited in tissue, usually as a result of inflammation.

eye injury Damage to the eye due to physical trauma caused by either a blunt object (e.g., a direct blow with a fist or ball), large sharp objects (e.g., sticks and rackets), small flying particles (e.g., a piece of grit), chemical burns (e.g., excessively chlorinated water), and physical burns (e.g., ultra-violet radiation which causes *snow-blindness). The eye is surprisingly tough, but any eye injury should be regarded as potentially serious and requiring expert medical attention. Direct blows to the eye, or penetration of the eye with a foreign body, can cause retinal detachment or blindness. Medical advice should be sought in all cases of eye injury, especially if signs of bleeding or impaired sight are present after a blow. Sports associated with a particularly high risk of eye injury are contact sports, those which involve projectiles (balls and pucks), and those which use rackets or sticks. The risk of eye injuries can be reduced by wearing appropriate protective gear (e.g., goggles when playing squash), obeying the rules of the sport and playing safely, and abstaining from high risk activities if there is a predisposing defect (e.g., those who have suffered retinal detachment should not take part in contact sports).

Eysenck personality inventory An inventory based on the assumption that personality can be measured best by studying two basic trait dimensions: the introversion–extroversion dimension, and the neuroticism–stability dimension. A questionnaire based on Eysenck's inventory has been used to assess the sociability, impulsiveness, emotionality, and toughmindedness of athletes.

 # F

facet to **fusiform muscle**

facet Smooth, nearly flat, articular surface of a bone.

facet joint (zygapophyseal joint) A *synovial joint between two vertebrae formed by processes on the inferior surface of one vertebra articulating with processes on the superior surface of the other vertebra. In the lumbar region, facet joints have important weight-bearing properties and play a major role in lumbar motion.

facial bone Part of the skull forming the framework of the face. The functions of the facial bones are to secure the facial muscles, support the teeth, maintain a nasal airway, and form the margins of the eye orbits.

facial injury Physical damage to the structures in and around the face, for example, the fracture of a facial bone caused by impact with a squash racket. Facial injuries are very common in sport. Many are superficial and heal very quickly, but serious facial injuries often require the urgent attention of a maxillofacial surgeon because of the risk of permanent deformity. Orofacial injuries (i.e., those involving structures around the face and mouth) make up a large percentage of injuries in contact sports. Many could be avoided by wearing a gumshield.

fact An event or thing which can be verified by experience, observation, or experiment.

factor A component, constituent part, or condition which contributes to a result.

factor analysis A complex statistical procedure in which the correlations between a large set of observed variables are explained in terms of a smaller number of new variables called factors. Factor analysis has been used especially in sociology and psychology. In the case of *personality analysis, it has been used to discover the constituent irreducible traits from a complex mass of data.

FAD *See* **flavin adenine dinucleotide.**

Fahraeus–Lindquist effect The effect of vessel diameter on blood flow. In very narrow vessels, blood behaves as if *viscosity was reduced. This makes it less demanding for the heart to pump the blood through the vessels. The effect is very important during intense physical activity when the blood flow through capillaries is very high.

fainting *See* **syncope.**

failure anxiety Anxiety associated with an anticipation of failure prior to performing a feared task.

faking good Colloquial term used by researchers for false answers given by interviewees and respondents to questionnaires in an attempt to present themselves in a favourable light.

fallen arches Loss of the arched shape of the foot, with a flattening of the longitudinal arch between the heel-bone and toes. Fallen arches usually result from excessive strain which weakens the tendons and ligaments supporting the arch. Standing still for long periods and running on hard surfaces without proper arch supports can contribute to the condition. Fallen arches may be treated with appropriate *orthotics or exercises. *See also* **flat feet**.

false consciousness An individual's or group's social perceptions which another individual or group define as not matching the objective features of a situation. It is applied especially to class consciousness and is often seen to act against the interests of oppressed groups or individuals.

false feedback Feedback that informs athletes that they are doing better than they really are (false positive feedback), or that informs athletes that they are doing worse than they really are (false negative feedback). Future performance may be enhanced by false positive feedback, but only slightly and even then only if athletes believe it. False negative feedback tends to have a demoralizing effect.

false ribs Ribs not attached to the sternum (breastbone) or attached only indirectly.

falsification The process of using an *empirical method to refute or disprove a scientific *hypothesis.

fan An individual who is devoted to and enthusiastic about a given sport.

fanning A form of *massage. The masseur starts fanning with hands together and then spreads them out to cover a muscle, moving away from a central point and out towards the edges. Fanning is used on muscles such as those of the chest and abdomen which radiate outwards from a central point. It provides equal pull and pressure over the whole muscle to improve circulation of blood and lymph.

faradism A form of electrotherapy to treat conditions such as muscle *strain. The affected muscle is supported in the shortened position. Then, a rapidly alternating current is used to produce alternate contractions and relaxations to discourage *adhesions and encourage drainage of *exudate. Differential faradism is the use of a selective machine which makes one muscle contract just ahead of another, so altering muscle balance. Faradism is still used where more modern methods are unavailable, but generally it has been replaced by *electric muscle stimulation.

fartlek training (speed play) A relatively unstructured type of *continuous training that originated in Scandinavia. It is performed over natural terrain. A typical session lasts about 45 mins. The route is predetermined but the pace is varied from fast bursts to jogging (or walking) according to the terrain and the disposition of the runner. Depending on the precise composition, fartlek training can improve both the aerobic and anaerobic capacity of the athlete. Fun is the main objective, with distance and time of secondary importance. Many coaches use fartlek training because it provides relief from highly structured types of training.

far-sighted *See* **hypermetropia**.

fascia A tough, white fibrous connective tissue which may be superficial or deep. Superficial fascia is fatty and underlies the skin, forming a lining separating the skin from the deep fascia. Deep fascia ensheathes muscles, blood vessels, nerves, and organs, providing protection and support. It contains dense elastic tissue.

fascia lata The deep *fascia that surrounds the muscle of the thigh. The fascia lata is particularly evident as a broad band, the *iliotibial tract, that passes down the lateral aspect of the thigh.

fascial hernia (muscle hernia) The protrusion of muscle through a discontinuity in the connective tissue surrounding the muscle. The protrusion occurs when pressure increases in the muscle. It is sometimes painful. A fascial hernia commonly affects the *tibialis anterior muscle in the lower leg. The protrusion can be felt as a definite bulge on the surface of the muscle during or immediately after exercise, and a hole can be felt in the *fascia when the muscle is relaxed.

fascicle *See* fasciculus.

fasciculus (pl. fasciculi; fascicle) **1** A bundle of muscle fibres separated from the rest of a muscle block by a sheath of connective tissue called the perimysium. **2** A bundle of nerve fibres.

fasciotomy Surgical incision into the *fascia, for example, to relieve the pressure associated with a muscle *compartment syndrome.

fast force A force identified on the basis of the following formula: force= mass × acceleration, in which the acceleration component contributes more than the mass. Fast force is important for the production of explosive power. *Compare* endurance force.

fast glycolytic fibre *See* fast twitch fibre.

fast oxidative glycolytic fibre *See* fast-twitch fibres.

fast-twitch a fibre *See* fast-twitch fibre.

fast-twitch fibre (FT fibre; Type II fibre) A type of *muscle fibre that can reach peak tension quickly. It has a low oxidative capacity (low ability to use oxygen for *aerobic metabolism), a high glycolytic capacity (high ability to respire without oxygen during *anaerobic metabolism), and it fatigues quickly. Each fast-twitch *motor unit consists of a single neurone and 300 to 800 muscle fibres (compared with only 100 to 180 muscle fibres in each slow-twitch motor unit). Fast-twitch motor units are therefore much stronger than slow-twitch motor units. Muscles with a preponderance of fast-twitch fibres appear white because of their low levels of *myoglobin and low density of mitochondria. There are at least two subtypes of fast-twitch fibres: FTa fibres (fast-twitch a fibres, fast oxidative glycolytic, FOG, or Type IIa fibres) and FTb fibres (fast-twitch b fibres, fast glycolytic, FG, Type IIb fibres). FTa fibres have a higher oxidative capacity and fatigue more slowly than FTb fibres.

FTb fibres have the highest levels of *phosphocreatine and special enzymes, giving the highest glycolytic capacity. Fast-twitch fibres are associated with speed or power activities. FTa fibres are used predominantly in short, high-intensity endurance events, such as the mile run or 400 m swim. FTb fibres are used predominantly in high explosive events, such as the 100 m sprint run. Some evidence suggests that endurance training may cause FTb fibres to be converted to FTa fibres, enabling speed to be sustained for longer periods. *Compare* slow-twitch fibres; *see also* muscle fibre.

fat A type of *lipid. A true fat, or neutral fat, is a triacylglycerol (triglyceride) made of glycerol and three fatty acids. It provides energy, heat insulation, mechanical cushioning, and buoyancy. Fat can also be used in the body to make certain other chemicals, such as *steroids. Fat is one of the basic nutrients and it is the body's most concentrated source of energy. Each gram produces about 9 kcal of energy at a cost of 2.031 l of oxygen (i.e. 0.255 litres of oxygen per calorie) and the fat stores in the body exceed 70 000 kcal. Fat is preferentially metabolized during low intensity, long duration exercise. However, it has to be converted to its basic components (glycerol and free fatty acids) before it can be used to make *adenosine triphosphate and this conversion is too slow to meet all of the energy demands of intense physical activity. High fat diets are associated with *obesity and heat disease, therefore it is generally recommended that fat should contribute less than 35 per cent of the total calorific intake in the diet. *See also* essential fatty acids.

fat cell *See* adipocyte.

fatfold test *See* skinfold test.

fat-free mass (lean body mass) The mass of all nonfat body tissue, including muscle, connective tissue, and bone. It is often estimated as total body mass minus total body fat.

fatigue Exhaustion of muscle resulting from prolonged exertion or overstimulation.

Endurance training can delay the onset of fatigue. *See also* **muscle fatigue; physiological fatigue;** and **subjective fatigue.**

fatigue fracture A type of *stress fracture caused by repeated loads whose effects exceed the ability of an otherwise normal bone to functionally adjust to the demands being placed on it. Consequently, the bone collapses partially or completely. *Compare* **insufficiency fracture.**

fatigue fracture *See* **stress fracture.**

fatigue index A concept used in the study of *fatigue during *anaerobic activities. The fatigue index is expressed as the power decline divided by the time interval in seconds between peak power and minimum power.

fatigue theory A theory which proposes that *stress fractures are caused by muscles not supporting repeated protracted activity loads adequately, therefore the loads are transferred directly to the skeleton. When the tolerance of the skeleton is exceeded, a stress fracture occurs.

fatigue threshold An indicator of the work rate that separates heavy exercises that can be sustained for a considerable time from severe exercises which, because of rapidly increasing fatigue, can be sustained for only a short time. It appears to correspond to critical power: the highest work rate above the *lactate threshold that can be sustained without blood lactate and hydrogen ion concentrations, and the rate of oxygen consumption continuing to increase throughout the work bout. Above the fatigue threshold, exercise becomes progressively anaerobic.

fat loading The consumption of extra amounts of fat in order to fill fat stores within muscle cells. It is suggested that the extra fat enables muscles to metabolize fat more efficiently during exercise, conserving muscle glycogen, and delaying fatigue. Fat loading may delay fatigue in athletes working at moderate intensities, but there is little support from sports nutritionists for fat loading because of the potentially harmful effects of a high fat diet on health.

fat mass The absolute amount of body fat.

fat mobilization The breakdown of stored fat into free fatty acids which can be transported in the blood stream. *Beta oxidation converts the free fatty acids into acetyl coenzyme A which can enter the *Krebs cycle and be used by respiring muscles to generate *adenosine triphosphate. Endurance training improves the ability to mobilize fatty acids which may be used by respiring muscle and delay fatigue (*see* **glycogen sparing**).

fat pad A pad of fatty tissue located between the fibrous capsule and membranes in and around a *synovial joint. Fat pads help to cushion the joint.

fat-soluble vitamins Vitamins A, D, E, and K. They dissolve in dietary fat and are absorbed along with the digested products. Anything interfering with fat absorption, such as bile deficiency, interferes with the uptake of fat-soluble vitamins. All except vitamin K are stored in *adipose tissue.

fatty acid Long linear chain organic acid with the general formula $CH_3(C_nH_x)COOH$, where the hydrocarbon chain is either saturated ($x = 2n$) or unsaturated. Fatty acids combine with glycerol to form triglycerides (triacylglycerols) which are the main type of lipid in the body.

faulty processes *See* **Steiner's model.**

fear An *emotion characterized by unpleasant feelings of tension evoked by a specific situation or object. Physiological changes associated with fear include increases in heart rate, blood pressure, and sweating. Behavioural changes can include an overwhelming desire to avoid the fear-evoking situation.

fear of failure *See* **motive to avoid failure.**

fear of success *See* **motive to avoid success.**

febrile Pertaining to or affected with fever.

feedback 1 In *cybernetics, feedback occurs when some of the output from a system is isolated and fed-back as input (*see* **feedback mechanism**). **2** The information provided to a performer during or after an activity which enables the performer to assess the success or failure of his or her performance. Feedback is regarded by many as the single most important factor in the acquisition of skills. *See also* **augmented feedback; false feedback; knowledge of results;** and **intrinsic feedback**.

feedback mechanism Mechanism by which the products or outcomes of a process are coupled to the input. Feedback mechanisms are important in regulating many physiological processes. *See also* **negative feedback;** and **positive feedback**.

feedforward control A mechanism within some control systems in which information is sent ahead in time to prepare a part of a control system for future action or to prepare the system to receive a particular kind of *feedback. Feedforward control mechanisms are important in the control of movement by the central nervous system.

feeling An affective experience reported by the individual as pleasantness, unpleasantness, excitement, calmness, sadness, happiness, etc.

female athlete triad The development of an eating disorder (e.g., *anorexia nervosa), menstrual disorder (e.g., *amenorrhea), and a bone mineral disorder (e.g., *osteoporosis) in a female athlete. It has been suggested that female athletes, especially those who compete in appearance sports, endurance sports, and weight-classification sports, are at higher risk from these disorders than the general female population. It has also been suggested that the triad starts with an eating disorder which may after a period of time lead to a menstrual disorder and then a bone mineral disorder.

femininity Physical and behavioural characteristics, such as tenderness and consideration, which tend to be perceived by society as being in greater abundance in women, but which many regard as qualities desirable in both sexes. *Compare* **masculinity;** *see also* **BEM sex role inventory**.

feminism 1 An ideology which opposes misogynous ideologies and practices. **2** A social movement which confronts the sex-class system. **3** A theory concerned with the nature of women's oppression and subordination to men. **4** A socio-political theory and practice which aims to free all women from male supremacy and exploitation and which demands equal rights for women.

feminization The social process which has resulted in certain occupations, such as nursing, being regarded as women's work.

femoral Pertaining to the *femur.

femoral anteversion The angle made by the *femoral neck to the *femoral condyles. It is a measure of the degree of forward projection of the neck from the coronal plane. Femoral anteversion may lead to medial *femoral rotation and squinting patellae (*see* **femoral torsion**) in adults. This increases the risk of overuse injuries in the lower leg.

femoral condyle A *condyle on the femur which forms part of the knee joint.

femoral hernia *See* **inguinal hernia**.

femoral neck Part of the *femur connecting the proximal head to the shaft. It is the weakest part of the femur because it is smaller in diameter than the rest of the bone and because it is made mainly of spongy bone.

femoral neck stress fracture A *stress fracture of the neck of the femur. It causes pain in the groin and down the front of the thigh, sometimes as far as the knee. If caused by compression, it usually affects the lower, medial margin of the neck. If caused by a distraction, it affects the upper margin of the neck. The compression type is more common in young athletes, especially long-distance runners. The distraction type tends to affect elderly people. It is potentially more dangerous because the fracture lines may disrupt the blood supply to the head; death of bone cells leads to *osteoarthritis and other complications. Treatment depends on the severity and precise location of the stress fracture. Conservative treatment (cessation of activity; bed rest, the use of crutches) is often sufficient for undisplaced fractures, but displaced fractures require surgical reduction and fixation.

femoral shaft stress fracture A stress fracture of the shaft of the femur, usually the upper third, characterized by a deep-seated diffuse pain in the groin and/or thigh or knee. Pain increases during exercise. It has been reported in runners, skiers, hurdlers, and basketball players. Treatment depends on the site of the stress fracture and the amount of damage done. Conservative treatment (e.g., complete rest from exercise for 3 to 6 months) may be sufficient, but surgery is sometimes necessary.

femoral stress fracture *See* **femoral shaft stress fracture**; and **femoral neck stress fracture**.

femoral torsion The nonalignment of the *femur and *tibia so that the *patellae face inward slightly instead of facing forward. Femoral torsion is thought to indicate an imbalance of the strength of the different members of the *quadriceps group of muscles. It is also associated with *femoral anteversion. Femoral torsion may be relieved by strengthening the lateral rotators of the hip joint and increasing the flexibility of the medial rotators.

femoral valgus A condition in which the *femur is curved outwards from its proximal to its distal end, giving the appearance of bow legs. It is an unusual condition usually caused by skeletal deformity rather than being mechanically induced. It places extra tensile stress on the medial aspect of the hips and the lateral aspect of the knee.

femoral varus A condition in which the *femur curves inwards from its proximal to its distal end. It contributes to a knock-kneed appearance. Femoral varus puts extra tensile stress on the lateral aspect of the hips and the medial aspect of the knees. The condition is relieved by strengthening the *adductors and *quadriceps muscles which stabilize the knee. Femoral varus is often accompanied by a compensatory *tibial valgus which puts even more stress on the knee.

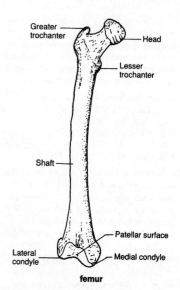

femur

femur The thigh bone; the largest, longest, and strongest bone in the body.

femur width In anthropometry, the distance between the medial and lateral epicondyles of the femur when the subject is seated with the leg bent at the knee to form a 90° angle. *See also* **body breadths**.

ferritin An iron-containing protein found mainly in the liver, spleen, and bone marrow. Serum ferritin levels reflect the amount of iron stored in these organs. It has been suggested that low serum ferritin levels can cause fatigue, even in the absence of *anaemia, but this suggestion is not accepted by most sports scientists. They regard serum ferritin only as an inert marker of iron stores.

feud Relations of continuing mutual hostility between groups where one group has been wronged, or perceives itself to have been wronged, by another and retribution is sought. Feuds are sociological phenomena observed in situations of kin solidarity. They also occur in sports teams where there is an assumed kin solidarity; thus, if one member of the team has been abused by the opposition, he or she can rely on support from other team members.

FEV *See* **forced expiratory volume**.

fever (pyrexia) A condition in which the core temperature is higher than normal (i.e. oral temperature more than 37 °C and rectal temperature more than 37.2 °C). Fever is usually due to an infection, but may also be linked to an emotional condition. It is usually accompanied by headaches, shivering, and nausea. Fever is caused by a rise in the set point in the temperature control centre in the *hypothalamus, so that heat-loss mechanisms (e.g., sweating) do not begin until core temperature exceeds that of the new set point. Fever can result in *dehydration and loss of muscle strength. Exercise during some febrile diseases can worsen the illness. This applies especially to enteroviral infections. It is a golden rule of sports medicine that an athlete should not compete or take part in strenuous physical activity when in a fever which raises body core temperature above 38 °C.

FFA *See* **free fatty acid**.

FG fibre *See* **fast-twitch fibre**.

fibre (roughage) **1** The indigestible part of plants consisting of cellulose, hemicellulose, gums, pectin, and lignin. Nutritionists divide fibre into two main types: insoluble fibre and soluble fibre. Foods high in fibre include cereals, fruit, and vegetables. Fibre is resistant to human digestion and therefore passes through the gut virtually unaltered, absorbing water, and helping to speed elimination of the faeces. A diet rich in fibre decreases the time taken for food to pass through the alimentary canal. It reduces the risk of constipation and some types of cancer. It may also help to reduce cholesterol levels, but a diet that has too much fibre may lead to diarrhoea, loss of body fluids, and dehydration. **2** A thread-like process such as a *muscle fibre, *collagen fibre, or *nerve fibre.

fibre splitting Longitudinal splitting of a muscle fibre which may increase the total number of muscle fibres. It has been suggested that fibre-splitting takes place in response to overload and contributes to muscle growth by *hyperplasia. However, although some animal experiments support the concept of fibre splitting, the general belief is that adult human fibre number is established at birth, or shortly after birth, and that no net increase occurs as a result of strength training. *See also* **myofibril splitting**.

fibrillation Rapid and irregular beating of the heart, or quivering of cardiac fibres, causing inefficient emptying of the heart chambers. Fibrillation in the ventricles causes cardiac arrest.

fibrin A fibrous, insoluble protein formed during blood clotting. Molecules of *fibrin form a network, trapping cells and debris, and sealing off damaged blood vessels.

fibrin deposit theory A theory suggesting that regular exercise reduces *fibrin deposits in the blood, thereby lowering the risk of *atherosclerosis.

fibrinogen A relatively soluble blood protein. It is converted to *fibrin during blood clotting.

fibrinolysis The process which removes blood clots from circulation by the break down of insoluble *fibrin. Vigorous exercise may increase fibrinolysis.

fibrocartilage A tough cartilage with a matrix consisting of dense bundles of fibres. *Intervertebral discs and *menisci are made of fibrocartilage which has great tensile strength and is able to absorb considerable loads. *See also* **cartilage**.

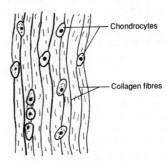

fibrocartilage

fibrosis Proliferation of fibrous connective tissue, usually as part of scar tissue formation.

fibrositis Inflammation of the fibrous connective tissue of muscles and tendon sheaths. The affected area is tender to the touch and painful. Although fibrositis is exacerbated by exercise, range of movement is not usually affected. The term is often applied loosely to any condition in the shoulder or upper back characterized by a dull ache. Fibrositis may result from chilling, toxins, chronic strain, or physical fatigue. It often responds well to heat treatment and massage.

fibrous cartilage *See* fibrocartilage.

fibrous connective tissue *See* **dense regular connective tissue**.

fibrous joint An immovable joint in which the ends of the bones forming the joint are dovetailed together and connected by tough fibrous tissue.

fibula Stick-like long bone in the lower leg which articulates proximally and distally with the *tibia. It is the outer and smaller of the shin bones. The lower end of the fibula forms the lateral malleolus (the protuberance on the outer side of the ankle). The fibula stabilizes the ankle joint, but it is nonweight-bearing.

Fick principle A principle first proposed by the German physiologist Adolf Fick. He established that the blood flow through the lungs can be calculated from the amount of oxygen absorbed by every 100 ml of blood during its passage through the lungs and the total oxygen uptake per minute. Since the blood flow through the lungs is equal to the output of the left ventricle, this knowledge can be used to calculate cardiac output (Q), which is given by: Q = (oxygen uptake in millilitres per minute/ $A - V$ oxygen difference) × 100, where $A - V$ oxygen difference is the difference in the oxygen content between the blood leaving the lungs and the blood arriving at the lungs expressed as millilitres of oxygen per 100 millilitres of blood.

Fiedler's contingency theory (Fiedler's contingency model of leadership effectiveness) A theory of leadership which suggests that a particular *personality disposition of leader that is effective in one situation may not be effective in another. Leaders are viewed as being either task-centred and autocratic, or athlete-centred and democratic. Task-centred leaders, high in task motivation, are believed to be more effective in both the least and most favourable conditions. Athlete-centred leaders, high in relationship motivation, are believed to be more effective in moderately favourable conditions. It is proposed that leadership effectiveness can be improved by changing either personality or situational features, with the latter being easier to control.

field experiment Experiment conducted in a natural setting (e.g., on a sports field during play). The conditions of field experiments are usually very difficult to replicate. *See also* **field test**.

field of vision The area that can be seen without moving the eyes or head. It is measured as degrees visible with both eyes while looking straight ahead. A wide field of vision reduces unnecessary head and eye movement. It is an important factor in many sports, especially team games.

field test In sports science, this is usually a measurement of a physiological function that is produced while an athlete is performing in a simulated competitive situation. Usually such tests are not as reliable as laboratory tests, but often have greater validity because of their greater specificity.

field theory A theory in which constructs from biology and physics have been borrowed to explain complex psychosocial behaviours and interactions. Field theory takes a holistic and dynamic view of psychological events as systems of psychological energy which can be represented mathematically; it holds that a person has *personality and reacts from the very beginning as a whole; and psychosocial behaviour is seen as the outcome of interacting forces (psychological, intellectual, emotional, and social) similar to those operating within the field theory of physics. *See also* **Gestalt psychology**.

figural after-effects A perceptual distortion produced after an extended period of exposure to a particular stimulus or combination of stimuli. For example, after a person has concentrated on curved lines for a while, straight lines may be perceived as being slightly curved.

figuration The network of mobile links which occurs between people in any social context, but which is typified by those taking part in a sports game. The figuration indicates the interdependencies and interactions of players, including tensions, which may result in both cooperation and conflict.

figurational sociology The sociological approach based on figuration of Norbert Elias (*see* **eliasian**) and those influenced by his writing.

fine motor skill A skill requiring delicate muscular control and in which certain parts of the body move within a limited area in order to produce accurate responses. Examples of fine motor skills are golf putting and rifle shooting. *Compare* **gross motor skill**.

finger dexterity A skill-orientated ability underlying tasks in which small objects are manipulated primarily with the fingers; for example, spin bowling.

finger extensor A muscle which effects extension (straightening) of one of the finger joints. Finger extensors include the extensor digitorum, extensor pollicis longus, and the extensor pollicis brevis.

finger flexor A muscle that effects flexion (bending) of one of the finger joints. Finger flexors include the flexor digitorum superficialis and flexor digitorum profundus, with the thumb flexor being the flexor pollicis longus.

finger joint *See* **interphalangeal joint**.

Finklestein's test A test used during the examination of wrist and forearm injuries. It involves the passive ulnar deviation of the wrist with the thumb forcibly opposed across the palm. Pain indicates de Quervain's disease (*see* **paddler's wrist**)

first class lever A lever which has its fulcrum (point of support or axis of rotation) between the point of resistance (load) and the point of effort (applied force). In the human body, a first class lever is used when the head is raised off the chest.

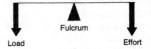

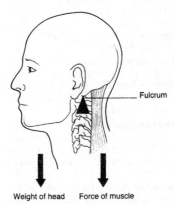

Weight of head   Force of muscle

first class lever

first law of thermodynamics *See* **conservation of energy**.

first order traits (first order factors; primary factors; source traits) Innate traits of behaviour. *Compare* **second order traits**.

fissure 1 A groove, crack, or cleft-like defect in the skin or mucous membranes (e.g., an anal fissure). **2** A groove or narrow slit-like opening in a bone through which blood vessels and nerves can pass. **3** A deep groove on the surface of the cerebral hemispheres.

fistula An abnormal connection between a hollow organ and the exterior, or between two hollow organs.

FIT A mnemonic for remembering the three main ways to achieve a training overload: you can increase training frequency (F); increase training intensity (I); or increase training duration (time T).

fitness The ability to live a happy and well-balanced life. Fitness involves not only physical factors, but it also has intellectual, emotional, social, and spiritual components. These components interact and are interdependent so that if any component deviates from normal it affects the overall fitness and ability of an individual to meet the demands made by his or her way of life. Clearly, fitness is a relative term which depends on an individual's circumstances and aspirations. Fitness is also specific to a particular physical activity: a person fit to run the marathon will not necessarily be fit to do gymnastics (*see* **physical fitness**).

fitness continuum A continuum used to describe a person's level of fitness. It extends from an optimal capacity to accomplish goals, through lack of disease, to severe disease and, finally, death.

fitness target zone A range of levels of exercise intensity from the minimum required to improve physical fitness to a maximum amount above which exercise may be harmful.

fitness test A test usually conducted to assess the level of *physical fitness, for example, of an athlete during rehabilitation from an injury. Fitness has several components, therefore there is no such thing as a single fitness test. Coaches continually make subjective assessments of their athletes, but an objective assessment of fitness usually requires testing each component independently under standardized laboratory conditions. The components commonly assessed are strength, speed, power, flexibility, and endurance. A test should be conducted only with the approval of the subject who should be fully informed of the purpose of the test. The primary consideration during the test must be the safety of the subject. It is important that the tester knows of any illness, injury, medication, or treatment that subject has had so that risk to health is minimized. Equipment and test procedures must be safe.

Fitt's law A mathematical expression of the trade-off between the speed of a movement and its accuracy. For a simple aiming movement, the average movement time (T) is linearly related to the $\log_2$ of the ratio of the movement amplitude (A) and target width (W), as follows: $T = a + b \log_2(2A/W)$. The law indicates that as speed of movement increases, accuracy tends to decrease. This law holds for a wide variety of movements.

fixation 1 A firm, stable, flexible aspect of behaviour. In childhood fixation may result from traumatic events preventing the child from progressing to the next stage of mental development. **2** Surgically fixing bones together with threads, pins, or screws. Fixation is used to stabilize a joint that has been repeatedly dislocated, or to fix a fracture.

fixator (stabilizer) During a particular movement, the role of a muscle which immobilizes one or more bones, allowing other muscles to act from a firm base. Fixators stabilize joints, preventing undesirable movements.

fixed action patterns (fixed pattern response) Patterns of movement which appear to be stereotyped, genetically defined, and triggered as a single programmed action. Fixed action patterns can be completed without the involvement of feedback.

fixed-choice questionnaire A questionnaire in which the questions posed are accompanied by a range of answers from which each respondent is asked to indicate which answer, out of the fixed choices, best applies to them. Such questionnaires are useful in gathering data and standardizing responses but there is a danger that none of the fixed-choice responses really applies to the respondent, and the researcher's own prejudices may be imposed on the respondent.

fixed joint *See* **fibrous joint**.

fixed-pattern response *See* **fixed action pattern**.

flat back A postural defect in which there is little or no lumbar curve. The lumbar region of the back is flat and the pelvis is pointed backward. It is usually associated with *kyphosis. It may be corrected by strengthening the back extensors (erector spinae), the gluteus maximus, and the abdominals, and improving the flexibility of the hamstrings.

flaccid Flabby; lacking muscular tone.

flame-out Fatigue experienced by athletes at the end of a hard season. Flame-out is a form of physical *burnout from which an athlete usually recovers quickly with a break or reduction in exercise.

flat bone A bone which is largely smooth, flat, and slightly curved (e.g., the scapula). Flat bones have two roughly parallel surfaces of compact bone with a layer of spongy bone between them.

flat feet (pes planus) A physical defect of the foot characterized by a lowering of the longitudinal arch so that the sole lies flat upon the ground and the foot becomes elongated. The gripping action of the toes is reduced or lost, causing mechanical problems during walking and running, and increasing the risk of overuse injuries (e.g., stress fractures, posterior tibial tendinitis, and compartment syndrome). Shoe inserts (see **orthoses**) may help an athlete who has flat feet by supporting the inside of the foot.

flavin adenine dinucleotide (FAD) An electron carrier in the *respiratory chain, important in *aerobic metabolism. FAD is derived from riboflavin.

flaw A systematic error in the performance of a motor skill. Flaws occur because of faulty learning and, according to some theorists, result in ingrained mistakes in the *motor program. Usually, in order to eradicate the flaw, the whole skill has to be relearned.

flexed-and-tensed arm girth Maximum circumference of the arm (usually the right arm) in supination when held at a 45 degree angle with the biceps tensed.

flexibility The ability to move a joint smoothly through its complete range of motion. Flexibility is determined by the nature of the joint structure, the condition of the ligaments and fascia that surround the joint, and muscle extensibility. Flexibility may also be limited by the skin, connective tissue, and bones around the joint. Flexibility is one of the main components of physical fitness and is believed to be important for optimum health. Flexibility exercises have been prescribed for the relief of dysmenorrhoea, general neuromuscular tension, and low back pain. However, an athlete who concentrates on flexibility exercises at the expense of strength training may reduce joint stability and increase the risk of dislocations. See also **dynamic flexibility**; and **static flexibility**.

flexibility test A method of measuring the range of motion of a joint or series of joints. Tests include the direct measurement of the angular displacement of a joint using a *goniometer, *flexometer, still-photography, or X-rays. There are many indirect methods which involve measuring the linear distances between two body segments, or between a body-part and an external object. These tests include the standing toe-touch test, and the sitting toe-touch test. Such indirect tests are quite easy to perform but difficult to interpret because the movements are quite complex and it is not clear which joints and muscles are involved.

flexion The bending of a joint so that the bones forming the joint are brought closer together. Compare **extension**.

flexion–relaxation phenomenon A phenomenon which occurs when the spine is in full flexion: the spinal extensors relax completely and the flexion torque is supported by the spinal ligaments. Therefore, during weight-training, it is especially important to use the correct technique when the spine is fully flexed because the tension in the spinal ligaments adds significantly to the anterior shear force on the lumbar vertebrae and increases the load on the facet joints.

flexometer Instrument which uses a gravity needle and compass to measure directly the range of motion about a joint (*see* **static flexibility**).

flexor A muscle that causes a joint to bend (*see* **flexion**).

flexor carpi radialis A muscle running diagonally across the forearm. Midway along its course, its fleshy belly is replaced by a flat tendon which becomes cord-like at the wrist. It has its origin on the medial epicondyle of the humerus and its insertion at the base of the second and third metacarpals. It is a powerful wrist flexor. It is also involved in wrist abduction and acts as a *synergist during elbow flexion.

flexor carpi ulnaris A two-headed muscle which is the most medial muscle of the forearm. It has its origins on the medial epicondyle of the humerus and the olecranon process of the ulna. It has its insertion on the pisiform, hamate, and fifth metacarpal bones. It is a powerful wrist flexor and hand abductor working in concert with the extensor carpi ulnaris. It stabilizes the wrist during finger extension.

flexor digitorum longus A long, narrow deep muscle in the posterior compartment of the lower leg. It has its origin on the posterior surface of the tibia and its insertion tendon runs along the medial malleolus and splits into four parts to insert onto the distal phalanges of the second to fifth toes. Its primary actions are plantar flexion, inversion, and toe flexion.

flexor digitorum profundus A muscle with its origin on the proximal part of the ulna and its insertion on the base of the distal phalanx of digits 2–5. Its primary actions are flexion at the distal and proximal interphalangeal joints and the metacarpophalangeal joints, digits 2–5, and the hand.

flexor digitorum superficialis A muscle which has its origin on the medial epicondyle of the humerus and its insertion on the base of the middle phalanx of digits 2–5. Its primary actions flexion of the wrist, the interphalangeal joints and metacarpophalangeal joints of digits 2–5, and the hand.

flexor hallucis longus A bipennate muscle in the posterior compartment of the lower leg. Its origin is on the lower two-thirds of the fibula and its insertion is on the distal phalanx of the great toe. Its primary actions are plantar flexion, inversion, and toe flexion.

flexor pollicis longus A deep muscle of the forearm, partly covered by the flexor digitorum superficialis. It has its origins on the anterior surface of the radius and its insertion on the distal phalanx of the thumb. Its primary actions include flexion of the interphalangeal and metacarpophalangeal joints of the thumb. It also acts as a weak wrist flexor.

flexor tendinitis 1 Inflammation of the tendons of the flexor muscles that run along the top of the foot. Flexor tendinitis is characterized by pain and a puffy swelling on top of the foot; the pain intensifies during running. It may be caused by lacing the shoes too tightly. The condition usually resolves itself within a week or two by resting the foot, immediately applying ice to the injury (for the first 72 hours, 20 minutes at a time), loosening the laces, and keeping direct pressure off the tendons. If the pain persists for more than two weeks, medical attention should be sought. **2** Inflammation of the tendons of the flexors that run from the forearm across the wrist and into the hand and fingers. It is characterized by pain, soreness, and stiffness in one or more finger, and pain in the palm of the hand at the site of the tendon. It commonly occurs in those who repetitively and forcefully bend their fingers (e.g., racket players, golfer, and baseball pitchers). Initial treatment is rest and ice (*see* **RICE**) and anti-inflammatories. If the pain persists, medical attention is required; the affected fingers may need to be immobilized in a splint for a few days and more powerful anti-inflammatories used. If treated early, flexor tendinitis usually clears up in a few days. However, if the condition is allowed to deteriorate by continuing to put pressure on the tendon, it can become chronic and difficult to resolve. *See also* **carpal tunnel syndrome**.

flexural rigidity The ratio of stress to strain in an elastic material when that material is being bent. *See also* **elastic modulus**.

flight path *See* **trajectory**.

flight time *See* **ltime of flight**.

floating ribs The eleventh and twelfth ribs. They are false ribs with no anterior attachment; their costal cartilage is embedded in muscle.

flooding A method of coping with *stress by exposing the subject to anxiety-provoking stimuli in the absence of the unpleasant experiences or feelings usually associated with those stimuli, in the hope that the *anxiety will be extinguished by *extinction.

floor effects A restriction on performance imposed by the physiological or psychological limitations of the performer or by the scoring system, that places a minimum on the score that a performer can achieve in a task. For example, there must be a score of more than 0 s for a test of reaction time. As a person approaches the floor, it becomes increasingly difficult to improve the performance. *Compare* **ceiling effects**.

flotation The ability of a body to float in a fluid. Flotation occurs if the body-weight is less than the maximum buoyant force of the fluid. Specific gravity is a measure of a body's capacity to float in water. When a swimmer breathes in, the lungs fill with air and flotation is increased. Although flotation is a distinct advantage to a swimmer, many people have learnt to swim without this ability, and some have broken world records.

flotation therapy (REST; Restricted Environmental Stimulation Therapy) A form of stress therapy which is becoming increasingly popular among athletes. The subject floats in a tank filled with warm, saline solution and experiences reduced sensory input due to the quiet environment. Physiological changes (reduced heart rate, blood pressure, muscle tension, and depression) associated with flotation help athletes recover from demanding training sessions.

flow A psychological state of extreme well-being which is sometimes experienced during the performance of an activity. A person experiencing flow has a feeling of great pleasure and satisfaction with his or her actual performance. The subjective experience of doing the performance is the primary reward rather than the outcome. Flow is similar to peak performance, but tends to be more voluntary in nature. Flow is thought to occur when there is a perfect balance between the demands of a task and the skill an athlete possesses.

fluctuation The characteristic feeling obtained by placing the fingers of one hand on one side of a swelling containing a fluid and, with the fingers of the other hand, tapping a distant point on the swelling. The sensation of wave motion transmitted from one hand to the other is an important sign of the presence of an abscess or the effusion of fluid into a joint.

fluid A substance which flows when subjected to shear stress. Gases and liquids are fluids with similar mechanical properties.

fluid balance *See* **water balance**.

fluid flow See **laminar flow**.

fluid friction *See* **fluid resistance**.

fluidity Reciprocal of viscosity; the SI unit for fluidity is the rhe, which is the reciprocal of the *poise.

fluid mechanics Study of the conditions which govern the movement of objects through fluids, such as a swimmer in water.

fluid resistance (fluid friction) Resistance to motion of a body in a fluid due to forces of friction being exerted between the body and the fluid. Fluid resistance is directly proportional to the cross-sectional area of a body at right angles to the motion, and directly proportional to the square of the velocity of the body relative to the fluid. *See also* **drag**.

fluid retention (water retention) The retention of fluid, mainly water, in the body. The amount of water in the human body is usually kept relatively constant by *osmoregulation: if excess water is taken into the body, extra water is usually eliminated in the urine (*see* **water balance**). However, water retention increases with increased storage of carbohydrates because the water binds to glycogen molecules (*see* **carbohydrate loading**).

fluoride A compound containing the element fluorine. Fluorides are found in bones and teeth. It has been added to water to harden teeth and protect them against decay. In the USA, the Recommended Dietary Allowance is 1.5–4.0 mg. Tea and seaweeds are good sources. Excess fluoride intake may increase the risk of *osteoporosis.

fluorine *See* **fluoride**.

flushing A method used by body-builders to improve the appearance of their muscles. The body-builder performs several different exercises one after the other with the same muscle group to fill the muscles with blood. Flushing tends to be avoided by competitive weight-lifters and those weight-training for sport because it does not usually improve muscle strength.

flutter A more rapid than normal heart beat, but not so rapid or chaotic as with fibrillation.

focal degeneration Deterioration in the function of a tendon due to the formation of a small lesion with a microscopic loss in the continuity of *collagen, and the presence of blood vessels and *granulation tissue. Healing is slow and disability may persist. It may require surgical decompression.

focus The degree to which an individual can integrate various factors and use them simultaneously to construct a more complete and balanced picture of his or her internal or external world. *See* **attentional style**.

focused attention *See* **narrowing**.

focusing Concentrating on relevant stimuli even in the presence of distractions.

FOG fibre *See* **fast-twitch fibre**.

foil *See* **aerofoil**.

folate *See* **folic acid**.

folic acid (folate; pteroylglutamic acid) A member of the B-complex of vitamins. Folic acid is a yellow crystalline substance that acts as a coenzyme in the synthesis of nucleic acids and is involved in haematopoiesis (formation of red blood cells). Deficiency causes macrocytic anaemia (enlarged red blood cells), diarrhoea, and other gastrointestinal disorders. Little is known about folic acid on physical performance, but deficiency is likely to hinder endurance athletes due to anaemia. In the UK, the daily Reference Nutrient Intake of folic acid (as folate) is 200 micrograms; in the USA, the Recommended Dietary Allowance is 180 micrograms for females and 200 micrograms for males. During pregnancy an additional 100 mg are recommended for growth of embryonic and maternal tissues. Deficiency has been linked to brain and spinal cord defects in the embryo. The richest source of folic acid is brewer's yeast.

foot 1 Part of the body containing a total of 26 bones and many articulations. The bones include the tarsus (ankle), metatarsus (instep), and phalanges. The foot supports the weight of an upright body and serves as a lever to propel the body forwards during walking and running. Its many bones give it a segmented, pliable structure which adapts well to uneven surfaces, unlike a single bone. **2** Imperial unit of length equal to 0.3048 m.

footballer's ankle An *impingement exostosis around the ankle joint which commonly occurs in footballers and others who repeatedly overstretch the ligaments and joint capsule of the ankle. Overstretching causes the edges of the bones which make up the ankle to knock against each other. This happens particularly to the front of the tibia which knocks against the upper talus (ankle-bone) causing spikes of bone to develop and, if large, break off. Symptoms of footballer's ankle include pain at the front of the ankle and loss of ankle flexibility. X-rays reveal the small fragments of bone (osteophytes) and, unlike osteoarthritis, the joint space is well maintained. Surgery is sometimes required to remove the osteophytes.

footballer's groin *See* **groin pain**.

footballer's migraine A headache and other unpleasant symptoms (e.g., visual defects, nausea, and vomiting) that develop after heading a football during soccer. It is thought that the migraine is due to distortion and spasm of basal cerebral blood vessels. This is more likely to occur if the ball is headed incorrectly on the parietal region instead of on the frontal region. Many soccer players head the ball several thousands of times during the course of their careers with no apparent ill-effect. However, a condition similar to punch-drunk syndrome has been reported in some footballers due to repeated minor head injuries.

football hooliganism Violent crowd disorder and associated soccer-related disturbance away from football grounds which first gained public attention in the 1960s. Attempts have been made to explain football violence in terms of the psychological characteristics of the hooligans, but more recent sociological explanations see it as a ritualized form of behaviour which is media amplified. The *civilizing process has resulted in a decrease in its acceptance. *See also* **deviance amplification, moral panic, labelling theory, ritualized behaviour, violence**.

foot injury Physical damage to the foot. The foot is the site of many acute injuries (e.g., *fractures, *strains, *sprains, and *dislocations) and overuse injuries (e.g., *tendinitis, *bursitis, and *stress fractures). Overuse injuries are usually caused by forceful repeated stress on the small bones and soft tissues which have to take the whole weight of the body during a sport. Good footwear is essential for protection (*see* **training shoe**). Many of the overuse injuries of the foot are associated with anatomical abnormalities which exaggerate the effect of the repetitive stresses of sports. The most common abnormalities that affect the lower leg are flat feet, feet that excessively pronate (roll inward when

an athlete runs), femoral anteversion (turned in thigh bones), high arches, genu valgum (knock-knees), and genu varum (bow legs).

foot length In anthropometry, the distance between the *acropodian and the *pternion.

foot-pound Unit of work. One foot-pound is the work done by a force of one pound acting through a distance of one foot.

foot-strike haemolysis *See* **haemolysis**.

foramen A round or oval hole or opening in a bone, or between bone cavities through which nerves and blood vessels pass.

force The effect one object has on another, such as a pull or push, which causes or tends to cause a change in motion. A force can cause a body at rest to move, or cause a moving body to slow down, stop, increase its speed, or change its direction. Forces can result in deformative movements, rotational movements, and translational movement. That is, they can change the shape of an object, cause it to rotate, or move it from one place to another. Therefore, forces include any agency which alters or tends to alter an object's state of rest or uniform motion. Force is measured in newtons and is the product of the mass of an object and its linear acceleration (i.e., force = mass × acceleration). On the basis of this formula, three different types of forces may be identified (*see* **shear force, fast force, and endurance force**). *See also* **compression**; and **tension**.

force arm *See* **moment arm**.

force couple (couple) Two equal but oppositely directed forces acting simultaneously on opposite sides of an axis of rotation. Since the translatory forces (forces which produce linear motion) cancel each other out, a force couple produces torque (rotatory forces) only. The magnitude of the force couple is the sum of the products of each force and its moment arm.

forced-choice scale A scale often used in questionnaires in which the respondent is instructed to pick the one response that

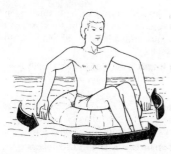

force couple

best describes his or her reaction. *See* **Likert scale**; **frequency scale**.

forced expiratory volume (FEV$_{1.0}$) The volume of air forcibly exhaled in the first second after maximal inhalation. The FEV$_{1.0}$ is a measure of the expiratory power of the lungs. It is reduced by asthma and decreases with age (*see also* **exercise-induced asthma**).

forced-pace task A motor skill in which the timing and manner of performance is dictated by the environment rather than the performer.

forced reps A method of weight-training in which a partner helps a lifter to continue training beyond the normal limit of fatigue. When the lifter has completed the number of repetitions that causes fatigue, the partner physically assists the lifter to perform more repetitions (usually 3–5 more). This form of training stimulates muscle growth and improves strength.

force–length relationship The relationship between a muscle's length and the force it can exert. In the human body, maximum force generation occurs when muscles are slightly stretched. Parallel fibred muscles (e.g., the biceps brachii) produce maximum tensions at just over resting length; pennate muscles (e.g., the deltoids) produce maximum tensions at between 120 to 130 per cent resting length.

force moment *See* **torque**.

force platform A device which measures the magnitude and direction of forces between a person and the ground. Force platforms are typically built flush to the floor.

force summation The combination of forces produced by different parts of the human body. When a person is moving or attempting to move an object, several different parts of the body act together to maximize the force. In theory, force summation occurs when all body parts act simultaneously. In practice, the strongest and lowest body parts around the *centre of gravity (e.g., trunk and thighs) move first, followed by the weaker, lighter, and faster extremities. This is known as sequential acceleration and results in successive force summation. To obtain a maximum force, summation also needs sequential stabilization of body parts, with some body parts having to be fixed at stable points while other parts produce the effective forces.

force vector A vector quantity in which direction and magnitude of a force is specified.

force–velocity curve A curve on a graph showing the relationship between muscle tension and the velocity of shortening or lengthening of the muscle. It is used to analyse the effects of training and to identify muscle fibre types used in different activities.

force–velocity principle A principle based on the force–velocity relationship. If training loads are high, movement velocity produced by a concentric muscle action (i.e. muscle shortening) is low and the training effect is primarily to improve strength. If the movement velocity is high and the load low, the main training effect is to improve speed.

force–velocity relationship The velocity of muscle shortening (concentric action) is inversely proportional to the load it must move. Conversely, as the velocity of a concentric action increases, the total tension produced by the muscle decreases. When the load (force) is minimal, muscle contracts with maximal velocity. As the force progressively increases concentric muscle action velocity slows to zero. As the load increases further, the muscle lengthens.

forearm (antebrachium) Region of the arm extending from the fingertips to the elbow point (olecranon process).

forearm extension *See* **elbow extension**.

forearm flexion *See* **elbow flexion**.

forearm girth The circumference of the arm when the hand is held palm up and relaxed.

forearm length The difference between *radial height and *stylion height.

forearm pronator *See* **elbow pronator**.

forearm supinator *See* **elbow supinator**.

forearm tenosynovitis An inflammation of the tendon sheath of any *tendon in the forearm that extends into the hand. Forearm tenosynovitis affects the fingers and wrist. It is commonly caused by a blow or forceful, repeated stresses. *See also* **tenosynovitis**.

forebrain The anterior part of the brain that gives rise to the cerebral hemispheres, olfactory lobes (concerned with the sense of smell), pituitary gland, pineal gland, and the optic chiasma which carries nerve fibres from the eyes to the brain.

forefoot valgus Condition in which the *metatarsals have an eversion misalignment (*see* **eversion of foot**); the first two metatarsals are in a more plantar flexed position than the third to fifth metatarsals. Forefoot valgus can cause compensatory misalignments in other joints, particularly inversion of the subtalar joint during weight-bearing. Orthotics may be used to treat the condition.

forefoot varus Condition in which the metatarsals have an *inversion misalignment; the first two metatarsals are in a more dorsiflexed position than the third to fifth metatarsals. It is often accompanied by a compensatory eversion of the subtalar joint at the ankle. Orthotics may be required to treat the condition.

foreperiod In measurements of *reaction time, the interval between the warning signal and the presentation of a stimulus to which the subject is expected to respond. It also refers to the period between a 'get set' command or signal and a 'go' at the start of a race. The duration and predictability of the foreperiod greatly influence reaction times.

form The manner of expressing a movement in time and space when performing a complex *gross motor skill. Form is unique from person to person, and though good form is usually associated with outstanding athletes, it is difficult to define exactly what constitutes good form. It is a factor taken into consideration when judging some sports, such as gymnastics, and relates to aesthetic value of performance. Judges consider factors such as balance, symmetry, rhythm, and composition which contribute to the finished shape and action of performance.

formal leadership theories Theories of *leadership behaviour which focus on the principles of good management and the formal aspects of the organization. Formal leadership styles have strong similarities with *initiating structure. *Compare* **human relations theory**.

form drag (frontal resistance; pressure drag; profile drag) The difference between the pressure acting on the front surface of a body moving through a fluid and the pressure acting on its rear surface. Form drag of an asymmetrical body depends on its orientation to the direction of free fluid flow. It increases with the cross-sectional area of the body aligned perpendicular to the flow. It is also affected by the shape and smoothness of the body; streamlining helps to minimize form drag. Cyclists and, to a lesser extent runners, reduce form drag by following closely behind another participant (a process called drafting).

forming *See* **team**.

fossa A rounded basin-like depression in a bone which often provides a surface for articulation (e.g., the acetabular fossa).

fovea A shallow pit in the retina of the eye in which cones are concentrated. It is an area of acute vision.

fovea capitis A small central pit in the femur from which the *ligamentum teres runs to the *acetabulum in order to secure the femur.

Fowler position A body position adopted at rest with the trunk supine and the legs raised and supported on a bench. This position helps to unload the spine, for example, prior to heavy physical training.

fracture A break in bone usually resulting from a more or less instantaneous application of an excessive load. A suspected fracture requires proper medical diagnosis which includes X-radiography. *See also* **avulsion fracture; comminuted fracture; compound fracture; depressed fracture; greenstick fracture; impacted fracture; simple fracture;** and **spiral fracture.**

frame of reference 1 In sociology, a set of standards that determines and sanctions behaviour. **2** Any set of planes or curves, such as the coordinates and axes used to define a set of points.

Frank–Starling law *See* **Starling's law.**

Frank–Starling mechanism *See* **Starling's law.**

Frankfort plane A line used in anthropometry which passes from the highest point of the ear canal through to the lowest point of the eye socket.

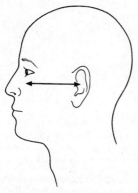

Frankfort plane

free active exercise An exercise in which muscle actions work only against the forces of gravity acting upon the part being moved. *Compare* **resisted active exercise.**

free body diagram A sketch showing all the force vectors acting on a defined system (e.g., human body or a projectile).

free energy Amount of energy available to perform biological work, such as growth and muscle actions. *Adenosine triphosphate is the most important source of free energy in the human body.

free fall The fall of an object which has only the gravitational pull of the earth acting on it. *See also* **acceleration of free fall.**

free fatty acid (FFA) A fatty acid that is only loosely bound to plasma proteins in the blood. Fatty acids are used by the body as a metabolic fuel (*see* **beta oxidation**). Endurance training usually results in an elevation of blood levels of FFA. This enables active muscle to use proportionately more fat, conserving carbohydrate stores (*see* **glycogen sparing**).

free phosphate Phosphate ions not bound tightly to an atom, molecule, or ion.

free radical A chemical group that has unshared electrons available for a reaction. Free radicals can damage the integrity of DNA and have been implicated as a cause of cancers. Antioxidants, such as vitamin C and vitamin E, neutralize free radicals.

free weight A weight, such as a dumb-bell or barbell, not attached to a specialized weight machine. Free weights allow the exerciser to move in any direction and provide a great variety of routines. However, they do not isolate individual muscle actions as effectively as weight-training machines, and the resistance remains constant throughout the range of movement of the muscle being exercised.

freezing spray *See* **aerosol administration.**

Freiberg's disease An *osteochondrosis affecting the toes: the articular surfaces of the second or third metatarsal heads collapse. It is commonest in girls aged 12–15 years. It causes pain on weight bearing and restricts physical activity. Rest and use of a metatarsal pad are usually sufficient treatment, but surgery is sometimes necessary. This entails removing fragments of articular cartilage and resectioning the dorsal aspect of the metatarsal head to allow the joint to move freely and painlessly.

frequency 1 In statistics, the number of members of a class or set (the absolute frequency), or the ratio of the number of members in a class to the total number of individuals under survey (the relative frequency). **2** Number of times an event occurs in a given period.

frequency code The code by which information concerning the nature of a stimulus is conveyed in the nervous system. The frequency code consists of the number of *nerve impulses transmitted per unit time along a neurone; changes in stimulus intensity cause a change in the frequency of the impulses. See also **population code**.

frequency curve A graphical representation of frequency distribution, with the values a variable may take forming the x-axis, and the number of times each value occurs (or percentage occurrence) forming the y-axis.

frequency distribution A way of representing observations in a table with at least two columns: the left hand column contains the values which a variable may take, and the right hand contains the number of times each value occurs or its percentage occurrence.

frequency of training See **training frequency**.

frequency scale A scale, often used in questionnaires, to measure behaviours or cognitions. The respondent circles the appropriate number indicating the frequency of a particular variable, and this number is used in the analysis of the results.

Freudian theory Theory concerning the structure and dynamics of personality derived from the works of Sigmund Freud (1865–1939), one of the most important figures in psychoanalysis. Practitioners of Freudian theory divide mental experiences into the conscious and the unconscious; and the personality into the *id, *ego, and *superego. Freud believed that people were driven by sexual and aggressive impulses struggling for expression. People who believe that sport participation is only appropriate for males because it allows them to express their 'natural' sexuality and aggression, appear to be adopting a Freudian approach to sport.

friction A force resisting the relative motion between two surfaces in contact with each other. Friction acts at the area of contact between the two surfaces in the direction opposite that in which a body is moving or tending to move. See also **coefficient of friction**; **limiting friction**; **rolling friction**; and **sliding friction**.

friction burn A burn caused by the skin rubbing against a surface such as synthetic turf. Friction burns range from a superficial redness to deep abrasions. They should be treated as any other *burn. See also **mat burn**.

frictional bursitis See **bursitis**.

friction, first law of A scientific law which states that for two dry surfaces in contact with each other, the frictional force is proportional to the *normal reaction, and is dependent on the nature of the surfaces: friction = normal reaction × coefficient of friction.

friendship A fluid, voluntary relationship, varying greatly in duration and intensity, between persons well known to one another which involves liking and affection, and may also involve mutual obligations such as loyalty. Forming friendships is an important part of the development of a *team.

frontal In anatomy, pertaining to the forehead.

frontal axis See **mediolateral axis**.

frontal plane (coronal plane) A *cardinal plane which divides the body from left to right into front (anterior) and back (posterior) halves of equal mass. It is the plane in which lateral movements of the body and body segments occur.

frontal resistance *See* form drag.

front region The public and open part of a social organization where its members may be viewed by nonmembers. *Compare* back region.

frostbite A collective name for the tissue damage resulting from exposure to very low temperatures. The affected parts should not be rubbed as blood circulation stops or is greatly reduced in the tissues. Instead, the tissues should be gently warmed in tepid water. The extent of the frostbite depends on the temperature, the exposure time, and the wind chill factor. For temperatures above freezing, dampness is also an important factor.

frostnip A mild, though still painful, case of *frostbite in which the tissues become numbed by the cold but remain pliable. Blood continues to circulate through frostnipped tissues.

frozen shoulder A *capsulitis in which portions of the joint capsule in the shoulder stick together and form *adhesions. It is characterized by chronic pain, inflammation, and restricted movement. It is a common overuse injury of those in the 50+ age group. It may be caused by wrenching the shoulder which induces a protective spasm in the subscapular muscles, but it is also associated with a stroke, cardiac infarction, or it may occur for no apparent reason. Treatment is by gentle massage and exercises, sometimes combined with corticosteroid treatment. Frozen shoulder is exacerbated by inactivity so it is important to maintain mobility by properly prescribed activities.

fructose A monosaccharide sugar found in honey and sweet fruits. It is often added to drinks as a sweetener because it is much sweeter and more readily absorbed than glucose. It can be converted to fat quickly.

frustration A psychological state which occurs when the satisfaction of motivated behaviour is rendered difficult or impossible.

frustration–aggression hypothesis The hypothesis that frustration leads to aggressive behaviour. Frustration develops when an aggressor is unable to attain a goal. Aggression is usually directed towards the cause of the frustration, but if this is not possible, the aggression may be displaced onto another person or object. It has been suggested that competitive sport is inherently aggressive because participants who are losing become frustrated. The original form of the frustration–aggression hypothesis, that frustration *always* leads to aggression, is not generally accepted. A revised version includes elements of *social learning theory. It suggests that frustration increases arousal and anger, but this leads to aggression only if the individual has learned to be aggressive in the particular situation. *See also* instinctual theory; and instinct theory.

frustration tolerance The ability to withstand frustration without developing inadequate modes of response, such as 'going to pieces' emotionally, becoming neurotic, or becoming aggressive.

FT fibre *See* fast-twitch fibre.

fulcrum A fixed point of support of a lever which acts as the pivot about which the lever turns. In biomechanics, when viewing the movement of the skeleton, the fulcrum is a fixed point, usually a joint, on which a bony lever moves.

function 1 A mathematical expression describing the relationship between variables. In the scientific literature, a dependent variable may be expressed as a function of one or more independent variables. **2** Applied to a group, the behaviour of the group and how it operates. **3** In sociology, the contribution to the working and maintenance of a social system made by a particular social occurrence.

functional activities Activities beneficial to society. *See* functionalism.

functional aggressive behaviour Aggressive or assertive behaviour (such as rebounding, stealing, shot-blocking in basketball) that facilitates a successful performance.

Compare **dysfunctional aggressive performance.**

functional capacity Maximal oxygen uptake expressed in METs or millilitres of oxygen per kilogram of body weight. *See also* **aerobic capacity.**

functionalism A major sociological perspective which views society as composed of parts or institutions. These parts include the family, the church, the military, the education system, sports organizations, and others. In a healthy society, all these parts work together to ensure that the society remains healthy.

functionalist explanation Explanation of the persistence of any feature of society in which this feature makes an essential contribution to the maintenance of the society or social system. Sometimes biological analogies are made in functionalist explanations in which the society or system is regarded like a biological organism and that its features persist merely to help that organism survive.

functionalist perspective A view of the relationship between sport and politics which suggests that sport is used to promote common values held essential to the integration and development of a society, thus sport helps to maintain social order. *Compare* **conflict perspective.**

functionalist perspective of social inequality A sociological viewpoint which argues that social inequality is necessary for the survival of any society or for any small or large organization. It is argued that without this inequality, division of labour would be difficult (not everyone can be team captain). It is also argued that to attract people to both the important and less important roles there must be variation in rewards which motivates individuals to make the effort needed to gain the top positions. *Compare* **conflict perspective of social inequality.**

functionalist perspective of sport A view of the relationship between sport and politics which suggests that sport is used to promote common values held essential for the integration and development of a

society. Thus sport helps to maintain social order. *Compare* **conflict perspective.**

functional model of attribution A model used by sport psychologists to study *attributions. It assumes that the main function of an individual's attributions of the causes for a particular performance is to maintain *self-esteem. Thus athletes tend to attribute positive outcomes to personal controls, (e.g ability) and negative outcomes to external controls, such as luck. The model assumes that athletes adopt a self-serving attributional bias.

functional model of leadership A leadership theory which proposes that it is difficult for a single leader to display both high levels of task and relationship behaviour at the same time. Therefore, a single coach cannot satisfy the needs of all athletes and might require the assistance of other coaches to complement his or her behaviour. For example, if a head coach is very task-oriented, an athlete-oriented assistant coach might be selected to complement the head coach's behaviour.

functional overload Training closely related to conditions experienced in competition, but with a greater workload than normal. For track events, for example, training might be carried out in heavy boots and a harness. During functional overload, care is taken to use the same muscle groups and patterns of movement as used during competition.

functional residual capacity The volume of gas remaining in the lungs after resting expiration; it is the sum of the *residual volume of the lungs and the *expiratory reserve volume, typically about 2.4 l.

functional short leg A condition in which the anatomical leg lengths are equal, but the legs are functionally unequal because of differences in *pronation or *supination of one foot relative to the other. Functional short leg may cause complications and joint dysfunctions in the lower back. *Compare* **anatomical short leg.**

fundamental motor skill A motor skill such as sprinting, jumping, and throwing which is used in many sports and games.

fundamental movement pattern A movement which forms part of a more complex skill. In some theories of motor control, fundamental movement patterns are represented in *motor programs as subroutines. There are three main types: locomotor (e.g., walking and skipping), nonlocomotor (e.g., balancing and stretching), and manipulation (e.g., kicking and throwing).

fundamental skill *See* **basic movements**.

fundus Part of an organ farthest from its opening; the base of an organ.

fungal infections Disease such as athlete's foot and dhobie itch, which are caused by a fungus. Fungi thrive in damp, warm, unclean environments. Infections can be prevented by keeping the skin dry and scrupulously clean. Antifungicides (e.g., miconazole cream) can be used to treat acute infections.

fungus A plant-like organism which, lacking chlorophyll, is unable to photosynthesize.

It obtains nutrients by absorbing organic matter from its surroundings.

funiculus A cord-like structure, such as a bundle of nerve fibres enclosed within a sheath (e.g., the column of white matter in each lateral half of the spinal cord).

furuncle A boil. A tender pus-filled area of skin usually caused by infection with the bacterium *Staphyllococcus aureus*. A furuncle is a very contagious skin infection and precludes participation in contact or collision sports.

fusiform muscle A spindle-shaped muscle, such as the *biceps brachii, with an expanded belly. The muscle fibres are arranged more or less parallel to each other and the long axis of the muscle. This strap-like arrangement provides the greatest degree of shortening and enables the muscle to produce a large range of motion quickly, but it is not a very powerful type of muscle. *Compare* **pennate muscle**.

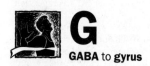

G

GABA to **gyrus**

GABA *See* **gamma aminobutyric acid**.

Gaenslen's test A test used in the differential diagnosis of pelvic disorders. The patient lies supine on a table with one leg over the edge of the table and the opposite knee pulled to the chest.

gain The relationship, usually expressed as a ratio, between the amount of input to a mechanical system and the output produced by it.

gait Style of walking. Gait is an important sign of health and disease. A person walking with toes turned out at right angles may be suffering from flat feet, or the gait may be due to stiffness (following disease of the knee-joint, for example).

galactose A simple sugar found in milk, yeast, and liver.

galvanic skin response The response of the skin to the passage of a small electric current. The ease with which the current flows between two points on the skin can be used to indicate *stress. When a person is tense or emotional, the sweat glands become more active, increasing moisture on the skin; this allows the electric current to flow more readily. The response may also be used in relaxation training: information about the galvanic skin response is fed back aurally or visually to the subject who can, with practice, learn to increase or decrease sweating on the skin by learning to relax or tense muscles (*see* **biofeedback**).

game A contrived competitive experience existing in its own time and space.

gamekeeper's thumb *See* skier's thumb.

gamesmanship (gamespersonship) The art of winning or defeating opponents by cunning practices without actually breaking the rules.

gamespersonship *See* gamesmanship.

game theory Mathematical theory concerned with the optimum choice of strategy in situations involving a conflict of interest. *See also* **theory of games**.

gamma-aminobutyric acid (GABA) An amino acid which functions as an *ionotropic neurotransmitter. It is secreted by some neurones in the cerebellum and spinal cord where its effects are generally inhibitory. GABA acts as a muscle relaxant. Some anti-anxiety drugs, such as *benzodiazepams, are thought to have their effects mediated by GABA. It is suspected that GABA has been used by some sports competitors to reduce *anxiety.

gamma globulin A class of specialized plasma proteins. Nearly all gamma globulins are immunoglobulins which recognize and deactivate bacterial toxins and some viruses; they function in the immune response which helps protect the body from invasive foreign substances.

gamma hydroxybutyrate (GHB) A substance that is claimed to release *growth hormone and act as an anabolic agent. It has been used in the USA by body builders. In 1990, it was associated with at least 57 cases of poisoning, and the Food and Drug Administration advised that it should be used only under experimental protocols for narcolepsy and is otherwise unsafe. Despite this advice, body builders still continued to use GHB.

gamma loop *See* gamma system.

gamma motor neurone A small neurone that innervates the ends of *intrafusal muscle fibres within a muscle spindle.

gamma system (gamma loop) A nerve pathway by which the central nervous system controls muscle actions. It carries nerve impulses from the motor cortex which stimulate *gamma motor neurones in a muscle, causing muscle spindles to be stretched. Sensory impulses are sent from the spindles to the alpha motor neurones, causing the muscle to contract. The sensory impulses also convey information to the CNS about the state of the muscle. This information is needed for the execution of smooth coordinated voluntary movements. *See also* **stretch reflex**.

Gamow bag A portable lightweight, rubberized bag which acts as a hyperbaric chamber into which a patient suffering *high altitude pulmonary oedema or high altitude cerebral oedema is placed. It increases the ambient pressure and provides oxygen for a patient awaiting evacuation to a lower altitude.

ganglion 1 A cyst-like mass of fibrous tissue on a *tendon or in an *aponeurosis. The ganglion is a fibrous sac which fills with fluid. It develops into a relatively painless swelling on the top of the wrist where its formation is triggered by irritation of the tendons that run across the top of the wrist joint. Ganglia also commonly occur on the top of the feet. If painless, they are usually left; if painful during an activity, for example during golf or racket sports, medical advice should be sought. The ganlion may be aspirated with a needle to release the viscous fluid, or surgically removed. **2** A collection of neurone cell bodies located outside the central nervous system.

gangrene Local death of body tissue due to a deficient blood supply. The dead tissue may decay through putrefaction by bacteria. Gangrene can be caused by disease, injury (such as a physical blow to a bone), *frostbite, or *burns.

gas chromatography An analytical technique used to detect drugs and their metabolites. The chemical constituents of the sample are absorbed onto a stationary phase of the apparatus. A gas then displaces these chemicals at different rates under different physical conditions. The molecules leaving the apparatus are monitored and recorded on a chart. The peaks on the chart are compared with those of known standard drugs.

gaseous exchange The transfer of gases, specifically oxygen and carbon dioxide, between a person and the environment, and between tissues and the blood. Gaseous exchange occurs between air in the alveoli and blood in the pulmonary capillaries, and between respiring tissues and capillaries.

gas exchange ratio *See* **respiratory exchange ratio**.

gas laws Laws which govern the physical state of a gas (e.g., its temperature, pressure, and volume). Knowledge of these laws is particularly pertinent to underwater divers and those active at high altitudes (e.g., skiers and mountaineers). *See also* **Boyle's law**; **Charles's law**; and **Henry's law**.

gastric emptying Movement of food and drink mixed with gastric secretions through the pyloric sphincter from the stomach into the duodenum. Nutrients (including water) are not absorbed in the stomach, therefore the benefits of drinking fluids to maintain water balance are obtained only after gastric emptying. Gastric emptying is delayed by fat, intense exercise, and by drinking strong carbohydrate solutions.

gastrocnemius A superficial muscle with two prominent bellies that form the proximal curve of the posterior calf. Its origin consists of two heads attached to the posterior medial and lateral condyles of the femur. Its insertion is on the tuberosity of the *calcaneus via the Achilles tendon. The primary action of the gastrocnemius are knee flexion when the foot is dorsiflexed, and plantar flexion when the knee is extended.

gate out To exclude or ignore irrelevant sensory information.

gelatin A jelly-like substance produced when tissues such as tendons and ligaments are boiled in water. Gelatin has been used as a source of dietary protein.

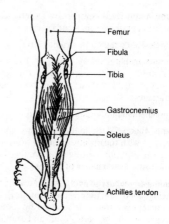

Femur
Fibula
Tibia
Gastrocnemius
Soleus
Achilles tendon

gastrocnemius

gemellus One of two small thigh muscles, the gemellus superior and gemellus inferior, which have a common insertion on the *greater trochanter of the femur. The origin of the gemellus superior is on the ischial spine and that of the gemellus inferior on the ischial tuberosity. The primary action of the muscles is lateral (outward) rotation of the femur.

gender In sociology, the social and cultural differences between men and women. Gender is a social division frequently based on, but not necessarily coincident with, anatomical differences; it refers to attributes which are categorized as masculine and feminine. Gender is not biologically determined but is socially and culturally determined. *Compare* **sex**.

gender differentiation The process of assigning social significance to biological differences between the sexes. Gender differentiation often results in gender inequality, with one gender being regarded as inferior to the other with regards to certain activities.

gender identity The subjective perception a person has of his or her own gender. It occurs as a result of a complex interaction between the person and others and results in the internalization of masculine and feminine traits.

gender inequality Social process by which people are treated differently and disadvantageously, under similar circumstances, on the basis of gender.

gender relations The social relations between males and females. In most social contexts, males have more power than females.

gender role conflict A conflict which may result from a male taking part in social activities which are ascribed as feminine, or a female taking part in activities ascribed as male.

gender role stereotyping The labelling of certain forms of behaviour and actions as being appropriate to one sex but not the other.

gender stratification See **sex stratification**.

gender verification The process of sex testing to confirm the sexuality of participants taking part in all-female sports. The first attempt at gender verification was by the International Amateur Athletic Federation who paraded naked female athletes before a panel of male doctors. In 1968, this rather dubious test procedure was dropped by the International Olympic committee who used the *buccal smear test or Barr test at the Winter Olympics in Grenoble. At the 1992 Barcelona Games, the Barr test was replaced the *Polymerase Chain Reaction Test.

gene The basic unit of inheritance by which hereditary characteristics are passed from parents to offspring. It is generally considered that one gene contains the information responsible for the synthesis of one polypeptide chain. See also **genetic endowment**.

genealogical method A method, based on the study of an individual's family history, of determining the effect of inheritance on any individual trait. It has been used to find out if sporting proficiency runs in a family.

general adaptation syndrome A set of characteristics which are manifested in the body as a response to *stress. The syndrome typically has three stages. Initially,

a stage called the alarm reaction occurs when there is an increase in resting heart rate and mobilization of muscle glycogen. This happens, for example, as an acute adaptation to exercise. During this stage, resistance to infection is temporarily lowered and defence mechanisms activated. This is followed by a resistance stage when the body shows maximum adaptation to the stress which includes an increase in the activity of the adrenal cortex and changes in muscle tone. If stress persists, a third stage of exhaustion occurs during which the defences of the body begin to break down. Overstress causes changes such as gastrointestinal ulceration; enlargement and hyperactivity of the adrenal cortex (which raises serum cortisol concentrations); low immunoglobulin A concentrations in the saliva (indicative of immunosuppression); and stiffness of muscles, tendons, and joints.

general avoidance skill A general awareness of danger and the ability to take avoidance measures when confronted with high risk situations. See also **escape training**.

generalization (stimulus generalization) Tendency of a person to respond to an unfamiliar stimulus or situation in a manner similar to a trained response to a familiar stimulus. Generalization is believed to be important in *transfer of training.

general motion A combination of angular motion and linear motion. It is the most common form of motion in sport. A racing cyclist, for example, uses a combination of several angular motions to produce the linear motion of the bicycle.

general motor ability The idea that the ability to perform different motor skills is determined by one general ability. Thus, a person with high general motor ability tends to learn motor skills more quickly than a person with low general motor ability. It is now thought that there are a large number of specific independent motor abilities.

general physical capacity A measure of the ability of active muscle systems to deliver, by *aerobic metabolism or *anaerobic metabolism, energy for mechanical work, and to continue working for as long as possible. This capacity increases through training.

general strength Whole-body strength. *See also* **conditioning**.

general trait anxiety *See* **trait anxiety**.

generation An age-based subgroup consisting of people in adjacent birth cohorts, in which most members have shared a similar sociohistorical event in a similar manner (e.g., the baby boom generation). This event often influences life chances and life styles throughout the life cycle. Different generations may experience different processes of socialization which may result in conflict due to what has been called the generation gap. A recent example in sport is the decline in popularity among young people of team sports in favour of individual activities, while many older people still retain their enthusiasm for team sports.

generator potential *See* **receptor potential**.

genetic Pertaining to a *gene.

genetic endowment The genes a person inherits from parents. Genes affect physical and physiological characteristics such as body build, cardiovascular traits, the proportion of different types of muscle fibre, and the capacity to improve physical fitness with training. It has been estimated that genetic factors account for 94 per cent of the variance in physical characteristics and maximum aerobic capacity.

genetic potential The limitations imposed by the genetic constitution (genotype) of a person. *See also* **genetic endowment**.

genital herpes A highly contagious infection characterized by painful lesions in the genital areas. *See also* **Herpes gladiatorum**; and **scrumpox**.

genu The knee or any anatomical structure similar to the knee.

genu recurvatum Hyperextension of the knee.

genu valgum Medical term for knock-knees. The condition usually accompanies *fe-

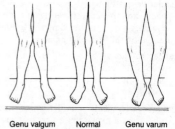

Genu valgum   Normal   Genu varum
genu valgum

moral varus and *tibial valgus. It increases the risk of knee injuries (especially *patellofemoral pain syndrome) because the abnormal angling of the thigh and lower leg imposes most of the athlete's weight on the inside of the knees.

genu varum Medical term for bow-legs. The condition is associated with lax ligaments which increases the risk of injuries on the outside of the knee (e.g., *iliotibial band syndrome). It usually accompanies *femoral valgus and *tibial varus.

geographical location In sport, the position and role of a player on a team which can be described in terms of *propinquity, *task dependence, and *centrality. The geographical location of an athlete seems to be correlated with leadership opportunities. Many of those players who are in highly visible, interactive and interdependent positions (e.g., quarterback in American football) are often perceived to have leadership skills and go on to be coaches or managers.

gerontological theories *See* **disengagement theory**; and **activity theory**.

gerontology The study of ageing and of elderly people. Some gerontological studies, such as adaptation to retirement, have had particular application to sports sociology. *See also* **ageism**; and **ageing process**.

Gerschler interval work *See* **interval training**.

Gestalt psychology School of psychology which disparages the partist, reductionist approach to experience and behaviour. Gestalt psychologists argue that people behave as whole individuals which are more than the sum of their parts. In learning, this school emphasizes the ability of a person to organize and interpret sensory experience; stimuli are not merely received by the sense organs, but meaning is imposed on the sensory data during the process of perception.

GH *See* **human growth hormone**.

giardiasis A relatively uncommon intestinal infection caused by the protozoan *Giardia lamblia*. It is of interest to participants of water sports because it can be transmitted in water contaminated with sewage effluents, from person to person, or by wild animals. It is characterized by chronic diarrhoea, loose greasy stools, and malabsorption. In 1985 an outbreak of giardiasis affected groups of swimmers who had been using an inadequately chlorinated pool in New Jersey, USA.

ginglymus *See* **hinge joint**.

ginseng A herbal root from the plant *Panax ginseng* which is made into a tea-like drink. It is the best known of the traditional Chinese medicines, and is claimed to give the consumer a long and happy life. Pharmacological analysis has identified saponins (ginsenosides) as the active substances. There is no concrete, irrefutable evidence that ginseng improves athletic performance, but it has been taken by élite athletes before major competitions. Reported side-effects of taking doses as low as 3 g per day include hypertension, insomnia, and depression. Some herbal products marketed as ginseng contain ephedrine-like drugs which are on the International Olympic committee list of *banned substances.

girdle An arch-like arrangement of bones that encircles a structure. *See* **pectoral girdle**; and **pelvic girdle**.

girth The distance around a structure; its circumference.

Gjessing–Nilsen ergometer An oar ergometer, used for specific functional evaluations of canoeists in a laboratory under controlled conditions.

glabella The elevated, smooth, rounded surface of the frontal bone, just above the bridge of the nose, between the eyebrows.

glare recovery The ability to adapt the eyesight to varying light conditions (e.g., in a sports stadium parts of which are exposed to the full glare of sunlight and parts of which are in shadow).

Glasgow coma scale A scale used for the extensive examination of head injuries. It is used to compare serial examinations of an injured athlete. The score is based on numerically grading eye opening, motor response, and verbal response. Changes in the score correlate well with the athlete's prognosis. Of those with a score of 3 to 4, 80 per cent die or remain in a vegetative state, as the score rises above 11, only 6 per cent die or remain in a vegetative state. *See also* **AVPU**.

glass jaw A colloquial term used to describe the susceptibility of an athlete, especially a boxer, to be knocked out or sustain a fracture of the mandible from a blow to the jaw.

glenohumeral joint The shoulder joint; a synovial, multiaxial, ball-and-socket joint in which the head of the *humerus articulates with the *glenoid cavity of the *scapula. Joint stability is sacrificed for flexibility and depends on the surrounding muscles; the ligaments contribute little to stability. This is the most freely movable joint in the body, permitting abduction, adduction, circumduction, extension, flexion, and rotation.

glenoid cavity (glenoid fossa) A shallow rounded basin-like depression in the scapula into which the head of the humerus is inserted.

glenoid labrum A rim of fibrous cartilage on the edge of the *glenoid cavity. It slightly deepens the cavity, adding a little to the stability of the glenohumeral joint.

glenoid labrum tear A rupture of the glenoid labrum commonly associated with dislocation of the shoulder. The condition, which can be confirmed by arthroscopy, is characterized by a deep pain and tenderness, a sensation of locking during movement, and a feeling of instability. Isolated tears, without instability, can occur in young athletes, particularly throwers, boxers, and tennis players.

glenoid fossa *See* glenoid cavity.

glia *See* neuroglia.

gliding joint (arthrosis; arthrodial joint) A *synovial joint, such as the *facet joints of the vertebrae and the intercarpal joints of the wrist, which allows only nonaxial gliding or twisting movements.

gliding movement A movement produced as one flat, or nearly flat, bone surface slips over another similar surface. The bones are merely displaced relative to each other. The movements are not angular or rotatory. Gliding movements occur at the intercarpal, intertarsal, and sternoclavicular joints.

global attribution A concept used in *attribution theory to describe attributions which are generalized and relate to many areas of sport. An individual who states that he or she is hopeless at sport, for example, is making a global attribution.

global self-esteem Generalized feelings of self-worth which are not specific to a particular situation but which apply to many activities or areas of life and predispose the subject to view new activities in particular ways.

glucagon A polypeptide hormone secreted by alpha cells of the islets of Langerhans in the pancreas. Glucagon increases the conversion of glycogen to glucose, causing blood glucose levels to rise (*compare* **insulin**). Glucagon levels generally increase in response to exercise, but this response is lessened by training.

glucocorticoid A class of *steroid hormones produced by the adrenal cortex that enable the body to cope with stressors by increasing blood glucose, fatty acid, and amino acid levels, and by raising blood pressure. Excessively high levels of glucocorticoids depress the immune system and inflammation response.

gluconeogenesis Synthesis of glucose from noncarbohydrate sources, such as amino acids, lactate, pyruvate, and fats. Gluconeogenesis occurs mainly in the liver and kidney when dietary sources of carbohydrate are insufficient to meet the demands of the body for glucose.

glucose A monosaccharide sugar. It is the main form of carbohydrate used by the human body. Glucose serves as the primary fuel of the brain, red blood cells, and muscles. Because the brain is very sensitive to glucose shortages, the blood glucose level (commonly referred to as blood sugar level) is kept constant. Excess glucose is either converted into *glycogen, metabolized to release heat, or turned into body fat. *See also* **carbohydrate-loading; diabetes mellitus**; and **glycogen overshoot**.

glucose–alanine cycle Chemical reactions preceding *gluconeogenesis which may be important in enabling blood glucose levels to be maintained during prolonged exercise. Protein, including muscle protein, is broken down and some of the amino acids transferred to pyruvic acid to form another amino acid called alanine. Alanine is then transported to the liver where it is converted back into pyruvic acid and eventually changed to liver glycogen and glucose.

glucose–fatty acid cycle *See* Randle cycle.

glucose phosphate An important intermediate in carbohydrate metabolism. Before glucose can be broken down into pyruvic acid during *glycolysis, it has to be first activated by ATP; glucose 6-phosphate is the product of that activation. In addition, when muscle glycogen is mobilized, glucose is split off in the form of glucose phosphate.

glucose polymers Short chains of glucose molecules sometimes added to sports drinks to provide more energy with less sweetness than normal glucose. It is claimed that they leave the stomach quickly (*see* **gastric emptying**) and do not cause as many gastrointestinal disturbances as some other sugary drinks.

glucose transporter Chemical which transports glucose into skeletal muscle. The most abundant glucose transporter is an insulin-regulated substance called GLUT4 . It occurs in the cell surface membrane of muscle fibres. After a single bout of exercise both the number of transporters and transporter activity increases.

glutamate *See* glutamic acid.

glutamic acid An amino acid, the salt (glutamate) of which functions as an *ionotropic neurotransmitter. Glutamate is secreted in many areas of the brain and by some neurones in the spinal cord where its effects are generally excitatory.

glutamine An amino acid derived from glutamic acid. It is a constituent of proteins and plays an important role in protein metabolism. Glutamine is classified as a nonessential amino acid, but premature infants cannot make it fast enough to satisfy their requirements for protein synthesis, so they must be provided with supplements. This has led to the idea (as yet unsubstantiated) that glutamine supplementation might stimulate muscle growth in adults. Plasma glutamine levels may reflect the ability of an athlete to repair muscles after intense exercise. Low plasma glutamine levels have been associated with *overtraining and exercise-induced muscle damage.

gluteal Pertaining to the buttocks.

gluteal girth (hip girth) The circumference of the hips at the level of the greatest posterior protuberance.

gluteal muscle One of the muscles in the buttocks which have their origin in the pelvis. See gluteus maximus, gluteus medius, and gluteus minimus.

gluteale An anatomical landmark in the midsagittal plane at the point where the sacrum and coccyx fuse.

gluteus maximus The very powerful, large buttock muscle which has its origins on the pelvic girdle (posterior ilium, iliac crest, sacrum, and coccyx), passes across the hip and has its insertion on the gluteal tuberosity of the femur and via a strong tendon on the *iliotibial band. The primary actions of the gluteus maximus are extension and lateral rotation of the femur. It swings the leg powerfully backwards. The muscle works more effectively if the body is bent forward at the hip (e.g., in a crouch start of a sprint). It is usually inactive during walking.

gluteus medius A thick buttock muscle covered by the *gluteus maximus. Its origin is on the lateral, posterior surface of the ilium, and its insertion is on the lateral aspect of the greater trochanter of the femur. Its primary actions are abduction and medial rotation of the femur.

gluteus minimus The smallest and deepest of the buttock muscles. It has its origin on

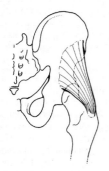 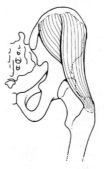 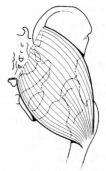

gluteal muscle

the lateral, posterior surface of the ilium, and its insertion on the anterior surface of the greater trochanter. Its primary actions are abduction and medial rotation of the femur.

glycaemic index A measure of the relative increase in blood-glucose level after eating a standard amount of a food. White bread is given a glycaemic index of 100 and other foods compared with it. Pure glucose has a glycaemic index close to 100. Eating foods with a high glycaemic index increases blood glucose rapidly, providing a quick energy boost. Foods rich in total glucose content but with a low glycaemic index, do not cause rapid changes in blood glucose levels. The glucose is absorbed into the blood stream over a relatively long period of time.

glycerol A 3-carbon sugar alcohol. Glycerol is a component of triacylglycerols (triglycerides or neutral fats).

glycine A simple amino acid which acts as an *ionotropic neurotransmitter in the spinal cord and retina. It is thought to be the main inhibitor of motor neurone activity in the spinal cord. Blocking its action with *strychnine results in uncontrolled muscle spasms, convulsions, and respiratory arrest.

glycogen A highly branched polysaccharide consisting of alpha glucose units. The liver stores most of the glycogen in the body. Liver glycogen is readily hydrolysed to glucose to maintain blood sugar. *See also* **muscle glycogen**.

glycogenesis The synthesis of *glycogen from glucose. Glycogenesis occurs in the liver and muscle. *See also* **insulin**.

glycogen loading *See* carbohydrate loading.

glycogenolysis The breakdown of glycogen to form glucose. *See also* **glucagon**.

glycogen sparing The use of noncarbohydrates as a source of energy during exercise so that the depletion of muscle glycogen stores is delayed. If fat, for example, makes a greater contribution to an athlete's efforts during the initial stages of a race, more glycogen will be available for the later stages and muscle fatigue will be delayed.

glycogen supercompensation *See* carbohydrate loading.

glycolysis The first stage of cellular respiration in which one molecule of glucose is broken down into two molecules of pyruvic acid. During the process, nicotinamide adenine dinucleotide (NAD) is reduced, liberating free energy which is used to synthesize ATP. Glycolysis takes place in the cytoplasm with or without oxygen.

glyconeogenesis Manufacture of glycogen from noncarbohydrate sources, such as fats and proteins.

glycosuria The presence of glucose in the urine; a symptom of *diabetes mellitus.

gnathion An anatomical landmark at the most inferior border of the mandible in the midsagittal area.

goal The end towards which an action, physical or mental, is directed, and towards which an individual consciously or unconsciously strives. A goal is a specific target that is either achieved or not. Well-defined goals play an important part in *motivation, providing athletes with something concrete towards which to direct their energies. The setting of appropriate goals (*see* **goal setting**) is regarded as critical for all performers in sport.

goal acceptance The agreement by an athlete to attempt to achieve a defined goal. Goal acceptance may change between training and competition: a goal set in training may well be regarded as too high for competition. *See also* **goal setting**.

goal difficulty A measure of the probability of a performer not achieving a goal. Goal difficulty is usually expressed as a percentage. Research indicates that as goal difficulty increases so too does performance, up to a critical point, thereafter performance decreases. The critical point varies, but some evidence suggests that it lies around the 70 per cent difficulty level, therefore goals which are only 30 per cent achievable should produce the best performance. It is

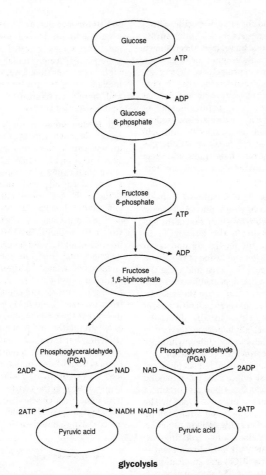

glycolysis

generally agreed that competition goals should be set at a level the performer expects to achieve about 70 per cent of the time during normal training.

goal displacement The process by which the means used to achieve a goal become more important than the goal itself. For example, runners who perform time trials in preparation for a competition may expend more energy on the trial than the actual competition.

goal image A mental image of a future goal. Goal images help direct and motivate ath-

letes so that they can overcome present difficulties to achieve a future goal.

goal keeper's thumb *See* **skier's thumb.**

goal orientation A motivational construct referring to personal definitions of success. Those defining success as winning, or defeating other, have an 'ego' goal orientation, whereas those viewing success as personal improvement and task mastering have a 'task' or 'mastering' goal orientation.

goal setting A motivational technique widely used in sport which involves the assigning and choosing of specific, object-ive, concrete targets or goals which an ath-lete strives to achieve. It has been shown that a systematic programme of goal set-ting and working to achieve these goals is highly effective in developing both phys-ical and psychological skills: well-defined goals improve performance, quality of practice, clarify expectations, relieve boredom, and increase pride and self-confidence. Ideally, goals should be spe-cific, realistic but challenging, and short term. Generally, individual goals are more effective than team goals.

golfer's elbow (javelin thrower's elbow; medial epicondylitis; pitcher's elbow; thrower's elbow) Inflammation of the ten-dons which attach the forearm flexor muscles onto the medial epicondyles of the humerus, on the inside of the elbow. The flexors curl the wrist and close the fingers into a fist. Repeated forceful curl-ing and gripping can strain the tendons, damage nerves, and even pull off a piece of bone. Golfer's elbow usually affects the right elbow of right-handed golfers (or the left elbow of left-handed golfers) who place excessive stress on the forearm flexors dur-ing the acceleration and impact phases of the swing; risk is increased when making large divots. Golfer's elbow also occurs in throwers who put too great a load on the elbow, for example when straightening the arm too forcefully. Weight-lifters ac-quire golfer's elbow when 'rotating out' during a snatch lift. Initial treatment is rest and ice (*see* RICE) and application of anti-inflammatories. Surgery may be nec-essary if bone fragments have been torn off the inner aspect of the elbow. Strength-ening exercises and correction of faulty technique reduces the risk of recurrence. In differential diagnosis, it is important to ensure that the symptoms are not caused by nerve entrapment.

golfer's toe An acute inflammation of the halux (great toe) which may develop into *arthritis causing a painfully rigid joint. It may develop in golfers (and others) who have a foot with structural imbal-ances.

Golf Performance Survey A survey based on a questionnaire devised specifically for golf. The survey revealed that skilled golfers have greater mental preparation, higher concentration, fewer negative feel-ings and thoughts, greater *automaticity, and more perseverance to practise golf than less skilled golfers.

Golgi tendon organ A small sensory re-ceptor, located at the junction between a muscle and tendon, that monitors ten-sion. Each Golgi tendon organ consists of small bundles of tendon fibres enclosed in a layered capsule with dendrites (fine branches of neurones) coiling between and around the fibres. The organ is activ-ated by muscular contractions which stretch the tendons. This results in an in-hibition of alpha motor neurones (special neurones that innervate the contractile elements of striated muscle), causing the contracting muscle to relax, thereby pro-tecting the muscle and connective tissue from excessive loading. It was once be-lieved that the Golgi tendon organs were only stimulated by prolonged muscle stretches, but it is now known that they are sensitive detectors of tension on local-ized portions of a particular muscle: they feed back information about force levels in the muscle to the central nervous sys-tem. Some research scientists believe that if the activity of Golgi tendon organs is re-duced during a muscle action, the muscle

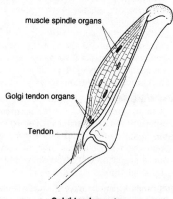

muscle spindle organs

Golgi tendon organs

Tendon

Golgi tendon organ

can exert more force (*see* **deinhibition training**).

gomphoses Fibrous joint represented only by the articulation of a tooth with its bony socket.

gonadotrophic hormone *See* **gonadotropin**.

gonadotropin (gonadotrophic hormone) A hormone, such as follicle-stimulating hormone or luteinizing hormone, that acts on the gonads (testes or ovaries) to stimulate production of sex hormones.

gonads Primary reproductive organs (i.e., the testes of males and ovaries of females) that produce the gametes (sperm and egg cells respectively).

goniometer A device containing a 180° protractor for measuring *static flexibility. The centre of the goniometer is positioned at the joint axis, and the arms of the goniometer are aligned with the longitudinal axis of the body segments to measure the angle present at stationary joint. *Compare* **electrogoniometer**.

gracilis A long, thin thigh muscle which has its origin on the anterior, inferior pubic symphysis, and its insertion on the medial, proximal tibia. Its primary action is adduction of the femur and flexion of the lower leg.

graded exercise test *See* **exercise stress test**.

graded potential A transient localized change (depolarization or hyperpolarization) in the potential difference across a cell surface membrane. A strength of the graded potential varies with the intensity of the stimulus and causes local flows of current which decrease with distance from the stimulus point. Graded potentials are given different names according to their function. *See also* **receptor potential**.

gradient Degree of inclination of a slope, usually expressed as a ratio or percentage of vertical distance to horizontal distance.

gram (gramme) Unit of mass (symbol g) equivalent to 1/1000 of a kilogram. One ounce is equal to 28.35 g. An average paper clip weighs approximately 1 g.

gram weight Unit of force; the pull of the Earth on a gram mass. A gram weight varies slightly according to the *acceleration of free fall at different points on the Earth, but a force of 1 gram weight equals approximately 981 dynes.

gramme *See* **gram**.

granulation tissue Florid, bright pink connective tissue and blood vessels which grow in a healing wound.

granulocyte White blood cell with granules in the cytoplasm. Granulocytes include polymorphonuclear leucocytes, eosinophils, and basophils.

graph A diagram, generally plotted on axes at right angles to each other, showing the relationship of one variable with another (e.g., the variation of oxygen consumption with time).

grass burn A form of friction burn due to abrasion of the skin on the grass. Grass burns are notorious for the ease with which they can become infected. Special care has to be taken when the grass has been treated with chemicals which may cause toxic reactions. This applies, for example, to cricket pitches which are often heavily treated.

gravitation, law of (attraction, law of) Newton's second law of motion which states that any two particles of matter attract one another with a force directly proportional to the product of their masses, and inversely proportional to the square of the distance between them. In sport, the forces between bodies are usually imperceptibly small, except for the force known as *gravity produced by the Earth.

gravitational field The region in which one body which has mass exerts a force of attraction on another body which has mass.

gravitational hypothesis Hypothesis which proposes that athletes have different personality traits from nonathletes because of a process of natural selection: individuals who are stable extroverts tend to gravitate towards sport, and competition causes all but the keenest competitors to withdraw so that those who adhere to sport tend to have the greatest levels of extroversion and stability.

gravitational movement A form of passive movement resulting from the accelerating force exerted by the gravitational field of the Earth. It is relatively constant in direction and magnitude (*see* **free fall**). Gravitational movements include pendulum swings of the limbs or the whole body in gymnastics.

gravity (gravitational field strength) The attraction between the Earth and an object on its surface or within its gravitational field. The rate of acceleration at which bodies are attracted toward the surface of the Earth is $9.806\,\mathrm{ms^{-2}}$. This figure is based on the Earth's mass and distance to the centre of the Earth. The Earth's gravitational force is very slightly less near the equator because the planet is not perfectly spherical, hence the performance of athletes in competitions involving jumping and throwing may be very slightly enhanced by being near the equator (for example, a world-class shot-putter would be able to put the shot 8 cm further in Quito, Ecuador than in Oslo, Norway because of the lower gravity).

gravity line Vertical line showing the line of action produced by an individual force acting on a body. It passes through the point of application of the force and through the point on the *fulcrum upon which the force is balanced.

greater trochanter A large protuberance on the lateral junction between the shaft and neck of the *femur. It acts as an attachment point for gluteal (buttock) muscles.

greater tuberosity A large rounded protuberance on the *humerus. It is an attachment point for a number of muscles, including the supraspinatus, infraspinatus, and teres minor.

great man theory of leadership *See* **trait theory of leadership**.

great toe *See* **hallux**.

Greek ideal A philosophical ideal of ancient Greeks who believed that each person should have a harmonious blend (sometimes called balance) of physical, mental, and spiritual aspects.

green stick fracture Fracture in which the bone breaks incompletely, in the same way that a green twig breaks. Children commonly have green stick fractures because their bones have more collagen and are more flexible than adult bones.

grey matter Region of the central nervous system containing a large density of nerve cell bodies and unmyelinated nerve fibres. *Compare* **white matter**.

grief reaction response The typical response of many athletes to a serious injury. It consists of five stages: denial, anger, bargaining, depression, and acceptance. The speed and ease with which an injured athlete moves through these stages varies widely. Generally, the denial and bargaining stages are more prominent than those of anger and depression.

groin Region of the body which includes the upper part of the front thigh and lower part of the abdomen.

groin itch *See* **dhobie itch**; and **scrumpox**.

groin muscle One of the adductor muscles of the groin which include the *gracilis, *pectineus, and *adductor longus. All these muscles originate from the pubic bones and are inserted into the posterior surface of the femur. The muscles work powerfully when, in a running action, the foot leaves the ground and begins to swing, and the leg rotates outward in relation to the hip.

groin pain (inguinocrural pain) A pain in the groin. In athletes, this is often assumed to be a strain or other sport-related injury of the muscles in the groin, but there are many other causes including osteitis pubis, hernias, disorders of the lymph nodes, various forms of arthritis, stress fracture of the thighbone or pelvis, and (rarely) tumours. Any persistent pain in the groin should be investigated by a doctor.

groin strain A strain of an *adductor muscle (usually the adductor longus) in the groin. The adductor longus runs the length of the pubic bone to the inside of the thigh, and draws the leg inwards from the hip.

Groin strain often occurs after a forceful movement, such as a broadside kick in football, turning quickly in hockey, or, bringing the free leg forward in skating. The strain is characterized by a sudden stabbing pain in the groin, the intensity depending on the severity of the strain. Except in the case of a complete rupture, treatment is nearly always nonsurgical and consists of rest and ice (*see* **RICE**), and sometimes crutches to relieve the load. Anti-inflammatories are often used, but cortisone injections are not administered for fear of weakening the muscle tendon. It is essential to allow the strain to heal completely before returning to sport; this usually takes a minimum of 3 weeks. Training should take place only if there is no pain. Premature resumption of activity will weaken the muscle and increase the risk of strains in the future. Groin strain can be avoided by developing the strength and flexibility of the adductor muscles. One useful exercise comprises holding a football between the knees and using the groin muscles to compress the ball.

groove A furrow in a bone which may act as a tract for blood vessels, nerves, and tendons.

grooving The process of establishing a behaviour as a conditioned reflex by specific and repeated training.

gross anatomy The study of large body structures, such as the heart and lungs, which can be examined easily without any type of magnification.

gross body coordination The coordination of the simultaneous movements of different parts of the body which are involved in whole-body actions. It is an important component of physical fitness.

gross body equilibrium An ability to maintain balance when blindfolded.

gross body movement Movement of the whole body or large segments of the body.

gross motor skill A skill that involves the action of many muscle groups and requires movement of the whole body e.g., running. *Compare* **fine motor skills**.

grounded theory A sociological theory which is formulated only *after* careful naturalistic observations of selected social phenomena. It is used in qualitative analysis of data, and allows categories to emerge from the data obtained, rather than imposing a theory upon data *before* research has begun.

ground reaction force A force exerted by the ground in response to the forces a body exerts on it. If the body is pushing down and forwards, the ground reaction force is up and backward; if the body pushes down and backward, the ground reaction force is up and forwards.

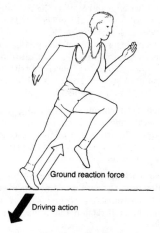

Ground reaction force

Driving action

ground reaction force

ground substance A relatively unstructured material, usually containing fibres, that fills the space between cells of connective tissue.

group A collection of individuals interacting with one another so that each person influences and is influenced by each other person to some degree. Group members are distinguished from a mere aggregate of individuals by having a shared purpose, by being aware of each other, and by interacting and communicating with each other. A team can be regarded as a special type of group which has a well-defined structure, organization, and communication patterns. Team assignments are usually designated before an activity whereas those of other types of groups are often assumed in the course of group interaction.

group cohesion An adhesive property or force that binds group members together. Group cohesion increases the significance of membership for those who belong to the group, motivates members to contribute to group welfare, and encourages a sense of loyalty and commitment.

group dynamics 1 The interactive processes within groups. Sports sociologists tend to focus on the shifting patterns of tension, conflict, adjustment, and cohesion within groups as well as the effect of different styles of leadership. **2** The study of the underlying features of group behaviour such as group motives and attitudes. Group dynamics is concerned with the characteristics of groups which change rather than those which are stable.

group environment The physical, psychological, and social surroundings of a group. The group environment especially refers to the social relationships between the members of the group.

group environment questionnaire A multidimensional questionnaire which directly measures *team cohesion in terms of individual attraction and group integration.

group integration The functioning of a group as a unit. The opportunity to belong to a cohesive unit is, according to the *conceptual model of team cohesion, one reason why individuals are attracted to join groups. Measures of group integration take into consideration an individual's perception of closeness, similarity to other group members, and bonding to the group as a whole. *See also* **individual attraction**.

group locomotion A motivational construct that represents the reason or purpose behind a group's existence and symbolizes the activity of the group in relation to achieving group objectives.

group mentality A characteristic reflecting the unanimous will of a group. Individuals may be unaware of the contributions they make to group mentality and they may influence other members negatively when they feel they are at variance with group principles, norms, and objectives.

group motives Motives which contribute to the success of a group. They include four which are very important: *conflict, *cohesion, *socialization, and expectation. Other group motives include *achievement need and *need to avoid failure. Groups behave in much the same way as individuals when goal setting and reacting to failure and success. However, the group as a whole tends to be more resistant to negative criticism and is less likely than an individual to adjust goals downwards after failure. *See also* **group personality**.

group performance (group productivity) The actual productivity of a group, that is, its achievements, such as scoring a goal, winning a game, or the potential productivity which consists of the group's best possible performance given its resources and task demands. Resources include all the relevant knowledge and skills of individual members. *See also* **Social loafing**; and **Ringelmann effect**.

group personality Characteristic of a group which is analogous to that of the *personality of an individual, in that the group behaves as a unit in certain circumstances; it possesses energy (*see* **synergy**), has drives and emotional states, and it engages in collective deliberations in much the same way as individuals. The group personality is relatively independent of those apparently possessed by the group members. *See also* **synality**.

group processes Everything a group does while transforming its group resources into a product or a performance.

group productivity *See* **group performance**.

group resources The combined relevant knowledge and skills of individual members of a group, including the level and distribution of talents.

growth Increase in size. The growth of human tissue may take place by hypertrophy (enlargement of individual cells), hyperplasia (increase in number of cells), or a combination of the two processes.

growth hormone *See* **human growth hormone**.

growth plate *See* **epiphyseal plate**.

growth spurt A period of accelerated physical development during which there is a rapid increase in height. Typically, there is a major growth spurt in males between 11 to 14 years, and in females between 9 and 11 years. During the growth spurt, the growth plates (physes) of bones are particularly susceptible to overuse injuries because the ligaments may be stronger than the physis during this period (*see* **gymnast's wrist**).

GSR *See* **galvanic skin response**.

guidance A series of techniques, used when practising a skill, in which the behaviour of the learner is limited or controlled by various means to minimize errors. The learner is in some way guided through the task that is to be learned; for example, gymnasts may have manual assistance and support-belts to ensure a mistake will not result in injury.

guide movement (tracking) A gross body movement requiring accuracy and steadiness, but not force or speed, in which both *agonist and *antagonist muscles contribute to the movement.

gum 1 A plant substance that contributes to dietary fibre. **2** Layer of tissue that covers the neck of the teeth.

gumshield (mouthguard) A protective device which fits around the teeth. A suitable protector acts against injury to the teeth; reduces the risk of lacerations to the lips, mouth, and tongue; and reduces the likelihood of *concussion and mandibular fractures during contact or collision sports. The best type of gumshield is one that

is designed by a dental surgeon. Poorly fitting gumshields are uncomfortable and can cause dental injury.

gut *See* **alimentary canal**.

gymnast's back A lower back injury due to vertebrae rubbing against each other when the back is arched during *hyperextension.

gymnast's fracture A supracondylar fracture of the elbow, most frequent in children. It results from excessive extension or flexion of the elbow (common movements in gymnastics) causing an indirect trauma to be transmitted through the radius and ulna against the distal humerus. Gymnast's fracture is often accompanied by injuries to the brachial artery and ulnar nerve.

gymnast's wrist Differential growth of the ulna and radius leading to a malalignment between the two bones. It is associated with activities, commonly performed by young gymnasts whose bones are still growing, which repeatedly place large compression loads on the wrist, injuring the growth plate of the distal radius. Because of the differential growth of the bones in the forearm, the load on the ulna and triquetrum (one of the carpal bones in the wrist) is increased. This compresses the thin, relatively unstable triangular fibrocartilaginous complex between the two bones, causing pain. The repetitive stress may also tear the fibrocartilaginous complex. Preventative treatment consists of young gymnasts (and other young athletes) avoiding weight-bearing when wrist pain occurs. If ulnar deviation occurs and pain persists after prolonged rest, surgical resectioning may be required.

gynaecomastia Development of breasts in a man. It may be due either to a hormonal imbalance or the administration of anabolic steroids. Gynaecomastia associated with steroid abuse is often irreversible.

gynoid fat distribution Distribution of *adipose tissue predominantly around the hips, buttocks, and thighs. Often called 'pear-shaped' obesity, it is more common in females than males. *Compare* **android fat distribution**.

gyroscopic stability The resistance of a rotating body to a change in its plane of rotation. The faster a body spins (the greater its angular velocity), the greater the stability of the body in its particular position or orientation. Gyroscopic stability accounts for the stability of a spinning discus or a spinning football in American football.

gyrus An elevated ridge of tissue on the surface of the cerebral hemispheres of the brain.

habit to **H-zone**

habit A learned, stereotyped response to a particular stimulus or stimuli. A habit results in the formation in the nervous system of a path of preferred conduction between the stimulus and response.

habitual skill A *motor skill requiring a fixed response to a given situation. Such skills are usually performed in a relatively stable environment and are acquired only after much practice. *See also* **perceptual skill; closed skill; self-paced skill**.

habituation A learning process resulting in the diminution and eventual loss of a normal behavioural response or sensation. Habituation results from continuous stimulation with a constant stimulus. It explains how, for example, cricketers become accustomed to uncomfortable sports equipment (such as protective helmets) and swimmers become accustomed to cold water.

habitus The general, outward physical appearance of a person, especially in the context of a medical examination.

HACE *See* **high altitude cerebral oedema**.

haem A ring-structured porphyrin group containing ferrous iron. It is the prosthetic (nonprotein) group of *haemoglobin. Haem gives the blood its red colour and its ability to transport large amounts of oxygen. *See also* **haem iron**.

haemarthrosis Presence of blood or bleeding in a joint, causing pain and swelling. It may be due to an injury or disease. Treatment includes immobilization, cold compresses, and withdrawal of the blood from the joint.

haematin An oxidized derivative of the iron-containing nonprotein portion of *haemoglobin.

haematocrit The volume of red blood cells, usually expressed as a percentage of the total blood volume.

haematoma A swelling caused by the accumulation of clotted blood in tissues. There are two common types of haematoma in sport caused by direct blows or muscle strains: intramuscular haematomas and intermuscular haematomas; they sometimes occur together and can be diagnosed using ultrasound. After treatment with relative rest and ice, a small haematoma may resolve itself. However, a large haematoma may never be reabsorbed (it may develop into a *fibrosis and scar). It may be aspirated under aseptic conditions, and hyaluronidase may be used to increase the absorption of residual blood. *See also* **black nail**; and **extradural haematoma**.

haematopoiesis *See* **haemopoiesis**.

haematuria Discharge of blood into the urine. The blood may come from diseased or physically damaged kidneys, urethra, or bladder. Haematuria is often due to trauma related to the shaking or agitation of the kidneys and bladder during strenuous exercise (*see* **runner's haematuria**).

haem iron Iron incorporated into the haem group of the blood pigment, *haemoglobin. Haem iron constitutes about 40 per cent of the iron in red meats and is the type of dietary iron most readily absorbed by the body.

haemobursa A bursa that fills with blood, usually after a single violent impact.

haemoconcentration An increase in the proportion of red blood cells in blood, usually due to a reduction in the volume of plasma; the absolute number of red blood cells remains unchanged. Haemoconcentration results in increased blood viscosity. It is caused by dehydration and may be artificially induced by *blood doping.

haemocytoblast A cell in the bone marrow which gives rise to blood cells and platelets.

haemocytometer A glass chamber used for examining and counting the cellular components of a known volume of blood viewed with a microscope.

haemodilution A decrease in the proportion of red blood cells in blood due to a relative increase in the volume of plasma; the absolute number of red blood cells remains unchanged. Haemodilution may take place as a result of endurance training.

haemodynamics Study of the physical laws which govern the behaviour of blood flow in the circulatory system. Haemodynamics uses and applies the principles of fluid dynamics to the special conditions pertaining to a living circulatory system which contains a fluid (blood) with unusual properties, and vessels which can change their shape.

haemoglobin A large conjugated protein consisting of four polypeptide chains, each with a prosthetic (nonprotein) haem group which contains ferrous iron, able to combine reversibly with oxygen. It is the oxygen transporting component of red blood cells.

haemoglobin saturation The number of oxygen molecules bound by each molecule of haemoglobin. The maximum number is four. *See also* **oxygen–haemoglobin dissociation curve**.

haemoglobinuria The presence of free *haemoglobin in the urine. It occurs when haemoglobin released from damaged or dead red blood cells is not taken up rapidly enough by blood proteins. It sometimes occurs after strenuous exercise (*see* **march haemoglobinuria**) and after repeated hand trauma in karate. Haemoglobinuria is also associated with some infectious diseases. *See also* **haematuria**; and **myoglobinuria**.

haemolysis Disintegration of red blood cells. The cell membrane ruptures, releasing the contents, including haemoglobin. Premature haemolysis can lead to anaemia. Haemolysis can result from physical trauma to capillaries, for example when the foot repeatedly strikes the ground during long-distance running (a condition known as exertional haemolysis or footstrike haemolysis). *See also* **march haemoglobinuria**.

haemopoiesis (haematopoiesis) The formation of blood; the production of blood cells and platelets. In healthy adults, it takes place mainly in the bone marrow.

haemorrhage Loss of blood through the ruptured walls of blood vessels. Bleeding from a major artery can result in so much blood loss that it leads to *shock, collapse, and death if untreated.

haemostasis The arrest of bleeding or stoppage of blood flow. It applies to the natural physiological processes of blood clotting and contraction of damaged vessels, and medical procedures aimed at stemming blood flow (e.g., ligatures).

haemothorax The accumulation of blood from the lungs into the pleural cavity. A massive haemothorax (i.e., accumulation of more than 1500 ml of blood in the pleural cavity) is exceedingly uncommon, but it does sometimes occur in athletes who have sustained a severe blunt trauma.

Haglund deformity A rounded protuberance at the back of the ankle (sometimes called a 'pump bump' because it coincides with the position of the heel counter in many training shoes) that forms part of a syndrome consisting of a *postcalcaneal bursitis and an *Achilles tendinitis at the point of insertion of the tendon.

half-reaction time The time taken for a chemical reaction to be half completed. For example, a half-reaction time of thirty seconds for restoration of phosphagen stores following an anaerobic activity, means that in thirty seconds half the total ATP stores and PC stores are replenished.

hallux In anatomy, pertaining to the great toe.

hallux rigidus A degenerative condition of a bone in the great toe causing stiffness and disability. It may occur after repeated minor injuries to the metatarsophalangeal joint of the great toe.

hallux valgus Permanent lateral (outward) displacement of the great toe in which the sesamoid bones under the head of the first metatarsal are displaced so that they lie between the first and second metatarsal. Normally the great toe can be angled outwards by ten degrees, but in hallux valgus the displacement is greater. It is a common disorder in those who wear pointed toes or who exhibit excessive pronation.

hamate (unciform bone) A bone which forms part of the *carpus (wrist). It articulates with the fourth and fifth metacarpals distally, and the triquetral posteriorly. The hamate has a hooked-shaped projection which can, rarely, become fractured after a fall, or when a golfer, for example, strikes a solid object (usually a tree root) with the club in mid-swing. The impact force is transmitted down the shaft of the club to the base of the palm of the hand over the hook of hamate. A hook of hamate fracture can also be caused by repetitive impact associated with sports activities such as cycling, baseball, and tennis. The fracture

causes pain and tenderness in the ulnar side of the palm (the 'karate chop' area), and the ulnar nerve may also be irritated or compressed. Confirmation of diagnosis requires a special radiographic view known as the carpal tunnel view. Early diagnosis usually involves immobilization in a cast for about 6 weeks; late diagnosis may necessitate surgical excision of the fracture fragment or internal fixation of the fracture.

hammer toe Deformity of the second toe which becomes buckled as the proximal interphalangeal joint of the first phalanx is pointed upwards in a flexed position. It is usually caused by repeated bumping of the toe against the front of a shoe. If not treated, it may develop into a permanent condition because the tendons under the toe tighten and those above the toe loosen. A corn often develops on the top of the toe. The incidence of hammer toe is higher in those with a weak anterior transverse arch. Hammer toe can be avoided by wearing shoes that fit properly. It can be treated in the early stages by toe exercises and the application of a doughnut pad to reduce friction. Chronic cases that cause pain may require surgery.

hamstring muscles Fleshy group of muscles at the back of the thigh. They consist of the *biceps femoris, *semitendinosus, and *semimembranosus. The hamstrings extend the hip and flex the knee.

hand dynamometer A dynamometer that measures hand strength.

handedness A tendency to prefer the use of either the right or left hand. Humans are predominantly right handed, but being left handed can have the advantage of producing novel and unexpected effects in sports such as tennis, fencing, and boxing. *See also* **cerebral dominance**.

handicapped Term used to describe individuals with some form of disability. Use of the term is regarded by some as a form of negative stereotyping which often leads to those with physical disabilities or learning difficulties from achieving their full potential.

hand injuries Physical trauma to the hand and fingers. The hands are the most commonly damaged part of the body in sports, but penetrating injuries are rare; most hand injuries are closed. Acute injuries include fractures, dislocations, and sprains that can occur from falls, twisting and bending movements, or impact with an implement (*see* **mallet finger**). Boxer's hands are particularly vulnerable to acute injuries (*see* **Boxer's fracture**). Overuse injuries mainly involve the tendons of the finger flexors. Other overuse injuries are usually transmitted upwards to the wrist and forearm (*see* **carpal tunnel syndrome, and handlebar palsy**).

handlebar neuropathy *See* **handlebar palsy**.

handlebar palsy (handlebar neuropathy) An ulnar neuropathy caused by repeated irritation of a deep branch of the ulnar nerve in the palm of the hand. Initial symptoms are tingling or numbness in the hands. It can lead to a chronic weakness of the muscles supplied by the nerve. It is an overuse injury common among cyclists which can be prevented by protecting the hands with padded gloves and frequently changing the position of the hands on the handlebars. Upright or aero bars may also reduce the stress. In the initial stages, conservative treatment (e.g., rest and anti-inflammatories) is usually successful, but once motor weakness is established, surgery may be required.

hand length In *anthropometry, the difference between the stylion height and the dactylion height.

HAPE *See* **high altitude pulmonary oedema**.

haptic perception Perception related to the sense of touch provided by cutaneous receptors and which combines with information from *proprioceptors to contribute to *kinaesthesis.

hard bone *See* **compact bone**.

hard/easy concept The concept that if you train hard or are competing on one day, you should rest or train at a low intensity the next day. Adherence to this concept would reduce the risk of *overtraining

and sustaining overuse injuries. The relatively easy day gives the body a chance to recover from the hard day.

hardening of arteries *See* **arteriosclerosis**.

harmonic motion Motion that repeats itself, usually in equal intervals of time, back and forth across the same path. During harmonic motion, energy is being transformed from kinetic energy into potential energy and back. Harmonic motion occurs when a trampolinist stretches the bed of a trampoline imparting potential energy to it. This energy is then converted to kinetic energy that projects the trampolinist up into the air, and so on.

Harter's competence motivation theory A theory of achievement motivation that is based on a person's feelings of personal competence. According to the theory, competence motivation increases when a person successfully masters a task. This encourages the person to master more tasks. *See* **perceived competence scale for children**.

Harvard step test A test of physical fitness devised at Harvard University during World War II. It involves a subject stepping on and off a bench 20 inches (50.8 cm) high, thirty times a minute at a steady rhythm for up to 5 minutes or until exhausted. The pulse rate is taken at rest before the test, then one minute, two minutes, and three minutes after the test. Fitness levels are estimated from the rate at which the pulse returns to its resting level. The test is not used in medicine any more because it is not very reliable.

Haversian canal A central canal within the lamellae of compact bone containing blood vessels, nerves, and lymphatics. It forms part of the *Haversian system.

Haversian system A cylindrical unit of compact bone consisting of a system of interconnecting channels (canaliculi) around a central Haversian canal. The canaliculi ramify through the concentric rings of bone matrix (*see* **lamellae**), supplying bone cells with nutrients.

Hawthorne effect A general improvement in performance which occurs when persons receive special attention. Successful coaches often show considerable respect for this effect, providing members of their group with as much support and sense of importance as possible.

hay fever *See* **rhinitis**.

H-band *See* **H-zone**.

HCG *See* **human chorionic gonadotropin**.

HDL *See* **high density lipoprotein**.

head 1 Part of the body which contains the brain and organs of sight, hearing, smell, and taste. **2** The rounded expansion of bone which fits into a cavity of another bone to form a joint. **3** The upperpart of a muscle closest to a tendon.

headache A pain felt deep within the skull. Headaches have a variety of causes, most are relatively trivial, including those associated with fatigue, emotional stress, and poor posture. Some headaches, however, have more sinister implications and may be due to poisoning, high blood pressure, or brain damage after a blow to the head. Anyone suffering from a persistent headache, or headaches following physical trauma, should seek medical advice. *See also* **effort headache**; **footballer's migraine**; and **weight-lifter's headache**.

head extension Movement of the head backwards, with the chin moving away from the chest.

head extensor A muscle that carries out head extension e.g., the *splenius and *erector spinae muscles.

head flexion Movement of the head forwards with the chin moving towards the chest. Head flexion usually results from the combined action of gravity and relaxation of the head extensors. It may also be carried out by the sternocleidomastoid muscle. Excessive flexion is prevented by the *ligamentum nuchae.

head flexor Muscle which effects *head flexion. Head flexors include the *sternocleidomastoid muscles and a number of deep muscles in the neck.

head injury Damage caused by physical trauma to the head. Acute head injuries are classified as *concussion, fractures, contusions, and haemorrhage (or haematoma). They are usually caused by a direct blow and can be serious because they involve the brain, spinal cord, and surrounding nerves and sense organs, or they may disfigure or disable delicate structures in the face. A blow to the skull is almost inevitable in contact and collision sports. Most athletes who sustain such a blow recover quickly and have no long-lasting ill-effects. Nevertheless, even a seemingly innocuous blow can have dire consequences (e.g., *see* **epidural haematoma**). Therefore, every head injury should be dealt with cautiously and any loss of consciousness should be medically investigated.

head louse A parasite, *Pediculosis capitis*, which lives in the scalp causing irritation and itching. Lice may induce eczema. They have little effect on physical performance, but they are very contagious and spread readily in contact sports (e.g., in a rugby scrum).

head protectors Headgear, such as helmets, that are designed to protect the head from injury. Protective headgear is used in several sports, including cycling, American football, ice hockey, horseriding, climbing, canoeing, and skiing. Amateur boxers also use headgear in the Olympic Games, significantly reducing the incidence of knock-outs. Head protectors have to be specific to the sport, and individual, light, yet good at absorbing energy. Cycling helmets, for example, have to be very aerodynamic. The helmets used by jockeys have a similar design to motor cycle crash helmets. Heavy or poor-fitting helmets can actually exacerbate an injury, exaggerating cervical flexion and increasing the risk of neck injuries. Some helmets have integrated eye and mouth protection. These are difficult to remove, especially after injury. Unless there is respiratory distress, removal should be delayed if an athlete has been knocked unconscious, or if there is a suspected cervical spine injury. If helmet removal is essential, it should be performed by trained personnel. Because helmets offer considerable protection, there is a danger that users take greater risks because they feel invulnerable. However, this sense of invulnerability is not justified. When helmets were first introduced into ice hockey, cervical injuries actually increased because the helmets offer little protection to forces applied to the neck.

head rotation Lateral movement of the head around its axis. Head rotation is effected by the unilateral action of the *sternocleidomastoids and deeper neck muscles, including the *scalenes.

head rotator A muscle that effects *head rotation.

health Ability of an individual to mobilize his or her resources (physical, mental, and spiritual) to the preservation and advantage of him or herself, and the dependents and society to which the individual belongs. Health is a state of complete, physical, mental, and social well-being. It is not merely freedom from disease and infirmity.

health history (medical history) Information about the health record of an individual.

health-related fitness Aspects of physical fitness which are associated with improving health. Emphasis is usually given to *aerobic endurance, *flexibility, muscle condition, and body composition.

health-risk appraisal An assessment tool used by health promoters to evaluate how healthy a person is. A health-risk appraisal usually takes the form of an extended questionnaire which enquires into personal lifestyle habits, and personal and family medical history. It may be accompanied by laboratory tests for blood analysis, blood pressure, and physical fitness levels. The outcome is a profile outlining areas of high risk, and this is usually accompanied by strategies and targets for lifestyle change.

healthy person A person who is not obviously ill, and whose physical and mental functions correspond to those of the average person of the same sex in the same age-group.

heart A hollow, four-chambered muscular organ lying in the thoracic cavity between the lungs. Its wall consists mainly of *cardiac muscle. The heart is divided by a septum into a right and left side, each of which has two chambers: an atrium and a ventricle. Deoxygenated blood from the veins enters the right atrium and is passed into the right ventricle. This contracts and pumps the blood through the pulmonary artery into the lungs. Oxygenated blood returns through the pulmonary vein into the left atrium and then into the left ventricle. This contracts forcefully to pump the oxygenated blood to the rest of the body.

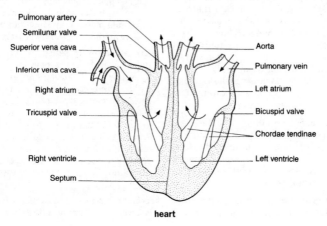

Pulmonary artery
Semilunar valve
Superior vena cava
Inferior vena cava
Right atrium
Tricuspid valve
Right ventricle
Septum
Aorta
Pulmonary vein
Left atrium
Bicuspid valve
Chordae tendinae
Left ventricle

heart

The unidirectional flow of blood is maintained by heart valves.

heart attack (myocardial infarction) Blockage of blood flow to a portion of heart muscle. If the block is towards the end of a coronary artery, the heart attack may not be severe since the amount of tissue deprived of oxygen would be minimal, but if the block is towards the beginning of the artery, the amount of tissue affected would be large and the heart attack severe. Much inferential evidence indicates that exercise, if properly prescribed and supervised, can reduce the risk of heart attack. Exercise rehabilitation is used on those who have suffered a heart attack. It may not reduce the chances of having a second attack, but it can reduce its seriousness. *See also* **coronary heart disease risk factor**.

heartbeat The events of a single *cardiac cycle.

heart block Impaired transmission of impulses from the pacemaker region in the sinoatrial node to the rest of the heart resulting in a slowing down of the heart rate. The condition may be congenital or caused by heart diseases such as *myocarditis.

heart burn (pyrosis) A burning pain behind the sternum that often seems to be rising from the stomach into the throat. It is usually caused by regurgitation of the acidic contents of the stomach into the oesophagus. It is sometimes confused with a heart complaint, but heart burns are very common and usually not serious. Heart burn appears to occur more often after intense exercise, but it can be alleviated or prevented by increasing fluid intake, limiting fat intake, and not eating solids immediately before exercise.

heart failure A condition in which the pumping action of the heart is insufficient to meet the demands of the body. Heart failure may result from overload, damage, or disease of the heart. The sufferer experiences breathlessness.

heart hypertrophy An increase in the size of the heart. Heart hypertrophy may be a pathological condition resulting from the need of the heart to pump more blood due to a defect in the circulatory or respiratory systems. In athletes, however, it can be a nonpathological training effect (*see* **athlete's heart**).

heart murmur Abnormal heart sound detectable with a stethoscope applied over the heart and particular blood vessels. Murmurs are heard in most athletes after severe exercise. They are usually benign and do not affect the athlete's performance or heart function. However, heart murmurs may need to be evaluated by a cardiologist to exclude serious conditions, such as defective valves, which might preclude athletic involvement.

heart overload A condition which occurs when the demand for oxygenated blood exceeds the ability of the heart to pump oxygenated blood around the body.

heart rate The number of heart beats per minute. The heart rate is commonly taken in four positions: sitting, supine, quick-standing, and after standing for one minute. An individual's resting heart rate varies by as much as 10 beats per minute according to the position in which it is taken.

heart rate method A method of determining optimal training intensities based on heart rate so that the *overload principle can be applied. Generally, heart rate increases with workload. *See also* **maximal heart rate method**; **maximal heart rate reserve method**; and **target heart rate**.

heart rate recovery period The period of time it takes for the heart rate to return to its resting rate following exercise. After regular aerobic training, the heart rate recovery period is significantly less than before the training. The period can be used to monitor changes in a person's *aerobic fitness, but it is an unreliable indicator for comparing the aerobic fitness of different people because individual factors other than fitness can influence the heart rate recovery period.

heart rate reserve (HRR; maximal heart rate reserve) The difference between maximal heart rate (HRmax) and resting heart rate (HRest). HRR = HRmax − HRrest. *See also* **maximal heart rate reserve method**.

heart sounds Normally, during one cardiac cycle, two heart sounds (usually described as 'lub-dub' or 'lub-dup') which can be heard over the chest through a stethoscope. The first sound is caused by closure of the atrioventricular valves towards the beginning of systole, the other is caused by the closure of the semilunar valves guarding the aorta and pulmonary artery at the beginning of ventricular diastole. *Compare* **heart murmur**.

heart valve A structure which restricts the flow of blood through the heart to one direction only. The heart valves are the tricuspid valve between the right atrium and the right ventricle, the bicuspid (mitral) valve between the left atrium and left ventricle, and the semi-lunar valves in the pulmonary artery and dorsal aorta.

heat Energy possessed by a substance in the form of atomic or molecular kinetic energy. Heat contained within a body is the product of the body's mass, temperature, and specific heat capacity. Heat is transmitted by radiation, conduction, and convection. Changes in the heat content of a body may result in changes of state of matter within the body (e.g., liquid water converted to vapour; *see* **latent heat of vaporization**) or changes of temperature. The SI unit for heat is the joule.

heat acclimatization Physiological adaptations associated with prolonged exposure to high environmental temperatures. The adaptations which improve heat tolerance include an increase in blood volume, increase in sweating rate with the sweat containing a lower concentration of sodium, decrease in heart rate and lowering of core temperature at a given work load, and a reduction in the perceived intensity of exercise. In addition, heat-acclimatized individuals tend to suffer less from nausea, dizziness, and discomfort in hot temperatures than those who are unacclimatized. Most athletes from temperate regions acclimatize in hot climates very quickly, but

a minimum of 7–10 days is advisable. Typically, acclimatization occurs after four to seven sessions of exercising 1–4 hours per session. The exercise should start gently with periods of about 15 minutes of work alternated with 15 minutes rest. The exercise intensity should increase as heat tolerance improves. It is important that athletes take plenty of fluids in a hot climate.

heat balance A condition reached when heat gained by a body is equal to heat lost from it. At heat balance, the amount of stored heat does not change and the body temperature remains constant. In humans, heat is exchanged with the environment by radiation, conduction, convection, and evaporation. In addition to external sources of heat, heat is also gained internally by metabolism. During exercise, metabolism increases dramatically and produces much heat. Evaporation of sweat is the major means of losing this heat.

heat collapse Loss of consciousness associated with hot environments or exercising in clothing which restricts heat loss and causes overheating. Excessive sweating and shunting blood to the skin and muscles, reduces blood flow to the brain, causing fainting. Heat collapse is one of the commonest medical conditions on a hot day and is exacerbated by standing for long periods. It is potentially dangerous because it can lead to *heat exhaustion and *heat stroke. Uncomplicated heat collapse often occurs when individuals stand for long periods in a very hot environment. Recovery is usually quick if the sufferer lies down with legs elevated, is given a watery drink, and is sponged with tepid water. However, if the sufferer loses consciousness and has a high rectal temperature (41 °C or above), heat stroke should be suspected until a medical diagnosis proves otherwise.

heat conduction The transfer of heat from the warmer to the cooler of two solid bodies that are in contact. In the human body, the rate of conduction depends on the temperature gradient between the skin

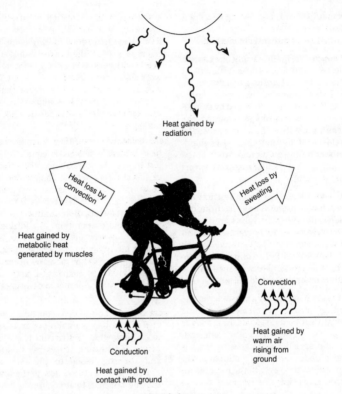

Heat gained by
radiation

Heat loss by
convection

Heat loss by
sweating

Heat gained by
metabolic heat
generated by muscles

Convection

Conduction

Heat gained by
warm air
rising from
ground

Heat gained by
contact with ground

heat balance

and the material with which the skin is in contact, and on the thermal properties of the material. *See also* **clo unit**.

heat content The total calories of heat contained within the body. Since each kilogram of body tissue requires about 0.83 kilocalories to raise its temperature by 1 °C, the heat content of the body can be estimated using the following equation: Heat content = 0.83 (body mass × mean body temperature).

heat cramps Painful muscular contractions caused by prolonged exposure to environmental heat. They probably result from electrolyte imbalances. Drinking plenty of watery fluids and obtaining adequate salt in the diet should prevent heat cramps.

heat equivalence (calorific equivalence) Energy produced by the oxidation of food in one litre of oxygen. Heat equivalence varies according to the mixture of food types (fats, carbohydrate, or protein) being oxidized. It is usually measured in kilocalories. *See also* **net oxygen cost of exercise**; and **respiratory quotient**.

heat exhaustion Fatigue caused by an inability of the cardiovascular system to satisfy all of the requirements of the body's tissues when blood is shifted to the skin for cooling. Typically, those suffering from heat exhaustion have a normal body core temperature, but their pulse rate is accelerated, their skin is cold and clammy, and they often experience drowsiness and vomiting. The condition can be alleviated by rest and cooling with tepid water, but if it persists there is a risk of *heat neurasthenia. Heat exhaustion can usually be prevented by regular water replacement.

Heath–Carter method *See* **somatotyping**.

heating pad *See* **hydrocollator**.

heat neurasthenia A progressive deterioration leading to chronic *neurosis brought about by prolonged heat exhaustion. Heat neurasthenia is characterized by feelings of apathy, hysteria, and aggression.

heat stroke A potentially fatal condition caused by prolonged overheating which may result from exercising in a hot environment or exercising in clothes which restrict the elimination of heat. Heat stroke is characterized by a high body core temperature (above 40.5 °C or 105 °F), and hot, dry skin which is usually flushed. Heat stroke patients show signs of mental confusion and loss of motor control, and may collapse into unconsciousness. The first priority of treatment is to lower the core temperature back to normal. This can be achieved by loosening clothing, fanning, and sponging with tepid water. However, iced fluids and iced baths should not be used because they may constrict blood vessels in the skin and reduce heat loss. Expert medical attention is necessary and hospitalization may be required as there is a danger of renal failure.

heat syncope Fainting or sudden loss of strength due to overheating. *See also* **heat collapse**.

heat treatment The use of heat to treat injuries and accelerate recovery. The heat may be applied superficially or directed to deep tissues. Superficial heat induces feelings of relaxation and comfort. Other therapeutic properties of heat (deep and superficial) include increasing blood flow through damaged tissue, increasing metabolism, and increasing the threshold of sensory nerve endings (therefore decreasing pain). Heat treatment should not be used immediately after injury, particularly if there is any bleeding. *See also* **diathermy**.

hedonism theory A theory which assumes that people are constant seekers of pleasure and avoiders of unpleasant stimuli. Therefore, according to the theory, human motives (including those associated with sport) can be understood with reference to whether the individual is moving towards pleasurable outcomes and consequences and/or avoiding unpleasant ones. *See* **social reinforcement**.

heel Part of the foot formed by the heel-bone (*see* **calcaneus**) which extends behind the ankle joint.

heel bone *See* **calcaneus**.

heel bruise *See* **heel pad contusion**.

heel bursitis *See* **Achilles bursitis**.

heel counter Rigid cup of material which wraps around the heel of a training shoe to hold the heel in place. A badly designed heel counter or one which does not fit properly, can rub against the soft tissue in the ankle, increasing the risk of overuse injuries, such as *Achilles tendinitis.

heel pad A pad of fatty fibroelastic tissue which acts as a shock absorber in the heel. With age, the thickness of the heel pad decreases, possibly predisposing athletes to injury.

heel pad contusion (heel bruise) Bruising of the *heel pad caused by striking the heel heavily on the ground. Repeated bruising (e.g., during distance running) can give rise to a precisely localized pain in the heel every time the foot strikes the ground. Rest usually resolves the condition quickly, but additional shock-absorbing heel inserts may be required to minimize a recurrence.

heel raise An insertion, usually made of rubber, in a training shoe which alters the angle of the foot as it strikes the ground during walking and running.

heel spur A growth of bony tissue that occurs at the attachment of the *plantar fascia to the calcaneus (heelbone). It is often associated with *plantar fasciitis.

heel tab A tab of material that extends from the top of the heel counter of a training or running shoe. If the material is hard and extends too far up the heel, it can damage the Achilles tendon. There is little danger of this with low, flexible tabs.

height of release The height above the ground level, or the height above the point of landing, of the *centre of gravity of a projectile immediately before it leaves the ground. The height of release affects the trajectory of the projectile and, for a given *speed of release and *angle of release, the horizontal displacement increases as the height of release increases.

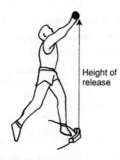

Height of release

height of release

Heimlich manoeuvre A technique to dislodge an obstruction from the trachea of a choking person. The arms are wrapped around the patient from behind. A tight fist is made with one hand which is grasped above the navel and just below the ribcage by the other hand. The patient hangs forwards and the fist is forcefully pressed upwards into the abdomen. It is a useful technique for coaches and officials to know, especially as many people foolishly chew gum while participating in sport.

helmets *See* **head protectors**.

Henry's law A gas law which states that the mass of a gas dissolved by a given volume of liquid at a constant temperature is directly proportional to its pressure. At a constant temperature, therefore, the volume of a gas absorbed by a given volume of liquid is independent of the pressure. The law applies only to sparingly soluble gases at low pressures.

Henry' memory drum theory Theory concerned with memorization of motor skills which postulates that neuromotor coordination patterns are stored in the form of neural patterns in the higher centres of the central nervous system on what is called a memory drum. The drum has been likened to a computer memory store which contains programs ready to function in a desired fashion upon the appropriate signal. Thus, in humans, whenever a specific movement pattern is needed, the stimulus causes the memory drum to 'play back' the particular learned skill. The theory supports the idea that learning motor skills is specific rather than general, and that there is little or no carryover from one skill to another unless the skills are nearly identical (*see* **transfer of training**).

heparin A complex organic acid found in mast cells (large cells in the connective tissue involved in inflammation response). It inhibits blood coagulation by interfering with the formation and action of thrombin (a blood clotting factor). A heparin drug can be prepared from snake venom. In addition to its anticoagulant properties, it has effects similar to caffeine, increasing free fatty acid levels. These effecct may be utilized during aerobic exercise, reducing the rate of muscle glycogen utilization and delaying fatigue.

heparinoid Ointment containing an anticoagulant used to treat contusions.

hepatic Pertaining to the liver.

hepatic artery Blood vessels supplying the liver with oxygenated blood.

hepatic portal system A system of blood vessels consisting of hepatic portal veins which carry nutrients absorbed from the intestines to the liver tissues for processing.

hepatic vein A major vein carrying deoxygenated blood away from the liver towards the heart.

hepatitis A highly infectious inflammatory disease of the liver commonly caused by viruses, but also by alcohol, drugs, and overexposure to toxic chemicals. Hepatitis comprises at least two very different illnesses. Hepatitis A (infectious hepatitis) is spread via viruses taken in with food and excreted in the faeces. Hepatitis B (serum hepatitis) is transmitted sexually or via infected blood or blood products. It is a very serious illness. Hepatitis B has been recorded in orienteers who run in woods and brush past undergrowth carrying the virus from an infected person who has been scratched. Rules specifying clothing to be worn in orienteering and other outside sports are aimed at minimizing the risk of these and other diseases (*see also* **Lyme disease**). Carriers of the hepatitis B virus are not excluded from sport, but it is important that any injury that causes bleeding is cleaned and secured immediately. Although hepatitis B is a relatively rare infection amongst athletes, it has a relatively high theoretical risk of transmission, therefore sensible precautions should be taken and good hygiene practised. Hepatitis C virus is transmitted primarily by blood and blood products. It is rare among athletes.

herbal preparations Substances extracted from naturally occurring plants. These may include banned substances. Ma Huang (Chinese ephedra), for example, contains *ephedrine. *See also* **ginseng**.

herding behaviour *See* **contagion theory of collective behaviour**.

Hering–Breur reflex A reflex action involving *muscle spindles within intercostal muscles which prevents overinflation of the lungs and helps maintain the normal rhythm of inspiration and expiration.

hermeneutics The science of interpretations. The word hermeneutics derives from a term for interpreting scriptural texts, but in sociology hermeneutics refers to a theory and method of interpreting cultures in general and literal texts in particular. One of its concerns is evaluating the veracity of multiple interpretations of a particular phenomenon. For example, hermeneutic research on the behaviour of soccer fans includes the different interpretations of the fans themselves, and the interpretations of other observers who may include the researcher.

hernia The protrusion of an organ through a weakness in its body cavity wall; it is commonly caused by weight-lifting, obesity, or muscle-weakness. Some hernias are quite easy to return to their normal site but others (irreducible hernias) may be impossible to replace. *See also* **fascial hernia**; **inguinal hernia**.

herniated disc *See* **prolapsed intervertebral disc**.

herniated muscle *See* **fascial hernia**.

herniography The use of a special technique to investigate the presence of an *inguinal hernia. A nonirritating contrast medium is introduced into the lower left quadrant of the abdomen, allowed to be taken by gravity into the lower pelvis, and viewed fluoroscopically.

herpes Inflammation of the skin caused by viruses. *See also* **herpes gladiatorum**.

herpes gladiatorum A very contagious skin infection characterized by multiple or single lesions caused by the herpes simplex type I virus. Its name derives from the ease at which an infected participant of combat, contact, and collision sports can transmit the virus to an uninfected opponent in practice and competition. In 1989, 60 participants (35 per cent) at a wrestling camp in Minnesota had herpes gladiatorum. Infected athletes should not take part in contact or collision sports. Treatment with acyclovir (an antiviral agent) often helps to resolve the infection. *See also* **scrumpox**.

herpes simplex *See* **herpes gladiatorum**.

heterotopia Displacement of an organ or part of the body, such as a bone, from its normal position.

heuristic device 1 In sociology, any general concept which is proposed merely as an aid to analysis. **2** A method of solving mathematical problems which cannot be solved in a finite number of steps. It involves progressively limiting the field of search by inductive reasoning from past experience. **3** A method of teaching where students are allowed to learn things for themselves.

hexose A simple sugar, such as glucose, containing six carbon atoms.

hexokinase An enzyme which catalyses the phosphorylation of glucose (glucose → glucose 6-phosphate). This phosphorylation provides the *activation energy required for *glycolysis. Hexokinase, therefore, enables glucose, taken up into muscle cells from the blood, to be used as an energy source for muscle actions.

hexose monophosphate shunt (pentose-phosphate cycle) A biochemical pathway which provides an alternative system to *glycolysis and the *Krebs cycle for the *metabolism of glucose. The hexose monophosphate shunt involves an intricate series of reactions in which glucose-6-phosphate is initially dehydrogenated and decarboxylated and then resynthesized in smaller amounts. The reactions generate reducing power in the form of NADPH (reduced nicotinamide adenine dinucleotide phosphate) for fatty acid and steroid synthesis, and ATP. The hexose monophosphate shunt can contribute between 10 to 90 per cent of energy supplied by carbohydrate metabolism; it is sometimes known as the direct oxidative pathway.

hGH *See* **human growth hormone**.

Hick's law Mathematical statement that choice-reaction time is linearly related to $\log_2$ of the number (N) of stimulus–response alternatives, or to the amount of information that must be processed in order to respond. It is expressed as follows: choice–reaction time = $a + b(\log_2 N)$, where a and b are constants. In simple experiments, reaction time is increased by nearly a constant 150 ms for every doubling of the stimulus–response alternatives.

hidden audience The audience not actually present at an event. The hidden audience includes parents, coaches, and others interested in the event and those who study the results in the media. The hidden audience can be a source of *anxiety which can disrupt the performance of an athlete. *See also* **audience effect**.

hidrosis Sweating; especially applied to excessive sweating.

hierarchy An organization of habits or concepts, in which simpler components are combined to form increasingly complex integrations.

high altitude cerebral edema *See* **high altitude cerebral oedema**.

high altitude cerebral oedema (HACE; high altitude cerebral edema) Accumulation of fluid in the cranial cavity at high altitudes. Most cases occur above 4300 m. It results in mental confusion that can lead to loss of consciousness, coma, and death. Its precise cause is unknown. Treatment is by administering supplemental oxygen and moving the patient to a lower altitude. *See also* **Gamow bag**.

high altitude pulmonary edema *See* **high altitude pulmonary oedema**.

high altitude pulmonary oedema (HAPE; high altitude pulmonary edema) Accumulation of fluid in the lungs at high altitude. It occurs most frequently in those who ascend rapidly to altitudes above 2700 m. The fluid interferes with ventilation and results in shortness of breath and fatigue. Oxygen transport to the brain is impaired, leading to mental confusion and loss of consciousness. The condition is potentially fatal. Its precise cause is unknown. HAPE is treated by administering supplemental oxygen and returning the patient to a lower altitude. *See also* **Gamow bag**.

high arches *See* **cavus foot**.

high blood pressure *See* **hypertension**.

high culture The moral, social, intellectual, and physical qualities which are perceived to be the most valuable to a *culture. High culture is thought by many to be developed and refined by training in the tastes and manners of society. It includes aspects of culture, such as classical music, ballet, poetry, and fine arts, which involve a relatively small segment of the population. These aspects are usually the domain of the upper class or well-educated social élite, particularly in Western countries. *Compare* **mass culture**; **taste culture**.

high-density lipoprotein (HDL) A *lipoprotein that carries *cholesterol in the blood and lymph. It transports the cholesterol from tissues (including the arterial walls) to the liver to be broken down and excreted. Thus, HDL seems to accelerate the clearance of cholesterol from the blood, reducing the risk of cholesterol deposition in arterial walls which leads to *atherosclerosis. Regular aerobic exercise increases the proportion of HDL in the blood. *Compare* **low-density lipoprotein**.

higher order conditioning The use of previously conditioned stimuli to condition further responses, in much the same way as unconditioned stimuli are used. *See* **conditioning**.

high-intensity continuous training Continuous training performed at work intensities equivalent to 85% to 95% of a person's maximal heart rate. High intensity continuous training is an effective way of developing endurance and, if performed at a sufficiently high intensity, will help develop the appropriate leg speed for competition. However, slower paced training (e.g., *LSD or *fartlek) should be incorporated into the training programme at least once or twice a week as a relief from the stress of exhaustive, high-intensity continuous training.

high means interdependence Relationship exhibited by team members in interactive sports that requires the members to depend upon each other to achieve team goals. *Compare* **low means interdependence**.

hill training Training which usually involves running, skiing, or cycling repeatedly up a hill. Hill training is an excellent way for runners, walkers, cross-country skiers, and cyclists to increase training intensity. A 10 degree incline, for example, can almost double the energy demands of a run. An equivalent increase in training intensity over a level course would necessitate running much faster and putting far greater stress on bones and joints. For runners, hill training is particularly good for developing buttock muscles.

Hill–Sachs lesion A fracture in the shoulder of the posterolateral aspect of the articular surface of the humeral head. It is caused by compression of the head (ball) against the anterior rim of the glenoid fossa (socket). It occurs in about 30 per cent of acute shoulder dislocations and 75 per cent of recurrent dislocations.

hind brain Part of the brain consisting of the medulla oblongata, the pons, and the cerebellum.

hinge joint (ginglymus) A *synovial joint that permits motions, such as extension and flexion, along a single axis only (e.g., the interphalangeal joints of the fingers, and the ulnohumeral joint of the elbow).

hip Region either side of the pelvis where the femur articulates with the *coxal bones.

hip abduction Movement of the *femur to the side, away from the midline or lifting the leg sideways.

hip abductor Muscle effecting hip *abduction. The major hip abductor is the *gluteus medius with the *gluteus minimus assisting.

hip adduction Movement of the *femur towards the midline or from a sideways position back to the anatomical position.

hip adductor A muscle which effects *hip adduction. The hip adductors include the *adductor longus, *adductor brevis, *adductor magnus, and the *gracilis.

hip bone *See* **coxal bone**.

hip extension Movement of the *femur backwards on the pelvis.

hip extensor A muscle which effects *hip extension. The hip extensors are the *gluteus maximus and the three *hamstring muscles.

hip flexion Movement of the *femur forwards.

hip flexor A muscle that effects *hip flexion. The major hip flexors are the *iliacus and *psoas major (often referred to jointly as the iliopsoas). Other hip flexors are the *pectineus, *rectus femoris, *sartorius, and *tensor fascia latae.

hip horizontal abduction (hip horizontal extension) Movement of the *femur in the transverse plane from an anterior position to a lateral position. This movement requires the coordinated actions of several muscles, including the hip abductors.

hip horizontal adduction (hip horizontal flexion) Movement of the *femur in the transverse plane from a lateral position to an anterior position. This movement involves several muscles, including the *hip adductors.

hip joint A multiaxial ball-and-socket joint between the *acetabulum and the head of the *femur. The hip joint is inherently strong because of the conformation of the articulating bones (the femur head fits snugly into the deep socket of the acetabulum) and the number and strength of the muscles and ligaments which cross it. The hip joint permits movement of the femur in all three planes.

hip lateral rotation Rotation of the *femur outwards around its longitudinal axis.

hip lateral rotator A muscle that effects *hip lateral rotation. Although a number of muscles contribute to the movement, six muscles function solely as hip lateral rotators: the *piriformis, *gemellus superior, *gemellus inferior, *obturator internus, *obturator externus, and *quadratus femoris.

hip medial rotation Inward rotation of the *femur about its longitudinal axis.

hip medial rotator A muscle that effects *hip medial rotation. The main medial rotators are the *gluteus medius, *gracilis, *semitendinosus, and the *semimembranosus. Medial rotators are weak in comparison to the lateral rotators because medial rotation does not usually require a substantial amount of muscle force.

hip movements Movements permitted by the hip, described with respect to the femur (thigh bone). Movements of the pelvic girdle are important in positioning the hip joint for effective femur movement (*see* **pelvic girdle**).

hippocampus A tract of nervous tissue in the lateral ventricle of the brain. Its function is uncertain. It may be involved in spatial and cognitive mapping, or it may screen novel sensory information about the environment in order to discard or store it. Damage to the hippocampus is associated with *amnesia.

Hippocrates manoeuvre A technique for immediately replacing an anterior dislocation of the shoulder when the head of the humerus comes out of its socket. An unshod heel of the practitioner is placed gently in the patient's axilla (armpit), the arm pulled and the head of the humerus levered in position. This manoeuvre should be used by medically trained personnel only; it is difficult to control the leverage and the pressure exerted by the heel can damage nerves and blood vessels in the axilla. A dislocated shoulder often requires a general anaesthetic.

hip pointer A painful contusion (bruise) of the iliac crest, the bony part of the pelvis that can be felt on either side of the waist. It is usually caused by a direct blow, sometimes accompanied by a popping sound, sustained in contact or collision sports. Ice and compression should be applied immediately after the injury and at intervals for the next 48 hours. Analgesics such as paracetamol (acetaminophen) can be taken to relieve moderate pain; aspirin or ibuprofen (if tolerated) can be taken to relieve pain and swelling. As soon as symptoms allow, this is usually followed by an aggressive rehabilitation programme of supervised stretching exercises of the muscles attached to the iliac crest. If treated correctly, a hip pointer is usually resolved within a few weeks, but a serious contusion or poor treatment will delay recovery.

His, bundle of Atrioventricular bundle of modified cardiac muscle fibres in the heart. The bundle of fibres run from the atrioventricular node down the septum to transmit the wave of stimulation which causes the ventricles to contract.

histamine An endogenous substance responsible for some allergic responses in the eyes, nose, and skin (e.g., during a bout of hay fever). It is formed in the body from histidine. Histamine is released by *mast cells in most tissues during inflammation. It is also secreted by some areas of the *hypothalamus and functions as a *metabotropic neurotransmitter belonging to the biogenic amines. It acts as a powerful vasodilator and increases the permeability of blood vessels.

histidine An essential amino acid in the diet of both adults and infants.

histogram A graph used in statistics in which frequency distributions of interval-level data are represented by contiguous rectangles. In a histogram, the area of each rectangle is directly proportional to the frequency of each class interval represented. *Compare* **bar chart**.

hitting the wall A phrase commonly used to describe the onset of fatigue during endurance events, such as the marathon. It is thought to coincide with the depletion of *muscle glycogen stores, the accumulation of metabolic products (e.g., hydrogen ions from lactic acid), and an increasing dependence on *anaerobic metabolism.

HIV *See* **human immunodeficiency virus**.

hold relax, agonist contract technique *See* **contract relax, agonist contract technique**.

holism The idea that the whole is greater than the sum of its parts. Thus a holistic view of behaviour is one in which a particular behaviour cannot be explained merely by reducing it to its simplest units. *See also* **Gestalt psychology**.

holistic Pertaining to *holism.

holistic training concept The idea that coaches and athletes should consider the whole 24–hour period in the day when devising a training programme, not just the short time devoted to exercise. The concept recognizes that everything that takes place outside training (especially the amount of sleep, type of rest and recreation, and eating patterns) affects the performance of athletes in competition. The concept also emphasizes the need to have a holistic attitude towards the actual training programme. The programme should achieve a balance between many factors so that the person is healthy, has good overall spiritual, physical, and mental fitness, and is well-trained in the specific skills needed.

hollow sprints Training in which one sprint is separated from the next by the so-called hollow period involving jogging or walking.

holocrine gland A gland that stores its secretions in its own cells. The secretions are released only when the cells disintegrate; e.g., a *sebaceous gland.

home court advantage (home field advantage) The notion that playing at home is an advantage because of audience support. *See* **self-attention**.

home-field advantage *See* **home court advantage**.

homeostasis Compensatory control mechanisms which maintain a constant physical or chemical state within a system. Physiological homeostasis is illustrated by the maintenance of a constant body core temperature and blood sugar levels. Psychological homeostasis is illustrated by the maintenance of self-respect through compensatory devices such as rationalization and blaming others for faults. In sociology, homeostasis has been applied to the controversial suggestion that social systems (including governing bodies of sport) tend to act in ways which are self-maintaining and self-equilibrating.

homophobia An irrational fear or intolerance of homosexuality, or behaviour that is perceived to uphold and support traditional gender role expectations. The prevalent assumption in Western society is that heterosexuality is the only acceptable sexual orientation. In sport, homophobia is expressed in ways ranging from telling jokes directed against homosexual activity, through harassment to physical violence against homosexual sportspeople.

hook of hamate fracture *See* hamate.

Hooke's law A law of mechanics which states that, within the *elastic limits of a material, a *strain is proportional to the *stress producing it. Therefore, the deformation imparted to a body is directly related to the magnitude of the distorting force. *See also* **elasticity**; and **elastic modulus**.

hooliganism Rough, antisocial behaviour commonly performed by a young person. Hooliganism has been used to describe the behaviour of lawless soccer fans who form a subcultural element of British soccer structure. The term is probably derived from an antisocial family named Houlighan who lived in the East End of London during the nineteenth century.

horizontal abduction (horizontal extension) Movement of the arm or thigh in the transverse plane from an anterior position to a lateral position.

horizontal adduction (horizontal flexion) Movement of the arm or thigh in the transverse plane from a lateral position to an anterior position.

horizontal displacement The distance a projectile has moved between its point of release and its point of landing, measured as a straight line parallel to the ground. *Compare* **vertical displacement**.

horizontal extension *See* **horizontal abduction**.

horizontal flexion *See* **horizontal adduction**.

horizontal plane *See* **transverse plane**.

horizontal projection The horizontal path of a projectile.

horizontal status The different but equal positions in an organization among individuals who are on approximately the same levels within a hierarchy. On a team, the horizontal status reflects comparisons of different team members. *Compare* **vertical status**.

horizontal velocity Component of a projectile's velocity which acts parallel to the ground and which does not lift the projectile in the air.

hormonal agent A *hormone believed to enhance athletic performance.

hormone A chemical produced in one part of the body which has its effects on another part (target cells). Endocrine glands are the sites of secretion. The bloodstream transports the hormones to their target tissues. Hormones act as chemical messengers, helping to regulate specific body functions.

horse power A British unit of power; one horsepower is equal to the work done at a rate of 550 foot-pounds per second. It is equivalent to 745.7 watts.

hostile aggression (reactive aggression; hostility) Aggression against another person with intent to do physical or mental harm; the goal or reinforcement is to inflict pain or suffering on the victim. It is always accompanied by anger. *Compare* **instrumental aggression**.

hostility *See* **hostile aggression**.

house-maid's knee (prepatellar bursitis) An inflammation of the *bursa in front of the patella. The inflamed bursa becomes tender and restricts knee mobility. Housemaid's knee is usually caused by repetitive friction or frequent pressure, such as when moving about on the knees (hence its common name), and among sports people whose knees come into regular contact with a hard surface (e.g., wrestlers and trampolinists). Immediate treatment includes rest, application of ice and a doughnut-shaped compression pad. A doctor may inject a local anti-inflammatory (e.g., cortisone) into the bursa and drain the excess fluid from the bursa. Recovery from prepatellar bursitis usually takes about one to two weeks. If it does not respond to simple treatment, surgical removal of the sac may be necessary.

HR *See* **heart rate**.

HRmax *See* **maximum heart rate**.

HRR *See* **heart rate reserve**.

Hull's drive theory *See* **drive theory**.

human chorionic gonadotrophin (chorionic gonadotrophin; hCG) A hormone produced by the placenta during pregnancy which stimulates the production of testosterone. Drugs containing hCG have been misused by athletes to increase testosterone levels artificially. hCG has also been taken by male athletes to prevent testicular atrophy associated with the use of *anabolic steroids. Consequently, hCG is on the International Olympic committee list of *banned substances. Small quantities of hCG have been found in the serum of men and nonpregnant women. It is also produced by different types of tumour. Unfortunately, the dope tests on urine samples of athletes do not distinguish between hCG from the different sources.

human competency A component of managerial competency which refers to a leader's or coach's power of persuasion and ability to establish harmonious relationships within a team. It is a critical component of leadership.

human development model (educational model) A framework around which the study of behaviour may take place. The model incorporates statements about desirable goals; focuses on sequential change; emphasizes techniques of optimization rather than remediation; considers the individual as an integrated bio-psycho-social unit and therefore amenable to a multidisciplinary focus; and views individuals as developing in a biocultural context. There is therefore more concern with development of a person's potential than with the therapeutic or remedial handling of a person's social or emotional problems.

human growth hormone (growth hormone; GH; hGH) A hormone secreted by the anterior pituitary gland which stimulates body growth generally, and the lengthening of long bones in particular. Whereas anabolic steroids act primarily on muscles, human growth hormone strengthens bones and tendons as well. Human growth hormone belongs to the peptide hormones, a group of hormonal agents banned by the International Olympic Committee. Natural production of human growth hormone increases during exercise, but the increase is not so fast in a

trained as an untrained person. Risks associated with taking extra human growth hormone include acromegaly (abnormal bone thickening), glucose intolerance, diabetes, and pathological changes in heart muscle.

human immunodeficiency virus (HIV) A virus transmitted sexually and by contact with infected blood or blood products. It is the virus responsible for AIDS, but many people carry the virus without developing AIDS. There is much concern about the risk of acquiring the virus in a sporting context. The risk is probably exceedingly small (much less than the risk of contracting hepatitis B), but several reports suggest that the virus might have been transmitted to athletes from contact with blood from opponents. It is important to maintain strict standards of hygiene on the sports field, and to give extra care when dealing with bleeding from wounds. It is unacceptable, for example, in football to use a communal bucket and sponge when treating an injured player. *See also* **acquired immune deficiency syndrome**.

humanistic Applied to beliefs which emphasize self and the power of individuals to realize their human potential.

human relations theory Theory of *leadership behaviour which focuses on the employee or, in a coach–athlete relationship, the athlete. It is consistent with the *consideration approach to leadership. *See also* **McGregor's theory X and McGregor's theory Y**.

human science model A theoretical approach to psychology based on the view that human psychological processes are qualitatively distinct from those of other forms of life. *Compare* **natural science model**.

humeroradial joint *See* **elbow joint**.

humeroulnar joint *See* **elbow joint**.

humidity The amount of water vapour in the atmosphere. It is usually expressed as either the absolute humidity (total mass of water vapour, kg or g, present in one cubic metre of atmosphere) or relative humidity (the ratio of the amount of water vapour in the atmosphere to the amount of water vapour required to fully saturate the same volume of atmosphere at the same temperature; it is usually given as a percentage). Generally in sport, relatively humidity is the more usual measurement because of its greater correlation with evaporation. Higher relative humidity decreases the capacity to lose heat by evaporation, the main avenue of heat loss during exercise.

humoral immune response Immunity provided by *antibodies present in blood plasma and other body fluids.

Humphrey's ligament A ligament connecting the posterior horn of the lateral meniscus (semi-lunar cartilage) in the knee to the femur. The fibres of this ligament are anterior to those of the posterior cruciate ligament.

hunchback *See* kyphosis.

hyaline cartilage Smooth, shiny *cartilage which covers the articular surfaces of bones. Hyaline cartilage contains whitish-blue elastic material with chondrocytes forming distinct cell nests, and a fine network of collagen fibres. Its smoothness reduces friction between opposing bones in a joint.

hyaluronic acid An acid mucopolysaccharide found in the *synovial fluid and nearly all types of connective tissue. Hyaluronic acid acts as a binding agent and affects the viscosity of the ground substance.

hyaluronidase An enzyme found in the testes, semen, and other tissues. Preparations of hyaluronidase have been used successfully to treat bruises.

hybrid system In cybernetics, a large control system that consists of smaller systems of various types. Most cyberneticians regard humans as such a hybrid.

hydrarthrosis A swelling in a joint, commonly the knee, caused by the accumulation of *synovial fluid.

hydrocollator (heating pad) A hot, moist pack used as a therapeutic aid in the treatment of *contusions, muscle sprains, and muscle spasms. A pack is heated to about 65 °C, placed in thick towels and applied to the injured region for 20–30 minutes per session. Care must be taken to prevent burning the skin. The pack has an *analgesic effect and increases surface circulation.

hydrocortisone (cortisol) The main *glucocorticoid hormone secreted by the adrenal cortex in response to intense exercise and *stress. It has a strong anti-inflammatory action and helps to regulate the metabolism of fats, carbohydrates, and proteins. It helps to make fuels more available for energy production by increasing *gluconeogenesis, the mobilization of free fatty acids, and the breakdown of proteins. Overtraining might impair cortisol levels and increase susceptibility to stress. Hydrocortisone is on the International Olympic Committee list of *banned substances. Its use in the treatment of Achilles

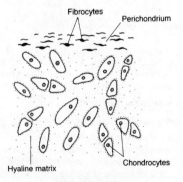

Fibrocytes Perichondrium

Hyaline matrix

Chondrocytes

hyaline cartilage

CH₂OH

hydrocortisone

tendinitis sometimes results in complete rupture of the tendon. There is also an increased risk of ligament rupture if heavy training or competition is carried out within 48 hours of pain-killing injections or a steroid injection. Steroids should never be injected directly into a tendon because this is likely to cause a rupture.

hydrodynamic drag force The drag force which resists the movement of a body through water.

hydrodynamic lift force A lift force developed in a liquid, especially water.

hydrodynamics The mathematical study of forces, energy, and pressure of liquids in motion. *Compare* **hydrostatics**.

hydrogen ion A positively charged hydrogen atom; a proton. Accumulation of hydrogen ions associated with lactic acid production during exercise changes the acid–base balance and contributes to fatigue.

hydrostatic pressure The pressure exerted by a liquid.

hydrostatics The mathematical study of forces and pressures of liquids at rest. *Compare* **hydrodynamics**.

hydrostatic weighing A technique used to estimate body volume. A person is weighed in air (normal scale weight) and then weighed when totally immersed in water (underwater weight). The difference between the scale weight and underwater weight is used to calculate body volume. In the calculation, the density of water and the gas trapped in the lungs is taken into account. *See also* **densitometry**.

hydrotherapy The use of water to treat disorders. Hydrotherapy has been used successfully to treat sprains, strains, contusions, tendinitis, and tenosynovitis. Water is also, often used as an exercise medium after surgery, immobilization, or illness (e.g., *chronic fatigue syndrome) to help athletes regain mobility and physical fitness. Because of the buoyancy provided by water, such exercises put less mechanical stress on the joints and bones than

land-based exercises. Usually low temperatures (8–12 °C) are used in the initial hydrotherapy of sports injuries because hot water may exacerbate bleeding.

hydroxyacyl coenzyme A dehydrogenase (3–hydroxyacyl coenzyme A dehydrogenase; HAD) An enzyme the level of which is commonly used in exercise physiology as a measure of the capacity for fat degradation (fatty acid oxidation).

hydroxyproline A chemical similar to an amino acid and found in connective tissue. An increase in urinary hydroxyproline is indicative of damage and breakdown of connective tissue.

hydroxytryptamine (5– hydroxytryptamine) *See* serotonin.

hydroxytryptophan *See* serotonin.

hygiene 1 The science of preserving health. **2** Clean or healthy practices. Personal and corporate hygiene are of considerable importance in sport to prevent the occurrence and spread of contagious disorders, such as *athlete's foot, *hepatitis, and *scrumpox, which can spread rapidly in communal changing facilities.

hygrometer An instrument for measuring the relative humidity of the atmosphere.

hyoid bone A small U-shaped bone in the neck which supports the tongue.

hyperaemia The presence of excess blood in a vessel or body-part. Hyperaemia may be caused by increased blood flow or blockage of the affected part.

hyperbaric bag A portable bag which produces a high-pressure environment, for example, around a mountaineer suffering from *high altitude cerebral oedema. *See also* Gamow bag.

hyperbaric environment An environment with a high atmospheric pressure, such as that underwater.

hyperbaric oxygen therapy A therapeutic procedure used to accelerate healing and enhance recovery from soft tissue injuries. Patients inspire pure oxygen while their whole bodies are subjected to a pressure greater than atmospheric pressure at sea level. The procedure has been used to treat leg injuries of professional footballers. Although its effectiveness has not been fully evaluated, hyperbaric oxygen therapy appears to accelerate recovery, especially if treatment is given within eight hours of the injury being sustained.

hypercapnia An abnormally high carbon dioxide concentration in the blood causing an overstimulation of the respiratory centres.

hypercholesteraemia An abnormally high *cholesterol level in the blood.

hyperextension Movement beyond the *anatomical position, in a direction opposite to flexion.

hyperextension test A diagnostic test for suspected spondylolysis. The patient stands on one leg and extends the spine. The test is positive if pain is felt on the weight-bearing side.

hyperextosis Excessive thickening of the outer layers of bone. *See also* **exostosis**.

hyperflexibility Excessive flexibility, either of one or a number of joints, resulting in joint laxity and an increased risk of dislocations. hyperflexibility of the lower limbs can lead to bow-legs (*see* **genu varum**) or knock knees (*see* **genu valgum**). It is sometimes due to abnormal development and ossification of bones, or, in young athletes, overtraining when the bones are still growing.

hyperglycaemia An abnormally high blood glucose level. It may occur as a result of an excessive dietary intake of carbohydrates or as a result of a disease, such as *diabetes mellitus.

hyperhidrosis Excessive sweating not directly related to exercise. It may be associated with a hot environment, wearing inappropriate clothing, fever, and certain hormonal conditions such as hyperactivity of the thyroid gland. Hyperhidrosis is not in itself a problem in sport as long as there is sufficient replacement of fluids. However, it can cause problems in gripping equipment, and may produce a moist environment for fungal infections of the skin.

hyperkinesis Condition characterized by excessive motor activity.

hyperlipaemia An abnormally high lipid concentration in the blood.

hyperlipoproteinaemia The presence of abnormally high levels of lipoproteins in the blood.

hypermetropia (far sighted; hyperopia; long sightedness) Eye defect resulting in light rays converging beyond the retina and an inability to focus on close objects.

hypermobile joint disease A condition in which the joints are excessively mobile ('double-jointed'). It may be congenital, but it also occurs in young athletes who do too much flexibility training. Some of these youngsters may suffer growing pains. In later life they may develop *osteoarthritis, joint pains, recurrent dislocations, and other musculoskeletal disorders.

hypermobility Excessive motion at a joint which lacks stability due to laxity of ligaments, muscles, or joint capsule.

hypernatremia An abnormally high sodium ion concentration in the blood (usually diagnosed as being greater that 150 mmol^{-1}). It may occur as a result of excessive sweating or inadequate fluid intake.

hypernoea A marked increase in pulmonary ventilation with both increased rate and depth of breathing that is related to increased levels of exercise or metabolism.

hyperopia *See* hypermetropia.

hyperplasia An increase in the number of cells. The number of muscle fibres within a particular muscle may increase by longitudinal splitting as a result of regular resistance training; this may contribute to an increase in muscle size. *See also* **hypertrophy**.

hyperpolarization A change in the potential difference (PD) across a cell surface membrane so that the PD becomes more negative than the normal resting potential (e.g., if the resting potential is -70 mV, hyperpolarization may change it to −80 mV). *See also* **after hyperpolarization**.

hyperpronation Excessive or prolonged *pronation of the foot during the support phase of running. Hyperpronation is indicated by excessive wear on the medial side of the heel of the shoes. Hyperpronation can increase the mechanical stress on the bones and tissues within the foot, and on the foot's extrinsic muscles. It often results in a compensatory increase in the internal rotation of the entire leg which exaggerates the twisting forces within the Achilles tendon and places abnormally high stress on the joint between the patella and the femur.

hyperreactivity A response, similar to an allergic reaction, to contact with an extremely small dose of an irritant substance.

hypersensitivity Abnormally high sensitivity, especially to a particular *antigen, which may result in conditions such as hay fever, asthma, or even *anaphylactic shock.

hypertension High blood pressure, both systolic and diastolic. In adults, blood pressure is abnormally high when the average of several supine measurements of systolic pressure is equal to or more than 140 mmHg, and the average of several measurements of diastolic pressure is equal to or more than 90 mmHg. Hypertension increases the risk of cardiovascular diseases and kidney failure because it adds to the workload of the heart, causing it to enlarge and, over time, to weaken; in addition it may damage the walls of the arteries. Arterial hypertension occurs in about 20 per cent of adults in western countries. Mild, regular aerobic exercise reduces the chances of developing hypertension and reduces blood pressure in those who have moderate hypertension, but seems to have little effect on those with severe hypertension.

hyperthermia An abnormally high body core temperature (more than 40 °C). *Compare* **hypothermia**. *See also* **heat stroke**.

hypertonic 1 Applied to muscles that are too tight. **2** Applied to a solution that tends to cause the volume of a cell to decrease. Thus the cell, when immersed in a hypertonic solution, tends to lose water and shrink. The term is applied to high-energy, concentrated drinks that have a higher total salt concentration than body fluids.

hypertrophic cardiomyopathy A structural abnormality of the heart in which the ventricular septum is uncharacteristically large. A person with hypertrophic cardiomyopathy (HCM) may not have any clear symptoms; about a half of those affected with HCM have a completely normal functional capacity when they take part in sport. However, the abnormality can stop the flow of blood from the left ventricle, with fatal consequences. HCM is a major contributory factor to sudden death in young sportspeople. Anybody with HCM should avoid all moderate or vigorous forms of physical activity. In most cases, HCM is a genetically transmitted disorder, so that anyone with a family history of the disease should be screened before participation in sport. *See also* **athlete's heart**.

hypertrophy An increase in the size of a tissue or organ due to growth of individual cells without an increase in the number of cells. Chronic hypertrophy of a muscle refers to a relatively permanent increase in its size, in contrast to temporary increases (transient hypertrophy) due, for example, to *muscle pumping. Chronic hypertrophy results from resistance training that is repeated over a long period whereas muscle pumping occurs during a single exercise bout. *See also* **hyperplasia**.

hyperventilation Excessive ventilation of the lungs caused by increased depth and frequency of breathing. It can occur voluntarily or as a result of impaired gas exchange in the lungs. It is also an important response to low partial pressures of oxygen at high altitudes. Voluntary hyperventilation helps eliminate carbon dioxide from the blood and reduces the main stimulus to breathe. It may provide a small advantage where a short burst of activity is needed (e.g., during a sprint) as more carbon dioxide is removed from the alveoli, possibly allowing more oxygen to combine with haemoglobin (*see* **Bohr shift**). However, hyperventilation is dangerous prior to underwater swimming because it may cause fainting. *See also* **alkalosis**; and **Valsalva's manoeuvre**.

hypervitaminosis A condition caused by the intake of excessive quantities of certain vitamins, such as the fat soluble vitamins A and D.

hypervolemia An increased volume of circulating blood.

hyphaema Bleeding in the anterior chamber of the eye. In sport, it is usually caused by trauma with a blunt object (e.g., elbow). *See also* **eye injuries**.

hypnosis An artificially induced, trance-like mental state in which the subject is more than usually receptive to suggestions. Hypnosis has been used in sport as a relaxation strategy in stress management and in dealing with various psychological problems, such as phobias. Hypnosis has also been used as an intervention strategy to improve the self-confidence of boxers. *See also* **autogenic training**; **posthypnotic suggestion**.

hypnotic 1 Pertaining to hypnosis. **2** Applied to a sedative drug; a sleeping pill.

hypobaric environment An environment with a low atmospheric pressure, such as that at high altitude.

hypocapnia A condition in which there is a deficiency of carbon dioxide in the blood, for example, after hyperventilation.

hypodermis (superficial fascia) Tissue lying immediately beneath the skin. The hypodermis is made of loose *connective tissue, containing areolar and adipose tissue. It anchors the skin to the underlying organs.

hypoflexibility A condition in which joint mobility is less than normal due, for example, to joint stiffness. Hypoflexibility may increase the risk of injuries such as *sprains and *strains.

hypoglycaemia Abnormally low blood glucose concentration. It causes loss of coordination, muscle weakness, sweating, and mental confusion. Severe hypoglycaemia is rare and dangerous; it may lead to a coma. It may be the result of severe physical exhaustion or an intake of medicines such as insulin. Diabetics are particularly prone to hypoglycaemia which is rapidly relieved by the administration of glucose. A form of hypoglycaemia called post-exercise delayed-onset hypoglycaemia, can occur in diabetics several hours or a full day after a bout of intense exercise. The exercise may increase the diabetic's sensitivity to insulin and deplete the muscle of glycogen stores which are replenished from glucose in the general circulation. This type of hypoglycaemia can be prevented by reducing pre-exercise insulin, and increasing pre-exercise and post-exercise carbohydrate intake. It is important that all diabetic athletes monitor their post-exercise blood glucose levels frequently.

hypohidrosis Abnormally low sweating rate.

hypokalaemia A condition characterized by a profound lowering of potassium levels in the blood and extracellular fluid. It may occur after repeated use of *diuretics or after severe dehydration.

hypokinesis Lack of, or insufficient, regular exercise and movement of the body. *See also* **hypokinetic disease**.

hypokinetic disease A disease brought on, at least in part, by insufficient movement and exercise. Hypokinesis has been identified as an independent risk factor for the origin and progression of several widespread, chronic diseases, including coronary heart disease, diabetes, obesity, and lower back pain.

hyponatremia Abnormally low concentration of sodium ions in the blood plasma (less than the normal range of 136 to 143 mmol l^{-1}. It may be caused by drinking too much water, particularly after excessive sweating. Symptoms of hyponatraemia include muscle weakness, disorientation, and seizures that may lead to a coma.

hypopnoea Condition in which the depth of breathing is shallow.

hyposensitization A method of reducing sensitivity to an allergen. *See also* **desensitization**.

hypotension An abnormally low arterial blood pressure. It occurs after excessive fluid losses and bleeding. *See also* **orthostatic hypotension**.

hypothalamus A small portion of the brain derived from the sides and floor of the forebrain. It is the main visceral control centre and is vitally important for *homeostasis. It regulates the activity of the *autonomic nervous system and a number of endocrine glands. It also contains centres of *thermoregulation, ionic regulation, and osmoregulation. The hypothalamus is involved in many other autonomic functions, including the control of thirst, sleep, and hunger. It plays a role in regulating the metabolism of fats, carbohydrates, and proteins, and is also concerned with motivation and emotions.

hypothermia An abnormally low body core temperature resulting in a rapid and progressive mental and physical collapse. When the core temperature goes below 34.5 °C, the body loses its ability to regulate temperature. Hypothermia is usually caused by prolonged exposure to cold, especially in wet and windy conditions when a person is suffering from physical exhaustion and lack of food. Immersion in water at temperatures below 32 °C, results in hypothermia developing at a rate proportional to either the duration of exposure or the temperature gradient. Sufferers have a weak pulse because heart rate and cardiac output are reduced. They often become irrational and slow to respond. They are cold to touch, and have speech and visual difficulties. Treatment of mild hypothermia includes warming in a controlled manner with warm blankets or a warm bath. Application of external heat direct to the body surface, enforced exercise, rubbing the skin, or taking alcohol can be dangerous because they can result in further heat losses. Severe hypothermia requires expert medical attention; it can be fatal if not treated properly.

hypothesis A conjectured statement which implies or states a relationship between two or more variables. A hypothesis is usually formed from facts already known or research already carried out and is expressed in such a way that it can be tested or appraised as a generalization about a phenomenon. *See also* **experimental hypothesis; Null hypothesis**.

hypotonia A condition characterized by deficient muscle tone.

hypotonic 1 Applied to an external fluid which causes cells to increase in volume. **2** Applied to sports drinks which have a salt concentration less than that of the body fluids. **3** Applied to conditions below normal tension or tone.

hypoventilation Reduced ventilation of the lungs due to reduced breathing-rate and *tidal volume.

hypovitaminosis A deficiency of vitamins which may result from lack of dietary vitamins or an inability to absorb vitamins from food in the alimentary canal.

hypoxaemia Deficient oxygen-content of the blood.

hypoxia A condition in which there is an inadequate supply of oxygen to respiring tissues.

hypoxic vasoconstriction Constriction of the blood vessels in response to low blood oxygen levels. Hypoxic vasoconstriction occurs in the lungs at high altitude, contributing to *pulmonary hypertension.

hysteria 1 A temporary state of tension or over-excitement in which there is loss of control over emotions. **2** A neurotic condition marked by emotional instability which may be converted into physical symptoms such as paralysis of an arm or leg.

H-zone The area in the middle of a muscle *sarcomere where actin and myosin filaments do not overlap; it contains myosin filaments only.

iatrogenic to IU

iatrogenic Applied to a disorder or disease caused by surgical or medical treatment, including the side-effects of drugs prescribed or administered inappropriately.

I-band A zone bisected by the *z-line within a *sarcomere of a muscle fibre. The I-band contains the contractile protein, *actin.

ibuprofen An *analgesic drug derived from propionic acid. Ibuprofen is commonly used in sport as a nonsteroidal anti-inflammatory drug (NSAID) to reduce swelling and pain, and accelerate recovery from soft tissue injuries. Its use is allowed by the International Olympic Committee (IOC) medical commission.

ICE *See* **RICE.**

iceberg profile The expected psychological profile of an élite athlete incorporating the six factors measured by *Profile Of Mood States in which the élite athlete scores low on all mood states except vigour. *See also* **gravitational hypothesis**; and **mental health model.**

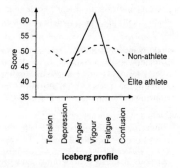

iceberg profile

ice massage *See* ice treatment.

ice treatment The most common form of cold therapy for the initial treatment of most sports injuries (especially contusions, sprains, and strains). Ice reduces swelling and internal bleeding, reduces the metabolism of injured tissue, and decreases the activity of pain receptors. Generally, the ice is applied for at least the first 24–48 hours after the injury, for periods no longer than 20 minutes and with intervals of at least 30 minutes between applications. Evidence now suggests that intermittent icing for up to seven days may be beneficial, particularly for severe bruises. There are many ways of applying the ice, but usually it is wrapped in a wet towel; if ice is applied directly to the skin, there is a risk of ice burns on the tissue or damage to superficial nerves. A very popular method of ice treatment is ice massage using a styrofoam cup. Water is frozen in the cup which is torn halfway down to expose the ice. The remaining styrofoam portion is used to hold the ice so that the injury can be ice massaged with gentle circular movements. The ice is held against a single position for no longer than 90 seconds. The total massage lasts about 5–10 minutes depending on the size of the injury and cold tolerance of the patient (thin athletes with little adipose tissue generally require less treatment time than fatter athletes). Usually, ice treatment is combined with compression and elevation (*see* **RICE**).

id One of the three elements of personality proposed by Freud (*see* **Freudian theory**). The id is the unconscious part of the mind and the basis of *personality, containing all the inherited resources, especially instincts. It has been referred to as 'the deepest part of the psyche'. It is from the id that the other two elements, the *ego and *superego, develop.

ideal Pertaining to a highly desirable and possible state of affairs.

idealization The representation of a general or particular phenomenon by, or, in accordance with our desires or ideals.

ideal model A hypothetical description of how an ideal performance can be attained by a particular individual. During coaching, an ideal model can be used as a standard against which the actual performance of an athlete can be compared. It is assumed that learning takes place as the performance of the skill more closely approximates to that of the ideal model. It is generally agreed that, if there is to be effective communication and good interpersonal relations, the ideal model must be formulated by both coach and athlete.

ideal performance (peak performance) The best performance an athlete can achieve on a specific occasion.

ideal performance feeling (IPF) A feeling created by an ideal performance. Conversely, an ideal performance feeling achieved prior to a competition (for example, by mentally repeating a successful performance) can help an athlete achieve an ideal performance during the competition.

ideal performance state (IPS) A mental state associated with a peak or *ideal performance. Typical features of the IPS include a trance-like state of consciousness, similar to hypnosis; selective or even total amnaesia; increased tolerance to pain; more intensive concentration on relevant stimuli; and a general inattentiveness to irrelevant stimuli. *See also* **peak experience**.

ideal self A concept of self which refers to the person one would like to be. The ideal self is usually based on moral principles acquired from significant others, especially family.

ideal type A representation of a phenomenon in its abstract or pure form.

ideal weight In medicine, the recommended body weight for good health and maximum life expectancy, usually expressed as a weight range based on height, body build, sex, and age. In insurance tables, it often refers to the average, but not necessarily the most desirable, weight for persons of a given height and sex.

identical-elements theory Theory which posits that transfer of learning between two tasks increases with the similarity between components of the tasks.

identification 1 The process of modelling one's behaviour after another individual, usually an older person. **2** A form of direct motivation used by a coach. It involves disguised *compliance. For example, a coach using identification may say to the athlete 'if you care about the team, you will do this for me'. Successful use of identification depends on a positive relationship between a coach and athlete in which the athlete wishes to please the coach.

identity The perception of self that develops as a child differentiates from parents and family and takes a place in society. *Play is regarded as an important element in the formation of identity.

identity crisis A condition which occurs when a person experiences great difficulties in acquiring a clear perception of self. It occurs especially with a young person who urgently seeks greater self understanding, or when a person undergoes psychological turmoil in attempting to formulate a *self-concept and decide upon future goals.

ideomotor training A term often used interchangeably with *mental practice and *imagery.

idioculture 1 A group, such as a sports team, that creates norms and behaviour patterns (for example, nicknames and rituals) that are different from those in the subculture of which it is a part. **2** The culture of a small group, such as a sports team. The idioculture consists of a system of knowledge, beliefs, behaviours, and customs shared by members of the group.

idiographic An approach to social enquiry which focuses on cultural and historical particulars rather than generalities. Methods, such as ethnography and biography are used to study individual and unique experiences.

idiopathic Applied to a disease or condition the cause of which is not known.

idiosyncrasy An unusual or unexpected sensitivity exhibited by an individual to a particular food or drug. Idiosyncrasy is usually determined genetically and it may be due to a biological deficiency (e.g., an inability to metabolize a drug).

IGF *See* **insulin-like growth factor**.

ileum Part of the alimentary canal between the duodenum and colon, in which food is absorbed and digestion completed.

iliac Pertaining to the *ilium.

iliac crest Thickened superior margin of the *ilium which terminates in the iliac spine; it forms an attachment point for muscles of the trunk, hip, and thigh. It is the part of the upper part of the pelvic girdle which you can feel either side of the waist.

iliacitis Inflammation of the iliac.

iliacus The large fan-shaped thigh muscle that has its origin on the iliac fossa and adjacent sacrum in the pelvis, crosses the hip, and inserts on the lesser trochanter of the femur. It works in close association with the *psoas major. Its primary action is flexion of the femur.

iliocostalis (sacropinalis) A lateral member of the *erector spinae group of muscles. The iliocostalis extends from the pelvis to the neck and divides into three regional parts: the iliocostalis lumborum, iliocostalis thoracis, and the iliocostalis cervicis. Its origins are on the *iliac crest and thoracic ribs. The insertions are on the ribs. The iliocostalis extends the vertebral column and helps to maintain an erect posture. When acting unilaterally, it bends the vertebral column sideways.

iliocastrale An anatomical landmark at the most lateral point of the iliac crest.

iliopsoas A composite of two closely related thigh muscles, the *iliacus and *psoas major, which share a common insertion on the lesser trochanter of the femur. It is a major hip flexor.

iliopsoas tendinitis Inflammation at the junction between the *iliopsoas and its tendon which inserts onto the femur. It is characterized by groin pain when attempts are made to raise the knee to the chest. The inflammation is caused by repeated hip flexion (e.g., doing a large number of squats during weight-training or repeatedly kicking a ball). Initial treatment involves replacing the precipitating activity with one that does not cause groin pain. Anti-inflammtories may be prescribed and, if the tendinitis is severe, a physician may administer a steroid. *See also* **bowler's hip**.

iliospinale An anatomical landmark on the inferior aspect of the tip of the anterior superior iliac spine. It is sometimes referred to inexactly as the spinale.

iliotibial band (iliotibial tract) Thickened portion of the *fascia lata that runs down the lateral aspect of the thigh. It extends from the iliac crest to the tibia, helping to stabilize the knee.

iliotibial band friction syndrome A condition that includes inflammation of the iliotibial band caused by friction of the band against the outer part of the knee joint. It is often associated with an overtight iliotibial band commonly found in patients with anatomical abnormalities, such as genu varum (bow legs). It is also common in long-distance runners who overpronate the foot and who run on heavily cambered roads. The syndrome is characterized by pain and tightness on the outside of the knee when running downhill or walking downstairs. The pain usually subsides when activity stops (*see* **Noble test**; and **Ober's test**). Iliotibial band friction syndrome can be notoriously difficult to resolve. Conservative treatment includes rest from the precipitating activity and correcting biomechanical or anatomical faults, ice treatment, and nonsteroidal anti-inflammatories. Steroid injections and surgery are used only when other treatment fails. Exercises which stretch the iliotibial band are an important part of successful rehabilitation.

iliotibial tract *See* **iliotibial band**.

ilium A large, flaring bone which forms the upper part of each side of the hip bone. The two ilium bones are separate in children but become fused in adults.

illogical model A model used in *attribution theory which is based on evidence that people are not always logical in making causal attributions but often make blatantly self-serving ones which are ego-enhancing or ego-protecting. *Compare* **logical model**.

illusion 1 A sensory perception considered as mistaken because it does not conform with an objective representation of a physical form or pattern. **2** A subjective falsification of past experience.

imagery A psychological technique involving the production of vivid mental experiences by the normal processes of thought. In sport, imagery is an extremely versatile technique used to learn and practise skills; to improve self-confidence; to acquire the right frame of mind before competition; to promote relaxation and recovery after competition; and to accelerate rehabilitation after an injury. Imagery is a purely mental process. Through imagery, an athlete recreates past positive experiences or creates new experiences without receiving any external stimuli or producing any overt body movements. Imagery can involve any sensory experience. In practising a skill, for example, imagery is especially effective if the athlete imagines the auditory, olfactory, tactile, and kinaesthetic sensations associated with performing the skill well.

imagery orientation The perspective of *imagery; that is, whether it is external or internal. *See also* **external imagery**; and **internal imagery**.

imagery rehabilitation Use of imagery to accelerate recovery from a sports injury. Imagery rehabilitation can be used to help an athlete recover mentally from a traumatic incident. For example, a cyclist injured in a crash might imagine riding a bike again before actually getting on it, so that anxiety associated with the memory of the crash can be reduced. Imagery rehabilitation can also be used to accelerate the physical healing process. An injured athlete could use internal imagery to imagine, for example, blood flowing to an injured knee, bathing it with the nutrients and warmth required for healing.

imagery relaxation A relaxation procedure which involves athletes imagining themselves in some environment or place where they always feel relaxed and comfortable. For example, Jackie Stewart, ex-world champion formula 1 racing driver, used to sit in his car moments before a race and imagine his body inflating like a balloon. Then he would let the air out and feel himself relax. This, he contended, helped him prepare physically and mentally for a race. Imagery relaxation is often part of flotation therapy. It is a form of *somatic stress management.

imbalance Lack of balance, for example, between antagonistic pairs of muscles, between water and electrolyte, or between the components of a diet.

immersion injury An injury caused by falling or jumping into very cold water. Sudden immersion into freezing or near freezing water can be fatal. Very cold water in the ears and/or nose can cause a vagal reflex with instantaneous cardiac and respiratory arrest.

immobilization Restriction of movement of a joint or bone by taping (strapping), splinting, or casting. Some forms of localized immobilization restrict joint movement in one plane but allow movement in other planes; a stirrup splint around a sprained ankle protects the ankle from lateral displacements, but allows it to move up and down. Prolonged immobilization can delay rehabilitation of sports injuries. Muscles may lose up to 20 per cent of their strength per week of immobilization, and joints may become chronically stiff. Many sports doctors promote early mobilization (*see* **aggressive rehabilitation**).

immune response A host reaction in response to foreign antigens. It involves the formation of antibodies by B-cell lymphocytes, or a cell-mediated response from T-cells.

immunity The ability of the body to resist many agents (both living and nonliving) that can cause disease; resistance to disease. Immunity is provided by antibodies and white blood cells (*see* **leucocyte**).

immunization The process of conferring *immunity by artificial means. Passive immunity may be conferred by the injection of antiserum. Active immunity is conferred by the administration, orally or by injection, of antigens in the form of a vaccine which promotes the production of antibodies. The vaccine may consist of dead or inactivated bacteria or viruses, or their toxins, which trigger the production of antibodies to a specific disease so that the individual is immune to it. All athletes should be immunized against tetanus, especially those who take part in activities in the countryside or on fields used by farm animals. All athletes travelling abroad should seek medical advice about the immunization they need, and the effects that this immunization is likely to have on their training and competition.

immunocompetence The ability of lymphocytes to recognize and deal effectively with specific antigens. Moderate exercise is thought to improve immunocompetence.

immunodeficiency disease Disease resulting from the deficient production or function of lymphocytes or certain molecules required for natural immunity.

immunogen Foreign substance which stimulates an immune response.

immunoglobulin A protein in the blood (e.g., gamma-globulin) which possess antibody activity. Immunoglobulin is an important part of the body's immune system. *See also* **salivary Immunoglobulin A**.

immunology The study of immunity and all the defence mechanisms of the body against disease and infection.

immunosuppression A reduction in the ability of the immune system to deal with infection. Strenuous exercise is thought to increase immunosuppression and the risk of infection. Immunosuppression during overtraining is indicated by raised serum cortisol concentrations, low serum glutamine concentrations, and low salivary immunoglubulin IgA.

impact The collision of two bodies characterized by the exchange of a large force or forces during a small time interval.

impacted fracture Fracture in which the opposite sides of the broken bone are compressed together. Impacted fractures are commonly associated with hip fractures, and with fractures which occur when a person attempts to break a fall with outstretched arms.

impact force (contact force) A force which reaches its maximum value earlier than 50 milliseconds after the first contact between two bodies. An impact force occurs during the take-off and landing phases of jumps; for example, when a long-jumper strikes the take-off board, the contact time is about 100 ms with the first 20–30 ms being the duration of the impact force. *Compare* **active force**. *See also* **coefficient of restitution**.

impact, Newton's law of A law formulated by Sir Isaac Newton (1642–1727) after his studies of the impact between elastic bodies. He observed that if two bodies move towards each other along the same straight line, the difference between their velocities immediately after impact has a constant relationship with the difference between their velocities at the moment of impact: $(v_1 - v_2)(u_1 - u_2) = -e$, where e is the coefficient of restitution, v_1 and v_2 are the velocities of the two bodies immediately after impact, and u_1 and u_2 are the velocities of the two bodies immediately before impact.

imperial unit A system of units based on the pound, yard, and gallon. It has been replaced by SI units for most scientific purposes.

impetigo A skin disorder caused primarily by the bacterium *Staphyllococcus aureus* or a streptococcus which infects a minor skin trauma, such as an abrasion. It is characterized by small pus-filled blisters and fever. It is extremely contagious and should preclude participation in all contact or collision sports until the lesions are dry. It is treated with a systemic antibiotic.

impingement Trapping of soft tissues, e.g., a nerve.

impingement exostosis A benign bony outgrowth where the surfaces of two bones rub against each other in a joint (*see* **footballer's ankle**).

impingement sign An indicator of an *impingement syndrome of the shoulder. An intense pain is felt when the patient's arm is held straight out in front and pushed upwards (i.e. when the greater tuberosity of the humerus is pushed upwards against the inferior aspect of the acromion process of the scapula).

impingement syndrome An overuse injury characterized by a number of symptoms and signs caused by repetitive pinching of soft tissue by bones in a joint, for example, the shoulder (*see* **shoulder impingement syndrome**), ankle (*see* **footballer's ankle**), and elbow.

impression management A person's management of his or her own behaviour and social actions so that the impressions he or she conveys to others can be controlled. The aim of impression management is for the person (e.g., a coach or team manager) to present himself or herself in a generally favourable way which is appropriate to the social setting, and it often involves the person adopting a particular role.

imprinting A form of *learning which occurs in young animals, usually during a critical, sensitive period of their lives. During imprinting, a young animal learns to direct some of its social responses to a particular object, usually a parent.

impulse In a human movement, the impulse of force is the area under a force–time curve which represents the amount of force applied to a bone at each moment of an action. For a constant force, impulse is the product of force and the time over which the force acts (impulse = force × time); for a variable force, the impulse is the integral of the force with respect to time. In either case, the impulse of an object is equal to the change in momentum that is produced by it, and the longer the time a force is applied to an object the greater the change in the object's momentum. Techniques have been developed in athletic throwing events to extend the length of time a thrower can apply a force to a projectile and thereby increase its change in momentum (*see* **O'Brien technique**). Athletic movements are often analysed in terms of two types of impulse: controlled impulse and transmitted impulse. A controlled impulse is due to direct muscle effort and joint leverage, as with the driving leg during a sprint start. A transmitted impulse occurs when, for example, a high jumper is about to take off. The take-off leg braces itself against the ground, but the magnitude and direction of impulse is determined by the free arms and leg, and not through the take-off leg.

impulse–momentum relationship An important relationship between *impulse and *momentum derived from Newton's second law, which shows that the impulse of force is equal to the change in momentum that it produces. It is basic to an understanding of many sports techniques, including starting in track and swimming events.

impulse-timing model A model of the control of limb movement which suggests that *motor programs time the onset, duration, and amount of electrical activity delivered to a muscle, thereby controlling the *impulse of forces from the muscles. Since the pattern of limb movement can be determined by the amount and duration of the forces applied to it, the impulse-timing model is viewed as one way in which the trajectory of the limb can be controlled.

impulse-variability theory A theory applied to simple, rapid aiming movements in which the variability of the impulse of forces leads directly to variations in the movement end-point of a limb. The impulse-variability theory maintains that as the distance from a target increases, more force must be exerted, leading to a greater variability in movement trajectory, decreasing the chances of hitting the target. To compensate for this, the movement time can be slowed down.

impulsion A motion produced by an *impulse.

inborn motivation (primary motivation) *Motivation which is part of an individual's inheritance, such as the need for food and drink, and rest. *Compare* **acquired motivation**.

incentive A more or less extrinsic motive for acting in a certain way. Incentives often act in addition to other motives. An incentive strengthens a drive towards an end or objective, such as food, drink, or money, by attaching additional values to that objective.

inch An imperial unit, equal to 0.0254 m.

incidental learning Learning without making a direct attempt to learn. Sometimes referred to as passive learning. *See also* **short term memory**.

included joint angle The smaller of the two relevant angles between two segments defining a joint.

incommensurability A relationship between two characteristics or two phenomena which cannot be directly compared in terms of the same unit, standard, or scale. Incommensurability applies especially to the relationship between two scientific theories which cannot be compared directly because of the nature of their different propositions or content.

incomplete protein Applied to a food that may be protein-rich, but which lacks one or more essential amino acids. Cereals, for example, are low in lysine, and leafy vegetables are low in methionine, but a well-balanced vegetarian diet containing cereals and leafy vegetables can provide all the essential amino acids.

increasing intensity test Test of *aerobic fitness in which the subject performs successive phases of activity at an increasing intensity with rest periods between one phase and the next.

incremental run A run which increases in intensity at predetermined fixed levels. Incremental runs are performed on treadmills as part of fitness tests and for determining aerobic capacity.

independent variable Variable which is manipulated, sometimes experimentally, in order to observe its effects on a dependent variable. For example, in a study of the effects of age on sports participation, age is the independent variable and sports participation the dependent variable.

indexicality The use of a word or expression which makes sense only from the immediate context of its use. Indexicality is an important feature of many explanations made by social *actors of social events.

index of difficulty A measurement of the theoretical difficulty of performing an aiming movement. It is based on *Fitt's law, and is expressed as $\log_2(2A/W)$, where A is the amplitude of the movement required and W is the width of the target. It indicates that the difficulty of a movement is jointly related to the distance a limb moves and the narrowness of the target at which it is aimed.

indication In medicine, a strong reason for believing that a particular course of treatment is desirable. *Compare* **contraindicated procedure**.

indirect calorimetry A method of estimating energy expenditure by measuring respiratory gases. Oxygen consumption and carbon dioxide release is measured (*see* **open circuit spirometry**; and **closed-circuit spirometry**) and the *Respiratory Exchange Ratio (RER) calculated to establish which type of food is being oxidized. It is assumed that each food type liberates a given amount of energy for each litre of oxygen consumed, and that the body's oxygen and carbon dioxide content remain constant. Total energy expenditure is estimated from the RER and total oxygen consumption.

indirect competition Competition against a standard rather than directly against other people. An individual strives to better an objective mark such as a record, a personal best, or climb a mountain. *See also* **parallel competition**.

indirect measure In sports psychology, a measurement in which individuals are asked indirect question. For example, in the assessment of *team cohesion, team members are asked questions about other team members, but not specifically about cohesion. *Compare* **direct measure**.

indirect motivation An alteration of the situation or environment, either psychological or physical, to enhance *motivation. Indirect motivation includes changing the location of practice and changing training partners.

indirect ossification Development of a bone by the transformation of fetal cartilage into bony material. After birth, the growth areas of the bone are confined to *epiphyseal plates of cartilage which generate new cells. At maturity, the plates themselves become ossified and the bone can no longer grow in length.

indirect trauma An injury which is not the result of a direct blow. *See also* **overuse injury**.

indisposition A deterioration in performance which may be caused by psychological factors (e.g., worry) or transitory physiological factors (e.g., muscle soreness) lasting a few hours or days. Indisposition may or may not be associated with *overtraining. It is a manifestation of *rundown.

individual attraction A factor which personally attracts an individual to a group, team, or another individual. Analysis of individual attractions take into account how team members feel about each other and the quality of team mate interaction. *See also* **conceptual model of team cohesion**.

individual differences Stable deviations of individuals from the average or from each other on some task or behaviour. The study of individual differences examines the factors that make individuals different from each other.

individual differences principle of training *See* **principle of individuality**.

individual differences scaling analysis (INDSCAL) A multi-dimensional form of *scaling analysis which allows the investigator to interpret how the characteristics of individuals and situations interact to determine behaviour.

individual differences theory A theory of mass communication which proposes that individuals respond differently to the *mass media according to their psychological needs, and that individuals consume the mass media to satisfy those needs. The need may be informational (e.g., providing statistics about players and teams), integrative (offering a sense of belonging to a group of similarly interested people), affective (e.g., by providing excitement), or escapist (helping to release pent-up emotions). *Compare* **social categories theory**.

individual difference variable (organismic variable) A variable peculiar to an individual which can be studied to see if it affects the performance of the individual. Individual difference variables are usually definable traits that can be measured, such as age, height, weight, sex, skin colour, etc.

individualism Any social doctrine which advocates the autonomy of the individual in social actions and social affairs. Advocates of individualism in sport emphasize the importance of allowing the free expression of an individual's skills. In many sports there is a tension between individualism and collectivism.

individualistic social situation A situation in which there is no correlation between the goal attainments of the participants. *Compare* **cooperative social situation**; and **competitive social situation**.

individual motive A motive which originates in unique individual experiences as contrasted with those that are inborn and those that are learned by most members of a particular culture.

indolamines A subclass of biogenic amines which can act as neurotransmitters. They include *serotonin and *histamine.

indomethacin A very effective nonsteroidal anti-inflammatory drug, used to treat soft-tissue sports injuries. However, side-effects of indomethacin include headaches, dizziness, and gastric inflammation.

INDSCAL *See* **individual differences scaling analysis**.

induction A process of reasoning in which a general statement suggesting a regular association between two or more variables is derived from a series of specific empirical observations.

induction time The time interval between the administration of a drug and manifestation of its effects.

inertia The tendency of a body to preserve its state of rest or uniform motion in a straight line. Inertia has no units of measurement, but the amount of inertia a body has is proportional to its mass. The more massive an object, the more it resists any change in its state of motion, whether motionless or moving with a constant velocity.

inertia, law of Newton's first law of motion which states that an object at rest tends to remain at rest unless acted on by an external force. Also, an object in motion tends to remain in motion and travel in a straight line with uniform velocity unless acted on by an external force.

inertial movement A form of passive movement, such as sliding into a base during a baseball run, in which there is a continuation of a previous movement but there is no concurrent propulsive force provided by muscle action. Inertial movements are affected by decelerating forces such as air resistance and tissue viscosity.

infarct A small localized region of dead, deteriorating tissue resulting from lack of blood supply.

infarction Formation of an *infarct. *See also* **myocardial infarction**.

infection 1 The process by which a disease is communicated from one person to another. **2** A disease which can be transmitted from one person to another. Such diseases always involve a microorganism, such as a virus, bacterium, or fungus which has a high capacity for reproduction (*compare* **infestation**). Sport offers many opportunities for the epidemic spread of infections due to the close contact of both spectators and performers. Contact and collision sports are notorious for spreading highly contagious infections, such as *scrumpox. Athletes with contagious infections should be precluded from participation in these sports, and all athletes should avoid very strenuous physical activity during the febrile stage of an infection. Although moderate exercise may stimulate the body's immune system and offer some protection from infection, overtraining is associated with an increased incidence of infections such as colds, sore throats, and influenza-like illnesses.

infectious mononucleosis An acute communicable viral disease that is an important and common infection in athletes, affecting mainly adolescents and young adults. The virus is transmitted by direct contact, airborne droplets, or shared utensils. The infection causes fatigue, sore throat, fever, liver disorder, and swollen lymph glands. A common complication is an enlarged spleen which can be ruptured easily by a blow to the abdomen. Owing to the symptoms, athletes are usually unable to train during the early stage of the infection, but, because of the high risk of splenic rupture, strenuous exercise and alcohol consumption should be avoided for the first months following infection. Participation in contact or collision sports should be resumed only if the spleen is not enlarged.

inference A guess or judgement derived by deduction or induction from certain data. *See also* **hypothesis**.

inferential statistics Complex statistical techniques used to infer cause and effect and to determine the degree to which the findings of a sample can be generalized to a larger population. For example, in a study of the effect of a pre-match pep-talk on performance, a researcher may design a study with appropriate control groups and use an appropriate statistical analysis to see if a significant difference occurs between the test and control groups. If a significant difference exists, the researcher would infer that the pre-match talk caused the effect. *Compare* **descriptive statistics**.

inferior (caudal) Pertaining to the lower or under part of a body structure.

inferiority complex A psychological disorder that may manifest itself during *achievement situations. The complex results from a conflict between a desire to seek self-recognition in the situation and the desire to avoid the feelings of humiliation frequently experienced in similar situations in the past. The disorder is characterized by compensatory behaviour such as aggressiveness and withdrawal.

inferiority feelings Feelings of worthlessness and inability to cope with situations. The individual usually has difficulty accepting the inferiority which may be real or implied.

infertility Inability of a woman to conceive or of a man to induce conception. Strenuous regular physical activity of more than 1 hour each day may be a factor contributing to the infertility of some women since such activity can disrupt menstruation (*see* **amenorrhoea**) and it may even prevent ovulation in some women. The abuse of certain drugs as *ergogenic substances may also lead to infertility. For example, anabolic steroids can cause testicular atrophy which may lead to infertility because of lack of sperm. Usually, this situation is resolved after withdrawal of the drugs, but the sperm count may remain abnormally low for 12–24 months.

infestation The presence of animal parasites such as fleas, mites, and tapeworms on the skin or in the body, or in the clothing or the home. *Compare* **infection**.

inflammation (inflammatory response) Nonspecific defensive response of tissues to a physical or chemical injury, or bacterial infection. The response includes dilation (widening) of blood vessels and an increase in vessel permeability, and is indicated by redness, heat, swelling, pain, and dysfunction. Inflammation destroys, dilutes, or isolates the injurious agent and the injured tissue. Nonsteroidal anti-inflammatories are often used to alleviate the symptoms and localize the inflammatory response. Some physical therapies (e.g., ultrasound) actually accelerate the inflammatory response, stimulating the activity of mast cells (large cells in connective tissue which produce inflammatory chemicals) and accelerating the normal repair process. Chronic inflammatory conditions caused by overuse injuries can be self-perpetuating and require strong anti-inflammatories (e.g., steroid injections) to resolve them.

inflammatory response *See* **inflammation**.

influence system An approach to *leadership in which influence or power between coach and athlete flows both ways. Coaches adopting such a system recognize the importance of interaction between themselves, the team, and the specific situation they are in. *Compare* **power system**.

information 1 Any unit of data or knowledge. **2** The content of a message that serves to reduce uncertainty. **3** In the information processing model or theory of behaviour, the data to which a person reacts, and which precipitates behaviour in a particular situation. *See also* **bit**.

information aspect In *cognitive evaluation theory, the extent to which extrinsic rewards provide positive feedback about an outcome and thereby increase *intrinsic motivation by enhancing feelings of competence. According to cognitive evaluation theory, people are intrinsically motivated to perform activities that make them feel competent. If a reward, such as 'best player' award, makes an individual feel more competent, it will increase intrinsic motivation. *Compare* **controlling aspect**.

information dependence Social situation occurring within a group, team, or dyad when knowledge from another person is needed by a performer to achieve some goal. *Compare* **performance dependence**.

information processing The storing and handling of information within a system as in a computer or a human being. In humans, the main processes involved include perception, memory, reasoning, and other forms of thinking.

information processing theory A theory which views humans as information processing systems which take in information from the *environment, process it, and then output information to the environment in the form of movement. The theory is based on the proposition that humans process the information they receive rather than merely responding to stimuli. Many cognitive processes are involved between the reception of a stimulus and the response of the individual, these include sensory input, perception, and the storage and retrieval of information. *See also* **black box model**.

information theory A branch of cybernetics (*see* **negative feedback**) that attempts to define the amount of information required to control a process of given complexity. The theory has been used in the study of learning processes and acquisition of skill. One of its most valuable contributions has been in the analysis of the processes associated with selection, perception, memory, and decision making in skilled performances.

infrared interactance A technique used to measure body composition. A probe directs electromagnetic radiation through the skin at the site to be measured. The energy reflected back is collected by optic fibres and analysed on a spectroscope; the amount of this reflected energy depends on body composition.

infrared radiation Invisible heat radiation which has a longer wavelength than the red of the visible spectrum.

infrared therapy The use of infrared radiation in physiotherapy to warm tissue, relieve muscle spasms, and increase circulation.

infrared thermography A method of measuring skin temperature by the amount of infrared radiation emitted at the skin surface. It may be used clinically to locate inflamed areas which are warmer than surrounding tissues. It is also used in

sports science research, for example, to study the dissipation of heat from the body during exercise.

infraspinatus A *rotator cuff muscle of the shoulder which is partially covered by the deltoid and trapezius muscles. The infraspinatus has its origin on the underside of the shoulder blade, on the infraspinous fossa, and its insertion on the greater tubercle of the humerus. Its primary actions about the shoulder are lateral rotation and horizontal abduction. It also helps to hold the head of the humerus in the glenoid cavity.

inguinal Pertaining to the groin.

inguinal canal One of a pair of openings connecting the abdominal cavity with the scrotum. The spermatic cord and blood vessels pass through the inguinal canal to the testes in males.

inguinal hernia (abdominal hernia; femoral hernia; rupture) A hernia which may develop during intense exertion due to the production of a very high abdominal pressure. A sac of peritoneum (the connective tissue lining the abdominal cavity and its organs) is forced through the inguinal canal. In men the hernia tends to descend along the spermatic cord into the scrotum. Sometimes an abdominal hernia descends through the point at which the femoral artery passes from the abdomen to protrude at the top of the thigh. This is called a femoral hernia. Presence of an inguinal or femoral hernia in athletes is potentially dangerous because an increase in intra-abdominal pressure accompanying physical exertion can cause strangulation, stopping blood flow and resulting in gangrene. Therefore, surgical repair is usually recommended. In the past, athletes with an inguinal hernia were precluded from participation in strenuous activity, especially contact and collision sports. Although this preclusion still applies to those with symptomatic hernias, many doctors now judge each case separately and make recommendations dependent on the desired sport and individual circumstances.

inguinal ligament (Poupart's ligament) Ligament connecting the anterior spines of the ilium to the pubis. The inguinal ligament is part of the *aponeurosis of the *external obliques.

inguinocrural pain *See* groin pain.

inhalation 1 The process of breathing air into the lungs though the mouth and/or nose. **2** Taking medication by breathing it in as a gas or vapour, or in aerosol form.

inhibiting factor A *hormone secreted by the *hypothalamus and transported to the anterior pituitary gland where it inhibits the release of some other hormone. Somatostatin (growth hormone-inhibiting hormone), for example, is the inhibiting factor for growth hormone secretion.

inhibition The complete or partial prevention of an activity or process. Muscle actions are inhibited by the actions of certain nerves. In psychoanalysis, specific commands may be given to prevent the subject from doing something forbidden or undesirable. In psychology, inhibition may be a central, cortical, or subcortical process restraining an instinctual drive. The extinction of conditioned reflexes is also regarded as inhibition.

inhibitory postsynaptic potential (IPSP) A transient *hyperpolarization of a post-synaptic membrane caused by an inhibitory nerve impulse, during which a stronger than normal excitatory stimulus is necessary to initiate depolarization and evoke the discharge of a *nerve impulse.

initiating structure A leadership style in which patterns of organization, channels of communication, and procedures are well established. Other descriptions of leadership style which are consistent with initiating structures include *autocratic leadership, *authoritarian leadership, *product-orientation leadership, and *task-motivation leadership. *See also* **leader behaviour description questionnaire**.

initial velocity For a projectile, a vector quantity incorporating both the *speed of release and the *angle of release of the projectile.

injection The introduction of fluid, usually containing medicines, into the body by means of a syringe. It is essential that injections are made at the correct site and that they are administered under aseptic conditions. Failing to do the first can damage tissue; failure to do the second can introduce infectious diseases, such as hepatitis.

injury A physical hurt or damage. Some sports carry such a high risk of a specific injury that the injury has acquired a sporting epithet, for example *tennis elbow, and *runner's knee. The region of the body at greatest risk of injury depends on the sport being played, but generally the lower limbs (especially the knees) are the most injured sites, followed by the upper limbs, the head, and trunk. Most sports injuries are not life-threatening, but if not treated properly they can prevent an athlete from performing well and may put an end to a promising athletic career. Some unpleasant and even potentially fatal conditions including multiple sclerosis, osteomyelitis, and bone cancer, first manifest themselves in what appears to be a sports injury. For this reason, if for no other, sports injuries should be taken seriously and medical advice sought if symptoms persist or recur. However, it is also important to remember that some signs and symptoms that appear to indicate a harmful condition, may be an innocuous result of strenuous activity (e.g., blood in the urine associated with march haemoglobinuria).

injury-prone *See* accident prone.

innate ability An ability that is inborn or instinctive. *See also* **born athlete**.

inner game The cognitive processes (thoughts, positive and negative) that take place during a game. Special mental strategies, so-called 'inner game' techniques, have been devised to enable an athlete to handle difficult game situations. One technique, popular among golfers and tennis players, uses the concept of relaxed concentration and identifies two Selfs: Self 1, the analytical problem solver; and

Self 2, the intuitive and emotional self. Athletes are trained to discriminate between the two Selfs and choose the most appropriate one to deal with a particular game situation.

inner range One of three parts to the *range of motion during which the muscle responsible for the movement is moving into full action. *See also* **midrange**; and **outer range.**

innervation The nerve supply to an organ or body part.

innominate bone *See* **coxal bone.**

inoculation Process by which infective material is introduced into a culture or the body through a small wound in the skin or in a mucous membrane. Inoculations are performed to give protection against infective diseases. Many athletes have inoculations during the off-season when they will have their least effect on performance. *See also* **immunization**; and **vaccination.**

inosine monophosphate An organic chemical belonging to the nucleotides. Some weight-lifters and body-builders claim that it delays fatigue and accelerates strength development. They also claim that it helps metabolize sugar, improves protein synthesis, and facilitates oxygen transport. Evidence for these claims is anecdotal, not scientific.

inositol A water-soluble substance similar to hexose sugar. Inositol is sometimes classified as a vitamin, but this is incorrect because it can be synthesized in the body.

INSAD CAGES A mnemonic for diagnosing depression. IN represents loss of INterest in pleasurable activities; S, Suicidal thoughts; A, change of Activity (usually decreased); D, Dysthymia (depressed feelings); C, decreased Concentration; A, loss of Appetite; G, Guilt feelings; E, change in Energy levels (usually decreased); S, changes in Sleep patterns (often insomnia). The simultaneous occurrence of six or more of the above criteria is highly indicative of a major depression.

insert *See* **insock.**

insertion The point of attachment of a muscle to a bone or other structure which usually moves during an isotonic muscle action. The insertion is usually distal to the *origin.

insock Insert of a training shoe. It is usually made of material which absorbs shock. The insock fits inside the shoe to form the part of the shoe in direct contact with the sole of the foot.

insoluble fibre Type of dietary *fibre that includes cellulose and lignin. It absorbs many times its weight in water and swells up in the intestines. By increasing the bulk of faeces, it promotes efficient waste-elimination from the colon and may help prevent colon cancer.

insomnia Difficulty in falling asleep or an inability to stay asleep. Although chronic insomnia is relatively rare, the nervous anticipation an athlete experiences before a major competition often causes sleep difficulties. The use of hypnotics, such as benzodiazepines, induce sleep, but they can be habit forming and have adverse side-effects (for example, drowsiness which decreases reaction times) that adversely affect physical performance. Relaxation techniques, such as progressive muscle relaxation, and sensible eating and drinking habits (e.g., avoiding a heavy or salty meal before going to bed) may help athletes overcome insomnia. Moderate exercise may also help some insomniacs, but strenuous exercise before retiring is likely to increase arousal and make sleep more difficult.

inspiration Breathing in or inhalation; the process by which air is drawn into the lungs through the mouth and nose, by the action of the *diaphragm and *external intercostals increasing the volume and decreasing the pressure within the thoracic cavity. Breathing through the nose helps to filter, warm, and humidify the air during inspiration.

inspiratory capacity Maximum volume of air inspired from resting expiratory level. A typical inspiratory capacity is 3600 ml; this increases during exercise.

inspiratory mechanism Mechanism by which air is drawn into the lungs. A combination of movements of the ribs upwards and outwards, and of the *diaphragm downwards reduces the intrapulmonary and intrapleural pressure which in turn causes air to rush into the lungs. During resting inspiration, the ribs are fixed by the *scalenus muscles, and contraction of the *external intercostals elevates the ribcage while the diaphragm contracts and flattens downward. Additional muscles become active during exercise when inspiration is a much more dynamic process: the scalenes elevate the first and second ribs, the sternocleidomastoids elevate the sternum, and the extensors of the back and trapezius muscle may also take part in the process.

inspiratory reserve volume Maximum volume of air inspired from the end of an unforced inspiration. The inspiratory reserve volume decreases during exercise.

instability Lack of stability in a joint, often through lax ligaments associated with *hyperflexibility. Joint instability predisposes an athlete to injuries such as recurrent dislocations.

instance theory A theory which attempts to explain how, during skill acquisition, responses change from being conscious to automatic. The instance theory suggests that, with practice, automatic performance develops because previously successful responses are retrieved instantly from memory rather than having to be constructed on an algorithm or set of rules.

instant centre The precise centre of rotation of a joint at a given instant in time. The centre of rotation changes during movement of a joint because of the asymmetry in the shapes of the articulating surfaces. The instant centre can be located using roentgenograms (X-rays).

instantaneous angular velocity The angular velocity of a body in rotation at any one moment of time. See also **average angular velocity**.

instantaneous power The ability of a body to explode into immediate action. It relies exclusively on the high energy phosphates stored within muscle cells.

instantaneous power test A test which indicates the ability to generate power instantly. Instantaneous power tests are of 10 seconds or less duration. They include the *Bosco jump test, *Margaria step test, *sargent jump test, 50-metre sprint test, and a 10-second sprint cycle test.

instantaneous speed The *speed of a body at a given moment in time. It is estimated as the average speed of a body over such a short distance or short period of time (starting from the position the body is in at the instant in question) that the speed will not have time to change. It can be determined by the gradient of a distance/time curve. The concept of instantaneous speed is useful when comparing different periods of performance, such as the different stages of a sprint.

instantaneous velocity The *velocity of a body at a given instant in time.

instinct A complex, unlearned adaptive response; an unlearned, fixed pattern of reflexes. If the responses are learned, the behaviour pattern is called a habit.

instinct theory of aggression The theory that human aggression is an innate biological drive similar to sex and hunger. As such, it cannot be eliminated but must be controlled, for the good of society. The theory is based on observations of non-human species in which aggression is used to maintain territory, and fighting is necessary for survival. The theory supports the contentious notion that sport acts as a catharsis providing a safe and socially acceptable outlet for aggression. Compare **frustration–aggression hypothesis; and social-learning theory**.

institution An established entity or activity in society comprising rule-bound and standard behaviour patterns. Institutions include any enduring activity by groups or organizations (e.g., the family, education system, law, polity, economy, or religion) which address some important and persistent societal problem. Many regard sport as a social institution because it has a distinctive kind of organization; it represents a unique form of social activity; it provides a basis of social identity; it serves as a link to other social structures; and it can act as an agent of social control.

institutional discrimination Control of social institutions by one social group to the disadvantage of another; applies to race, gender, and age.

institutionalization The process by which social units and social activities become organized in a relatively permanent and enduring way. *See also* **ludic institutionalization**.

instructional goal A general statement given by a coach of what he or she expects of his or her athletes. The statement commonly incorporates the following: a description of the performance goal in observable and measurable terms; the conditions under which the performance is to occur; and an indication of the standard upon which goal attainment can be evaluated.

instrumental Applied to something which is useful and can serve a purpose (like an instrument).

instrumental aggression A form of *aggression against another person in which the aggression is used as a means of securing some reward or to achieve an external goal such as a victory. Unlike *hostile aggression, harm to others is incidental and is not the perceived goal.

instrumental conditioning *Conditioning in which the response achieves some end such as obtaining a tangible reward or escaping punishment. It is often used as a synonym for operant conditioning but some psychologists make a distinction in the usage in these two terms.

instrumental error A constant error due to a defect in an instrument or piece of equipment.

insufficiency An inability of muscles which span two or more joints to produce a complete range of movements in all the joints simultaneously. *See also* **active insufficiency**; and **passive insufficiency**.

insufficiency fracture A *stress fracture caused by repetitive loads on bones which are weakened by pathological conditions such as *osteoporosis, osteoarthrosis, osteomalacia, Paget's disease, and bone tumours. A fracture of the femoral neck is a typical insufficiency fracture which affects elderly people. *Compare* **fatigue fracture**.

insulin A *hormone secreted by the beta cells of the Islets of Langerhans in the pancreas in response to elevated blood glucose levels. Insulin stimulates the liver, muscles, and fat cells to remove glucose from the blood for use or storage; it stimulates liver cells to convert glucose to glycogen; it promotes the conversion of glucose to fats; and promotes *glycolysis. Reduced insulin production or a decrease in the insulin-sensitivity of target cells causes blood glucose levels to increase. Insulin secretion is reduced by adrenergic impulses in the sympathetic nervous system, and by epinephrine (adrenaline). Insulin production falls during acute bouts of exercise, but insulin sensitivity of target cells increases. In trained individuals, insulin does not fall as much during exercise as in the untrained. This allows more energy to be derived from free fatty acids.

insulin-like growth factors (IGF; somatomedins) Small polypeptide hormones which mediate the actions of *human growth hormone. Growth hormone (GH) promotes the release of IGF from the liver and some other tissues, including muscles. In muscle fibres, most of the growth-promoting actions attributed to GH appear to be mediated by IGF.

insulin rebound A physiological response caused by ingesting too much sugar. Blood glucose levels rise quickly and induce an exaggerated insulin response which overcompensates for the rise, and causes the blood sugar level to fall to a level lower than it was before sugar ingestion. Although not everyone experiences insulin rebound, athletes should not consume simple carbohydrates during the period 15 to 45 minutes before an activity because it may cause *hypoglycaemia which could accelerate the onset of muscle fatigue. Carbohydrates consumed during or a few minutes before an exercise does not lead to hypoglycaemia.

insulin resistance A decreased sensitivity of target cells (e.g., muscle fibres) to *insulin. Insulin resistance is one cause of *diabetes mellitus (Type II diabetes which usually occurs in adulthood and develops gradually). Acute bouts of aerobic exercise improves the responsiveness of target cells to insulin, reducing the cells' requirements and reducing the insulin dosages some diabetics require.

integrating motor pneumachytagraph An instrument that measures energy expenditure in *indirect calorimetry.

integrator Part of the brain which controls the way an athlete integrates individual components of a skill into a complex whole. The integrator takes the analyser's blueprint of step-by-step instructions and converts it into a single image rather than a series of complex verbal instructions. It has been suggested that *imagery may guide the integrator in the same way as verbal instructions direct the analyser.

intellectualization An *ego defence mechanism by which unacceptable emotions are transformed by explanations which provide excuses for the undesirable behaviour.

intelligence There is no universally accepted definition of intelligence, but it is generally regarded as an ability to act purposefully, to think rationally, and to deal effectively with the environment; it is often measured by an intelligence test. A person of high intelligence has the ability to adapt to new situations which often involves the ability to utilize abstract concepts and to learn to grasp novel relationships. See also **sport intelligence**.

intelligence quotient (IQ) The ratio of mental age to chronological age expressed as a percentage. It is used as an index of intellectual development.

intelligence test A standardized procedure for measuring *intelligence. It is usually expressed as an intelligence quotient. No intelligence test has gained universal acceptance.

intensity The quantitative rather than the qualitative aspect of stimulation and experience; for example, the magnitude or amplitude of sound waves as distinguished from their frequency.

intensity of training The total training workload; training effort. According to the principle of progressive overload, in order to improve physical fitness, exercise must be intense enough to require more effort than normal. The method of determining which training intensity gives maximum benefits varies with each fitness component. Flexibility, for example, requires that muscles are stretched beyond their normal length; cardiovascular fitness requires elevating the heart rate above normal (see **Karvonen method**); and strength-training requires increasing resistance above normal loads (see **repetition maximum**). See also **minute ventilation method**.

intentionality A dimension in some *causal attribution models that refers to the extent to which an act was done on purpose.

interaction The combined effect of two or more independent variables acting simultaneously on a dependent variable. *Analysis of variance is used to assess the effect of the interaction between the variables as well as the specific effect of each. **2** The interplay which occurs between two or more persons or groups. Sport psychologists are interested in how members of teams interact and how that interaction can be made more productive. In some sports, such as basketball, the need for interaction is high and requires a lot of co-operation, while in other sports, such as athletic field events, interaction is not important.

interactional model A model proposing that an individual's behaviour is determined by the interaction between the individual's *personality traits and the environmental situation in which the behaviour occurs. Most sport psychologists adopt the interactional model in their studies of athletes' behaviour.

interactionism A behavioural viewpoint that adopts the *interactional model.

interaction orientation An approach to the study of behaviour which focuses on the interaction between people and their situations. Coaches who adopt an interaction orientation believe that motivation of their athletes does not result only from personal factors (e.g., the needs, interests, goals, and personality of the athletes), nor does it result from only situational factors (e.g., the leadership style of the coach, and the win–loss record of a team), but depends on the interaction of these two sets of factors. According to this approach, there is no one type of leadership style which suits all situations, and effective coaches adopt a leadership style which matches their specific situation.

interactive audience An audience which interacts verbally and emotionally with performers.

interactive sport A sport, such as soccer and volleyball, in which team mates must interact with each other to be successful.

interbrain Region of the brain that includes the thalamus, hypothalamus, and basal ganglia.

intercalated disc A junction between *cardiac muscle cells.

intercarpal joint A synovial diarthrotic joint between adjacent carpals. Intercarpal joints are mainly gliding joints.

intercellular Pertaining to the region between cells.

intercept The value (usually designated as 'a') on the y-axis when x is zero; one of the constants for linear empirical equations.

intercostal muscle Muscle lying between the ribs. The superficial external intercostals pull the ribs upwards and outwards, increasing the volume of the thoracic cavity and drawing air into the lungs during inspiration. The deeper, internal intercostals, draw the ribs downward and inwards, decreasing the volume of the thoracic cavity, forcing air out of the lungs during expiration.

intercostal space The space between two ribs. The fifth intercostal space is one of the positions in which a stethoscope is placed during a chest examination.

interdependent task A task to which all members of a group apply themselves simultaneously. The contribution of each group member may be added together to produce the final outcome (known as summary independence) or the group members may constantly adjust their performance so that errors of others in the group are either corrected or reduced. *Compare* **delegated performance**.

interference 1 Conflict which occurs when two tasks are performed simultaneously, resulting in the quality of performance of the tasks decreasing. **2** Difficulty in learning or remembering a task or event due to confusion between the material that needs to be remembered and another experience occurring before or after the task or event in question. *See also* **proactive inhibition**; **retroactive inhibition**; **capacity interference**; **structural interference**.

interferential A medium-frequency electrical apparatus for heating injured muscles and joints. It can increase circulation in damaged tissue, stimulating repair.

interferons A group of proteins that provide resistance against many viral infections. Interferon activity is increased by certain types of submaximal endurance exercise (e.g., 1 hour cycling at 70 per cent VO_2 max).

interleukin A product of macrophages and T-lymphocytes involved in inflammation and immunity. Certain types of interleukin activity increases after submaximal acute endurance exercise. This may increase cell-mediated immunity in peripheral tissues.

intermediate In anatomy, between a more medial or more lateral structure.

intermediate anaerobic performance Exercise lasting about 30 s. This type of exercise is supported mainly by *anaerobic metabolism with only a small contribution from *aerobic metabolism.

intermediate anaerobic performance capacity The total work output during a maximal exercise lasting 30 s.

intermediate cuneiform The middle of three cuneiform bones in the tarsus (ankle bone). The intermediate cuneiform articulates anteriorly with the second digit and posteriorly with the navicular bone.

intermediate-term anaerobic test A test of physical performances which lasts 20–50 s and which depends primarily on *anaerobic metabolism (see **Wingate 30-second test**).

intermittent claudication A term derived from the latin word 'claudicare' meaning to limp. A patient suffering with intermittent claudication experiences cramping in the legs due to a reduction in the arterial blood supply to the muscles, causing him or her to limp. It is commonly associated with *arteriosclerosis. It is induced by exercise and relieved by rest. Controlled exercise programmes, such as walking, are often recommended to improve circulation.

intermittent exercise Short bursts of intensive exercise (usually less than 1 minute) alternated with periods of rest. See also **interval training**.

intermittent training Training which incorporates periods of physical exertion interspersed with periods of rest. Compare **continuous training**. See also **interval training**.

intermittent yo-yo endurance test A test based on the same principles as the shuttle test, but with a 5 second recovery period at the end of every pair of 20 metre shuttles so that it more closely simulates the exercise pattern within a team game such as soccer. As with the shuttle test, the aim is to complete as many shuttles as possible while keeping up with the required pace.

intermuscular Applied to the region between muscles. Compare **intramuscular**.

intermuscular haematoma Internal bleeding between muscle fascia and interstitial spaces when muscles and fascial vessels are damaged. An intermuscular haematoma usually causes greater loss of function and more persistent swelling than an *intramuscular haematoma. See also **haematoma**.

internal axis of rotation An axis which passes through the human body, usually at a joint. Compare **external axis**.

internal controls (internals) People who are more likely to see events in their lives as being dependent on their own behaviour. They believe that if they perform well or poorly, appropriate consequences will follow. They do not consider luck as having much effect on their performance outcomes, and do not see their fate as being always in the hands of other people. Good athletes tend to be internal controls because they have learned that their abilities and efforts bring them reward and success. Compare **external control**.

internal environment The medium in which all cells are bathed; tissue fluid.

internal feedback See **intrinsic feedback**.

internal fixation Surgically rendering structures such as a fractured bone immovable by implanting a support, such as a Kuntscher nail, inside the body.

internal force A force internal to the system under consideration. Whether a force is regarded as internal or external depends on how the system is defined and classified, and is largely a matter of convenience. In biomechanics, the human body is generally regarded as the system and any force exerted by one part of the body on another is an internal force. Muscle contractions produce internal forces which move a joint. Compare **external force**.

internal imagery (kinaesthetic imagery) A form of *imagery in which subjects imagine what they would feel inside their own bodies by kinaesthetic feedback if they performed a particular skill. Compare **external imagery**; see also **mental practice**.

internal intercostal One of eleven pairs of muscles lying between the ribs. The fibres run downward and posteriorly, and are deeper than the *external intercostals. Each muscle has its origin on the inferior border of the rib above and its insertion on the superior border of the rib below. The internal intercostals take part in expiration by drawing the ribs together and depressing the rib cage, and may work as antagonists to the external intercostals but opinion is divided on this.

internalization 1 The acceptance and incorporation of the beliefs or standards of others. For example, internalization occurs when individual team members adopt the mores of the team in which they play. *Compare* **conformity**. **2** A form of direct motivation in which a coach seeks to motivate players by appealing to the players' own beliefs and values, not by administering rewards and punishments. A coach may, for example, praise an athlete for the preparation work he or she has completed, express confidence that the athlete will perform to the best of his or her ability, and reassure the athlete of continued support whatever the outcome of the performance.

internal locus of causality The *attribution of performance outcomes to causes which are perceived as being inherent and under personal control, such as ability and effort, state of health or fitness etc. *Compare* **external locus of causality**; *see also* **internal controls**.

internal locus of control *See* **internal controls**.

internal oblique muscle One of four pairs of *abdominal muscles lying under the external obliques. They have their origins on the lumbodorsal fascia, iliac crest, and inguinal ligament; they have their insertions on the *linea alba, pubic crest, and lowest three or four ribs. They function with the *external obliques to flex and rotate the trunk, and compress the abdomen.

internal overload An *attentional style in which an individual tends to become confused when having to deal with several ideas at the same time. *Compare* **broad internal**.

internal reinforcement *Reinforcement emanating from an increase in personal satisfaction and pride in an achievement.

internal respiration The exchange of gases between the tissues and the blood. *Compare* **cellular respiration**; and **external respiration**.

internal rotation Movement around the long axis of the body, towards the midline. *Compare* **external rotation**.

internals *See* **internal controls**.

internal sprain of ankle An ankle sprain in which there is little outward sign of injury except, possibly, a slight swelling, but there is great pain and limited movement. Internal bleeding in the damaged joint causes the blood-filled joint capsules to bulge outwards on either side of the Achilles tendon. The condition can lead to permanent stiffness if it is not treated quickly and properly (e.g., by aspiration). *See also* **ankle sprain**.

International Olympic Committee (IOC) The governing body of the Olympic Games. The IOC is a permanent committee entrusted with the control and development of the modern Olympic Games. It is responsible for ensuring that the Olympic Games are celebrated in the spirit that inspired their revival in Athens in 1896. The IOC elects its own members. Each member speaks either French or English and resides in a country which has a National Olympic Committee accepted by the IOC to promote the Olympic movement and amateur sport in that country.

International Olympic Committee Medical Commission (IOC Medical Commission) A body created in 1966 to combat doping. It is now divided into four subcommissions with responsibilities which include, in addition to combating doping, helping athletes to improve their performance without contravening basic principles, enabling athletes to avoid injury, and disseminating information, such as a code of ethics, to doctors treating athletes and to other interested people.

International Unit (IU) A unit used to measure the vitamin content of food, based on the vitamin's biological activity. Although IUs are still used, vitamin content is usually expressed as equivalent amounts of a pure standard form. For example, in the UK vitamin A content is given in microgrammes of pure retinol equivalent.

interneurone (association neurone; connective neurone; internuncial neurone) A *neurone within the central nervous system that connects an afferent neurone to an efferent neurone, or makes connections between any two neurones.

internuncial neurone *See* **interneurone**.

interoceptor (visceroceptor) An internal sense-organ composed of nerve endings which respond to stimuli, such as changes in pH of the blood, which arise inside the body. *See also* **proprioceptors**.

interosseus membrane A flexible membrane connecting two bones (e.g., the radius and ulna).

interosseus muscle One of eight muscles in each hand (*see* **dorsal interossei**; and **palmar interossei**).

interparietal bone A bone between the parietal bones and the occiput in the cranium.

interpersonal communication Communication between a minimum of two parties in which meaningful exchange is intended with the sender trying to effect a response from a person or group. The message may be received by the person for whom it was intended or by people for whom it was not intended, or both. The message may be distorted during transmission so that the sender's intentions are not perceived by the recipient and the intended effect is not achieved. Effective interpersonal communication is essential for successful relationships between coach and athletes.

interpersonal relationship Interactions between one group and another. *Compare* **intrapersonal relationship**.

interphalangeal joint A synovial, hinge-joint between adjacent phalanges, permitting flexion and extension.

interpolation The process of estimating intermediate values or terms between known values or terms. *Compare* **extrapolation**.

interpretation The process of giving an explanation.

interpretivism A sociological approach which emphasizes the need to understand or interpret the beliefs, motives, and reasons of social actors in order to understand social reality.

interquartile range In statistics, the range obtained by subtracting the value for the first quartile (i.e. the value which lies at the boundary between the values in the first and second quarters of the range when the values are arranged in ascending order) from that of the third quartile (i.e., the value which lies at the boundary between the values in the third and fourth quarters of the range when the values are arranged in ascending order). The interquartile range gives a measure of the spread represented by half of the entire sample, and has the advantage of excluding extreme values.

interrater reliability Reliability of a test or measurement based on the degree of similarity of results obtained from different researchers using the same equipment and method. If interrater reliability is high, results will be very similar.

intersection syndrome A *tenosynovitis of the forearm; an *overuse injury of the tendons that pass through the forearm and cross the wrist to insert into the hand. It is characterized by crepitating swelling of the tendon sheaths of the extensor pollicis brevis and abductor pollicis longus, about 5 cm proximal to the wrist where they cross over the tendons of the extensor carpi radialis. Treatment consists of rest from the precipitating activity, and anti-inflammatory procedures including NSAIDS, ice, and ultrasound. Steroid injections made into the tendon sheath parallel to, but definitely not into, the tendon usually resolve the condition rapidly. *See also* **de Quervain's disease**.

intersocietal systems Any social arrangement or social system which spans the dividing line between different societies. The intersocietal nature of sport is illustrated by the 1996 summer Olympic games in Atlanta, USA, in which over 190 countries took part.

interspinales *See* **deep spinal muscles**.

interstitial Pertaining to the area or space between cells.

interstitial cell-stimulating hormone *See* **luteinizing hormone**.

interstitial fluid Fluid bathing the intercellular spaces between cells and through which material is exchanged between the blood and the cells.

interstitial haematoma An accumulation of fluid and blood into interstitial spaces from a split in a muscle envelope. An interstitial haematoma is often accompanied by bruising which makes its way along tissue planes causing discoloration at the skin surface. This has sometimes been referred to as the bruise 'coming out'. Treatment is similar to that for an intramuscular haematoma; rapid recovery is usual.

interstitial tear A rupture in the fascial envelope of a muscle, muscle fibre, or connective tissue.

intertarsal joint A synovial, gliding joint between two tarsal bones.

intertask transfer A form of transfer of skill acquisition in which the learning and/or performance of one skill influences the learning and/or performance of a new skill.

intertransversari *See* **deep spinal muscles**.

intertubercular groove *See* **bicipital groove**.

interunit training ratio The ratio of the number of training units to recovery units within a microcycle (*see* **periodization**).

interval diet A diet and exercise regime designed to increase muscle glycogen stores in the body for a particular endurance event. It consists of four stages: (i) depleting muscle glycogen stores by a severe exercise session; (ii) reducing other carbohydrate stores by starving the body for 3 to 4 days; (iii) further reducing carbohydrate stores by another vigorous exercise session; and (iv) eating carbohydrate-rich food two to three days prior to replenish carbohydrate stores. This diet may boost muscle glycogen to double its normal level, but it must be used cautiously because it can cause fatigue and, in a few cases, chest pains, and myoglobinuria which may lead to kidney failure. *See also* **carbohydrate loading**.

interval goal setting A form of *goal setting in which past performances are used to compute target intervals of time or distance in which a future performance should be achieved. A performance falling within the interval is considered successful regardless of the outcome in terms of win and loss. Interval goal-setting can provide incentives for accomplishing both short-term goals and long-term goals.

interval measurements Measurements based on placing variables in rank order with the distances between categories fixed and equal. Interval measurements are artificial, and the zero point is arbitrarily determined; negative values may represent real values. The Celsius temperature scale is an example of an interval measurement.

interval scale A scale in which the distance or interval between any two numbers on the scale is of known size.

interval sprinting Training in which an athlete alternately sprints 50 m and jogs 50 m for a distance up to 5000 m.

interval training A system of training that alternates short to moderate bouts of intense activity (the work interval) with short to moderate periods of rest or reduced activity. By optimally spacing the periods of work and relief, a person can accomplish more total work than would be possible in a continuous training session. Interval training can be used in almost any sport, but it is most often used by track athletes, cross-country runners, and swimmers. Interval training can be adapted to fit individual requirements by adjusting the following: rate and duration of the work interval (load and duration of resistance training); number of repetitions and sets during each training session; frequency of training per week; duration of rest (recovery) interval; and type of activity during the rest interval. Gerschler interval work, devised for runners by the famous German coach Woldemar Gerschler, consists of a large number of repetitions run at a short distance (typically, 200–400 m) with a relatively long rest period (2–3 mins). Each repetition is run at or above race pace in order to develop a sense of race pace. In the controlled interval method, work and rest periods are related precisely to a physiological measure of the athletes condition (e.g., pulse rate). A typical programme of a runner may consist of a warm-up raising the pulse rate to about 120 beats per minute (bpm), a set of repetition runs which raises the pulse to about 170 bpm, and a rest of a jog or walk between each run which allows the pulse to return to about 120 bpm. The session stops when the recovery takes more than 90 seconds.

interval training prescription Written instructions containing pertinent information for an interval training session. The prescription indicates the number of sets and repetitions, training distance, work load (e.g., time taken to run a certain distance), and recovery period. A typical set for a runner is written as: Set 1 6 × 200 at 0.30 (1:40 jog); that is, the first set contains six repetitions of 200 metres in a time of 30 s and a recovery jog taking 1 min 40 s.

intervening variable A variable that brings about the effect of an independent variable on a dependent variable. For example, a study may reveal that social class has an observed effect on the ability to play golf, but this effect may be mediated by an intervening variable, such as income or proximity of a person's home to the golf course.

intervention strategy (intervention technique) Various cognitive and physiological strategies for altering existing levels of *anxiety, *arousal, and *self-confidence. Intervention strategies are used by sport psychologists to modify particular psychological sets or thought processes that may be inhibiting an athlete's performance. Through various techniques such as biofeedback, behaviour modification, anxiety management training, and attentional control training, an athlete can be trained to identify and modify undesirable psychological responses that may occur before and during competition.

intervention technique *See* intervention strategy.

intervertebral disc A cushion-like pad between adjacent vertebrae. It is composed of an inner semifluid material (nucleus pulposus) and a hard outer ring of fibrous cartilage (the annulus fibrosus). The disc acts as a shock absorber during walking, running, and jumping. Lumbar discs are the thickest because they have to be able to resist the greatest forces. For children of up to 8 years of age, discs have a blood supply, but after that age body movements are required to mechanically pump nutrients into, and wastes out of, the discs. Immobility prevents the pumping action and can adversely affect disc health; regular exercise can improve it.

intervertebral foramina Gaps between the dorsal processes of adjacent vertebrae through which the spinal nerves can pass.

intervertebral joint A cartilaginous *symphysis joint between adjacent vertebrae.

interview Research technique involving face to face verbal interchange in which an interviewer or interviewers attempt to obtain information, opinions, or beliefs from another person or persons. Highly structured interviews, in which the interviewer poses set question, are not so liable to interviewer bias and easier to analyse than unstructured interviews, but the latter often generate a greater depth of data.

intestinal absorption The process by which digested products pass from the small intestine into the blood or lymph.

intestine Region of the alimentary canal between the stomach and rectum.

intra-abdominal pressure Pressure within the abdominal cavity. Increases in intra-abdominal pressure during lifting stiffen and support the lumbar vertebrae to help prevent the spine from buckling under compressive loads. The action of the abdominal muscles can increase this pressure and contribute to spinal support.

intra-articular Pertaining to the inside of a *joint.

intracapsular Pertaining to the inside of a *joint capsule.

intracellular fluid The watery fluid contained within cells. Intracellular fluid makes up about 60–65 per cent of the total body fluids.

intracompetition Competition against oneself, for example, by attempting to improve on one's own previous level or score, or particular standards. Intra-competition is used in training as part of motivation strategy, but it needs to be used wisely as it can have negative effects.

intrafusal fibre A small muscle fibre lying inside a muscle spindle. The middle portion of the intrafusal fibre is noncontractile. When it is stretched, sensory nerve endings convey the information to the central nervous system. The ends of the intrafusal fibres can contract when stimulated by their motor neurones, the *gamma-motor neurones. See also **stretch reflex**.

intra-individual approach An approach to testing which compares how an individual performs on different occasions or in different situations, rather than how an individual performs in relation to others. Many applied sport psychologists use an intra-individual approach when testing athletes for anxiety and confidence.

intramembranous ossification Direct development of bone (e.g., an irregular bone such as the clavicle, and a flat bone of the skull) in one stage from connective, fibrous tissue. *Compare* **endochondral ossification**.

intramuscular haematoma An accumulation of blood that clots within a muscle. It may be caused by a muscle strain, tear, or bruise. The muscle fascia and the epimysium remain intact, trapping the blood within the injury site. The intramuscular haematoma results in pain and tenderness, and it limits the ability of the affected muscle to contract or to be passively stretched. In order to avoid long-term problems, it requires quick initial treatment by *RICE, followed by a method which increases blood flow, such as diathermy or ultrasound. An intramuscular haematoma is more painful than an intermuscular haematoma and requires more rehabilitation, with emphasis on stretching and strengthening the affected muscle. Occasionally, a cyst develops in an intramuscular haematoma that requires surgical removal.

intrapersonal communication Communication a person has with him or herself (e.g., self-talk). In coaching, it is generally less important than interpersonal communication.

intrapersonal relationship Interactions between members within a group and the resultant influence on individual members. See also **interpersonal relationship**.

intrapulmonary pressure Pressure within the lungs. It is usually greater than intrathoracic pressure, causing the lungs to remain slightly inflated after expiration.

intratask interference The mutually negative effects on performance of certain aspects of a task with other aspects of the same task.

intratask transfer A form of transfer of skill acquisition in which the learning and/or performance of a skill in one set of conditions influences the learning and/or performance of the same skill in another set of conditions.

intrathoracic pressure Pressure within the thoracic cage. This is usually less than the pressure in the lungs.

intratraining unit The ratio of exercise duration to recovery duration within a *training unit.

intravenous administration The introduction of medication directly into a vein.

intrinsic factor 1 A glycoprotein produced by the stomach that is required for the absorption of vitamin B_{12} (the extrinsic factor) across the intestinal membrane into the blood stream. A lack of intrinsic factor results in vitamin B_{12} deficiency and pernicious anaemia. **2** *See* **intrinsic risk factor**.

intrinsic feedback The feedback athletes receive as a natural consequence of their performance. For example, the *kinaesthetic feedback arising from sensory receptors in muscles, tendons, and joints which provides performers with information about their movements. *See also* **augmented feedback**.

intrinsic injury An injury derived directly from something the victim has done. It is a form of *primary consequential injury. Intrinsic injuries are usually caused by relatively low forces. *Compare* **extrinsic injury**.

intrinsic motivation *Motivation derived from engaging in a sport for its own sake, for the satisfaction and the sheer enjoyment that it brings, and for no other reason. Such intrinsic motivation is often associated with great persistence and high levels of achievement. It is thought to be reflected by an athlete's motive to achieve success and to be roughly equivalent to *self-confidence and *self-efficacy. *Compare* **extrinsic motivation**.

intrinsic muscle A small deep muscle found entirely within the body-part upon which it acts. In the hand, one often muscles that have both points of attachment (origins and insertions) distal to the wrist.

intrinsic reward Reward derived from feeling competent and satisfied with a performance. For example, when a person plays soccer for the sheer joy of playing the game, and then experiences that joy, the motive to play soccer is reinforced. *See also*

intrinsic motivation. *Compare* **extrinsic reward**.

intrinsic risk factor An internal factor that predisposes an athlete to an *overuse injury in his or her sport or activity. Intrinsic risk factors include age-related factors, such as growing bones, or bones weakened with age; anatomical abnormalities (e.g., one leg shorter than the other, flat feet, and overtight muscles); gender-related factors, such as breast development (*see* **bouncing-breast syndrome**); and **unfitness**. *Compare* **extrinsic risk factor**.

intrinsic value The value of doing something for its own sake rather than for any external reward. *See* **intrinsic motivation**.

intropunitive behaviour Aggression directed against oneself.

introspection The process of looking inward and describing one's own experiences.

introversion A *personality trait characterized by a tendency to be preoccupied with oneself; to be shy, cautious, and to be inwardly reflective more than overtly expressive. *Compare* **extroversion**.

introvert A person who exhibits high levels of *introversion.

invariant features Applied to aspects of movement that appear to be fixed (or invariant) even though other more superficial features can change. Invariant features are regarded as important features contained in *motor programs for sports skills.

invasion game Games such as American Football, which involve the occupation and defence of territory.

inventory A detailed description, list, or catalogue.

inverse stretch reflex A *reflex action mediated by the *Golgi tendon organs which, when the organs are stimulated by a prolonged stretch, cause the stretched muscle to relax. *Compare* **stretch reflex**.

inversion of foot Inward rotation of the foot so that the sole turns medially, inwards and sideways. Inversion during running and walking results in the body weight

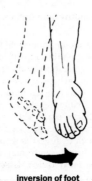

inversion of foot

being applied mainly on the outer edge of the foot. The muscles which effect inversion include the tibialis posterior, flexor digitorum, flexor hallucis longus, and the tibialis anterior. *Compare* **eversion**.

inverted-U hypothesis Hypothesis which states that performance improves with increasing levels of *arousal up to an optimal point beyond which further increases in arousal produce a detrimental effect on performance. Therefore athletes may perform badly because they are overaroused or underaroused. The hypothesis is qualitative and does not attempt to quantify the relationship between arousal and performance. The optima vary between people doing the same task and one person doing different tasks. A basic assumption in the hypothesis is that arousal is unidimensional and that there is consequently a very close correlation between

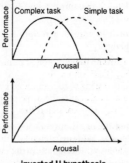

inverted-U hypothesis

indicators of arousal; this is not the case. *See also* **catastrophe theory**.

inverted-V pattern The observed relationship between precompetitive *state anxiety and amount of time before the competition. The inverted-V pattern appears when anxiety (y-axis) is plotted against time (x-axis) on a graph. It indicates that anxiety experienced prior to competition is typically more than that experienced during competition.

investment model A model of sport participation which predicts the conditions that promote continued participation, burnout, or withdrawal. The model is based on how five conditions (rewards, costs, satisfaction, alternatives, and investments) are perceived by an athlete. Athletes with high commitment to sport participation and low withdrawal tendencies, perceive the rewards and satisfaction of participation as being high, and the costs and alternatives as being low. They also perceive that the long term investments that they have made in the sport (including time, friendship, money, and physical and emotional energy) will be lost if they withdraw.

in vitro Applied to conditions outside the living body, such as in a test tube or other artificial environment.

in vivo Applied to a biological process or experiment occurring in a living body.

involuntary muscle Muscle, such as smooth muscle and cardiac muscle, which is not normally under voluntary, conscious control. However, the term is a misnomer because many so-called 'involuntary' muscles (e.g., the anal sphincter muscle) can be brought under conscious control by training.

involuntary nervous system *See* autonomic nervous system.

involvement Applied to different forms of participation in sport.

IOC *See* **International Olympic Committee**.

IOC Medical Commission *See* **International Olympic Committee Medical Commission**.

iodine A trace element required for normal growth and development. It is a component of thyroid hormones which help regulate growth, development, and metabolic rate. Deficiency results in an underactive thyroid gland and a lower metabolic rate; excess may suppress the secretion of thyroid hormones. In the UK, the Reference Nutrient Intake for adults is 140 micrograms per day; in the USA, the Recommended Dietary Allowance is 150 micrograms.

ion An atom or molecule which carries a charge due to the gain or loss of an electron.

ionotropic neurotransmitter A chemical substance, such as acetylcholine and amino acid transmitters, which opens channels through which ions (electrically charged particles such as sodium, Na$^+$, and potassium, K$^+$, ions) can flow in a postsynaptic membrane causing a change in the postsynaptic membrane potential. *Compare* **metabotropic neurotransmitter**.

iontophoresis A method by which ionized medication (e.g., the steroidal anti-inflammatory dexamethasone combined with xylocaine) is driven through the skin by an electric current so that it reaches deep tissues. Iontophoresis is used to treat acute and subacute inflammation. It is a relatively painless and sterile procedure, but the passage of the electric current through the skin sometimes causes galvanic burns. The most dangerous complication is an adverse reaction to the medication.

IPF *See* **ideal performance feeling**.

IPS *See* **ideal performance state**.

ipsative data analysis The analysis of data so that individual differences can be identified. In sport psychology such an analysis may be used to recognize the idiosyncratic nature of a particular athlete's behavioural responses. It includes the analysis of the variety of responses among individuals and how an individual's response varies in different situations.

ipsilateral In anatomy, situated on, or affecting the same side of the body.

IPSP *See* **inhibitory postsynaptic potential**.

IQ *See* **intelligence quotient**.

iron A mineral element essential for health. It is a component of haemoglobin, myoglobin, cytochromes, and other chemicals involved in vital metabolic activities. Dietary sources of iron include red meat, liver, dried fruit, nuts, molasses, and legumes. The best sources contain haem iron (i.e., iron contained within haemoglobin) because it is easily absorbed from the intestine. Vitamin C improves iron absorption, but tannic acid (e.g., in tea) and phytates (e.g., in wholemeal bread) interfere with it. In the UK, the daily Reference Nutrient Intake for adult males is 8.7 mg and 14.8 mg for females who do not have heavy menstrual losses. In the USA, the Recommended Dietary Allowance is 10 mg for males and 15 mg for females. Excessively high iron intakes can damage the liver, heart, and pancreas. A deficiency may lead to anaemia, decreased oxygen transport, and feelings of lassitude. Athletes training very strenuously may require higher than normal iron intakes to avoid iron deficiency, but supplementation of iron in those who are not deficient seems to have no benefit.

iron-deficiency anaemia A reduction in the quantity of haemoglobin in the blood due to the iron supply not meeting the demands of the body (iron is an essential component of *haemoglobin). Iron-deficiency anaemia may result from an iron-deficient diet, an inadequate absorption of iron through the intestinal wall, or an increased demand for iron. Most athletes are probably no more susceptible to iron-deficiency anaemia than the general population. Iron deficiency can be prevented by increasing dietary absorption by eating more lean red meat or dark meat of poultry, avoiding an excessive intake of caffeine-containing drinks, and having drinks rich in Vitamin C (this improves the absorption of iron). Some women athletes are particularly susceptible to iron-deficiency anaemia because of heavy menstrual bleeding. Female athletes who repeatedly develop iron-deficiency anaemia are often treated with iron supplements.

irreducible hernia A hernia that will not return to its normal position in the body cavity, even with gentle manipulation.

irregular bone A bone with an irregular shape (e.g., a vertebra).

irritability The responsiveness of an organism to changes in its immediate environment.

ischaemia Local and temporary deficiency of the blood supply to tissues, chiefly due to constriction. of blood vessels. Oxygen deficiency may cause pain in the tissue (ischaemic pain).

ischaemic pain *See* ischaemia.

ischaemic heart disease Myocardial ischaemia in which there is an insufficient blood supply to heart muscle. Endurance training is an effective measure in primary and secondary prevention, and aids rehabilitation in cases of ischaemic heart disease.

ischium One of three bones which make up the coxal bone of the pelvic girdle. Each ischium forms the lower part of each side of the hip bone. During sitting, the body weight is borne entirely by the tuberosities of the ischium, which are the strongest parts of the hip bone.

islets of Langerhans Endocrine tissue in the pancreas which secretes *insulin and *glucagon.

isokinetic action The action of a muscle that produces a movement at a constant speed or constant angular velocity over a joint's full range of motion. The muscle develops maximum tension over the complete range of motion. Some sports scientists suggest that the term isokinetic should not be used to describe a muscle action because isokinetic actions do not normally occur during sport or exercise performance; usually the linear movement of muscles varies in such performances. Furthermore, there is not even a guarantee that isokinetic actions occur on isokinetic machines. Although the controlled movement of the machine may be at a constant velocity, the velocity of the muscles generating the forces to produce the movement may vary.

isokinetic machine A weight-training device that produces a movement, controlled either hydraulically or electronically, at a constant velocity. It is designed to keep the speed of movement of the muscles being exercised constant, irrespective of the force being applied. Theoretically, this enables a well-motivated individual to contract the muscles at maximum force at all points in the range of motion. Exercises on isokinetic machines help to develop uniform strengthening of active muscles, improving muscle strength, endurance, and cardiovascular fitness. *See also* **isokinetic action**.

isolation stress A form of stress modelling which has been used by coaches of international athletes especially in Eastern Europe. Isolation stress involves placing the competitor in a situation that requires self-coaching for a period. It is imposed when it is thought that a top competitor might be shifted to a new team and coach, unfamiliar with his or her unique characteristics, just before encountering international competition. It is hoped that voluntarily breaking away from an accustomed coach under controlled conditions may be less traumatic than would otherwise be the case.

isoleucine An essential amino acid found in beans and other legumes but only in small amounts in corn and other grains, indicating the need for vegetarians to include legumes in their diet.

isometric exercise *See* static action exercise.

isometric action *See* static action.

isometric strength *See* static strength.

isometric training *See* static action exercise.

isosmotic Applied to two solutions having the same *osmotic pressure.

isotonic exercise An exercise which usually involves raising and lowering a weight. The muscles are used in a normal dynamic way, contracting at a speed controlled by the subject (*see* **isotonic muscle action**).

Ideally, the isotonic exercises should involve the same movements and muscles used in the subject's chosen sport. Isotonic exercises are good for developing strength and cardiovascular fitness.

isotonic muscle action A muscle action in which muscle tension purportedly remains constant while the muscle changes its length as it overcomes a constant resistance. Isotonic means 'equal in tone' and implies constant force development. However, no dynamic muscle action in sport or exercise performance involves constant force development because of variations in mechanical advantage as a joint angle is changed, as well as differences in maximal force capability of a muscle through its range of length. It has therefore been suggested that the term 'isotonic' should not be used in relation to human exercise performance. *See also* **concentric action**; and **eccentric action**.

isotonic solution A solution which has no effect on the volume of tissues and cells.

Thus a cell, when placed in an isotonic solution tends neither to gain or lose water. Isotonic sports drinks have the same concentration as the body fluids.

isotonic testing Performance tests using isotonic muscle actions. They usually involve dynamometers which, in addition to measuring absolute strength, may also measure acceleration, peak velocity, work, and power of isotonic muscle actions at various preset loads.

issue-oriented riot Spontaneous collective behaviour initiated by a specific event, as in a sport crowd rioting after a disputed decision by an official. *Compare* **issueless riot**.

issueless riot A collective behaviour which occurs spontaneously and does not appear to originate from a specific issue, as when a crowd celebrating a home team victory produces large scale property damage. *Compare* **issue-oriented riot**.

IU *See* **International Unit**.

 J

javelin thrower's elbow to **juxtaglomerular apparatus**

javelin thrower's elbow *See* **golfer's elbow**.

jaw Facial bone in which the teeth are embedded. The jaw consists of the maxilla (the upper jaw) and the mandible (lower jaw).

jejunum Part of the *alimentary canal between the duodenum and ileum.

jerk The sudden contraction of a muscle. Some jerks, such as the knee-jerk, are used to test nerve reflex actions.

jersey finger injury An *avulsion fracture of the flexor digitorum profundus tendon, usually affecting the ring finger, causing an inability to flex the interphalangeal

joint. It is common among Rugby players and American footballers who grab the jersey of an opponent during a tackle. It has also been reported in ice hockey players who remove their gloves to grab hold of an opponent's jersey during a fight. Jersey finger is treated by surgical reattachment of the tendon.

jet lag Disorientation, fatigue, and disrupted sleep patterns associated with long-distance jet aeroplane flights. Jet lag can impair the performance of athletes competing abroad. Apparently, it desynchronizes major *circadian rhythms which require time to readjust before an athlete's condition returns to normal. On the basis of empirical studies on runners crossing the Atlantic, athletes are generally advised to allow 1 day to readjust for each time zone shift.

jock itch A contagious infection of the skin around the groin, thigh, and buttocks usually caused by the fungus *Tinea cruris*. Typically, it causes the skin to become itchy and red, and pus-filled blisters may develop. It is spread rapidly in contact and collision sports, and where washing facilities, towels, and clothing are shared. It is much more common in male than female athletes. It is particularly common in male athletes who wear an athletic support (jock strap). It can be prevented by ensuring scrupulous personal hygiene, keeping the skin clean and dry. It is usually treated with antifungal creams after gently washing the affected area with unscented soap and water (ensuring that the area is thoroughly rinsed and dried). Transmission of the infection during contact sports can be prevented by covering the affected area of skin.

jogger's nipple Soreness of the nipple due to chafing by clothing, commonly experienced by male and female long-distance runners. The condition may be very painful and accompanied by bleeding. It can usually be avoided by applying petroleum jelly to the nipples before running. Treatment may include application of a mild topical steroid (e.g., 1 per cent hydrocortisone) three times daily for a few days.

jogger's nephritis *See* **athletic pseudonephritis**.

jogging A training technique involving slow, relaxed continuous running. It cannot be defined in terms of minutes per mile or kilometre, but the running pace should be slow enough to enable the jogger to continue holding a conversation. People considering jogging, particularly those over 35-years old unused to exercise, should check their fitness with their doctor. Jogging is regarded by many people as the foremost *aerobic exercise. It requires no special skill, little expenditure, and can be done almost anywhere. Since the 1970s, it has caught the imagination of the public and made exercise generally acceptable. However, excessive jogging can result in musculoskeletal problems arising from the stress and shock of running on hard surfaces such as roads and pavements.

joint The junction of two or more bones; an articulation. The joint is an anatomical structure which constitutes a functional unit biologically and biomechanically. It is composed of cartilage-lined extremities of the articulating bones (*see* **articular cartilage**), a layer of bone directly beneath the cartilage (known as the subchondral layer), a fibrous capsule with ligaments, and the joint capsule and associated musculature. The different parts of a joint are functionally interdependent; damage to one part usually affects all other parts. *See also* **amphiarthrosis**; **ball-and-socket joint**; **condyloid joint**; **gliding joint**; **hinge joint**; **pivot joint**; **saddle joint**; **synarthrosis**; **syndesmosis**; and **synovial joint**.

joint aspiration (tapping a joint) Withdrawal of fluid from a joint. Aspirations are performed to relieve pain and remove purulent fluid from a grossly swollen joint (most commonly the knee), and as a diagnostic procedure, for example, to distinguish between different types of arthritis. The presence of small fat globules on the surface of fluid aspirated from a joint usually indicates a fracture.

joint capsule (articular capsule) A double layered sleeve of fibrous tissue surrounding the joints of limbs and enclosing the joint cavity of a synovial joint.

joint cavity Cavity filled with synovial fluid within a *synovial joint. It is enclosed by a joint capsule.

joint flexibility *See* **joint mobility**.

joint mice *See* **loose bodies**.

joint mobility (joint flexibility) A term indicating the relative ranges of motion in different planes that can be performed at a joint. Joint mobility is determined by the ligaments, fibrous capsule, musculature, and the shape of the articulating surfaces. *Compare* **joint stability**; *see also* **flexibility**.

joint receptor A group of sense organs, such as *Ruffini's corpuscles and *Pacinian corpuscles, located in the capsules of *synovial joints. They are sensitive to pressure and may be involved in kinaesthesis, providing information to the central nervous system about the position of a joint.

joint stability The ability of a joint to withstand mechanical shocks and movements without becoming dislocated or otherwise displaced and injured. Stability is provided by the support of the surrounding bones (osseous stability) and the soft tissues, including the joint capsule, ligaments, and muscles. Stability varies according to whether the joint is moving (dynamic stability) or stationary (static stability). The bones contribute mainly to static stability; the ligaments and capsule to both static and dynamic stability; while the muscles contribute only to dynamic stability. Different joints vary greatly in their stability, and the different types of stability may vary within a single joint. The hip, for example, has a high osseous stability while the knee has a low osseous stability but high ligamentous and muscular stability. Excessive flexibility may reduce stability and make an individual accident prone.

joint stiffness 1 A measure of the resistance of a joint to movement defined as the change in joint angle divided by a change in joint *torque or moment. Joint stiffness depends on the resistances offered by joint structures (including muscles and ligaments), skin, and subcutaneous connective tissue. **2** A condition, characterized by difficulty in moving a joint, which is usually accompanied by discomfort and pain. Joint stiffness often follows a joint injury when muscles go into a protective spasm which reduces movement. Joint stiffness should be treated cautiously and no attempt should be made to move the joint forcibly. Persistent, painful stiffness requires medical investigation and treatment.

Jone's fracture A fracture of the fifth metatarsal within 1.5 cm distal of the tuberosity where the peroneus brevis muscle is inserted in the foot. It is usually caused by forceful landing of the forefoot when the load is concentrated over the fifth metatarsal. It is common among basketball players and other athletes who frequently perform lateral movements and sudden forceful jumping that imposes high impact forces on the fifth metatarsal. A Jone's fracture is often disabling and may require surgical fixation.

jostling Massage stroke in which a muscle is grasped at its point of origin and shaken gently back and forth while the athlete relaxes. The stroke continues all the way down the muscle to the point of insertion and then back again. Jostling is used mainly to relax muscle (for example, between deep stroking) and is claimed to reduce the *stretch reflex.

joule The derived SI unit of *work or *energy. One joule is the amount of work done when the point of application of a force of one newton is displaced through a distance of one metre in the direction of the force.

judgement The ability of an individual to assess a situation, consider the choices of action available, and to arrive at conclusions which best satisfy the needs of the situation. Sound judgement is an integral part of most sports. It is influenced by knowledge, experience, attitude, motivation, ability, and psychological and social factors, such as belief. The ability to make sound judgements is compromised by taking drugs such as marijuana and alcohol.

judo elbow A sports injury in which the ligaments either side of the elbow joint are torn. It occurs, for example, when a judo player resists an armlock by clenching the fists too tightly.

jumper's heel An injury to the heel characterized by pain between the *Achilles tendon and the back of the ankle bone. It is commonly associated with explosive jumping, stamping down, or blocking the foot as a ball is kicked. These actions compress the fat pad between heel-bone and shin-bone, causing the pad to become inflamed and painful. *See also* **Achilles bursitis**.

jumper's knee (patellar tendinitis) Inflammation of the tendon which connects the kneecap to the shin-bone. This injury is associated with any athletic activity which involves repeated jumping (such as basketball, volleyball, and triple jump), or activities which impose heavy loads on the knee (e.g., when a weight-lifter performs squats). It is extremely common among high-jumpers because they have to perform excessive knee extensions during take-off. Jumper's knee is characterized by pain just below the knee cap. Initially, the pain is felt only during exercise, but if untreated the symptoms may become progressively worse and more prolonged. An athlete with jumper's knee who continues to participate in explosive activities risks completely rupturing the tendon attachment. Thankfully, this catastrophic injury is rare. In the early stages, ice treatment, relative rest, and nonsteroidal anti-inflammatories usually resolve the condition. Surgery may be recommended for severe, chronic conditions and for tendon ruptures. The tendons have a poor blood supply, therefore recovery can take a long time, from two weeks to several months depending on the severity of the injury. A progressive exercise programme to strengthen the patellar tendon is an essential part of rehabilitation (*see also* **aggressive rehabilitation**).

jump height A measure of the difference between the standing height of an athlete and the height attained in a jump. For jump heights to be comparable, the type of jump (e.g., countermovement jump, drop jump, or squat jump) must be standardized.

junctional feet Knob-like structures in muscle fibres connecting *transverse-tubules (T-tubules) with the sarcoplasmic reticulum. It has been hypothesized that the junctional feet undergo a conformational change on the arrival of an electrical impulse at the T-tubule, causing adjacent calcium channel proteins to open. This allows calcium ions to diffuse inside the muscle fibre, enabling a muscle action to take place (*see* **sliding filament theory**).

jury A group of people appointed to judge a competition and, sometimes, to award prizes.

just-noticeable difference The smallest difference between stimuli which can be perceived.

juxta In anatomy, a prefix denoting near to.

juxtaglomerular apparatus Cells located near to the glomerulus of the kidney that play a role in blood pressure regulation by releasing the enzyme *renin.

K
kallidin to kyphosis

kallidin *See* **kinins**.

Karvonen method A method of calculating the training heart rate which is equivalent to a desired percentage VO$_2$ max. It involves adding a given percentage of the maximal heart rate reserve (maximal heart rate−resting heart rate) to the resting heart rate (usually assumed to be 220−age in years). Therefore, the following equation is used to calculate the training heart rate for a work rate equivalent 75%

VO_2 max: training heart rate = resting heart rate + 0.75 (maximal heart rate–resting heart rate).

karyogram *See* **karyotyping**.

karyotyping The determination of an individual's karyotype, the total chromosome complement of typical body cells, as seen on a photomicrograph (karyogram). Karyotyping can be used for gender verification (sex testing) because the Y chromosome (one of the pair of chromosomes that determine sex) in males has a very distinctive appearance.

kcal *See* **kilocalorie**.

kelvin SI unit of temperature. It has the symbol K. The unit interval of the kelvin temperature scale is the same as that for the Celsius scale. A temperature expressed in degrees kelvin is equivalent to degrees Celsius plus 273.15. Absolute zero is equal to 0 degrees kelvin or–273.15 degrees Celsius.

keratin Water-soluble fibrous protein found in the epidermis. Keratin is the main constituent of hair and nails, and contributes to the waterproofing of skin.

keratitis Inflammation of the cornea of the eye. It may be caused by trauma, exposure to dust or ultraviolet light, or extreme cold. Participants of winter sports such as skiing are particularly at risk. Keratitis can be avoided by wearing appropriate protective glasses. *See also* **snow-blindness**.

keratoiritis Inflammation of both the cornea and iris.

ketone An organic chemical containing a carbonyl group (C=O) and having the general formula RR'C=O, where R and R' are hydrocarbon groups.

ketone bodies Ketones formed in the liver from acetyl CoA as breakdown products of fat oxidation. They include acetone, aceto-acetic acid, and beta-hydroxybutyrate. Ketone bodies can be used in the brain as an alternative fuel.

ketonuria The presence of ketone bodies in the urine. Ketonuria may occur as a result of starvation, or *diabetes mellitus.

kg *See* **kilogram**.

kg-m *See* **kilogram-metre**.

kidneys The major excretory and osmoregulatory organs in the body. A pair of kidneys lie dorsally (at the back), in the abdomen. The kidneys also act as endocrine organs releasing *erythropoietin, a hormone which regulates red blood cell production.

Kienbock's disease Softening and eventual death of the lunate bone in the wrist due to disruption of its blood supply. It is characterized by pain and tenderness of the lunate bone, just in front of the wrist crease and behind the little finger. It can be caused by repeated microtrauma to the bone. Although conservative treatment sometimes works (e.g., RICE followed by immobilization and anti-inflammatories), surgery is often necessary to replace the lunate bone with a silicone implant.

kilocalorie (Cal; kcal) The amount of heat needed to raise the temperature of 1 litre of water by 1 °C. Energy changes associated with biochemical reactions are often expressed in kilocalories although the SI unit is the *joule. Sometimes the term 'calories' used to describe the energy content of foods, is really kilocalories; 1 kilocalorie equals 1000 calories.

kilocalorie/minute Unit of *power.

kilogram SI base unit of *mass, defined as the mass of the international prototype kilogram: a particular cylinder of platinum-iridium alloy kept at the International Bureau of Weights and Measures, at Savres, Paris. One kilogram is equivalent to 2.2 pounds.

kilogram-metre Unit of work.

kilojoule (kJ) Unit of energy equal to 1000 joules.

kinaesthesis The sense by which motion, weight, and position of various body parts are perceived. Kinaesthesis depends on the sense organs, especially *proprioceptors, skin receptors, and the vestibular apparatus providing information about the state of contraction of muscles and the position of the limbs and the body in space.

kinaesthetic Pertaining to *kinaesthesis.

kinaesthetic feedback *Feedback about the position and movement of the body, provided especially by *proprioceptors in muscles and joints.

kinaesthetic imagery *See* **internal imagery.**

kinaesthetic perception Awareness of body and limb position and movements. Tests of kinaesthetic perception include asking a blind-folded subject to attempt to distinguish between objects according to their weight, or asking the blind-folded subject to maintain balance under controlled conditions.

kinanaesthesia An inability to perceive body positions and movements of the body, resulting in impaired physical activity.

kinanthropometrics The study of human body size and *somatotypes, and their quantitative relationships with exercise, sport performance, and nutrition.

kinase An enzyme that catalyses the transfer of a phosphate group from ATP to an acceptor (*see* **phosphofructokinase**).

kinematic chain *See* **kinematic couple.**

kinematic couple (kinematic chain) In the human body, a system involving the contact of two rigid body-segments which transmit forces. Kinematic couples may connect successively or they may connect by branches to form chains of several kinetic links. If the final link of the chain is free, it is able to move independently of the other links and the chain is known as an open chain; if the final link is not free to move, the chain is known as a closed chain. A closed chain does not permit isolated movements but it does facilitate the transmission of muscle actions to adjacent or distant articulations. *See also* **kinetic link principle.**

kinematic feedback *Feedback about a person's movement pattern or movement characteristics, without regard to the forces involved. *Compare* **kinetic feedback.**

kinematics A branch of mechanics concerned with the descriptive study of motion, including the pattern and speed of movement of different body segments. Kinematics deals with the appearance of motion; it does not refer to the mass or forces causing the motion. *Compare* **kinetics.**

kinesics Body language; a form of nonverbal communication by physical appearance (especially changes in facial and eye movements), posture, gestures, and touching behaviour.

kinesiology Study of the art and science of human movement.

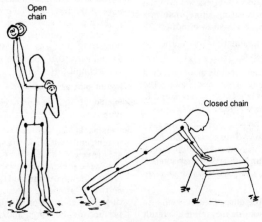

kinematic chain

kinetic Pertaining to motion.

kinetic energy The capacity to do work by virtue of a body's motion. Kinetic energy is measured in joules. A mass m (kilograms) moving with a velocity v (metres per second) has a kinetic energy of $0.5mv^2$. Compare **potential energy**.

kinetic feedback Feedback about the force characteristics of a movement. Compare **kinematic feedback**.

kinetic friction Friction generated between two surfaces in contact during motion. Kinetic friction is a product of the *coefficient of kinetic friction and the *normal reaction force. It assumes a constant value regardless of the amount of applied force or the speed of the motion. Its value is always less than the *limiting friction between the same two surfaces. See also **rolling friction**; and **sliding friction**.

kinetic link principle The principle that body segments generate high end-point velocity by accelerating and decelerating adjacent links, using internal and external muscle torques applied to the body segments in a sequential manner from proximal to distal, from massive to least massive, and from most fixed to most free. The kinetic link principle is applied when different body segments rotate during throwing and kicking. These actions have been likened to the motion of a bullwhip. If segmental rotations are free to occur at the distal end, the body's base-segments in contact with the ground act like the handle of a bull-whip. Just as the tip of the bullwhip can be made to travel at supersonic speed, the small distal segments of the hand and foot can be made to travel very fast by the sequential acceleration and deceleration of the body segments.

kinetic mobility The ability to swing a limb into a desired position at speed, using its own momentum. See also **ballistic movement**.

kinetic mobility exercise See **ballistic mobility exercise**.

kinetics 1 Study of the forces acting on a mechanical system and responsible for its motion. Kinetics is concerned with the causal analysis of motion. Compare **kinematics**. **2** The study of the rates at which chemical reactions proceed.

King Kong arm Nickname for the overdevelopment of the dominant arm and shoulder in tennis player. See also **unilateral muscular hypertrophy**.

kinins A group of endogenous polypeptides, including kallidin, *bradykinin, angiotensin, and *substance P, that cause smooth muscle to contract. They also act as powerful *vasodilators, lowering blood pressure. They are not normally present in the blood but occur, for example, when tissue is damaged. Kinins are thought to play a role in the inflammatory response and may contribute to ischaemic pain.

kiss of life Emergency mouth-to-mouth resuscitation in which the operator blows air into the victim's lungs to inflate them, allowing air to be exhaled automatically.

kJ See **kilojoule**.

kneading A form of *massage similar to kneading dough. It involves gently grasping a group of muscles between the thumb and finger and, alternating hands, squeezing the thumb and fingers together while working the muscle up and down. Kneading is used to assess the state of muscle tension. It may also aid deep circulation and remove metabolic wastes from muscles.

knee The *knee-joint and surrounding region.

kneebrace See **brace**.

kneecap See **patella**.

knee extension Straightening of the lower leg about the tibiofemoral joint of the knee: an action used during climbing, running, and rising from a seated position.

knee extensor A muscle that effects *knee extension. The major knee extensors are the four *quadriceps muscles. The rectus femoris is the only one of these which crosses the hip. It is an especially powerful extensor when the hip is extended but is weak when the hip is flexed.

knee flexion Bending of the lower leg about the tibiofemoral joint of the knee.

knee flexor A muscle that effects *knee flexion. The major flexors are the *hamstrings, but before flexion occurs from the fully extended position, the knee has to be 'unlocked'. This is achieved by the *popliteus muscle.

knee injury Physical damage to the knee. The knee is the largest joint in the body and subjected to enormous loads during many sports activities. However, it is a relatively unstable joint making it especially vulnerable to injury. Between one quarter and one third of all sports injuries involve the knee. The knee is a very complex structure and injuries often affect more than one component making diagnosis notoriously difficult. Many knee injuries are due to overuse (e.g., *chondromalacia patellae), but misalignments of muscles and bone in the lower leg also increases the risk of knee injury (see **unhappy triad**).

knee instability Excessive knee laxity; a reduction in the stability of the knee joint. It may be caused by direct injury to the joint, or to a weakening of the muscles (especially the quadriceps and semimembranosus) and/or ligaments (e.g., the anterior cruciate and collateral ligaments) supporting the joint.

knee jerk A reflex kick of the lower leg following a tap on the tendon just below the patella.

knee joint A complex, large *synovial joint that includes the two condylar articulations of the tibiofemoral joint and the articulation of the patellofemoral joint. Although the knee behaves mainly as a hinge joint, some rotation is essential for locomotion. The articulating surfaces of the tibiofemoral joint (around which most movement takes place) are shallow but deepened by the *menisci. The joint cavity is enclosed by a joint capsule only on the lateral and posterior aspects. Several capsular ligaments help to prevent displacement of the joint surfaces: two collateral ligaments, and the intracapsular anterior and posterior cruciate ligaments.

knee movements Movements of the lower leg about the knee joint. These include extension, flexion, and (to a lesser extent) rotation.

knee plica syndrome (plica syndrome; synovial plica syndrome) A tightening of the synovial plica (bands or folds of tissue) that may form in the knee joint. Many people have plicae in three or four places in the knee, with no adverse symptoms. However, when the plicae tighten (for example, as a result of an athletically related knee trauma) they can become hard and damage the knee. A tightened mediopatellar plica (the plica most likely to tighten) behaves like a bowstring, eroding the medial facet of the patella and the medial femoral condyle, causing anteromedial knee pain and a clicking noise as the plica snaps over the end of the femur. The symptoms mimic other knee disorders, so that knee plica is notoriously difficult to diagnose. Rest and ice are the most useful forms of treatment, but sometimes localized steroid injections are used. In cases which do not respond to conservative treatment, the plicae may be removed arthroscopically.

knee rotation Rotation (movement about the longitudinal axis) of the tibia with respect to the femur.

knee rotator A muscle that effects *knee rotation. Lateral rotation of the tibia is effected mainly by the *biceps femoris; medial rotation is effected mainly by the *semimembranosus, *semitendinosus, and *popliteus when the knee is in flexion and not bearing weight. When the knee is fully extended, the popliteus 'unlocks' it by medially rotating the tibia.

knockout See **concussion**.

knowledge of activity The kind of knowledge about an activity that can be demonstrated in a paper and pencil test. Knowledge of activity may also include the ability to utilize information from various types of *feedback, including *knowledge of results and *knowledge of performance. Studies of the value of knowledge of activity on performance are equivocal, but it is generally agreed that a complete physical education includes a knowledge, understanding, and appreciation of the factors that influence physical activity.

knowledge of performance (KP) A form of *augmented feedback given, for example, verbally by a coach at the end of a performance of a skill. The feedback contains information about the nature of the movement pattern produced during the performance and may include identification of the parts of the skill which were performed correctly and the parts performed incorrectly. *Compare* **knowledge of activity; knowledge of results**.

knowledge of results (KR) A form of *augmented feedback where verbal (or verbalizable) information is given to an athlete at the end of the performance of a skill; the feedback is about the outcome of the performance rather than about the movements which brought about the performance (*compare* **knowledge of performance**).

Kocher manoeuvre A procedure for treating an anterior dislocation of the glenohumeral joint in the shoulder. The elbow is flexed and traction applied to the humerus while it is in lateral rotation. The arm is then adducted and rotated medially allowing the head to return to its socket. The procedure is quite difficult to perform because it requires rotation in two different directions. It can also be dangerous because the articular cartilage can be damaged during leverage when the humerus is still in contact with the glenoid fossa.

Kohler's disease An *osteochondrosis affecting the navicular bone in the tarsus (ankle) of children, causing pain and limping.

KP *See* **knowledge of performance**.

KR *See* **knowledge of results**.

Krause's end-bulbs Bulbous capsules in the skin containing sensory nerve endings which may be mechanoreceptors, but which are also thought to be thermoreceptors sensitive to cold and activated by temperatures less than 20 °C. They occur more superficially in the skin than heat receptors.

KR delay The interval between the production of a movement and the presentation of *knowledge of results. Evidence concerning KR delay on performance indicates that it has negligible effect on the performance of motor tasks.

Krebs cycle (citric acid cycle; tricarboxylic acid cycle) A series of aerobic chemical reactions occurring in *mitochondria, in which carbon dioxide is produced and hydrogen is removed from carbon molecules; a process known as oxidative decarboxylation. The cycle is named after Sir Hans Krebs, the 1953 Nobel prizewinner in Physiology and Medicine. The reactions are exothermic, enabling one molecule of ATP to be generated during each cycle.

Kuntscher nail A long steel nail inserted down the cavity of a long bone to fix a fracture.

kurtosis A measure of the extent to which the curve derived from a set of values is flatter or more peaked than a normal distribution which has a kurtosis value of 0. A curve that is more peaked, has a positive value, a flatter curve has a negative value.

kwashiorkor A protein-deficiency disease in children characterized by apathy, impaired growth, skin ulcers, an enlarged liver, and mental retardation. The concentration of plasma proteins is inadequate to keep fluid in the bloodstream, resulting in *oedema and a bloated abdomen.

kymograph A revolving drum which carries a piece of paper onto which a trace is produced by a lever connected to a physiological preparation, such as a nerve or muscle. Kymographs are used to measure the time course of muscle contractions.

kyphosis (hunchback) A dorsally exaggerated thoracic curvature of the spine. It has also been called swimmer's back because it is common in adolescent swimmers who have trained heavily with the butterfly stroke. It is common in people suffering from *osteoporosis. It may also develop from poor posture or an unequal muscle pull on the spine. The condition is usually treated by bracing.

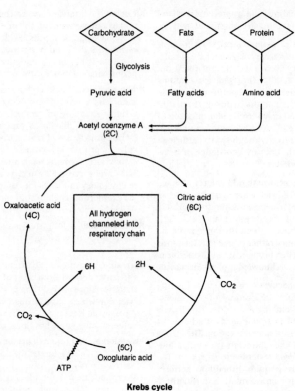

Krebs cycle

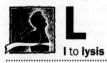

L

l to lysis

l *See* **litre.**

labelling theory A theory applied to the social processes involved in attributing positive or (more commonly) negative characteristics to acts, individuals, or groups, and the effects such labelling has on behaviour. Labelling theory has been particularly influential in the study of deviance.

laboratory test In sport, usually a measure of a physiological function that is conducted in a controlled environment and which uses protocols and equipment that simulate a sport or activity. *Compare* **field test.**

labrum A lip-like structure, such as that around the margins of the *acetabulum.

labyrinth A system of interconnecting bony cavities and membranes of the inner ear which comprises the organs of hearing and balance. The labyrinth includes the cochlea and semicircular canals.

laceration Damage to the skin producing a wound; known colloquially as a cut. A laceration may be superficial or deep. Long, shallow lacerations may cause no great problems and require simple cleaning and closure. Sometimes scrubbing is required if the laceration if contaminated with gravel or some other substance. If an implement such as arrow or javelin is involved, deep structures are likely to be damaged and surgery may be required. Blood flowing from a laceration should be treated with care because of the danger of bloodborne pathogens, such as *hepatitis B and HIV. The bleeding must be controlled and the wound covered before the patient returns to sporting activity. Any laceration sustained during an outdoor sport carries with it the risk of *tetanus, and all sportspeople should be immunized against this disease.

Lachman's test A test to diagnose an anterior cruciate ligament injury of the knee. With the patient in a supine position and the knee flexed about 30 degrees, the examiner stabilizes the femur with one hand and applies an anterior force to the tibia with the other hand. Excessive movement of the tibia forwards beneath the femur is indicative of an anterior cruciate ligament injury.

lactacid excess post-exercise oxygen consumption The portion of oxygen consumed after exercise that removes excess lactic acid from the blood. A small amount of the excess lactic acid is excreted in urine and sweat; a little contributes to the manufacture of protein; some is converted to glucose or glycogen in the liver and muscle; but most of the lactic acid produced during exercise is reconverted into pyruvic acid and used in *aerobic metabolism to form carbon dioxide and water. Approximately five to ten litres of oxygen forms the lactacid post exercise oxygen consumption; it is usually higher in highly trained athletes, especially sprinters.

lactacid system *See* **lactic acid system**.

lactase Enzyme that catalyses the breakdown of lactose (milk sugar) to glucose and galactose. *See also* **lactose intolerance**.

lactate A salt or ester of lactic acid in which a metal or organic radical has replaced hydrogen in the carboxyl group. Lactate is a dissociation product of lactic acid which occurs in the blood. Blood lactate levels vary but are usually 1–2 mmol/l and increase during anaerobic metabolism as lactic acid is produced. It has been suggested that lactate is not a useless by-product of anaerobic metabolism, but that it may be an important metabolic fuel used by muscles, especially during exercise. *See also* **lactic acid**.

lactate analyser An instrument used for the rapid, automatic analysis of lactate levels in blood samples from a single fingerprick. Although easy to use and reliable, lactate analysers are expensive and should be used only by trained medical staff.

lactate dehydrogenase (LDH) An enzyme, the level of which is commonly used in exercise physiology as a measure of the capacity of *glycolysis. It catalyses interconversions of pyruvic acid and lactic acid. It is found in many cells, but especially in muscle cells. There are different forms of LDH. One form called heart-specific LDH (H-LDH) preferentially catalyses lactate oxidation to pyruvate and predominates in slow-twitch muscle fibres. Another form, muscle-specific LDH (M-LDH), preferentially catalyses the reduction of pyruvate to lactate and predominates in fast-twitch muscle fibres. With endurance training, the relative activity of H-LDH increases in slow-twitch fibres, improving the ability of muscles to oxidize lactate. The amount of LDH in muscle fibres appears to decrease or not change in response to heavy resistance training.

lactate paradox The observation that during exercise, peak blood lactate concentration is lower in individuals acclimatized to high altitude, but, at any given exercise intensity, the blood lactate concentration of an individual is greater at high altitude.

lactate threshold The point during exercise of increasing intensity at which blood lactate begins to accumulate significantly above resting levels. There are several different methods of estimating the threshold. They include specifying a given value of blood lactate (usually between 2.0 to 4.0 mmol lactate l⁻¹) and using this value as a common reference point (known as Onset of Blood Lactate Accumulation or OBLA). Another method identifies graphically the onset of an exponential increase in lactate concentration. The assumption that the lactate threshold represents the *anaerobic threshold has been challenged recently, but the lactate threshold is generally accepted as being useful in identifying a specific intensity of exercise below which endurance is mainly a function of fuel supply, body temperature, or soft tissue trauma, and above which there is a significant reduction in endurance, probably due to metabolic disorders such as acidosis. Appropriate training (e.g., regular intensive aerobic activity) can enable an athlete to postpone lactate accumulation until higher intensities of exercise are reached. This is beneficial to an endurance athlete because lactate formation contributes to fatigue.

lacteal A central, blind-ended lymph vessel in a villus into which neutral fat is passed from the columnar epithelium of the small intestine where the fat has been re-synthesized from fatty acids and glycerol. The fat is in the form of a white, milky emulsion (hence the name lacteal) and is carried to all parts of the body.

lactic acid An organic acid with the chemical formula $CH_3CH(OH).COOH$. Lactic acid is a product of anaerobic glycolysis (*see* **lactic acid system**). Most of this lactic acid quickly dissociates into hydrogen ions (protons) and lactate. For this reason, the terms lactic acid and lactate are often used interchangeably. An excessive production of lactic acid is associated with muscle fatigue and certain forms of muscle soreness. It appears, however, that muscle fatigue during high intensity exercise is associated with the protons increasing the acidity in muscles and is not due to a direct effect of lactate.

lactic acid system (lactacid system) An anaerobic energy system in which ATP is manufactured from the breakdown of glucose to pyruvic acid. The acid is then converted to lactic acid. High-intensity activities lasting up to about two or three minutes use this energy system during which the reduction of nicotinamide adenine dinucleotide (NAD) is coupled

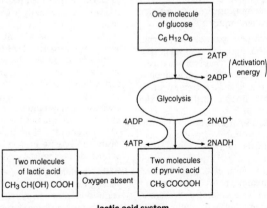

lactic acid system

with a net production of two ATP molecules for each glucose molecule metabolized.

lactogenic hormone *See* **prolactin.**

lactose A disaccharide sugar made from galactose and glucose; milk sugar. Although lactose is potentially a rich source of energy, many people suffer from lactose intolerance because they lack the enzyme (lactase) required to digest it.

lactose intolerance An intolerance to milk or milk products because of an inability to digest lactose (milk sugar) due to deficiency of the enzyme lactase. It is characterized by abdominal cramps, flatulence, and diarrhoea. The diarrhoea appears to be more pronounced during competitive sports that involve running. This can seriously impair performance. Some people do not produce lactase past adolescence, and most people tend to produce less of the enzyme as they age. Consequently, a large proportion of the population suffers lactose intolerance. Anyone who regularly develops diarrhoea during competition, should initially stop consuming dairy products for 24–48 hours before competition to see if milk is the precipitating factor.

lacuna A small cavity or space, for example, one of the many spaces between the lamellae of bone cells, or the space occupied by a cartilage cell.

laddergraph A technique for displaying data in which two test scales are orientated vertically with an individual's scores joined by a line.

laetrile (vitamin B_{17}) A water-soluble compound often found with members of the vitamin B complex. It is sometimes marketed as a vitamin, but it is not a true vitamin.

laevator scapulae *See* **levator scapulae.**

lambda In anthropometry, the point on the cranium at the junction of the sagittal and lamboid sutures.

lame brain jockey Term used to describe a jockey who has suffered repeated blows to the head from falls off a horse. It is described clinically as post-traumatic encephalopathy (*see* **encephalopathy, traumatic**).

lamella A thin layer, membrane, or plate of tissue. For example, the concentric ring of hard bone in compact bone.

lamellar bone *See* **compact bone.**

lamina 1 Thin layer or plate, especially of bone. **2** The part of a *vertebra which lies between the transverse process and the neural spine.

laminar flow (fluid flow; streamline flow) The smooth flow of a fluid in which adjoining layers of the fluid flow parallel to one another. During laminar flow, all the fluid particles move in distinct and separate layers; there is no mixing between adjacent layers. *Compare* **turbulent flow.**

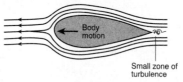

Small zone of
turbulence

laminar flow

landmark (anatomical landmark) A specific point on the human body from which measurements are taken. *See also* **anthropometry.**

large intestine Part of the alimentary canal consisting of the colon, caecum, appendix, and rectum.

laser An acronym for light amplification by stimulated emission of radiation. The laser is a device able to produce a very fine, continuous beam of highly concentrated light which can cut through materials. It is used in surgery to operate on very small structures. Lasers can also produce safe levels of photons in pulses which accelerate the healing process in damaged tissue. These so-called cold or soft lasers have been used to treat *overuse injuries.

latent function of sport A function of sport which is hidden, unintended, and unacknowledged by the participants.

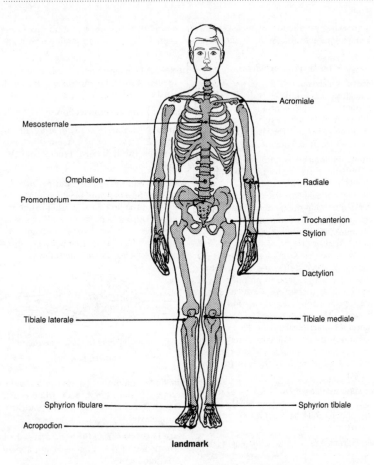

Acromiale

Mesosternale

Omphalion

Promontorium

Radiale

Trochanterion

Stylion

Dactylion

Tibiale laterale

Tibiale mediale

Sphyrion fibulare

Sphyrion tibiale

Acropodion

landmark

latent learning Type of learning which may not be immediately apparent. For example, a delay may occur between practising a skill and improvements in the performance of the skill. The delay may be due to the integration of the different components of the skill.

latent period The period of time between the presentation of a stimulus and the moment a response occurs. For example, the latent period between stimulation and the onset of muscle contraction is about 0.01 seconds and is an irreducible component of *reaction time.

lateral In anatomy, applied to structures away from the midline or on the outer surface of the body.

lateral axis (x-axis) In anthropometry, the axis formed by the intersection of a *frontal plane and *transverse plane.

lateral collateral ligament Knee ligament attached superiorly to the lateral femoral epicondyle and inferiorly to the head of the fibula. It forms part of the lateral ligamentous complex.

lateral compartment syndrome Pain in the lateral side of the lower leg caused by an increase in pressure in the lateral muscle compartment during exercise. *See also* **compartment syndrome**.

lateral cuneiform One of three cuneiform bones in the tarsus (ankle bone). It articulates with the third digit.

lateral epicondylitis *See* **tennis elbow**.

lateral flexion Sideways bending of the trunk, involving the actions of the **iliocostalis and *quadratus lumborum on one side of the trunk.

laterality A component of body awareness by which a person perceives that he or she has two distinct sides capable of independent movement.

lateral ligamentous complex 1 Structures in the lateral aspect of the knee which contribute to its stability. The complex includes the lateral collateral ligament, the iliotibial tract, biceps femoris tendon, the popliteus tendon, and the arcuate ligament. **2** Structures within the lateral aspect of the ankle which contribute to its stability. They include the anterior talofibular ligament, the posterior talofibular ligament, and the calcaneofibular ligaments intimately bound to the peroneal tendon sheath. *See also* **ankle sprain**.

lateral malleolus Lower end of the *fibula which articulates with the talus and forms the prominent bulge on the outer side of the ankle. *See also* **medial malleolus**.

latissimus dorsi (lats) A broad, flat triangular muscle occurring on both sides of the lower back, covered superiorly by the *trapezius and contributing to the posterior wall of the axilla (armpit). This is the broad back muscle which swings the arm backwards and rotates it inwards. It has its origins on the lower six thoracic vertebrae and all lumbar vertebra, the posterior sacrum, the iliac crest, and the lower three or four ribs. Insertions are on the intertubercular groove of the femur. The lats primary actions about the shoulders are extension, adduction, and medial rotation. The lats play an important part in bringing the arm down in a power stroke, as in striking a blow, swimming the front crawl, and rowing.

lats *See* **latissimus dorsi**.

law 1 A norm established by a legislative body and often sanctioned by punishments for violations. Generally, the governing body of each individual sport establishes its own laws. **2** In science, a statement which describes a stable dependency between an independent variable and a dependent variable.

law of acceleration *See* **acceleration, law of**.

law of diminishing returns A law which states that improvements in sporting skills are quite pronounced in the early stages of skill acquisition but then diminish as an athlete reaches a higher level of performance. *See also* **arrested progress**.

law of effect A law which states that rewarding a behaviour increases the probability that the behaviour will be repeated, and punishing a behaviour decreases the probability that the behaviour will be repeated. Thus, the law suggests that the effect of a particular behaviour, whether it is pleasing or displeasing, influences the chances of its recurrence: behaviours resulting in pleasant sensations tend to be repeated, while those associated with unpleasant sensations tend to be avoided. *See also* **law of exercise**.

law of exercise A law which states that, in *learning, the more frequently a stimulus and response are associated with each other, the more likely the particular response will follow the stimulus. The law implies that one learns by doing and one cannot learn a skill, for instance, by watching others. It is necessary to practise the skill, because by doing so the bond between stimulus and response is strengthened. In applying this to motor learning, the more often a given movement is repeated, the more firmly established it becomes. The performance of drills attempts to utilize this law. *See also* **law of effect**; and **Thorndike's stimulus–response theory of learning**.

law of gravitation *See* **gravitation, law of**.

law of inertia *See* **inertia, law of**.

law of mass action Law which states that the rate of chemical reaction is directly proportional to the concentration of the reactants.

law of motion *See* **Newton's laws of motion**.

law of reaction *See* **reaction, law of**.

law of readiness A law which states that *learning is dependent upon the learner's readiness to act, which facilitates the strengthening of the bond between stimulus and response. Thus an athlete who is highly motivated and eager to learn is more likely to be receptive to learning than one who is poorly motivated. *See also* **Thorndike's stimulus–response theory of learning**.

law of use and disuse A law which states that the size of a structure is modified by how much it is used. It applies especially to bones and muscles. Those which are used regularly are suitably stressed (*see* **principle of progressive overload**) and respond by hypertrophy. Those which are not regularly used respond by atrophy. *See also* **Wolff's law**.

laxity Looseness or slackness of the muscles and soft tissue surrounding a joint.

LDH *See* **lactate dehydrogenase**.

LDL *See* **low-density lipoprotein**.

leader 1 A role conferred on the basis of personal characteristics, experience, or through tradition by virtue of the position a person occupies in a group (e.g., team captain or coach). A leader generally takes a major role in making group decisions, motivating the group, and effecting group actions. *See also* **leadership behaviour**. **2** An individual or team occupying first position in a sports event.

leader behaviour description questionnaire A detailed questionnaire designed to describe how leaders behave. Results of many questionnaires have shown that *consideration and *initiating structure were the two most important factors in leadership behaviour. They are independent and a leader can be high in both, low in both, or some other combination.

leadership The exercise of authority over another person or persons. Leadership implies that someone is willing to follow and confer power and status on another person. Good leadership is the art of influencing individuals and groups so that they achieve set goals. *See also* **leader**.

leadership behaviour The behaviour associated with the exercise of authority. Effective leadership behaviour is characterized by the ability of the leader to influence the activities of a group, by initiating structures (such as goal setting) which enable the group to successfully overcome mutual problems and to achieve their group goals. The leadership behaviour exhibited by leaders may or may not reflect their personalities. *Compare* **situational behaviours; universal behaviours**. *See also* **consideration**; and **initiating structure**.

Leadership Scale for Sports (LSS) A scale developed to measure leadership behaviours of sport coaches. It includes the coaches' perceptions of their own behaviour, the athlete's preferences for specific behaviours, and the athlete's perceptions of the coaches' behaviour. The scale has five dimensions: instructional (training) behaviour, democratic behaviour, autocratic behaviour, social support behaviour, and motivational behaviour (in the form of positive feedback given).

leadership style The way a leader acts and the type of relationship he or she has with followers in particular situations.

leadership trait A relatively stable personality disposition, such as intelligence, assertiveness, and independence, associated with a *leader.

lead-up A task or activity which prepares learners for an important goal response. Lead-up activities usually consist of simpler tasks which are thought to be fundamental to the learning of more complex tasks. For example, gymnasts are often taught a number of subroutines which eventually lead to a complex routine.

lean body mass *See* **fat-free mass**.

learned effectiveness A state of mind of individuals who feel that they can control their own success or failures. Learned effectiveness often occurs in those who have been supported and encouraged during childhood and have a history of success at a sport. *Compare* **learned helplessness**.

learned helplessness A mental state in which people feel that they have no control over their failures, and that failure is inevitable. Learned helplessness often occurs in children who are raised in harsh social environments where success is difficult to achieve. They suffer motivational losses and are very resistant to training.

learning An internal neural process, associated with practice or experience, leading to relatively permanent changes in behaviour which are not due to growth or fatigue. Learning is often assumed to occur when relatively stable changes in performance occur.

learning curve A curve on a graph which shows performance changes against practice time or number of practice sessions. The term implies that changes in performance mirror changes in learning. Many scientists believe that this idea is an oversimplification (*see* **latent learning**). Learning curves (or, more correctly, performance curves) are used to depict the acquisition of skill. For many sports they are negatively accelerating, that is, show the fastest rate of improvement in the early stages of practice and the slowest rate as individuals approach the limits of their ability. However, accurate learning curves are difficult to obtain and are very variable since fluctuations are imposed by many factors, such as motivation, health, and concentration.

learning method A procedure used for learning and teaching a *skill. No one method is best for every skill. In fact, even the best method to learn a particular skill seems to be dependent on the individual learner. *Compare* **training**. *See also* **backward chaining method**; **part-method of learning**; **part-whole method of learning**; **progressive-part method**; **repetitive method**; **whole method**; **whole-part-whole method**.

learning objective An outcome a learner is expected to achieve at the end of a given unit of instruction. From the point of view of a coach, it is called an instructional objective. Learning objectives can be established at different levels of difficulty and in three domains: cognitive, usually concerned with verbal learning; motor, concerned with physical skills; and affective, concerned with attitudes, feelings, and values. Commonly, learning objectives in sport involve all three domains, although the motor domain may be the most obvious.

learning score A score computed as the difference between the initial and final levels of a variable, sometimes used in estimating the changes in performance as a result of practice.

learning variable An independent variable that affects both the performance of a skill when it is present and the learning of the skill after it has been removed.

least preferred co-worker scale A scale which measures the empathy of leaders for their least preferred team member. The scores are used to identify the type of motivation a leader tends to use. A high score indicates that a leader has positive feelings towards a weak member of the group and thus has high relationship motivation; a low score indicates the leader has high task motivation.

lecithin A phospholipid present in large amounts in egg yolk and soya beans. It is involved in fat metabolism and is a component of cell membranes and the myelin sheath of nerves. It has been claimed that inclusion of lecithin in a postcompetition diet accelerates recovery.

Le Fort fractures Fractures of the *maxilla that result in a backward displacement of the tooth-bearing portions so that the upper teeth are positioned behind the lower incisors.

left spin *See* side spin.

leg *See* **lower limb**.

leger test *See* **shuttle run test**.

leg-length discrepancy *See* anatomical short leg.

leg-overuse compartment syndrome A condition associated with excessive exercise. It is characterized by a dull, generalized ache in the anterior, lateral, or posterior compartments of the leg (*see* **muscle compartment**). *See also* **compartment syndrome**.

leisure A time in which individuals are not compelled to do anything, and are free to choose to relax or to take part in a leisure activity. Leisure has important social functions, including relief from the demands and restrictions of work.

leisure activity An activity, distinct from the routine obligations of work, family, and society, in which an individual voluntarily takes part. Leisure activities may or may not be physically demanding. They include watching and taking part in sport. It is generally agreed that many leisure activities have strong socializing influences (*see* **socialization**).

length A linear measurement of an object, end-to-end; it is usually the longest dimension. The SI unit of length is the metre.

length–tension diagram A graph of the tension produced by a contracting muscle as a function of its length. *See also* **length–tension relationship**.

length–tension relationship The relationship between the length of a muscle and the contractile tension which it can exert. A muscle can usually exert its greatest contractile tension when it is at its resting length, but in normal muscle, a greater overall force is produced when the muscle is stretched, which seemingly contradicts the general length–tension relationship. However, the apparent increase is due to the contribution of the elastic components of the joint tissues and not to an increased muscle tension.

leptospirosis *See* **Weil's disease**.

lesion Any discontinuity in a tissue, or loss of function of a body-part, as a result of damage by disease or wounding. Lesions range from sores and ulcers to tumours.

lesser trochanter A bony protuberance on the inner side of the neck of the *femur which acts as an attachment point for some of the muscles of the thigh and buttocks.

lesser tuberosity An elevation of the *humerus which acts as the insertion point for muscles such as the *subscapularis.

leucine An essential amino acid found in corns and legumes. It plays an important role in protein metabolism and is vital for growth of infants. Leucine may also promote muscle growth during recovery after prolonged exercise or after hard training sessions. It is one of the branch-chained amino acids which can be used by muscles as an energy source

leucocyte A white blood cell. Leucocytes include monocytes, granulocytes, and lymphocytes, all derived from the same type of cell in bone marrow. They protect the body against infection by engulfing foreign material (phagocytosis) and producing *antibodies. They also take part in bone-remodelling.

leukotrienes Endogenous chemicals derived from *arachidonic acid. They are released from *mast cells as part of the inflammation response. They attract white blood cells (*see* **leucocyte**) to sites of tissue damage and cause smooth muscle to contract. Large amounts are released during an allergic reaction or asthmatic attack when their effects on the smooth muscle can make it very difficult to breathe.

levator scapulae (laevator scapulae) A muscle with its origins on the transverse processes of the four upper cervical vertebrae and its insertions on the top of the scapula, close to the spine. It works with the trapezius to elevate and adduct the scapula. When the scapula is fixed, it slightly rotates the cervical spine.

levatores costarum *See* **deep spinal muscles**.

levelling effect The effect observed when highly skilled athletes compete with less skilled athletes. There is a tendency for the performance of the more skilled athletes to decline while performance of the less skilled athletes improves.

level of expectation *See* **aspirational level**.

levels of processing framework A framework for memory research that views *memory as continuous rather than discrete. The level of processing framework is a rival to the *black box theory of memory which regards memory as consisting of three compartments: STS, short term memory, and long term memory. The levels of processing framework attempts to explain the nature of processing which an item has received, without postulating discrete memory compartments. *See also* **depth of processing**.

lever A bar or some other relatively rigid structure hinged at one point so that it can do work by rotating about an axis (the fulcrum or pivot) when a force is applied to it. In the human body, bones act as levers. The axis of a bone passes through a joint and it is moved by muscle forces (the effort) at the point of muscle attachment. The load consists of any resistance to movement. Sports implements, such as golf clubs and rackets, become levers when held in the hand. The usual function of a lever is to gain a *mechanical advantage whereby a small force applied over a large distance at one end of the lever produces a greater force operating over a smaller distance at the other end of the lever, or whereby a given speed of movement at one end of the lever is greatly increased at the other end. *See also* **first class lever; second-class lever;** and **third class lever**.

lever arm *See* **moment arm**.

Leydig cell Testosterone-secreting cell in the interstitial area, between the seminiferous tubules, in the testis.

libido A store of vital energy, mental in nature, which is conceived as being derived solely from sexual energy. The idea of the libido was developed by Sigmund Freud and used in psychoanalysis. It is a component of Freudian theory.

lidocaine *See* **lignocaine**.

life chances The advantages and disadvantages, such as access to sports facilities and coaching services, of an individual or group which provide opportunities in life for changing status.

life course The sociohistorical process occurring from infancy to old age.

life-cycle The process of change and development that a person, institution, or other entity undergoes in relation to chronological age. Use of the term implies that different people or institutions share common features (such as growth, maturity, and decay) related to age.

life-cycle model of cohesion A model of *cohesion which suggests that teams and groups have a life cycle from creation or formation, to dissolution, and that cohesion follows this same pattern. In one model, five main stages have been identified: encountering, boundary-testing, role creation, producing or constructing, and dissolution. Thus cohesion increases after the creation of a group, levels off when the group is well established, and then decreases until members of the group finally separate. *See also* **team**.

life-cycle theory of leadership A theory suggesting that the type of leadership (or coaching style) appropriate for a given situation depends on the maturity of the athlete being coached. The need for coaching behaviour consistent with *initiating structure, for example, tends to decrease with age. The need for coaching styles consistent with *consideration tends to be low for very mature and immature athletes, and high for those with moderate levels of maturity.

life event Any significant event in a person's life which may have beneficial or detrimental effects on social relationships and status. Disruptive events, such as loss of job, disability, and bereavement, are called life crises. However, both the apparently beneficial events (such as selection for an international team) and the detrimental events may increase *stress and anxiety, and are implicated in the development of some diseases. Many people think that highly stressed athletes are more likely to be injured, but the results from research on links between significant life events and the susceptibility to sports injury are inconclusive.

lifestyle management training Training designed, usually with the help of a sport psychologist, to help an athlete cope with stress, manage time, and organize life to optimize performance potential.

lift A force acting on a body in a fluid in a direction perpendicular to fluid flow. Lift may assume any direction as determined by the direction of fluid flow and the orientation of the body; it is not necessarily directed vertically upward. Lift is affected by the relative velocity of the fluid; the density of the fluid; and the size, shape, and orientation of the body.

lift–drag ratio The magnitude of lift force divided by the magnitude of total *drag forces acting on a body at any given time as it moves through a fluid. The lift–drag ratio is affected by the angle of attack. When throwing a projectile such as a discus or javelin, the optimum *angle of attack for maximizing performance is the angle at which the lift–drag ratio is maximum.

lifter's fracture A stress fracture of the ulnar shaft. It is called a 'lifter's fracture' because it commonly occurred in farmers who frequently lifted heavy objects with a pitchfork. Among sportspeople, it has been reported in volleyball and tennis players, weight-lifters, and baseball pitchers. Four to six weeks, rest from the precipitating activity usually resolves the condition.

ligament A band of tough fibrous tissue joining two bones together. Ligaments may be capsular, extrinsic, or intrinsic. Capsular ligaments are thickenings within a fibrous joint capsule. Extrinsic ligaments run between bony joints, around the outside of a synovial cavity. Intrinsic ligaments occur within a synovial cavity and are generally less common than the other types. Ligaments are relatively nonelastic, but flexible enough to allow movement. Their main tasks are to bind bones together, to strengthen and stabilize joints (especially joints, such as the knee and shoulder, where the articulating bones do not fit very tightly together), and to limit joint movement to certain directions. If a ligament is ruptured or subjected to prolonged tensile stresses (e.g., through the performance of over-enthusiastic flexibility exercises), *joint stability may be reduced.

ligament injury In sport, usually physical damage to a ligament that deforms or tears the collagen fibres that make up the ligament. Ligament injuries are classified according to the degree of damage: in a grade I injury or sprain, there is no macroscopic tear in the fibres; in grade II, or partial tears, some fibres are torn or partly torn, causing joint instability; in grade III or complete tears, most or all of the fibres of the ligament are torn and the joint may be dislocated or substantially disrupted. Assessment of a ligament injury is by stress testing in various positions of the joint.

ligament tear A tear in a *ligament which may be partial or complete. *See also* **sprain**.

ligamentum flavum A ligament which connects the laminae of two adjacent vertebrae. The ligamentum flavum has an unusually high elasticity and is in tension even when the trunk is in the anatomical position. This tension creates prestress, a slight constant compression on the intervertebral discs which enhances stability.

ligamentum nuchae Ligament of the neck; an enlarged cervical portion of the supraspinous ligament which attaches to the neural spines throughout the length of the vertebral column.

ligamentum teres A flat intracapsular ligament running from the *femur head to the lower lip of the *acetabulum. It is not important in stabilizing the joint since it is slack during most hip movements.

light adaptation A term usually employed for the process which occurs when the eye is exposed to normal conditions for daylight vision, but it is used sometimes for the decreasing visual sensitivity which occurs when the eye remains in conditions of bright light.

light stroking Form of *massage, usually carried out with the palms of the hands, to apply oils and soothe muscles. The strokes are performed towards the heart to enhance blood circulation. Contact is maintained with the skin to help the subject relax.

lignocaine (lidocaine) A local *anaesthetic commonly used in minor surgery, including dental surgery. It is also prescribed for the treatment of conditions involving abnormal heart rhythms.

Likert scale A measure of *attitude consisting of a series of attitude statements, such as **1** 'Jogging is a good activity for most people'; **2** 'jogging is boring', each rated on a five-point scale (strongly agree, agree, undecided, disagree, strongly disagree).

Likert-type scale A scale used in many structured questionnaires. As in a Likert scale, an attitude statement is given, such as 'During a football match I find myself getting very tense and worried as the match progresses.'; the respondent then makes a scale reflecting his or her attitude to the statement. The scale might be shown as follows: definitely false 1 2 3 4 5 6 7 8 9 10 definitely true

limb *See* **upper limb**; and **lower limb**.

limbic system Functional brain system mainly associated with the forebrain and concerned with emotional or affective behaviour, learning, and memory. Extensive connections with higher and lower centres of the brain allow the limbic system to respond to a wide range of environmental stimuli.

limen *See* **threshold**.

limiting factor Any factor that tends to inhibit growth or activity of an individual or a population, either by being below the level necessary for normal growth and activity, or by exceeding the limits of tolerance.

limiting friction (maximum static friction) The maximum amount of *friction that can be generated between two static surfaces in contact with each other. Once a force applied to the two surfaces exceeds the limiting friction, motion will occur. For two dry surfaces, the limiting friction is a product of the *normal reaction force and the *coefficient of limiting friction.

line Narrow ridge, less prominent than a crest, which runs along the shaft of a bone. It is a site of muscle attachment.

linea alba The narrow tendinous area extending from the xiphoid process of the *sternum to the *pubic symphysis in the centre of the abdominal wall onto which the *transversus abdominus and part of the external and internal oblique muscles insert.

linea aspera A rough ridge on the posterior aspect of the shaft of the *femur. It acts as a site of muscle attachment.

linear Pertaining to a straight line.

linear model of cohesion A model which originated in psychotherapy but has been applied to development of *cohesion within a group. The model suggests that cohesion develops through well-defined progressive developmental stages. The stages have been referred to as forming, storming, norming, and performing. The forming stage occurs when the group members first meet and is characterized by orientation problems; the storming stage follows and is characterized by conflict; during the norming stage the group comes together and cohesion is enhanced; and finally the performing stage is characterized by the group working together to achieve its goals and directives.

linear momentum (quantity of motion) The product of the *mass and *velocity of an object. The greater the linear momentum of a moving object, the greater the force needed to stop it or alter its direction. Hence a rugby player or American footballer of large mass and velocity is harder to stop than one of less mass running more slowly.

linear motion Motion in which all parts of a system move in the same direction at the same *speed (e.g., a motorcyclist maintaining a motionless posture on a bike that moves in a straight line). Pure linear motion (also called translation) in which a body moves as a unit with different parts not moving relative to each other, is unusual in sport. Different limb movements are usually necessary to produce movement of the whole body. *See also* **curvilinear motion; and rectilinear motion**.

linear relationship A relationship which occurs when variable quantities are directly proportional to one another. A linear relationship can be represented on a graph as a straight line.

linear velocity Rate at which a body moves in a straight line from one location to another. Average linear velocity = displacement/time taken. The linear velocity of a point on a turning body, such as a lever, is directly proportional to its distance from the axis. Therefore, the maximum linear velocity of a moving lever (such as a limb) occurs at its distal end, and the longer the radius of the lever, the greater its linear velocity.

linear vibration Back and forth motion along a straight line. *See also* **angular vibration**.

line of action (line of force) The straight line extending indefinitely through the point of application of a force and along the direction of the force. *See also* **line of gravity**.

line of force *See* **line of action**.

line of gravity An imaginary vertical line passing from the *centre of gravity of an object down to the ground. It is also known as the line of action of the force of gravity.

liniment Preparation applied externally to the body in the belief that it warms and protects. A liniment, by providing a warm sensation, may have psychological benefits but it does not affect the deep muscles (except, possibly, by diverting blood from deep to superficial muscles) and is no substitute for a proper warm-up routine.

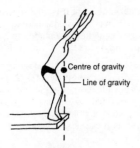

Centre of gravity

Line of gravity

line of gravity

link In a biomechanical system, a straight line through a body segment between adjacent hinge-joints.

linoleic acid A yellow oily polyunsaturated fatty acid. Linoleic acid is an essential fatty acid. It is a component of lecithin and may be used to synthesize *arachidonic acid and linolenic acid. It was once known as vitamin F but is no longer regarded as a vitamin.

linolenic acid A fatty acid ($C_{17}H_{29}COOH$) which can be synthesized from *linoleic acid.

$$CH_3CH_2CH = CHCH_2CH = CHCH_2CH(CH_2)_7COOH$$
linolenic acid

lipase An enzyme secreted by the pancreas. It catalyses the breakdown of fat into fatty acids and glycerol.

lipid Organic compound, insoluble in water, but which dissolves readily in other lipids and in organic solvents such as alcohol, chloroform, and ether. Lipids contain carbon, hydrogen, and oxygen, and sometimes phosphorus. They are classified according to their solubility. They include neutral fats (triacylglycerol or triglyceride), phospholipids, and steroids.

lipid deposit theory Theory which suggests that regular exercise can reduce lipid deposits and atherosclerosis, and thus reduce the risk of coronary heart disease.

lipolysis The hydrolytic breakdown of lipids into fatty acids and glycerol.

lipoprotein An organic compound formed from lipid and protein that transports fats

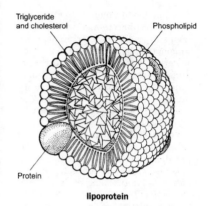

Triglyceride and cholesterol

Phospholipid

Protein

lipoprotein

and cholesterol through the bloodstream and lymph. *See also* **high-density lipoprotein**; **low-density lipoprotein**; and **very low-density lipoprotein**.

lipoprotein lipase An enzyme produced in fat cells (adipocytes) and bound to the walls of capillaries. It breaks down triacylglycerols (triglycerides) into free fatty acids and glycerol which can enter cells for storage or energy production.

liposis The accumulation of abnormally large amounts of fat in the body; also known as adiposis. *See also* **obesity**.

Lisfranc's joint The second metatarsal–tarsal joint in the foot. Female gymnasts doing floor exercises are predisposed to stress fractures of the bones of this joint because it is less mobile than the other metatarsal–tarsal joints.

litre (l) A unit of volume formerly defined as the volume occupied by a mass of 1 kg of pure water at its maximum density and standard atmospheric pressure. It is equal to 1.000 028 decimetres cubed. It has subsequently been defined as a special name for a decimetre cubed. This has caused some confusion.

Little Leaguer's elbow Recurrent pain on the inner aspect of the elbow of children and adolescents caused by damage to the *epiphysis (cartilaginous growth plate). The forces produced by repeatedly throwing a baseball can pull off a portion of the cartilage on the humerus (technically called a traumatic avulsion fracture of the medial epicondyle). If treated early by rest, ice, and immobilization in a splint, the separated growth cartilage can reattach. However, if treatment is delayed and the condition deteriorates, surgical fixation may be required. Little Leaguer's elbow is quite common in children in the USA because of the popularity in that country of baseball; the Little League is a junior baseball league. Young baseball players who make more than 350 forceful throws a week are at particular risk of developing Little Leaguer's elbow. Young pitchers are advised to restrict their pitching to less than 250 throws each week. *See also* **epiphysitis**.

Little League shoulder An injury affecting the proximal growing ends of the humerus due to excessive throwing. *See also* **Little Leaguer's elbow**.

liver One of the largest organs of the body. The liver has many functions including detoxication, glucose metabolism, urea formation, bile production, storage of fat-soluble vitamins and some minerals (e.g., iron), and the manufacture of the clotting agents, prothrombin and fibrinogen. The liver also plays an important role in thermoregulation; changes in metabolism of its cells varies the heat produced by the body.

load The sum of all the forces and moments acting on a body. In a human movement, the load is the bone, the overlying tissue, and anything else resisting that particular movement.

loading In strength training, the load or resistance used.

loading intensity The strength of a training stimulus or the work executed per unit time during a training session. Loading intensities for endurance training and speed-training are calculated from the athlete's speed in metres per second and frequency of movement; for strength training, loading intensity is reflected by the amount of resistance (*see* **repetition maximum**); for jumping or throwing, loading intensity depends on the height jumped or distances thrown.

loafer's heart theory The theory that the heart of an inactive person is less able than that of an active person to cope with stress and increases in demands, thereby making it more susceptible to a heart attack.

lobe A major division of an organ such as brain, liver, pancreas, and lung. Lobes are often separated from one another by fissures or bands of connective tissue.

lobule Subdivision of a lobe of an organ, such as the lungs, and pancreas.

local anaesthetic A drug which temporarily blocks the passage of *nerve impulses, removing the sensation of pain when applied locally to nerve tissue. Although local anaesthetics do not damage nerves, they may aggravate injuries, therefore the International Olympic Committee (IOC) restricts their use. Certain types of injectable local anaesthetics (e.g., procaine, xylocaine, and carbocaine, but not cocaine) may be used by athletes as long as the use is medically justified and the route of administration is either local or by intra-articular injection. Where appropriate, details of diagnosis, dose, and route of administration of local anaesthetics must be submitted in writing to the IOC Medical Commission or the relevant Sports Federation. Intravenous injection and the use of cocaine are always banned. There is no ban on the topical application of local anaesthetics.

local cross-fibre stroke Gentle but deep *massage applied with the thumb and or fingertips across muscles in which problem areas feel hard and knotted. It is used during rehabilitation rather than on newly injured areas.

local muscular fatigue Reduction in the effectiveness of a muscle or muscle group reflected by a decline in peak tension. Local muscular fatigue may be due to one or more reasons, such as failure of a motor nerve to transmit nerve impulses to the muscle; fatigue at the neuromuscular junction through depletion of neurotransmitters; inability of the contractile mechanism (the actin and myosin myofilaments) to generate force; accumulation of protons from lactic acid in the muscle; depletion of ATP and phosphocreatine; or failure of the central nervous system to initiate and relay nerve impulses to the muscle. The most probable sites of local muscular fatigue are the neuromuscular junctions, the contractile mechanism of the muscle itself, and the central nervous system. Fatigue at the neuromuscular junction, which might be more common in fast twitch fibres, is probably due to depletion of *acetylcholine. Fatigue within the contractile mechanism may be caused by accumulation of protons, depletion of ATP and phosphocreatine; depletion of muscle glycogen; dehydration; or lack of oxygen and inadequate blood flow.

locking Inability to move a joint through its full range of motion due to a mechanical defect or obstruction within the joint. It may result in an inability to fully extend the joint, or the fixation of a joint in one position. Locking or inability to move a joint can be caused by extreme pain due to a muscle spasm or by interference from a foreign body or torn cartilage. Locking of the knee-joint, for example, may be due to a spasm of the hamstrings, a meniscal tear, or loose bodies (joint mice).

lockjaw *See* **tetanus**.

locomotives A form of *pyramid training used especially in swimming. A typical session in a 25 m pool might consist of swimming four lengths hard, four lengths slowly; three hard, three slowly; two hard, two slowly; one hard, one slowly. Then back up the ladder, starting with one hard, one slow; two hard, two slow, etc.

locus of causality A dimension used in *attribution theory which relates to a competitor's perception of the cause of success or failure. The locus of causality may be internal (i.e., based on the competitor's own characteristics, such as ability or effort) or external (i.e., due to factors such as luck, outside the control of the competitor).

locus of control A psychological construct that refers to whether individuals believe that their behaviour or, more correctly, the reinforcements from behaviour, is under their own control (internal locus of control; *see* **internals**) or not (external locus of control; *see* **externals**).

logical model The notion that people make logical attributions about behavioural outcomes. *Compare* **illogical model**.

loin The area of the back between the pelvis and the thorax.

log-linear analysis Statistical technique used on cross-tabulations of data. It transforms nonlinear models into linear models by log transformations. This is required in some studies of sport sociology where measurements are *nominal and *ordinal, and therefore do not meet the assumptions needed by many statistical techniques. It is a *causal modelling technique.

loin The area of the back between the pelvis and thorax.

lombardianism View promoted by the American Football coach, Vincent Lombardi, which endorses the statement that only winners matter in sport. He is reputed to have the coined the phrase 'winning isn't the most important thing—it's the only thing'.

Lombard's paradox A situation which arises when a muscle spanning two joints contracts and affects the joints in two opposing ways. During running, for example, the *rectus femoris produces movements at two joints when contracting. While one movement, knee extension, is required in a particular phase of the activity, the other movement, hip flexion, is contrary to the desired action during that phase.

long biceps tendon A tendon which runs from the *biceps brachii through the bicipital groove over the head of the humerus to attach onto the supraglenoid tuberosity of the scapula. It is susceptible to degenerative changes and rupture in athletes over 40 years old.

long bone A bone consisting of a long hollow, roughly cylindrical shaft (the diaphysis) of compact bone, with bulbous ends (the epiphyses) of spongy bone. Examples include the tibia, humerus, and the femur. The long bones are so named because of their elongated shape, not because of their size; the three bones in each finger are long bones even though small. Long bones are adapted for weight-bearing and can withstand considerable stress; they also serve as levers for sweeping, speedy movements.

longevity The length of a person's life. There is some evidence that people who engage in regular, moderate aerobic exercise throughout life may increase their longevity by about 2 years but the evidence is limited.

long–fast duration training A relatively high intensity, relatively long duration form of training in which a distance or middle-distance athlete works at about 80–85 per cent VO_2 max (i.e. at about race pace or just below). This type of training is psychologically demanding. It also puts considerable stress on the bones and joints. Too much reliance on long–fast duration training can lead to *overuse injuries, but used properly, it can provide greater improvements than long–slow duration training (*see* **LSD training**). A typical session of long–fast duration training for a good middle distance runner would be 5 miles (8 km) at 5:30 per mile pace (about 3:15 per km).

longissimus A three-part muscle of the *erector spinae group which extends from the lumbar region to the skull. The longissimus consists of the longissimus cervicis, longissimus thoracis, and the longissimus capitis. The thoracis and cervicis act together to extend the vertebral column and, acting on one side only, bend it laterally. The capitis extends the head and turns the face to one side.

longitudinal axis An imaginary line (one of the anatomical reference axes) running down the centre of the body perpendicular to the transverse plane, around which rotations in the transverse plane (e.g., a body spin during pirouette) occur.

longitudinal research design A basic type of research method in which subjects are tested one or more times after initial testing. Typically, subjects are assigned randomly to an experimental group (e.g., a group that performs a specific type of training) and a *control group after the initial testing. Both the experimental and the control groups are tested again simultaneously one or more times during the period of the study. In this way, the effects of an experimental procedure can be measured over a period of time.

long loop reflex A *stretch reflex with a latency of 50–80 ms, modified by instructions mediated by a higher centre of the brain.

long–slow duration training See LSD training.

long-term anaerobic performance Exercise lasting about 90 s. It is supported by both anaerobic and aerobic metabolism, but depends more on the capacity of the former than the latter.

long-term anaerobic performance capacity The maximum total work output of exercise lasting about 90 s.

long-term anaerobic test A fitness test lasting between 60–90 s. It is designed to evaluate total *anaerobic capacity and the ability to maintain a high power output using mainly anaerobic metabolism. Tests include the *Cunningham and Faulkner treadmill test; the *Quebec ninety-second test; and the *Bosco jump test.

long-term endurance The ability to sustain a strenuous activity for 10 minutes or longer. Such endurance is associated with recruitment of mainly slow-twitch muscle fibres, and the energy is supplied mainly by the aerobic system. The contribution of the aerobic system becomes greater as the duration of the activity increases, and the activity becomes increasingly reliant on *free fatty acids as a source of fuel.

long-term memory According to the *black-box theory of memory, an almost relatively permanent memory compartment capable of storing very large amounts of information for long periods of time. The long-term memory is presumed to include a store of movement programs which are recalled during the execution of complex manoeuvres. It is believed that new information is added to the long-term memory from the *short-term memory, and that prior to the execution of movements, information from the long-term memory is processed together with that from the short-term sensory store in the short-term memory.

long-term motor memory A memory for relatively well-learned *motor skills with retention intervals of months or even years.

longus capitis See prevertebral muscles.

longus colli See prevertebral muscles.

loose bodies (joint mice) Small pieces of bone or cartilage floating within a joint capsule. Loose bodies may include pieces of articular cartilage. Their occurrence probably reflects a joint trauma or the wearing away of the articular cartilage which exposes the surface of the bone beneath, causing it to die and separate. Symptoms include painful catching or locking of the joint. Loose bodies may promote *osteoarthrtitis if not removed or, if the loose bodies consist of articular cartilage and bone, reattached.

loose-packed position See close-packed position.

lordosis (lumbar lordosis; sway back) An accentuated curvature of the spine in the lumbar region. Lordosis places compressive stress on the posterior elements of the spine which commonly leads to *low-back pain. Lordosis may result from rickets or some other disease, but it is more commonly caused by poor posture, weakened abdominal muscles, or an unequal muscle-pull on the spine, as when carrying a large mass in front of the body in pregnant women or obese people. There is also a tendency to develop lordosis during a growth spurt. There is a wide ethnic variation in the shape of the back, and lordosis may be quite marked and normal in some people.

loudness The intensity aspect of auditory experience, scaled in decibels.

low-back pain Localized pain or discomfort in the lumbosacral region of the back. Low-back pain is a frequently encountered complaint of athletes and the general population. It is often caused by postural defects when the normal relationship between muscles, bones, and other tissues is distorted. Low-back pain may also be caused by shortening of the hamstrings following vigorous exercise which puts a strain on the back. Sometimes the origin of low-back pain may involve the vertebral column and its nerves, or it may be a referred pain from damaged or diseased organs in the pelvis and abdomen. Back pain resulting from postural defects, or overtight or strained muscles can be treated by analgesics and anti-inflammatories in the acute stage. When pain is relieved, exercises should be performed which improve posture, strengthen the abdominal muscles, and improve the flexibility of the hamstrings. *See also* **ankylosing spondylitis**; **prolapsed intervertebral disc**; **spondylolisthesis**; and **spondylolysis**.

low-density lipoprotein (LDL) A specific kind of *lipoprotein which transports *cholesterol in the blood. LDLs contain a larger proportion of cholesterol than high-density lipoproteins. They release the cholesterol at sites in the body where it can be used (e.g., for synthesis of steroids), but continue to carry the cholesterol if it is not used. High concentrations of LDLs in the blood may result in excess cholesterol being deposited in the walls of blood vessels. This may lead to cardiovascular diseases such as *atherosclerosis. Regular exercise and a balanced diet can decrease the amount of LDLs relative to high density lipoproteins, and reduce the risk of cardiovascular heart disease.

low-intensity aerobics Aerobic exercise performed at low intensity. Many people believe that this types of activity is a quick way to become lean because it uses a higher percentage of fat for energy when compared with a high-intensity activity. However, the total energy expenditure for a given period of time is much less for the low-intensity activity, and the actual amount of fat lost may be the same for both types of activity. Nevertheless, low-intensity aerobics does have the advantage of being less stressful on the joints and, although it may not contribute greatly to aerobic fitness, it probably does provide a sufficient stimulus to the heart to reduce the risk of cardiovascular diseases.

lower leg extension *See* **knee extension**.

lower leg movements *See* **knee movements**.

lower limb (leg) Region of the body containing three functional segments: the thigh, the lower leg (knee, tibia, and fibula), and the foot. The lower limb carries the entire weight of the erect body and is subjected to exceptionally high forces during jumping and running. It contains thicker and stronger bones than the upper limb, and is specialized for stability and weight-bearing.

lower leg flexion *See* **knee flexion**.

lower means interdependence Relationships exhibited in coactive sports that do not require team mate interaction for success. *Compare* **high means interdependence**.

LSD training Long–slow duration training performed at 60 per cent to 80 per cent of maximal heart rate (seldom above 160 beats per minute for a young athlete and 140 beats per minute for an older athlete). This form of *continuous training is designed to improve *aerobic endurance. It places emphasis on distance rather than speed. Serious distance runners may run 16–32 km (10–20 miles) each day, with weekly totals exceeding 160 km (100 miles). LSD training is especially suitable for older or less fit individuals because it puts less stress on the cardiovascular and respiratory systems than high intensity exercise. If performed too often, however, it can result in *overuse injuries to the muscles and joints. People who use LSD training for health-related purposes, or athletes using it to maintain endurance condition during the off-season, usually reduce the training distance (e.g., 5 to 8 km, or 3–5 miles, for runners).

LSS *See* **Leadership Scale for Sports**.

LTM *See* **long term memory**.

lub-dub Heart sounds heard through a stethoscope applied to the chest. The first sound, a lub, coincides with the beginning of ventricular systole and closure of the atrioventricular valves. The second sound, dub, coincides with the beginning of diastole and the closure of valves in the aorta and pulmonary artery.

luck An external attribution, lack of which is often offered as an excuse for poor sports performance.

ludic activity Social interaction based on games and play. Ludic activities and sport share at least two elements: uncertain outcomes and sanctioned displays. The uncertain outcomes provide suspense and excitement; the sanctioned displays give participants socially acceptable opportunities to exhibit physical prowess.

ludic institutionalization The process by which simple, informal play and games develop into formal, highly regulated sports.

lumbago Acute pain resulting from inflammation of tissues in the lower back. It has many causes. The acute onset of lumbago may result from a herniated disc, a strained muscle, or a sprained ligament; any of these can be sustained during a sporting activity. *See also* **low-back pain**.

lumbar Pertaining to the lower back.

lumbar curvature *See* **spinal curvature**.

lumbar lordosis *See* **lordosis**.

lumbar pelvic rhythm Smooth simultaneous combination of lumbar flexion (a reversal of lumbar lordosis) and pelvic rotation around the transverse axes of the hip joints during trunk flexion.

lumbar region The region of the lower back defined by the five vertebrae situated between the *thoracic vertebrae and the *sacrum. The lumbar region forms the largest natural curve in the back and is sometimes referred to as the small of the back.

lumbar vertebra A vertebra of the lower back between the thoracic and sacral vertebrae. There are five lumbar vertebrae, designated L1–L5. Each lumbar vertebra has a sturdy, large, kidney-shaped centrum enabling it to carry out its important weight-bearing function; lumbar vertebrae take much of the strain during locomotion.

lumbosacral angle The angle between the plane of the upper border of the sacrum and the horizontal in a standing position. Poor posture can exaggerate the lumbosacral angle and contribute to static back pain. The angle can be reduced by doing corrective exercises involving the abdominal and gluteal muscles.

lumbosacral joint The articulation between the lumbar and the sacral bones in the back.

lumbosacral stress test A diagnostic test performed on a supine subject by passively raising both legs simultaneously, thereby stressing the *sacroliliac and lumbosacral facet joints. Pain and restricted range indicate dysfunction of the lumbosacral spine.

lumbricales Four muscles that lie between the *metacarpals in the palm of the hand. They have their origins on the tendons of the flexor digitorum profundus at digits 2–5, and their insertions on the tendons of the extensor digitorum at digits 2–5. Their primary action is flexion at the metacarpophalngeal joints (knuckles) of digits 2–5.

lumen Any cavity, such as that of a blood vessel or the alimentary canal, enclosed within a cell or tissues.

lunate bone A wrist bone that articulates with the triquetral and scaphoid, the hamate and capitate in front, and the radius behind. *See also* **carpus**.

lung One of a pair of respiratory organs in the thorax. The lungs consist of a system of

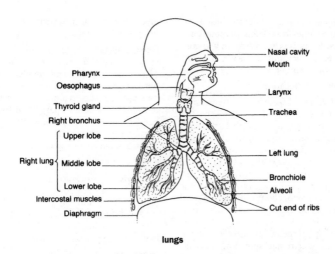

lungs

air tubes terminating in *alveoli where gaseous exchange takes place. The tubes are connected to the air by way of the bronchi and trachea. The lungs are fibrous elastic sacs which can be expanded and compressed by movements of the diaphragm and ribcage during ventilation. The lungs and its airways are a site of water evaporation, an important factor in water balance and thermoregulation.

lung compliance *See* compliance.

lung volumes The volume of air inspired, expired, and remaining in the lungs at different stages and rates of ventilation. Lung volumes can be measured using a *spirometer.

luteinizing hormone (LH) **1** An endogenous hormone produced by the anterior lobe of the pituitary gland. In females, LH stimulates ovulation and formation of the corpus luteum. In males, it stimulates secretion of *testosterone by interstitial cells in the testes. LH is also known as interstitial-cell stimulating hormone (ICSH). **2** A drug belonging to the peptide hormones which are on the International Olympic committee list of *banned substances. Its use is considered to be equivalent to the administration of testosterone.

luxatio erecta An exceedingly rare type of shoulder dislocation in which the humeral head dislocates directly inferiorly and

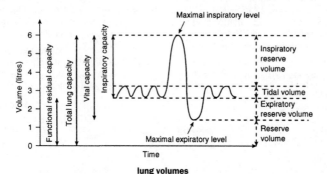

lung volumes

becomes inverted, so that the head is directed downwards and the humeral shaft upwards. Reduction is usually accomplished easily using a traction–countertraction technique.

luxation *See* **dislocation**.

Lyme disease A disease transmitted by ticks belonging to the genus *Ixodes*. The tick occurs throughout the world, particularly in woodland and grassy areas. The tick penetrates the skin, sucks out blood, and, in doing so, allows the causative agent *Borrelia burgdorferi* (a spirochaete bacterium), to gain entry. Unless removed, the tick clings on for about 4 to 5 days, until it is fully satiated and bloated with blood (at this stage it is about the size of a pea). Symptoms of the disease are variable, but typically a circular spreading rash develops around the tick's point of entry, along with stiffness, swelling, and fever. The infection may cause secondary complications which include chest pains, neurological complications, and arthritis. These start to develop one to four weeks after the bite. The infection usually responds well to antibiotics if caught in its early stages, before the onset of secondary complications. Cross-country runners, orienteers, and anyone active in the countryside are particularly vulnerable to this disease. They should either cover up areas of exposed skin, or use an insect repellant on exposed areas and check them every three to four hours. If a tick is found on the body, it should be removed as soon as possible by grasping the head with forceps or fingers (application of alcohol may ease removal). The tick should be kept in a container so that it can be identified by a doctor if symptoms of Lyme disease develop.

lymph The interstitial fluid within lymph vessels. It has a composition similar to blood plasma, but it is richer in fat and lymphocytes.

lymphatic system A system of blind-ending vessels which drain excess fluid from the extracellular spaces. The lymphatic system contains lymph nodes and produces macrophages and *lymphocytes. Groups of nodes occur in most parts of the body, but particularly in the groin, armpits, and behind the ears and neck. They often become inflamed during an infection.

lymphatic A vessel in the lymphatic system.

lymphocyte A type of leucocyte (white blood cell) formed in the bone marrow which plays a vital part in the immune defence system of the body. Lymphocytes divide to form T-cells, which destroy *antigens, or B-cells, which produce *antibodies.

lymphocytopaenia A decrease in the number of *lymphocytes in the blood. This occurs in a number of diseases, and also from 30 min to 3 h following continuous endurance exercise. Exercise-related lymphocytopaenia is usually moderate (20 to 25 per cent) and short-lived (lymphocyte counts return to normal after 6 h of recovery). The decrease in circulating lymphocytes may be due to lymphocytes invading muscle tissues to accelerate repair of cells damaged by the exercise.

lymphokine A substance produced by lymphocytes involved in cell-mediated immune responses that play a part in the body's defence system.

lymph vessel *See* **lymphatic system**.

lysine An essential amino acid found in all animal proteins but which is low in some plant proteins (e.g., cereals).

lysis 1 The breakdown of a cell surface membrane usually by hydrolytic enzymes which results in the cell releasing its contents. **2** The gradual decline of a disease.

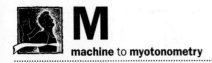

M

machine to **myotonometry**

machine A device which helps to perform work. Machines use energy in one form, modify it, and deliver it in a form more suited to its desired purpose. A simple *lever can be regarded as a machine.

macrocycle *See* **periodization**.

macromineral A mineral, such as *calcium, required by the body in relatively large amounts (more than 100 mg per day).

macronutrient A nutrient required in large amounts to maintain health. Macronutrients include *carbohydrates, *fats, and *proteins.

macrophage A large scavenger cell common in connective tissue and certain body organs where it engulfs and destroys bacteria and other foreign debris. Macrophages are also involved in the *immune response.

macrosociology The study of whole societies, the totality of their social structures, and their social systems.

macrotrauma A force produced by a single incident (e.g., a rugby tackle) sufficiently large to cause an acute injury. *Compare* **microtrauma**.

maculae Sensory receptors of static equilibrium which occur in the utricle and saccule of the inner ear. Each macula consists of hair cells sensitive to linear movements which initiate action potentials in the nerve fibres of the *vestibular apparatus.

magnesium A metallic element essential for good health. Magnesium is a constituent of coenzymes that play a role in the conversion of ATP to ADP. It also helps muscles and nerves function efficiently. Magnesium is absorbed and stored in the bones. Good dietary sources include milk, dairy products, wholegrain cereals, nuts, legumes, and, especially, leafy green vegetables. Excessive intakes may cause diarrhoea; a deficiency can result in neuromuscular problems. In the UK, the daily adult Reference Nutrient Intake is 270 mg in females and 300 mg for males. In the USA, the Recommended Dietary Allowance is 280 mg for females and 350 mg for males. Serum magnesium levels can fall dramatically after intense activity in heat and during endurance activity (for example, decreases of 20 per cent have been recorded after a marathon). However, this appears to be due to a redistribution of the magnesium in the body. The magnesium lost in sweat represents only a small proportion of the magnesium stored in the body, suggesting that magnesium replacement by supplementation after exercise is probably not necessary.

magnetic resonance imaging *See* **nuclear magnetic resonance**.

magnitude Term used in science to specify size or amount.

Magnus effect The deviation in the trajectory of a spinning projectile caused by the *Magnus force. The deviation is toward the direction of the spin and results from pressure differentials in the spinning projectile. The Magnus effect can be observed when a golfer hooks or slices a shot; when a footballer executes a 'banana shot'; and when a baseball pitcher throws a curve ball. The Magnus effect is greatest when the axis of spin is perpendicular to the direction of relative fluid velocity.

Magnus force A lift force which acts on a spinning projectile. The spin creates a region of relative low velocity and high pressure on one side of the projectile, and a region of relatively high velocity and low pressure on the opposite side. The pressure differential creates the Magnus force, a lift force directed from the high pressure region to the low pressure region. The Magnus force causes the trajectory of the

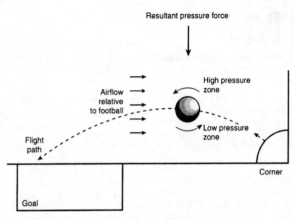

Magnus effect

projectile to deviate in the direction of the spin. Therefore, the Magnus force of a top spin is directed downwards, causing a tennis ball, for example, to rebound low and fast. The Magnus force of a backspin is directed upwards, causing the tennis ball to rebound high and slow. *See also* **Magnus effect**.

MAHR Maximum attainable heart rate; *see* **maximal heart rate**.

maintenance synergy *See* **synergy**.

Maisonneuve's fracture A combination of an ankle sprain involving the *deltoid ligament and a fracture of the proximal *fibula. It occurs, for example, when a skier falls on the ankle and rotational forces twist the tibia on the talus. The forces are so great that their damaging effects extend from the ankle up the *interosseus membrane to fracture the proximal fibula. Maisonneuve's fracture results in the ankle being very unstable. Surgery is usually required to fix the instability. A Maisonneuve's fracture should always be suspected if a medial ankle sprain is accompanied by tenderness high up the fibula. These injuries are seen in less than 2 per cent of all ankle sprains.

making weight Acquiring a particular body weight in order to compete in a specific weight category. To make weight in sports such as horse racing, boxing, and wrestling, competitors often try to lose weight very quickly by using a combination of methods: restricting food intake, depriving themselves of fluid, increasing their physical activity, and by thermal dehydration. In so doing, the athletes may be compromising their health. Weight losses (or gains) should be gradual, no more than 1 to 2 pounds (0.5 to 1 kg) per week. This can usually be achieved by reducing calorie intake by about 200 to 500 Calories per day. More rapid weight losses can lead to loss of fat-free mass and eating disorders.

malabsorption Impaired ability to absorb one or more substances from digested food within the small intestine.

malacia Abnormal softening of tissue, such as bone (osteomalacia) or cartilage (chondromalacia).

malalignment An abnormal position of a structure in relation to others. Malalignment of bones may be congenital, or caused by an injury or chronic postural defect. Malalignment, such as *femoral anteversion, genu varum (bow legs), and genu valgum (knock knees) can predispose athletes to sports injuries.

malate dehydrogenase A respiratory enzyme involved in the *Krebs cycle. It catalyses the interconversion of pyruvate or oxalo-acetate to malate using nicotinamide adenine dinucleotide (NAD).

malignant Any condition that is life-threatening. The term pertains especially to cancers that may spread and lead to death.

malignant melanoma *See* melanoma.

malleolus Either of two protuberances on the ankle. The lateral (outer) malleolus is formed from the lower end of the fibula and articulates with the talus. The medial (inner) malleolus is formed from the lower part of the tibia. The malleoli act as pulleys channeling muscles anterior or posterior to the axis of rotation at the ankle.

mallet finger An injury resulting from a sudden forced flexion of the terminal joint of the finger. It results in the bony insertion of the tendon being stripped off, leaving the patient unable to extend the affected finger. The attachment of the tendon to bone is so strong that the bone itself may be damaged, and the bony fragment may be torn away with the tendon (an avulsion fracture). A mallet finger is quite common in ball games when a hand is slightly closed before the ball is caught. The ball therefore strikes the end of a finger forcing it into flexion and tearing the tendon. If untreated or treated improperly, the finger can become permanently deformed, and a severe avulsion fracture may lead to arthritis in later life. Immediate self-treatment consists of immobilizing the finger and applying ice (*see* **ice treatment**). Subsequent treatment by a doctor depends on the severity of the injury. In an adult, mild injuries may need no special treatment but most mallet fingers require permanent immobilization of the finger in a fully straightened position in a plastic splint for 6–8 weeks; serious avulsion fractures sometimes require surgical reduction and internal fixation.

malnutrition Condition caused by an unbalanced diet with nutrients being deficient, in excess, or in the wrong proportions. Many people, including athletes, suffer from mild malnutrition that adversely affects their physical performance.

maltodextrin drinks Drinks containing maltodextrins, polysaccharides formed during the incomplete breakdown of starch. They can provide as much as ten times the energy of glucose drinks with the same *osmolality without slowing the rate of *gastric emptying. They are quite popular with athletes because they are not as sweet-tasting as glucose drinks and they provide quite a palatable way to consume a lot of carbohydrate. Maltodextrin drinks taken three hours before, or during, an endurance activity may delay fatigue, but their value has not yet been fully evaluated.

maltose A *disaccharide made from two glucose molecules. It occurs in malt extract, an energy-rich food used by some athletes.

manager A person who is responsible for the *leadership, coordination, and control of a sports team.

managerial competencies The personal characteristics or traits required by a coach to manage athletes successfully. Managerial competencies (also known as coaching competencies) include technical competency, conceptual competency, and human competency. A good coach requires these competencies to coach a team successfully.

managerial grid A grid on which the leadership style of managers is scored on two scales, one related to concern for production, and the other related to concern for people. The managerial grid has been adapted for coaches, where the two scales are concern for the athlete and concern for performance.

mandible The lower jaw-bone.

mandibular Pertaining to the lower jaw.

manganese An essential trace element required for the efficient functioning of a number of enzyme systems. Manganese deficiency causes tremors and convulsions. Good sources include nuts, legumes, wholegrains, leafy green vegetables, and fruit. In the UK, the daily adult Reference Nutrient Intake is not established, but a Safe Intake is set at 1.4 mg. In the USA, the Recommended Dietary Allowance is 2.5–5.0 mg.

manipulation Any technique using the hands to produce a desired movement of a body-part, or to return bones, joints, and other body structures to their normal position after displacement. Manipulation may be used by physiotherapists to relieve joint stiffness. It is more vigorous than mobilization; indiscriminate manipulation by an untrained person can cause extensive damage to athletes.

manipulative passive movements Movements performed by external forces exerted, for example, by a therapist on a subject. Manipulative passive movements are sometimes carried out on a subject who is under anaesthetic, to break down *adhesions that are limiting joint mobility.

manipulative skill A gross motor skill involving the use of the hands to control the movement of other objects.

manometer A device for measuring the pressure of a fluid.

mantra A key phrase or mental device used in transcendental meditation and as an intervention strategy by athletes to focus *attention internally and to reduce anxiety.

manual dexterity A skill-oriented ability which underlies tasks for which relatively large objects are manipulated, primarily with the hands.

manual guidance A technique used by coaches to show athletes how to perform a skill. Typically, the coach stands behind the athlete and, using his or her hands, manipulates the athlete to perform the correct movements, for example, of a golf swing or tennis stroke.

manual resistive muscle testing A test of muscle function. A body-part is placed in the desired position and the athlete maintains the position while a firm, constant resistance (not an overpowering force) is applied by the examiner in order to detect muscle dysfunction or weakness.

manubrium The upper part of the *sternum which articulates laterally with the clavicular notches of the *clavicle and the first two pairs of ribs.

manumometer A dynamometer which is placed in the hand and squeezed to measure strength of the gripping muscles. *See also* **muscle strength**.

MAO *See* **monoamine oxidase**.

MAOI *See* **monoamine oxidase inhibitor**.

marasmus A severe form of *malnutrition caused by deficiencies of protein and calorific intake, accompanied by progressive wasting, especially in infants.

march fracture A *stress fracture, typically of one of the long metatarsal bones (usually the second, but sometimes the third, fourth, or fifth) of the forefoot. March fractures were originally described in military recruits who marched a lot; they often result from overtraining among long-distance runners. Pain is felt in the central bone in the front of the foot when walking or running. Treatment consists of immobilization and rest.

march haemoglobinuria (exertional haemolysis; foot-strike haemolysis; runner's haemolysis) The presence of free *haemoglobin in the urine associated with prolonged walking or running. March haemoglobinuria may be due to the breakdown of muscle (*see also* **myoglobinuria**) in the legs or to mechanical trauma on the soles of the feet damaging red blood cells which release their contents of haemoglobin into the blood stream. The occurrence of blood in the urine of swimmers and rowers shows that exertional haemolysis (the splitting open of red blood cells during intense activity) may occur without obvious impact against an external surface. No treatment is needed for mild haemolysis, but in runners the condition can be minimized by avoiding hard running surfaces and wearing well-padded shoes.

Marfan's syndrome An inherited connective tissue disorder that can affect several organ systems. It may cause sudden cardiac death if the heart is affected. Anyone with a family history of Marfan's syndrome should be screened before taking part in sport or a strenuous activity.

Margaria staircase test A short-term anaerobic test or power test in which the subject stands 2 m from a staircase and then sprints at top speed up the staircase, taking two steps at a time, each step being 175 mm high. Pressure pads on the eighth and twelfth step act as switches recording time taken to run between the pads. It is assumed that all the external work of the subject is used to raise the centre of mass of the body, and that this rise is the same as the vertical distance between the eighth and twelfth step. The power output (P) of the subject is calculated as follows: $P = (W \times 9.8 \times D)/t$, where W is the body weight of the subject in kg; 9.8 is the normal acceleration of gravity in ms^{-2}; D is the vertical height in metres between the eighth and twelfth steps; and t is the time taken from the first pressure pad to the second pad. This test is also known as the Margaria step test.

marginal Applied to a role that is considered unimportant in a team or group. Those occupying marginal roles may be disadvantaged. An injured team player, for example, may become marginalized if the team continues to be successful in his or her absence, and the player may be in danger of losing a place in the team.

marijuana (cannabis) A drug obtained from the hemp plant (*Cannabis sativa*). Its active ingredient is tetrahydrocannabinol. The psychological effects of marijuana include sedation, euphoria, and relaxation. It is often used as a means of relaxation and escape from tension. It is generally ergolytic, disturbing the sense of balance and blunting assertiveness. Persistent use of marijuana is incompatible with serious sport participation because it tends to demotivate athletes, taking away their will to win. Marijuana is not on the International Olympic committee list of *banned substances, but it is prohibited by the governing bodies of some sports. Tests for the presence of its metabolites may be carried out at the Olympic Games if so requested by an International Federation. In many countries, marijuana is a controlled drug; it is illegal to possess such drugs except where the user is a registered addict and has obtained their drug legally or by prescription.

marrow cavity In adults, a medullary cavity containing fat (yellow marrow).

masculinity A quality characterized by physical and behavioural features, such as physical strength, which is commonly associated with males. *Compare* **femininity**.

masculinization (virilization) Development of male secondary sexual characteristics, such as growth of a beard. Masculinization in females and prepubertal males who take androgenic steroids or who suffer from hypersecretion of androgens, is known as androgenital syndrome.

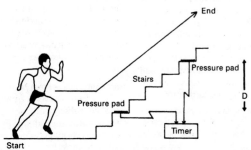

Margaria staircase test

masking agent An agent taken to hide the use of a *banned substance. *Diuretic drugs, for example, have been misused to flush out drugs from, and reduce the concentration of, anabolic steroids in urine samples.

Maslach Burnout Inventory A twenty-two item inventory designed to measure three aspects of burnout: emotional exhaustion, depersonalization, and lack of personal accomplishment. The inventory has been used to identify burnout symptoms in athletes.

mass The quantity of matter composing an object. Mass depends on the density and volume of an object and is constant regardless of where it is. The SI unit of mass is the kilogram (kg).

massage A form of physical therapy involving rubbing, kneading, and tapping body parts. Massage is used to accelerate healing of sports injuries and to prepare athletes for competition by improving muscle tone and circulation. Its benefits, depending on which form of massage is being used, include relaxation, neural stimulation, increased blood flow, and improved drainage from lymph vessels. It requires experienced application because of the risk of damage; massage of a recently traumatized muscle may disturb a clot and cause further haemorrhaging. Massage is not advised for those with circulatory, dermatological, or cardiac problems.

mass centroid *See* **centre of mass**.

massed culture Aspects of culture, including sports products and services, which are transmitted to many in society through the *mass media, and which are designed to appeal to the mass of the population. An important aspect of services and goods produced for the mass market is that they are often standardized, homogenous, and associated with inferior experiences or low quality. *See also* **popular culture**.

massed practice A form of practice of a motor skill in which there is relatively little or no rest between repeat performances of the skill. Massed practice sometimes refers to practice sessions in which the amount of practice time is greater than the amount of rest time between repetitions. Massed practice tends to have less positive influence on skill acquisition than *distributed practice.

masseter Thick cheek muscle attached to the mandible and the zygomatic arch; it closes the jaw during mastication (chewing).

mass media Techniques and institutions including television, radio, and newspapers which can convey information and other forms of symbolic communication rapidly and simultaneously to large, geographically remote and socially distinct audiences. The mass media have great economic, political, and social influences and have made significant contributions to sport.

mass spectrometer An apparatus used in exercise physiology to measure the composition of respired gases. In the fixed collector type of mass spectrometer, samples of gases are ionized, accelerated by an electric field, and, because the directions taken in this field depends on the mass of the ions, the fractions of oxygen, nitrogen, and carbon dioxide in the gas can be measured. The technique, known as mass spectrometry, is also used in dope testing to analyse the chemicals in a urine sample.

mast cells Large cells, often capable of amoeboid movement, found in connective and fatty tissue. They release substances such as *leukotrienes, *histamine, and *heparin during allergic reactions and the inflammation response.

mat burn A friction burn or an abrasion which often occurs among wrestlers when the skin over bony joints rubs against the unyielding surface of a canvas mat. Mat burns are notorious for becoming infected.

match analysis system An objectively compiled record of events in a match which can be subsequently analysed (usually statistically) to evaluate individual and team performance. Methods employed range from very simple paper and pencil records to highly complex event recorders, video recordings, and computerized analysis. Paper and pencil records typically involve identifying key features of play which are recorded by the use of frequency tallies.

matrix 1 A substance, situation, or environment which encloses something or from which something originates. **2** The extracellular substance secreted by cells that determines the specialized function of each type of connective tissue. **3** The rectangular array of elements presented in rows and columns, used to facilitate the solution of problems.

maturation The process of acquiring the adult form and function of a body structure or system.

Matveyev's six phases A training system based on six periods. Periods one and two are preparatory, consisting of general body conditioning and some specific training elements; periods three and four involve more competition-specific training during which athletes take part in some early competitions and prepare for a peak performance; period five is the major competitive period during which athletes attempt to achieve their goals; and period six is a transition period in which the athletes recuperate from a competition season before preparing for the next season.

maxilla (pl. maxillae) One of the pair of upper jaw bones in which the upper set of teeth are embedded. The maxillae also contribute to the bony structure of the orbits, nasal cavity, and the roof of the buccal cavity (palate). *See also* **Le Fort fracture**.

maxillary Pertaining to the jaw.

maxillofacial Pertaining to the upper jaw, face, and associated structures.

maximal Pertaining to the highest possible level.

maximal aerobic power *See* **maximal oxygen uptake**.

maximal expiratory volume (VE max) The maximal volume of air that can be breathed in one minute. It is the highest amount of ventilation that can be achieved during exhaustive exercise. In males VE max increases until physical maturity (from about 40 l min^{-1} at age 6 to more than 110 l min^{-1} at maturity) and then decreases with ageing (to about 70 l min^{-1} for a 65-year-old). Females have a similar pattern of change but generally have a smaller maximal expiratory volume at each age.

maximal heart rate (maximum attainable heart rate; MAHR; HRmax) The highest heart rate value attainable during an all-out effort to the point of exhaustion (i.e. during maximal exercise). Maximal heart rate is often used to compute training heart rates. It can be determined directly using maximal workloads but this is not always a safe or practical procedure. Therefore, it is generally estimated using the formula (220–age in years), since HR max decreases with age. This is only an approximation and may be subject to errors of 10 per cent or more. For example, maximal heart rates of 250 beats per minute have been recorded for brief periods in skiers subjected to stress and intense isometric control. Maximal heart rate varies according to the type of exercise: for example, it is about 13 beats per minute less in an upper body exercise such as swimming, than in a lower body exercise, such as cycling. The lower HRmax is probably due to the relatively smaller amount of muscle mass involved in the upper body exercise.

maximal heart rate reserve The difference between maximal heart rate and resting heart rate. It is used to calculate optimal training heart rates (*see* **Karvonen method**).

maximal oxygen uptake (aerobic work capacity; cardiorespiratory endurance capacity; peak aerobic power; VO$_2$ max) The maximum amount of oxygen that a person can extract from the atmosphere and then transport and use in tissues. Maximal oxygen uptake is estimated as the maximum volume of oxygen voluntarily consumed per unit time, during a large muscle group activity of progressively

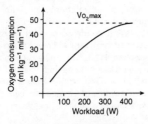

maximal oxygen uptake

increasing intensity that is continued until exhaustion. It is often expressed as VO_2 max: the maximum volume of oxygen consumed per minute. It may also be expressed as the absolute volume of oxygen consumed (l/min) to indicate total work capacity, or volume of oxygen consumed per minute per kilogram body weight $(ml^{-1}kg^{-1}min^{-1})$. The average VO_2 max for a 20-year old female is between 32–38 millilitres per kilogram per minute; for a 20-year-old male it is 36–44 millilitres per kilogram per minute. Endurance athletes tend to have a higher VO_2 max than those involved in power activities. The highest VO_2 max value recorded for a male is 94 millilitres per kilogram per minute for a champion Norwegian cross-country skier. Aerobic training may improve VO_2 max by 15–20 per cent or more. Such increases are due to changes within the cardiopulmonary transport system and tissue chemistry.

maximizing tasks Tasks which require an all-out effort (e.g., sprinting, the tug-of-war, and a power lift).

maximum active range Range of motion through which a joint can go under the direct pull of the muscles. It is greater than the normal active range, but less than the *maximum passive range.

maximum attainable heart rate *See* maximal heart rate.

maximum breath-holding (maximum inspiratory breath-holding) A component of some physiological tests of endurance (e.g., the *cardiopulmonary index). The subject inhales fully, exhales completely, and then takes another full inhalation and holds the breath as long as possible.

maximum expiratory pressure A test of cardiorespiratory function in which the subject takes a deep breath and blows as forcibly as possible into a manometer; the highest pressure maintained for at least 3 seconds is used in the *cardiopulmonary index and some other tests of cardiorespiratory endurance. Since expiratory pressure is more or less equal to intrathoracic pressure at an instant in time, when maximum expiratory pressure exceeds systolic pressure, no blood leaves the heart. This results in relative hypoxia and may cause fainting.

maximum heart rate The highest heart rate reached during a specified period of time or during a submaximal exercise. *Compare* maximal heart rate.

maximum inspiratory breath-holding *See* maximum breath-holding.

maximum passive range The greatest range of motion that can be produced by any means before significant joint damage occurs. It is always greater than the *maximum active range.

maximum static friction *See* limiting friction.

maximum strength The greatest force that can be exerted in a single maximum voluntary contraction.

maximum sustained ventilatory capacity (MSVC) The highest level of ventilation that can be sustained for long periods. When ventilation exceeds the MSVC, respiratory muscles fatigue. In moderately fit individuals the MSVC is between 55 to 80 per cent of the maximum voluntary ventilation (MVV); in highly trained athletes it may be as high as 90 per cent MVV.

MVO_2 *See* maximal oxygen uptake.

maximum voluntary ventilation (MVV) The maximum volume of air that can be breathed voluntarily by an individual in one minute; it is estimated from an extrapolation of the volume breathed in 15 s of rapid, deep breathing. Unlike *maximum sustained ventilatory capacity, the MVV is largely independent of fitness and training.

McArdle's disease A defect in cellular metabolism regulating ATP regeneration. Those with McArdle's disease are deficient in *phosphorylase or *phosphofructokinase and have an impaired ability to utilize intramuscular glycogen as an energy substrate.

McClelland–Atkinson model A mathematical model which proposes that peoples' motives to achieve and their fear of failure are the primary factors determining whether they will approach or avoid an achievement situation. The model proposes that: need to achieve = motive to achieve success–motive to avoid failure. That is, if the *motivation to achieve success is stronger than the motive to avoid failure, the athlete will enter into the achievement situation, otherwise he or she may withdraw. *See also* **extrinsic motivation**.

McCutchen's weeping lubrication theory A theory which proposes that when a joint is exercised, synovial fluid is squeezed in and out of the articular cartilage at the points of contact, providing the articular surfaces with nutrients and oxygen.

McGregor's theory X A management theory consistent with an *initiating structure approach to leadership behaviour, in which workers are regarded as being lazy and irresponsible and therefore need motivation and direction. The theory has been applied to coach–athlete relationships. *Compare* **McGregor's theory Y**.

McGregor's theory Y A management theory which is consistent with the *consideration approach to leadership behaviour, in which workers are regarded as being naturally self-motivated and responsible and therefore need only encouragement. The theory has been applied to coach–athlete relationships. *Compare* **McGregor's theory X**.

McMurray's test A diagnostic test for traumatic knee injuries. The test is designed to trap or catch a torn ligament between the femoral condyle and the top of the tibia. It is carried out with the patient's thigh flexed to 90° and the knee maximally flexed. The examiner then externally rotates the knee and, maintaining the rotation, moves the knee gradually from the fully flexed position to the fully extended position. The test is repeated using internal rotation. A palpable, audible, or painful click over the medial or lateral joint line indicates a meniscal tear. The test is useful when positive, but is unreliable when negative. It is difficult to perform on an acutely painful knee.

M-creatine kinase *See* **M-line**.

mean Statistical value computed from the sum of a set of numbers divided by the number of terms. *See also* **descriptive statistic**.

mean arterial pressure The average arterial blood pressure during a complete *cardiac cycle. The mean arterial pressure determines the rate of blood flow through the circulatory system. It is difficult to measure but is approximated using the following equation: mean arterial pressure = diastolic pressure + $\frac{1}{3}$ (systolic pressure–diastolic pressure).

mean body temperature An average body temperature which takes into account temperature variations throughout the body. It is not a mathematical mean, but is a weighted average often estimated using the equation: mean body temperature = $(0.4 \times T_{skin}) + (0.6 \times T_r)$; T_r is rectal temperature and T_{skin} is the skin temperature estimated as a weighted average of the temperatures recorded from different parts of the body. For example, the skin temperature can be estimated from recordings from temperature sensors on the arm (T_a), trunk (T_t), leg (T_l), and head (T_h) using the following equation: $T_{skin} = (0.1 T_a) + (0.6 T_t) + (0.2 T_l) + (0.1 T_h)$.

meaningful action Any conscious action determined by an actor's motives, reasons, or purposes, and directed towards others.

meaningfulness Often used with reference to the value of a test of physical performance and to experimental designs used in sport science. For a test or experiment to be meaningful to a particular athlete competing in a particular sport, it must be relevant, valid, reliable, standardized, and repeated sufficiently to minimize the effect of chance factors.

measure of association Type of descriptive statistic used to determine the degree to which one variable changes in relation to another variable. *See also* **correlation coefficient**.

measure of central tendency A descriptive statistic used to conceptualize average values from a series of observations, numbers, etc. *See also* **mean**; **median**; and **mode**.

measure of dispersion A statistical measure of the extent to which a set of observations, numbers, etc., cluster round a central value. *See also* **kurtosis**; **range**; **skew**; **standard deviation**; **standard error**; and **variance**.

measure of relationship *See* **measure of association**.

measure of variability A descriptive statistic describing the spread or dispersion of data. *See also* **range**; **standard deviation**; and **variance**.

mechanical advantage For a lever, the ratio of the perpendicular distance of the line of action of the effort from the fulcrum, to the perpendicular distance of the line of action of the resistance or load from the fulcrum. That is, mechanical advantage = force arm/resistance arm. When the mechanical advantage ratio is less than one, a force that is larger than the resistance must be applied to cause motion of the lever. Most skeletal levers appear to be relatively ineffective because they are third-class levers with a mechanical advantage of less than one, but this low mechanical advantage means that a small movement of the lever at the point of force application moves the load through a relatively large range of motion.

mechanical efficiency The ratio of the work output to work input. Conventionally, the mechanical efficiency (*ME*) of human movements is expressed as the ratio of external work performed to the extra production of energy during the movement: $ME = W \times 100/E-e$, where W is the external work performed, E is the gross energy

output during the movement, and e is the resting metabolic rate. Mechanical efficiency for muscle movements is generally low because of the loss of free energy as heat. Values vary for different muscles and for the different types of muscle action. The general opinion that mechanical efficiencies for muscular work are less than 25 per cent has been challenged in recent years. A mechanical efficiency of up to 40 per cent has been claimed for some runners. This level of efficiency was unexpected and is thought to be due to part of the energy of descent being absorbed by elastic components of joints, providing a store of free energy that can be used in the next stride (*see* **stretch-shortening cycle**). Training has a marked effect on efficiency. For example, the net efficiency of a novice swimmer may be as low as 1 per cent while that of an élite swimmer may be more than four times as great.

mechanical energy Type of energy which a body has by virtue of its motion (*see* **kinetic energy**), position (*see* **potential energy**) or state of deformation.

mechanical kinesiology The study of the mechanical factors affecting the human body at rest or in motion.

mechanics The study of the actions of forces acting on particles and mechanical systems. The mechanics of human movement involves the study of internal and external forces acting on the body during movement and rest. *See also* **biomechanics**.

medial Toward the midline of the body.

medial calcaneal nerve A nerve passing from the deep connective tissue to superficial layers at the inner edge of the heel.

medial calcaneal nerve entrapment Pain felt on medio-inferior aspect of the heel due to entrapment of the *medial calcaneal nerve. It often occurs as a result of *overpronation in distance runners. It is sometimes confused with *plantar fasciitis.

medial capsular ligament A deep layer of the *medial collateral ligament of the knee.

medial collateral ligament A knee ligament composed of a deep and a superficial layer, attaching the femoral condyle to the tibia. A collision, blow, or twist that forces the knee inwards, often sprains the medial collateral ligament (*see* **ligament injuries**).

medial cuneiform A bone of the tarsus immediately behind the hallux in the foot.

medial epicondylitis *See* **golfer's elbow**.

medial malleolus Inferior projection of the *tibia; it forms the inner bulge of the ankle. *Compare* **lateral malleolus**.

medial rotation *See* **rotation**.

medial tibial pain syndrome *See* **medial tibial stress syndrome**.

medial tibial stress fracture A *stress fracture of the inner aspect of the shin-bone. It causes pain and tenderness which, unlike the pain of *medial tibial stress syndrome, does not usually get less during exercise.

medial tibial stress syndrome (medial tibial pain syndrome) A periostitis of the medial margin of the tibia (shin-bone). Medial tibial stress syndrome (MTSS) is characterized by a cramping or aching pain, tenderness, and possibly swelling on the inner side of the shin. Unlike compartment syndrome, the pain starts with the onset of activity, decreases as the activity continues, but returns after the cessation of the activity. The main cause of MTSS is repeated loading of the leg on hard surfaces. On examination by palpation, there is always a tender area in the lower third of the inner aspect of the tibia. Athletes with high arches, tight calf muscles, and weak Achilles tendons are predisposed to this condition. Treatment is by rest, ice, compression, and elevation (*see* **RICE**); rest from the precipitating activity being the most important component. If the condition becomes chronic, surgical separation of the periosteum from the inner side of the tibia is sometimes performed. *See also* **anterior compartment syndrome**; **medial tibial stress fracture**; and **shin splints**.

median 1 Statistic derived from the middle value in a frequency distribution on either side of which lie values with equal total frequency. It is the middlemost score of a series arranged in rank order. **2** In anatomy, applied to a structure in a central body position, or situated towards or in the plane that divides the body or body part into left and right halves.

median cubital vein A principal vein in the elbow.

median nerve The central of three nerves supplying the lower arm and hand. The median nerve runs in front of the elbow joint and passes the *pronator teres muscle.

median plane The plane which runs vertically, dividing the body into right and left halves.

medical history *See* **health history**.

medicalization in sport The extension into sport of medical expertise about subjects such as sports nutrition, training, and rehabilitation, which were once the domain of a lay person.

medical screening Procedure used to examine an individual for the presence of disease or disorder. In sport, medical screening is usually performed to establish a person's ability to undertake strenuous exercise. Usually, its prime objective is to find abnormalities likely to present a risk of sudden death or injury to the individual, or to detect any condition that would be aggravated seriously by exercise. Routine screening of athletes is not common in the UK (except for boxing), but in the USA there is an increasing demand for medical certification for many sports and recreations. Anybody aged over 35 who intends taking part in vigorous activity should have a comprehensive medical examination to identify potential risks. Most deaths in sport are associated with individuals who have identifiable risks that have not been corrected.

medicine 1 The discipline dealing with the prevention, cure, and alleviation of disease, and with the restoration and maintenance of health. **2** A product which can be applied internally or externally to demonstrate, relieve, or cure disease, or the symptoms of disease.

medicine ball A large, heavy ball used for physical training.

medicine ball exercises Strength-training exercises that involve lifting or throwing a medicine ball. The exercises often include movements of the trunk, assisted by those of the shoulders, arms, hips, and legs.

medio-lateral axis (frontal axis; transverse axis) An axis of the body which runs from side to side.

medium-term endurance The ability to sustain a strenuous activity which has a duration of two to ten minutes. Electro-encephalographs and electromyographs indicate that medium term endurance is associated with a high level of activity of the brain and slow twitch muscle fibres. The energy for the activities is supplied by both anaerobic and aerobic energy systems.

medulla 1 The central part of an organ. **2** The myelin portion of some nerve fibres. Such a fibre is called medullated.

medulla oblongata Part of the brain stem which joins onto the spinal cord below and the pons above. The medulla oblongata contains several important control centres, including the cardiac centre, respiratory centres, and the vasomotor centre, which control autonomic reflexes involved in *homeostasis. The medulla oblongata has nuclei which regulate vomiting, swallowing, coughing, and sneezing.

medullary artery *See* **nutrient artery**.

medullary canal *See* **medullary cavity**.

medullary cavity Central cavity of long bone and spongy bone through which medullary canals allow blood vessels to pass. In adults, the cavity is filled with fat.

medullated nerve fibre A nerve fibre with a myelin sheath.

mega- 1 Prefix denoting large size or an enlargement. **2** In scientific measurements using metric units, denotes one million. **3** In computing, denotes 2^{20} (1 048 576), as in one megabyte of information units.

megadose A quantity of vitamin or mineral that exceeds the Recommended Daily Amount (RDA) by a factor of ten or more. Megadoses may be used to treat nutrient deficiencies and are sometimes prescribed for those with particular diseases. However, megadoses should be used cautiously because some vitamins and minerals are toxic in large doses.

Meissner's corpuscles Mechanoreceptors sensitive to gentle pressure in the skin particularly of lips, nipples, external genitalia, eyelids, and fingertips.

melaena Faeces which appear black and tarry because of the presence of blood.

melanin A dark pigment which imparts colour to skin and hair. Melanin is produced by cells in the skin called melanocytes, and its production increases in response to sunlight, causing the skin to become darker. This offers some protection against ultraviolet light. The population of melanocytes and ability to produce melanin decreases with age, increasing the risk of sun damage.

melanoma A dark pigmented mole on the skin, some forms of which can be very invasive and malignant. Malignant melanoma is a cancerous tumour of melanocytes that usually occurs in the skin and sometimes in the retina of the eye. It is often associated with intermittent excessive exposure to ultraviolet light from the sun, especially in youth. Malignant cells often spread quickly to other parts of the body. Melanomas usually have an irregular shape and irregular border; they are often multicoloured and measure more than 0.5 cm (quarter of an inch) in diameter. Anyone with a suspicious skin growth should contact their doctor immediately. Superficial malignant melanomas can often be treated successfully by surgery, but once the disease spreads the prognosis is poor. Anyone who spends a lot of time outdoors, and that includes most sportspeople, should be aware of the potential risk and wear protective clothing and high factor sunscreen on areas exposed to sunlight. *See also* **cyclist's melanoma**.

melting-pot theory A theory which suggests that it is socially beneficial to encourage ethnic groups to assimilate into a host society. Sporting contacts between different ethnic groups may facilitate this assimilation when members of a team come from different backgrounds, but if the team members come from the same background, assimilation is less likely. *Compare* **cultural mosaic theory.**

membership group The group to which an individual is assigned by others on the basis of education, age, sex, place of residence etc. Teams consisting of a relatively homogeneous membership group include school and college teams. The membership may or may not be the same as the reference group, that is the group with whom the individual actually identifies. *See also* **role theory.**

membrane A thin sheet of tissue lining a cavity. *See also* **cell membrane.**

memory The mental faculty which facilitates storage and retrieval of information that has been learned, such as sport knowledge or a motor program. According to the *black-box theory, memory has been viewed as consisting of three components *short-term sensory store *short-term memory, and *long-term memory. The hippocampus of the limbic system plays an important part in memory. The exact way in which the brain stores information is unknown, but it may involve chemical or structural changes. *See also* **engram; memory-drum theory.**

memory-drum theory (Henry's memory drum theory) A theory which proposes that unconscious neural patterns acquired from past experience are stored in the central nervous system as a memory storage drum, analogous to a drum which is used to store music in old-fashioned roll pianos.

memory storage Retention of information in a place so that the information can be recalled for later use. *See also* **memory.**

memory trace A modification of neural pathways in the central nervous system which, it is hypothesized, underlies *memory. *See also* **engram.**

menarche The onset of *menstruation defined by the appearance of the first menstrual flow. Regular high-intensity exercise may delay menarche in female athletes with long, lithe bodies. It is not clear what long-term effect that this delay has. *See also* **amenorrhoea.**

Meniere's disease A disease affecting the inner ear in which a build-up of fluid causes deafness, buzzing in the ears (tinnitus), and vertigo. Meniere's disease is a

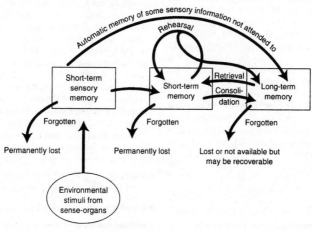

memory

contra-indication to underwater diving because an attack of vertigo could totally disorientate a submerged diver.

meningitis Inflammation of the meninges, the membranes surrounding the brain and spinal cord. Meningitis may be of bacterial or viral origin. It can be associated with a head injury, such as a depressed skull fracture, sustained during a contact or collision sport. Symptoms include headache, fever, and neck stiffness.

meniscal tear (torn cartilage) Damage of a meniscus (semi-lunar cartilage) in the knee. The cartilage is usually detached by a rotatory stress, for example, when the knee is twisted. Meniscal tears may occur as a result of a single traumatic event or they may be the cumulative effect of repeated twisting, turning, and compression forces on the knee over a long period. A tear is characterized by recurrent pain located along the affected joint margin (joint-line tenderness); intermittent catching, locking, or clicking (these can usually be demonstrated by the *Apley test and *McMurray's test); and weakened or atrophied quadriceps muscles. Radiography, magnetic resonance imaging, CT scanning, and arthroscopy have all been used in the diagnosis of tears. Meniscal tears are named according to their shape, for example, 'parrot beak' tear and 'bucket handle' tear. As the blood supply to most of the meniscus is very poor, it was once thought that this type of injury could never resolve itself. An athlete with a meniscal tear usually had the choice between retiring from active sport or surgical removal of the whole cartilage. Once removed, the space that was occupied by the meniscus is filled by replacement material, but not of the same type or quality as the original meniscus. Consequently, joint mobility becomes marginally worse and the likelihood of arthritis in later life is increased. It is now realized that parts of the meniscus have quite a good blood supply, and the formation of blood clots can encourage meniscal healing. Current treatments of meniscal tears depend on the extent and precise location of the tear.

They include partial *meniscectomy, meniscal repair, and leaving the tear alone. Total meniscectomies are rare. Most athletes return to activity within four to eight weeks of arthroscopic repair. Experimental work is being done on meniscal transplantations; initial results are encouraging. No short-term rejections have been reported, so the meniscus appears to be 'immunologically privileged'.

meniscectomy Surgical removal of meniscus cartilage in a joint. A meniscectomy is generally done using arthroscopy.

meniscus (pl. menisci) A semilunar disc of fibrocartilage separating articular cartilage of some joints. In the knee, menisci are located between the tibial and femoral condyles. They modify the shape of the articular cartilage, improving the fit between the articulating bones and increasing knee stability during complex movements. They also spread the load at the knee over a wider area, helping to absorb shock.

menopause The period during which ovulation and menstruation ceases. It usually occurs in women between 45 and 55 years. Menopause is associated with changes in the balance of sex hormones which can lead to emotional and physical changes. It is during menopause that bone density often falls significantly and may go below the fracture threshold (the density at which fractures occur easily). Regular weight-bearing exercises (provided they do not induce *amenorrhoea) and a calcium-rich diet, especially during the teens and early twenties, can increase peak bone density and decrease the risk of bone fractures in later life. During menopause, exercise intervention to reduce the rate of bone loss has little effect unless it is combined with hormone replacement therapy. *See also* **osteoporosis**.

menorrhagia (menorrhoea) Abnormally heavy bleeding during menstruation.

menorrhoea *See* **menorrhagia**.

menstrual adjustment The use of hormones (e.g. oestrogen and progesterone found in contraceptive pills) or their synthetic analogues, to adjust the time of menstruation in a female athlete so that important competition dates coincide with the time of maximum efficiency. Optimal performance varies between individuals. It is frequently in the pre-ovulation phase of the menstrual cycle (days 9–12) or post-ovulation phase (days 17–20), but some women perform best during menstruation.

menstrual cycle The cycle of changes associated with ovulation (release of an egg cell from an ovary) in sexually mature, non-pregnant females. It occurs at approximately monthly intervals and is characterized by menses (often called menstruation, the period during which blood is lost from the genital tract), changes in the wall of the uterus, and changes in the breasts. The cycle also often involves considerable variations in body weight, total body water, body temperature, metabolic rate, heart rate, and stroke volume (amount of blood leaving the heart at each contraction). These variations may have dramatic effects on the ability to perform exercise, therefore many female athletes use contraceptive pills containing steroids to control their menstrual cycle so that it does not coincide with important events. However, such pills are not very popular among endurance athletes because they sometimes cause weight increases and reduce *maximum oxygen uptake. Regular, intensive exercise can disrupt the menstrual cycle (see **athletic amenorrhoea**).

menstrual dysfunction Disruption of the normal menstrual cycle. It includes *oligomenorrhoea and *amenorrhoea.

menstruation The process or the instance of discharging blood and tissue fragments from the uterine wall. Some sportswomen may be particularly susceptible to iron-deficiency *anaemia during menstruation because of heavy blood losses combined with the high oxygen demands of their physical activity. Menstruation does not necessarily preclude exceptional athletic performances. World and Olympic titles

have been won during all stages of the menstrual cycle. See also **menstrual adjustment**.

mental Pertaining to the mind.

mental age A measure of an individual's level of intellectual development: for example, a person with a mental age of 5 years will function intellectually at the same level as an average 5-year-old child.

Mental Attributes of Performance in Sport (MAPS) A questionnaire initially designed to monitor the coping strategies of players of Australian Rules Football. MAPS refers to things a player might do, feel, or experience during a match or when preparing for a match. MAPS has also been used on other athletes.

mental device A word, phrase, object, or process used to help a person relax. Two commonly used mental devices are the *mantra and the process of taking deep breaths and exhaling slowly.

mental fat A colloquial expression for the loss of motivation that often occurs as an athlete ages, and which is responsible for retirement from sport before it would have been required by physical deterioration.

mental fatigue See **subjective fatigue**.

mental health A mental state marked by the absence of personal discomfort and socially disruptive behaviour. Those in good mental health have the capacity to adapt to environmental stresses and they work productively with others or alone. They are usually able and willing to attempt to improve society's condition as well as their own personal condition.

mental health model A model proposing that successful élite athletes generally have greater mental health than unsuccessful athletes. It is based on the observation that many (but by no means all) élite athletes exhibit the psychological profiles of mentally healthy individuals. See also **iceberg profile**.

mental illness A disorder of one or more functions of the mind resulting in the patient or others suffering. It does not include those conditions where the only problem is that the individual does not conform to the behavioural norms of society, nor does it include conditions of subnormality, where the individual has a general failure of normal intellectual development.

mental practice (mental rehearsal) A form of practice in which subjects produce a vivid mental image of actually performing a technique; that is, they do not imagine that they are watching themselves perform, but they actually carry out the activity in their imagination without overt physical movement. Some research evidence suggests that, for a skilled person, mental practice can be as effective as actual practice. See also **imagery**.

mental preparation Mental procedures, acquired by systematic mental training, which can be used on certain predetermined occasions (e.g., prior to a competition) to achieve an *ideal performance state.

mental preparation strategies Procedures, such as *psyching-up, *self-talk, and relaxation methods, which deal with psychological factors that can adversely affect a performance.

mental rehearsal See **mental practice**.

mental stamina The ability to maintain a high level of *motivation for long periods, despite discomfort and discouragement; a component of endurance.

mental training Systematic, long-term developmental training of mental skills which enable athletes to achieve peak performances in special events such as sport competitions.

meralgia paraesthetica Condition caused by trapping the lateral cutaneous nerve which supplies the outer part of the thigh. It may be caused by repetitive pressure or direct trauma. Symptoms include a burning sensation and numbness felt over the anterolateral aspect of the thigh. The condition usually resolves itself with rest.

mere presence Used in *social facilitation theory to describe the facilitative effect of a noninteractive audience or coactors on performers.

merocrine gland A gland that secretes substances intermittently and does not accumulate secretions. Compare **apocrine gland**.

meromyosin Either of two components obtained when *myosin is broken down by trypsin (a proteolytic enzyme): light meromyosin contains the tail of myosin; and heavy meromyosin contains the globular head, myosin cross-bridge which contains ATPase and attaches onto actin.

mesenchephalon See **midbrain**.

mesial Pertaining to the median line or median plane.

mesocycle See **periodization**.

mesomorph An individual who tends to be stocky, of medium height with well-developed muscles. See also **somatotype**.

mesomorphism The pattern of beliefs and values that defines the preferred body shape as being that of a mesomorph. Advocates of mesomorphism believe that muscularity and slimness are good attributes, and they assume that a mesomorphic body shape reflects control, efficiency, discipline, health, and beauty.

mesomorphy A *somatotype dimension characterized by well-defined skeletal and muscular development, and a rugged stocky appearance. Many sportspeople have a large element of this component.

MET See **metabolic equivalent**.

meta-analysis A statistical technique for summarizing and comparing results of independent samples. Meta-analysis has been used, for example, to analyse the results of many studies carried out by different research teams on the effects of exercise on depression.

metabolic acidosis Abnormally high acidity of body fluids caused by loss of base, or an excessive production or ingestion of acid other than carbonic acid. One of the main causes of metabolic acidosis is the accumulation of organic acids, especially lactic acid, during heavy exercise. Metabolic acidosis may lead to muscle fatigue. *Compare* **respiratory acidosis**.

metabolic alkalosis Abnormally high alkalinity of the body fluids caused by ingesting excess alkalis or loss of large amounts of acid (for example, by vomiting the stomach contents).

metabolic equivalent A unit used to estimate the metabolic cost (energy expenditure as reflected by oxygen consumption) of physical activity. One Met equals the resting metabolic rate, which is approximately 3.5 millilitres of oxygen per kilogram body weight per minute. METs are used to compare the energy costs of different activities.

metabolic fuel *See* **body fuel stores**.

metabolic load The amount of energy required to complete a task.

metabolic rate The energy expended by a person, usually expressed in units of energy per unit body mass, per unit time.

metabolic water production Water released into the tissues during the metabolism of foodstuffs. For example, during cellular respiration water is a by-product of the oxidation of carbohydrate and free fatty acids. In addition, water chemically bound to glycogen is released when glycogen is oxidized. Approximately 3 grams of water is released for each gram of glycogen broken down. Metabolic water production can contribute significantly to an athlete's fluid needs during exercise so that the ideal volume of fluid replacement is somewhat less than the total sweat loss.

metabolism The sum total of all of the chemical reactions which take place in the body to sustain life. Metabolism includes *ana-bolism and *catabolism.

metabolite Any substance produced by a metabolic reaction (i.e., a chemical reaction in the body) including chemicals formed by the metabolic transformations of a drug.

metabotropic neurotransmitter A neurotransmitter, such as a biogenic amine or neuropeptide, which affects the postsynaptic membrane potential indirectly and through a second intracellular chemical messenger in the postsynaptic membrane.

metacarpal 1 One of five small, long bones forming the metacarpus of the hand which join the fingers to the wrist. The metacarpals radiate from the wrist like spokes, forming the palm of the hand. **2** An adjective pertaining to the metacarpus.

metacarpale radialis An anatomical landmark on the most lateral point on the distal head of the second metacarpal of the outstretched hand (i.e., on the radial side of the body).

metacarpale ulnare An anatomical landmark on the most lateral point on the distal head of the fifth metacarpal of the outstretched hand (i.e., on the ulnar side of the body).

metacarpophalangeal joint Condyloid joint between the rounded distal head of a metacarpal and the concave proximal end of a phalanx that forms a knuckle in the hand. The movements normally performed by this joint are extension, flexion, abduction, and adduction.

metacarpus The skeletal part of the palm of the hand, between the wrist and fingers. Typically, it consists of five metacarpal bones.

metamotivational states Pairs of opposite motivational states (e.g. excitement seeking and anxiety avoiding), with only one of the pair operating at a time.

metaphor A descriptive phrase or term applied to an object or to a phenomenon to which it does not literally denote. Metaphors are used extensively in science and are of great value in suggesting new relationships or new explanatory mechanisms, but there are problems when they are interpreted too literally or when they are not supported by objective evidence. *See also* **model**.

metaphysis The most recent growing portion of bone between the epiphysis and the diaphysis of a long bone.

metatarsal One of five arching bones joining the tarsus to the phalanges of the toes of each foot.

metatarsalgia An aching pain in the metatarsal bones of the foot. It has a number of causes, including foot strain, plantar interdigital neuroma (*see* **Morton's syndrome**), stress fracture (*see* **march fracture**), Freiberg's disease, and sesamoiditis. Claw toe, hammer toe, and their associated callosities can all lead to metatarsalgia.

metatarsophalangeal joint A synovial condyloid joint formed between the rounded head of a metatarsal bone and the cavity of the proximal end of a phalanx in the toe. The joint permits abduction, adduction, extension, and flexion.

metatarsus The five bones which form the instep of the foot, uniting the *tarsus with the phalanges of the toes. The metatarsals are relatively large and strong foot-bones which play an important part in supporting the body weight. Distally, the metatarsus forms the ball of the foot.

methandrostenolone A synthetic anabolic steroid similar in structure to testosterone, which has enhanced tissue-building properties and less androgenic effects than testosterone. Methandrostenolone, a banned substance, was administered as dianabol to the disqualified 1988 Olympic 100 m champion, Ben Johnson. Johnson's coach, Charlie Francis, claimed that dianabol could allay fatigue, increase muscularity, and enhance self-image and confidence.

method of successive approximations *See* **shaping**.

methylxanthines Drugs related to caffeine which include theophylline and aminophylline. They are bronchodilators which have side-effects on the cardiovascular and nervous systems. Although the use of caffeine is restricted, methylxanthines are not banned by the International Olympic Committee.

metre The base unit of length in the SI system.

metric system A decimal system of measurements based on the metre which was intended to be 1/10 000 000 of a quadrant of the Earth through Paris. For scientific purposes, it has been superseded by the SI system.

Michigan studies Studies which identified two main kinds of orientation in leadership behaviour: *employee orientation and *product orientation.

microanatomy The study of structures too small to be seen without the aid of a microscope.

microcirculation The flow of blood through arterioles, capillaries, and venules of an organ or a body-part.

microcycle *See* **periodization**.

microdialysis technique A technique used to study muscle metabolism. A hollow probe is inserted into tissue and continuously perfused with blood so that the tube acts as an artificial blood vessel. Chemicals can be added to the extracellular fluid of muscles via the probe. The chemicals diffuse into the tissue along a concentration gradient. Subsequently, the extracellular fluid can be collected for analysis so that the effect of the chemicals on muscle metabolism can be monitored.

microfilament A cellular protein filament 0.4–0.8 nm in diameter.

microgravity An environment, such as a spacecraft, in which gravitational forces exerted on the body are less than normal. Prolonged exposure to microgravity results in effects similar to *detraining in athletes (e.g. loss of muscle and bone mass). These changes can present problems when returning to a normal gravity. Regular in-flight exercise, including resistance training and aerobic activities, may counteract some of these effects.

micrometre (micron) A unit of length equal to 1/1 000 000 metre (10^{-6} m)

micromineral (trace element) A mineral required by the body in relatively small amounts (less than 100 mg per day). Microminerals include chromium, cobalt, copper, fluorine, iodine, molybdenum, nickel, selenium, silicon, tin, vanadium, and zinc.

micron *See* **micrometre**.

micronutrient A component of a balanced diet required in only small quantities. *See also* **minerals**; and **vitamins**.

microorganism An organism which cannot be seen with the naked eye. Microorganisms include bacteria, some fungi, protozoa, and (in some classifications) viruses.

microsociology A branch of sociology which focuses on interpersonal interactions and on behaviours of groups. *Compare* **macrosociology**.

microtrauma The causative mechanism by which repetitive or chronic loading over a period of time produces an injury at the microscopic level. The force produced by a single application of the load is insufficient to cause injury. *See also* **stress fracture**.

microvilli Microscopic folds in the cell surface membrane which increase the surface area to volume ratio of some cells.

microwave diathermy *See* **diathermy**.

midbrain (mesencephalon) A short region of brain between the *diencephalon and the *pons. The midbrain carries a number of tracts of nerve fibres, including the pyramidal tract, involved in the performance of motor skills.

middle ear Part of the ear through which sound vibrations are transmitted from the ear drum to the inner ear via three small bones. The middle ear is air-filled and connected to the pharynx via the Eustachian tube through which air pressure can be equalized. If the tube is blocked as a result of an infection, it may not be possible to equalize the pressure either side of the eardrum during, for example, an underwater dive.

midrange That third of the range of movement of a joint in which the muscle is around its midpoint of contraction. The midrange separates the *inner range from the *outer range.

midsole A shock-absorbing layer of a *training shoe, between the outsole and the insole. It is the heart of the shoe, determining its degree of hardness or softness.

Athletes with a heavy footstrike and rigid lower-limb structure, generally benefit from having softer midsoles; those with a lighter more mobile footstrike, benefit from harder midsoles. The midsole must combine two conflicting properties: it must be strong enough to resist the compression and rotational forces produced by the foot striking the ground, and it must be flexible enough to allow the toes to bend during the push-off phase of running and jumping. Midsoles which do not have these properties, or which lose them through wear and tear, may increase the risk of sports injuries such as stress fractures.

migraine A severely painful type of headache believed to be caused by the constriction of blood vessels in the head. A migraine typically affects one side of the head and is accompanied by visual disturbances, nausea, and numbness or tingling of the limbs. *See also* **footballer's migraine**.

mild strain Overstretching of a muscle resulting in rupture of less than 5 per cent of the muscle fibres with no great loss of strength or deleterious effect on movement.

mile (statute mile) Unit of length equal to 1760 yards and equivalent to 1609.34 m. Although the use of miles has been replaced by metres for most purposes, the mile is still retained for certain sporting events, particularly in running.

miliaria *See* **prickly heat**.

milk sugar *See* **lactose**.

milli Prefix which, when attached to units, denotes the basic unit $\times 10^{-3}$; thus a milligram is 1/1000 of a gram.

Mills' manoeuvre A manipulative procedure used to treat tennis elbow. The examiner fully pronates the affected forearm, flexes the wrist, and then forcibly extends the elbow. The manoeuvre should be performed only by a trained person, since if it is carried out too vigorously, it can lead to traumatic synovitis of the elbow joint.

mind A hypothetical term representing the mental faculties in an individual responsible for intelligent behaviour, including memory, thought, and perception. There is much debate, particularly in philosophy and psychology, concerning the relationship between mind and matter in human functions.

mineralocorticoid A member of a class of *steroid hormones produced by the adrenal cortex, that regulate salt and water balance. The most important mineralocorticoid is *aldosterone.

minerals Natural inorganic substances that are components of the Earth's crust. They also occur in the human body where they play a vital role in a number of activities including enzyme synthesis, regulation of heart rate, nerve and muscle activity, bone formation and digestion. Major minerals required in quite large amounts in a balanced diet include calcium, chlorine (usually as sodium chloride), magnesium, phosphorus, potassium. and sodium. Minerals required in small amounts include chromium, cobalt, copper, fluorine, iodine, iron, manganese, molybdenum, and selenium.

mineral supplementation Substances usually taken in tablet or powder form to boost the dietary intake of minerals. They are commonly taken by athletes as an insurance against mineral deficiency and/or to enhance performance. However, there is little scientific evidence to support the value of taking such supplements (with the possible exception of calcium and iron) since the minimum daily requirements are usually easily met through a normal balanced diet. However, athletes on a low energy weight-reducing or weight-maintenance diet, may be at risk of mineral deficiencies and should seek the advice of a sports dietitian. Supplements should never be taken as an alternative to eating a well-balanced diet.

minimum effective strain Hypothetically, the lowest mechanical strain necessary to maintain constant bone remodelling and to preserve bone values. The concept of minimum effective strain is based on the observation that adult bone changes density in response to the stresses and strains it encounters (see **Wolff's law**).

Minnesota Multiphasic Personality Inventory (MMPI): An inventory which includes twelve scales designed to measure the personality of abnormal subjects, but which has also been used successfully on normal subjects. The twelve scales are: hypochondriasis (Hs); depression (D); hysteria (Hy); psychopathic deviate (Pd); masculinity–femininity (Mf); paranoia (Pa); psychasthenia (Pt); schizophrenia (Sc); hypomania (Ma); lie (l); validity (F); and correction (K)

minor league Any nonprofessional baseball league in the USA.

minute 1 Unit of time. **2** Unit of angular measurement equivalent to 1/60 of a degree.

minute ventilation The volume of air inspired into or expired out of the lungs in one minute. It usually refers to the expired amount and can be calculated using the following equation: $VE = VT \times f$; where VE represents the minute ventilation in $l\,min^{-1}$, VT represents tidal volume l), and f represents respiratory frequency in breaths per minute. A typical resting value of minute ventilation is 6 $l\,min^{-1}$, but it may rise to as much as 6 $l\,min^{-1}$ during intense exercise. The change in minute ventilation has been used to identify the anaerobic threshold (see **minute ventilation method**).

minute ventilation method A method for estimating the *anaerobic threshold. The minute ventilation and oxygen consumption of a subject is monitored during a progressive exercise test on a treadmill or bicycle ergometer. The running or cycling speed at which minute ventilation increases disproportionately compared to oxygen consumption is called the respiratory threshold, ventilatory breakpoint, or ventilatory threshold. This is sometimes taken as being equivalent to the lactate threshold and to indicate the point at which there is a substantial switch from aerobic metabolism to anaerobic metabolism (see **anaerobic threshold**). The basis of this assumption is that increases in blood lactate levels are associated with a lowering of blood pH (i.e. blood becomes more acidic), stimulating chemoreceptors which effect an increase in pulmonary ventilation through the action of the respiratory centres. However, this assumption has been seriously questioned because factors other than pH can contribute to the nonlinear increase in minute ventilation.

miserable malalignment syndrome A combination of malalignments of the leg that include excess *femoral anteversion with internal rotation of the hip, genu valgus, squinting patellae, external tibial torsion, and flat feet. Athletes with miserable malalignment syndrome are predisposed to overuse injuries and are often advised not to take part in certain sports, for example, long distance running.

mistake An occasional error that can occur in almost any sport no matter how experienced or expert the performer. *See also* **error**; and **flaw**.

mitochondrion (pl. mitochondria) A double-membraned structure within a cell concerned with aerobic metabolism. Mitochondria are sometimes referred to as the 'powerhouses' of the cell because they are the sites in which the *Krebs cycle and electron transport system generate large amounts of ATP. Muscle fibres of endurance athletes have a higher density of mitochondria than those of non-athletes. Resistance training decreases mitochondrial density but increases the overall number of mitochondria because of muscle growth.

mitral valve The bicuspid valve between the left atrium and left ventricle of the heart. The valve prevents backflow of blood from the ventricle to the atrium during ventricular systole.

mixed nerve A nerve containing sensory and motor fibres which carry information in the form of nerve impulses to and from the central nervous system.

mixed pace Training consisting of continuous work performed at varying pace. *See also* **fartlek**.

mixed sport *See* **alternate aerobic–anaerobic metabolism**.

mixed venous blood Blood, usually extracted from the pulmonary artery, which has returned from all the tissues and been mixed together in the right atrium of the heart.

M-line A line in the centre of the *H-zone of a muscle *sarcomere. Its name derives from the German word mitteline, meaning midline. The M-line contains at least three proteins: M-protein, which helps to hold the thick filaments in regular array; myomesin, which forms a strong anchoring point for the elastic filaments made of titin; and M-creatine kinase, which is located close to the myosin heads and catalyses the formation of ATP from creatine phosphate. The name 'M-line' is derived from the German word *mitteline*, meaning midline.

mobility 1 (joint mobility) The ease with which an articulation, or series of articulations, is able to move before being restricted by surrounding structures. Mobility is difficult to measure. Sometimes measurements of the end-position achieved by the extremity of a limb or limb-segment are used to reflect mobility, but these measurements are dependent on the positional relationships of other segments of the body. *See also* **active mobility exercise**; and **passive mobility exercise**. **2** *See* **social mobility**.

mobilization During rehabilitation from a sports injury, the return of a limb to full mobility by carefully applied pressure to a joint or muscle so that it will move through its normal range of movement. Mobilization maintains and then improves muscle tone, reduces joint stiffness, and strengthens ligaments and tendons. It is a graded process, starting gently with *passive mobility exercises when injuries are in the acute and painful phase, and becoming more forceful with both passive and *active mobility exercises during the recovery phase. Mobility exercises should be designed to restore full mobility by strengthening and stretching muscles. *See also* **aggressive rehabilitation**.

mode 1 The type of exercise; one of the main variables in an exercise programme. **2** In statistics, the most frequent scores of a series; the peak in a frequency distribution.

model A mathematical, physical, pictorial, or computer representation, of one phenomenon by another. Models are often used to simplify complex phenomena for analytical purposes. *See also* **metaphor**.

modelling A technique used in behaviour modification and the acquisition of a skill, whereby a person learns a behaviour or skill by observing and imitating someone else doing it.

model training (quality training) Training in which the external conditions and/or the state of mind of the athlete are similar to those during competition so that the benefits of the training can be maximized (*see* **state bound learning**).

moderate strain (second degree strain) A partial muscle tear involving a significant number of muscle fibres (more than 5 per cent), but not all of them. Pain may be aggravated by muscle movements.

modulus of compression The ratio of mechanical *stress to *strain in an elastic material when that material is being compressed; it is the *modulus of elasticity applied to a material under compression: modulus of compression = compressive force per unit area/ change in volume per unit volume.

modulus of elasticity The ratio of stress to strain for a body obeying *Hooke's law. There are several moduli corresponding to different types of strain (*see* **modulus of compression**; **modulus of rigidity**; and **Young's modulus**).

modulus of rigidity The ratio of mechanical *stress to *strain in an elastic material when that material is subjected to shear forces; it is the *modulus of elasticity of a body under a shearing strain: modulus of rigidity = tangential force per unit area/angular deformation.

molar 1 Applied to a solution in which one litre of the solution contains an amount of solute equal to its molecular weight in grams. **2** Back tooth used for grinding food.

molarity Measurement of the strength of a solution expressed as moles per litre; that is, the weight of dissolved substance in grams per litre divided by its molecular weight.

mole The SI unit of amount of a substance expressed as its molecular weight in grams. Thus one mole of glucose, which has the formula $C_6H_{12}O_6$, weighs 180 g, where the atomic weight of carbon is 12, hydrogen 1, and oxygen 16.

molybdenum A trace element that is an essential component of many enzymes. Deficiency is rare. There is no Reference Nutrient Intake in the UK, but in the USA Recommended Dietary Allowance is 75–250 micrograms.

moment arm (lever arm) The shortest perpendicular distance between a force's line of action and an axis of rotation (e.g., a pivot). In a lever, the moment arm of the force is often referred to as the force arm, and that of the resistance is referred to as the resistance arm.

moment of force *See* **torque**.

moment of couple *See* **torque**.

moment of inertia A physical property, measured in kg m^{-2}, defining a body's resistance to rotational forces. For the human body, the moment of inertia of each body segment is the product of the mass of the segment and the square of the *radius of gyration of the segment. The moment of inertia of the whole body is the sum of the moments of inertia of all its segments.

momentum The amount of motion possessed by a moving object. The linear momentum of a moving body is a product of its mass and velocity: $M = mv$; where M is linear momentum, m is the mass, and v the velocity of the body. Thus, an object's momentum can be changed by altering either its mass or its velocity. Linear momentum is a *vector quantity directed through the body in the direction of motion. *See also* **angular momentum**.

monoamine oxidase (MAO) An important endogenous enzyme responsible for the metabolic breakdown of monoamines, such as *serotonin, *adrenaline, and *noradrenaline. Monoamine oxidase is found in many tissues but especially in the liver and nervous system.

monoamine oxidase inhibitor (MAOI) A drug that blocks the action of monoamine oxidase and results in an increase in *serotonin, *adrenaline, and *noradrenaline, which leads to an increase in mental and physical activity. MAOI is sometimes used to treat affective disorders such as depression.

monoamines A group of organic, nitrogen-containing compounds to which adrenaline, noradrenaline, and serotonin belong.

monocyte A large, white blood cell with a single nucleus. Monocytes engulf bacteria by phagocytosis.

mononucleosis An abnormally high number of monocytes in the blood. Mononucleosis may indicate an infection, such as glandular fever.

monosaccharide A simple sugar; a crystalline, sweet-tasting, very soluble carbohydrate consisting of a single chain or a single ring structure. Examples are fructose, galactose, and glucose.

monosynaptic stretch reflex A *reflex action of striated muscle produced by stretching the muscle and its muscle spindle organ which are connected, via a single synapse, to an *alpha-motor neurone which terminates in the same muscle. *See also* **stretch reflex**.

monounsaturated fatty acid *See* **unsaturated fatty acid**.

Monteggia's fracture-dislocation A combination of an ulnar fracture and dislocation of the ulna at the elbow.

mood An emotional condition which persists for some time, such as irritable, cheerful, or aggressive mood.

moral Pertaining to human behaviour, especially the distinction between what is right and wrong.

moral development The development of the capacity to distinguish between behaviour which society generally regards as right and wrong. Some claim that sport and physical education promote moral development.

morale The degree of mental confidence, self-control, and discipline of a person or group.

moral panic A social reaction to relatively minor acts of social deviance which have been exaggerated and amplified by the media. It is claimed that moral panic has resulted in an exacerbation of some deviances such as *football hooliganism. *See also* **deviance amplification**; **labelling theory**.

morals Principles of behaviour based on the concepts of right and wrong.

morbid Applied to an abnormal, diseased, or disordered condition.

morbidity rate The incidence of a particular disease or disorder in a population, usually expressed as cases per 100 000 or per million in one year.

mores The socially approved forms of behaviour, promoted by laws and customs, which are generally regarded as essential for the maintenance of a society or a group.

Moritani and de Vries model A model used to estimate the relative contributions of muscle growth (*see* **hypertrophy**) and neural factors to strength gains. Moritani and de Vries measured force production and neural activity simultaneously. The model is based on the assumptions that strength gains due solely to neural factors should be associated with increases of neural activity within a muscle without any change in force production per motor unit, and that strength gains due solely to muscle growth should occur without any increases in neural activity.

morphology The study of shape, general appearance, or form of a person's body, as distinct from *anatomy which requires dissection to reveal structure. *See also* **somatotype**.

mortality rate The death rate in a population expressed as the percentage dying in a year, or the number of deaths per 1000 population.

Morton's foot Anatomical abnormality in which the foot consists of an abnormally short first metatarsal bone and an abnormally long second metatarsal bone. It is not usually disabling, but it can result in mechanical problems during running, causing the foot to over-pronate because of lack of stability. Those with Morton's foot are more likely to sustain *stress fractures if they overtrain.

Morton's metatarsalgia See **Morton's syndrome**.

Morton's syndrome (Morton's metatarsalgia) A condition characterized by pain and tingling that radiates between the second and third or fourth toes. It is usually caused by a neuroma (benign tumour) on any of the plantar digital nerves situated in the web between two toes. The neuroma may develop because ill-fitting shoes press against the nerve. The condition is accentuated in athletes who spin on the ball of the foot (e.g., golfers, tennis players, and bowlers). Morton's syndrome is temporarily relieved by removal of shoes and rest. Sometimes special padding in the shoes and anti-inflammatories help resolve the condition, but usually surgical excision of the neuroma is necessary.

motion The continual change of relative position of an object in space. An accurate analysis of the motion of a body requires a description of its successive positions and the time taken to move between these positions.

motion segment The functional unit of the spine. Each motion segment consists of two adjacent vertebrae and their associated soft tissues.

motivation The internal state which tends to direct a person's behaviour towards a *goal. The person may or may not be conscious of the motivation. It can occur independently of any external stimulus and is not due to fatigue, learning, or maturation. Many psychologists consider that motivation has two dimensions: intensity and direction. Intensity is concerned with the amount of activation and arousal the person has; that is how much effort is being given to reach a certain goal. Direction is concerned with movement towards a particular goal: psychologists talk about people approaching or avoiding a task, and understanding why they do so. In sport, coaches are frequently interested in knowing why a talented youngster will not play a particular sport, or why someone quits a team. Others want to know why some players are so doggedly persistent in playing a sport when they apparently would be better off doing something else. The study of motivation covers these issues. 2 The willingness to persevere with a long and arduous training program, a desire to excel in competition, and persistence in the face of discomfort and discouragement. See also **extrinsic motivation**; **intrinsic motivation**; **negative motivation**; **positive motivation**; **primary motivation**; and **secondary motivation**.

motivational hierarchy A hierarchy of human needs which are, in ascending order of importance: physiological needs; need for safety; need for love and belonging; need for *self-esteem and recognition; and the need for *self-actualization. Coaches are mainly concerned with enabling their athletes to fulfil the higher needs, but the concept implies this can only be achieved when the lower needs, such as the fundamental physiological need for food and shelter, have been met.

motivational sequence A series of related events involved in motivation, namely need, drive, incentive, reinforcement.

motivational strategy Technique used to improve or maintain the *motivation of a sports person or team. Motivational strategies include providing appropriate goals and competition, and giving pep talks, praise, or constructive criticism.

motivation principle The principle that a certain amount of fatigue, effort of expenditure, boredom, and discomfort has to be endured if training is to be successful.

motive A latent, relatively persistent cause which determines a particular course of action.

motive to achieve success A relatively stable disposition which underlies a person's desire to be successful. Those with a high motive to achieve success usually have high self-esteem and a keen desire to take part in competition. *See also* **McClelland–Atkinson model**.

motive to avoid failure (fear of failure) A relatively stable disposition which causes a person to tend to avoid competition because of a fear of failure. It is related to a person's anxiety. A highly anxious person is more likely to avoid competition than one who is low in this construct. *See also* **McClelland-Atkinson model**.

motive to avoid success (fear of success) A motive which results in a self-inflicted decrement in performance because of a fear of loss of status if a person succeeds. For example, an otherwise highly motivated and highly competent woman performer may purposely perform badly against men because she fears that success will result in a perceived loss of her femininity and social rejection by members of both sexes.

motor Pertaining to or connected with movements produced by muscle actions.

motor ability A genetically defined personal characteristic or trait, such as manual dexterity and reaction time which contributes to proficiency in a number of motor skills. Motor abilities cannot be easily modified by practice or experience (*compare* **motor skill**). *See also* **ability**, and **general motor ability**.

motor area Region of cerebral cortex which controls voluntary movements. *See also* **motor cortex**.

motor behaviour An area of study concerned mainly with the behavioural analysis of human skilled movements. It is similar to the study of motor control and motor learning.

motor capacity The genetically determined, maximum potential of an individual to succeed in the performance of a motor skill. Motor capacity is believed to be little influenced by the environment or learning. *See also* **motor ability**; **motor fitness**; **physical fitness**; and **motor educatability**.

motor control The study of the neural, physical, and behavioural aspects of the control of movement. Motor control is often used alongside the terms motor behaviour and motor learning, but it is not synonymous with them.

motor coordination *See* **coordination**.

motor cortex Region of the cerebral cortex in the brain which controls the actions of voluntary muscles. Different regions of the motor cortex are responsible for controlling different muscle of the body.

motor development 1 The changes in skilled movement associated with growth, maturation, and experience. **2** The study of changes in skilled movements associated with growth, maturation, and experience.

motor educatability The inherent ability to learn new motor skills easily and well. Tests of motor educability incorporate novel stunts which have not been practised or learned previously by the performer.

motor endplate The junction between a motor nerve and a muscle cell. *See also* **neuromuscular junction**.

motor engrams Memorized motor patterns used to perform a movement or skill, that are stored in the motor area of the brain. *See also* **engrams**.

motor fitness The neuromuscular components of fitness which enable a person to perform successfully at a particular motor skill, game, or activity. Specific motor fitness components include *agility, *balance, *coordination, *power, *reaction time, and *speed. Motor fitness is sometimes referred to as skill-related fitness. *See also* **physical fitness**.

motor imagery Imagery involving body movements, such as imagining hitting a golf ball or kicking a football.

motor learning 1 The acquisition of skills or skilled movements as a result of practice.

Motor learning involves a set of internal processes associated with practice or experience leading to relatively permanent changes in motor skill. **2** The study of acquisition of skills. *See also* **learning**.

motor nerve *See* **nerve**.

motor neurone A nerve cell which conveys nerve impulses from the central nervous system to an effector organ, such as skeletal muscle.

motor neurone pool Collection of *alpha motor neurone cell bodies in the grey matter of the spinal cord which serve *motor units in the same, or related muscles.

motor outflow time The time period between the change in electrical activity in the *motor cortex and the start of electrical activity prior to a movement. It is a component of *reaction time.

motor pattern A particular sequence of muscle movements directed to accomplishing an external purpose. It is similar to a *motor skill, but the term motor pattern is usually used to describe acts performed with less skill, and in which movement is stressed.

motor program An abstract code or structure, representing one or more skilled movements, stored in the central nervous system. The motor program resembles a computer program because it appears to consist of a series of neural commands which when initiated result in the production of a particular sequence of coordinated movement.

motor reaction time The interval between the first change in electrical activity in a muscle and the initiation of a muscle movement. It is a component of reaction time.

motor reflex A rapid, unlearned, involuntary motor response to a given stimulus. *See also* **reflex arc**.

motor skill A skill associated with muscle activity. Skills performed in sport form a continuum from fine motor skills to gross motor skills. Some sports scientists object to the prefix 'motor' being used on its own because it implies the skill is largely a motor reflex. They prefer to use terms such as perceptual motor skill, psychomotor skill, or sensorimotor skill because such terms emphasize the mental components of movement skills. A skilled movement can be defined as a product of four different elements: force, velocity, accuracy, and purposefulness. In a skilful performance, all four elements must be performed at the same time in exactly the right combination and amount.

motor unit A single motor neurone and all the muscle fibres it stimulates. Each motor unit supplies from four to more than a hundred muscle fibres. Generally, small muscles capable of precise actions

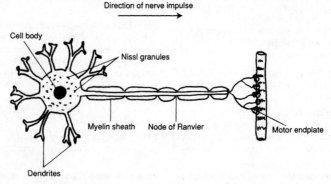

Direction of nerve impulse →

Cell body

Nissl granules

Myelin sheath   Node of Ranvier

Motor endplate

Dendrites

motor neurone

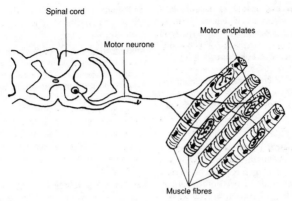

Spinal cord

Motor endplates

Motor neurone

Muscle fibres

motor unit

(e.g. intrinsic hand muscles) are composed of motor units with few muscle fibres, whereas trunk and proximal limb muscles contain motor units with a large number of muscle fibres. Each motor unit obeys the *all-or-none law: all the muscle fibres in a single motor unit receive the same neural stimulation, so they all act maximally when the *threshold of stimulation is met.

mountain sickness *See* **altitude sickness**.

mouthguard *See* **gumshield**.

movement The change in position of a whole body, body part, or centre of mass in relation to a reference system.

movement form A type of physical activity such as an exercise, a game, or a sport.

movement generator A component of the *information processing model which, when loaded with the appropriate *motor programs by the decision-making mechanism, is responsible for organizing and initiating these programs to bring about particular movements.

movement pattern A general series of anatomical movements that have common elements of spatial and temporal configuration, such as movements of body segments occurring in the same plane. Examples of motor patterns are walking, jumping, and kicking.

movement time The time that it takes to complete the movements of a particular action, from its initiation to its termination. *See also* **response time**.

M-protein *See* **M-line**.

MRI *See* **nuclear magnetic resonance**.

MSVC *See* **maximum sustained ventilatory capacity**.

mucopolysaccharides A group of polysaccharides which are a constituent of bone and other connective tissue. Mucopolysaccharides consist of repeating units of disaccharides, one of which is derived from an amino sugar, glucosamine. Mucopolysaccharides include *heparin and *hyaluronic acid.

mucus The slimy, viscous liquid secreted by mucous membranes that lubricates and protects the external surfaces of the membranes.

multiaxial movement Movement of a joint in three planes: transverse, frontal, and sagittal.

multidimensional anxiety theory Theory which predicts that an increase in cognitive state anxiety (worry) has a negative effect on performance. The theory is based on the premise that state anxiety is multidimensional with its two components (cognitive anxiety and somatic anxiety) influencing performance differently.

multidimensional model of leadership A model of *leadership which views athlete satisfaction and performance as the product of three components of behaviour: *actual leader behaviour, *preferred leader behaviour, and *prescribed leader behaviour. Discrepancies between an athlete's preferred coaching behaviour and the actual or prescribed behaviour has a measurable effect on an athlete's performance and satisfaction.

multidimensional model of self-esteem A model in which *self-esteem is seen as a global construct underpinned by increasingly differentiated aspects of the self, including physical, social, and academic self-perceptions.

multidirectional instability Laxity of multiaxial joint in all directions. Some swimmers, for example, have highly flexible shoulder joints which are lax in all directions in the absence of any trauma. This instability appears to be mainly due to an anterior glenohumeral inferior laxity which can cause pain in different phases of an overhead stroke, such as the front crawl or butterfly. Diagnosis is by downward traction on the humerus which causes a sulcus (downward infolding of soft tissue) to appear between the humeral head and the *acromion process.

multidisciplinary study A study carried out by a team of specialists from different disciplines. For example, a study of running efficiency carried out jointly by a team of physiologists, psychologists, and biomechanics.

multifactorial study Experimental investigation of the simultaneous influence of several variables. These variables may be summative, with their total influence equal to the sum of the separate influences, or interactive, in which case the influence of any one variable depends on the presence, absence, or level of another variable. Multifactorial studies are usually more complex than traditional single-factor studies.

multifidi *See* **deep spinal muscles.**

multi-joint muscle Muscle which passes over, and affects the action of, more than one joint.

multilayering The practice of wearing several layers of clothing when training in cold weather. Multilayering has the advantage that it provides more insulation than an equivalent thickness of a single garment of the same material. Also, clothing can be removed easily before the athlete becomes too hot during intensive exercise and is replaced before the athlete becomes too cold during rest periods or the cool-down.

multi-limb coordination An ability which underlies tasks for which the movements of a number of limb segments must be coordinated simultaneously. The simultaneous use of hands and feet in a gymnastics floor exercise is one example.

multipennate muscle *See* **pennate muscle.**

multiple motor unit summation The combined effect of a number of *motor units acting within a muscle at any given time. *See also* **recruitment**; and **spatial summation.**

multiple regression analysis A form of regression analysis used to explain the variations in one variable by means of the variation in two or more independent variables. *See also* **multivariate analysis.**

multiple sclerosis A medical condition in which the *myelin sheath gradually disappears around nerve cells, impairing the transmission of nerve impulses and resulting in sufferers gradually losing control over their muscles. Up until the 1980s, people with multiple sclerosis (MS) were generally advised that physical activity would exacerbate their condition, and that they should live a quiet life. In 1970 an American international alpine skier, Jimmie Huega, following this advice began to deteriorate physically and mentally. In order to stem the deterioration, he decided to develop a cardiovascular endurance programme that included stretching and strengthening exercises. His programme helped him regain health within the constraints of MS. His results have inspired hundreds of other MS sufferers to incorporate exercise into their treatment at a nonprofit making centre he established in Avon (Colorado USA).

multiple sprint sport A sport, such as hockey, basketball, tennis, and soccer, which involves a mixture of brief periods of exercise of maximum intensity followed by recovery periods of rest or light activity.

multiplicative principle The notion that *intrinsic motivation and *extrinsic motivation are interactive and not additive. The principle is based on the observation that, in some circumstances extrinsic motivation in the form of awards and trophies enhances *achievement motivation, but in other circumstances extrinsic motivation may diminish achievement motivation. *Compare* **additive principle**.

multi-poundage system A strength training schedule in which the *repetition maximum (usually 10 RM) is established for each exercise and the first set is worked with the full number of repetitions. Then, 5 kg is removed from the bar and, after a rest, the weight-lifter attempts as many repetitions as possible. The procedure is repeated by removing 5 kg each time for as many sets as possible.

multi-set system Strength training schedule in which several different exercises, with slightly different effects, are used to develop the same muscle group.

multi-stage fitness test *See* **shuttle run test**.

multivariate analysis A statistical technique in which several dependent variables are analysed simultaneously. For example, in a study of muscle strength, data may be collected on the age, type of training, and sex of the subjects being studied. In multivariate analysis, the effect of each of these variables can be examined, and also the interaction between them.

murmur *See* **heart murmur**.

muscle 1 Fleshy contractile tissue which moves parts of the body relative to each other. The three main types of muscle are cardiac muscle, smooth muscle, and striated muscle. **2** A body structure composed of numerous striated muscle cells wrapped in connective tissue, and supplied with nerve fibres and blood vessels. There are approximately 600 muscles in the human body.

muscle action The generation of tension within a muscle. The term muscle action is generally preferred to muscle contraction because the latter implies shortening. This does not always take place. In *striated muscle, there are three types of action: the muscle may shorten (*see* **concentric action**), it may remain the same length (*see* **static action**), or it may lengthen (*see* **eccentric action**). In many activities, such as running and jumping, all three types of action may occur in order to perform a smooth, coordinated movement.

muscle atrophy A wasting-away of muscle tissue due to lack of stimulation or malnutrition resulting in reduced muscle function. Muscle atrophy begins immediately after a muscle injury and occurs progressively as a result of disuse.

muscle belly The fleshy central part of a muscle.

muscle biopsy Withdrawal of a tiny sample of muscle tissue. A hollow biopsy needle is inserted, through a small incision made with a scalpel, into the belly of a muscle. The needle with its sample of muscle is withdrawn and the muscle is weighed, cleaned of blood, mounted, and quickly frozen. It is then cut into thin sections, stained, and mounted for microscopical examination and biochemical analyses. The technique enables exercise physiologists to conduct studies of the microscopical structure and biochemistry of human muscle before, during, and after exercise.

muscle bound A common colloquial term used to describe the condition of a person with well-developed muscles that limit the range of movement of a joint. The ligaments, tendons, and muscles touch the joint and restrict its movement. The idea that weight-training always results in a person becoming muscle-bound, is a myth. There is a risk of muscle bulk developing at the expense of joint mobility only with

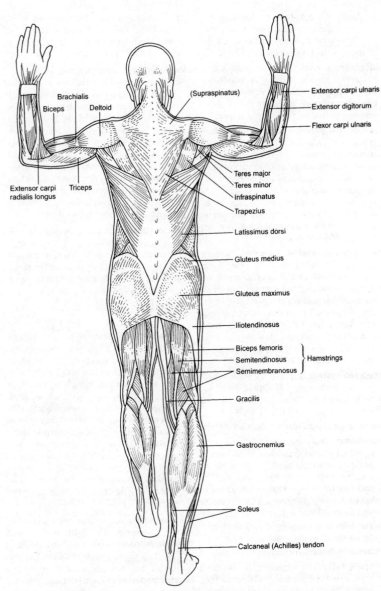

muscles: back view

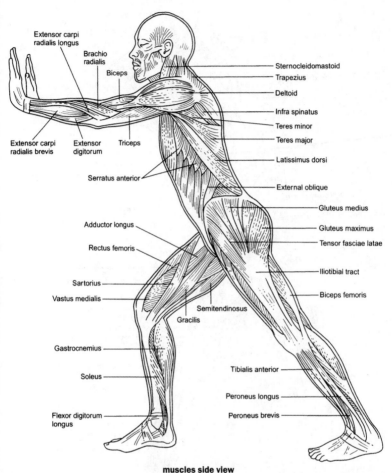

Extensor carpi
radialis longus

Brachio
radialis

Biceps

Extensor carpi
radialis brevis

Extensor
digitorum

Triceps

Serratus anterior

Adductor longus

Rectus femoris

Sartorius

Vastus medialis

Semitendinosus

Gracilis

Gastrocnemius

Soleus

Flexor digitorum
longus

Sternocleidomastoid

Trapezius

Deltoid

Infra spinatus

Teres minor

Teres major

Latissimus dorsi

External oblique

Gluteus medius

Gluteus maximus

Tensor fasciae latae

Iliotibial tract

Biceps femoris

Tibialis anterior

Peroneus longus

Peroneus brevis

muscles side view

a high-resistance, low-repetition exercise programme that does not incorporate a stretching routine.

muscle buffering capacity The ability of muscles to neutralize the acid that accumulates in them during high-intensity exercise, thus delaying the onset of fatigue. Muscle buffering capacity is improved by regular anaerobic training but apparently not by aerobic training.

muscle bulk The absolute volume of muscle in the body. A large muscle-bulk is advant-

ageous in contact sports and some collision sports to provide protection against opponents and to provide momentum to dislodge opponents.

muscle bundle *See* **fasciculus**.

muscle cell *See* **muscle fibre**.

muscle compartment A well-defined region which contains a group of muscles within a particular segment of the body. For example, the lower leg contains four muscle compartments: the anterior compartment,

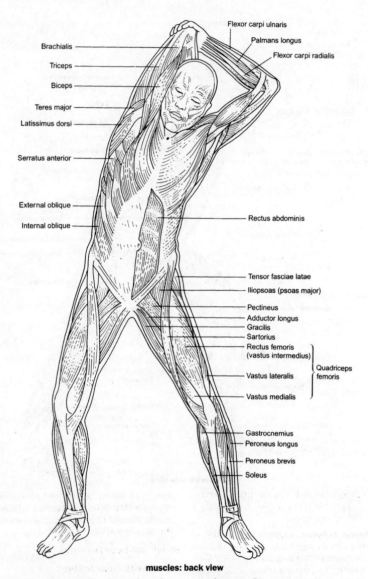

Brachialis

Triceps

Biceps

Teres major

Latissimus dorsi

Serratus anterior

External oblique

Internal oblique

Flexor carpi ulnaris

Palmans longus

Flexor carpi radialis

Rectus abdominis

Tensor fasciae latae

Iliopsoas (psoas major)

Pectineus

Adductor longus

Gracilis

Sartorius

Rectus femoris
(vastus intermedius)

Vastus lateralis

Vastus medialis

Quadriceps
femoris

Gastrocnemius

Peroneus longus

Peroneus brevis

Soleus

muscles: back view

lateral compartment, posterior deep compartment, and posterior superficial compartment. *See also* **compartment syndrome**.

muscle contraction *See* **muscle action**.

muscle cramp *See* **cramp**.

muscle endurance *See* **muscular endurance**.

muscle enzymes Enzymes, such as *succinic dehydrogenase (SDH), and *lactate dehydrogenase (LDH), present in the cytoplasm of muscle.

muscle fatigue A decreased capacity to perform a maximum voluntary muscle action or a series of repetitive muscle actions. A fatigued muscle is unable to continue working even when the type of activity is changed. Muscle fatigue may result from depletion of phosphocreatine or glycogen, accumulation of protons generated by lactic acid, exhaustion of neurotransmitters, or some other mechanism. *Compare* **subjective fatigue**.

muscle fatigue theory A theory that *stress fractures associated with weight-bearing activities result from progressive exhaustion of the muscles. Exhausted muscles are less effective as shock-absorbers. Consequently, abnormally high loads may be concentrated repeatedly on small areas of bone, causing microfractures.

muscle fibre In skeletal muscle, a single, multinucleated cell which appears banded or striated when viewed under a light microscope. A single muscle contains between 10 000 and 450 000 fibres. Each muscle fibre is less than 0.1 mm in diameter but most extend the length of the muscle. This means that a fibre in the thigh may be more than 35 cm long. Several systems have been used to classify muscle fibre type, but they all recognize three main types: two types of *fast-twitch fibres (FT) and one type of *slow-twitch fibre (ST). FT fibres can reach peak tension in about 50 ms and are associated with speed and power activities; ST fibres take approximately 110 ms to reach peak tension, and are associated with endurance activities. Élite marathon runners have more than 90 per cent ST fibres in their gastrocnemius muscle. Élite sprinters,

however, have only about 25 per cent ST fibres in this muscle. Muscle fibre composition appears to be determined early in life, but as we age our muscles tend to lose FT fibres which increases the percentage of ST fibres. Extreme and prolonged training may enable one fibre type to take on characteristics of the opposite type or it may even convert one fibre to the other type.

muscle fibre recruitment *See* **recruitment**.

muscle force The force generated by a *muscle action. The development of muscle force depends on the following: number and type of motor units activated (*see* **recruitment**); the size of the muscle (large muscles have more muscle fibres and can generate more force than smaller muscles); the initial length of the muscle when activated (muscles are elastic so that stretching results in energy being stored which can be released during an action; maximal force is generated when the muscle is stretched to a length approximately 20 per cent greater than its resting length); the angle of the joint (each joint has an optimum angle of force application which depends on the relative positions of the tendinous insertions on the bone and the load being moved); and the muscle's speed of action (during concentric contractions, force generation increases as the movement becomes slower; during eccentric contractions faster movement allows more force production).

muscle glycogen Glycogen stored in the muscles. Muscle glycogen does not contribute to the maintenance of blood glucose. It is used only in the muscle in which it is stored. Muscle glycogen is the main metabolic fuel during heavy and prolonged exercise. Fatigue is associated with its depletion, even when fats are still available as fuel. Typically, a person has about 1.5 g of glycogen for every 100 g of wet muscle. On its own, this provides enough fuel for about 80 minutes of activity.

muscle group Different muscles which contribute to the same action at a particular joint.

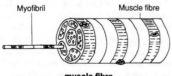

Myofibril · · · Muscle fibre

muscle fibre

muscle growth An increase in muscle volume which may occur by *hypertrophy and/or *hyperplasia.

muscle hernia See **fascial hernia**.

muscle hypertrophy Growth of a muscle due to an increase in the size of individual muscle fibres and an increase in the capillary density in the muscle.

muscle imbalance A condition resulting from the unequal development of the individual members of an antagonistic pair of muscles, with one being very much stronger than the other. Muscle imbalances sometimes result from enthusiastic but poorly scheduled weight-training programmes, and can increase the risk of injuries such as muscle strains.

muscle jerk See **myoclonus**.

muscle poops A fascial hernia in which a muscle protrudes through a hole in the *fascia creating a bump in the skin, with no breakage or tearing of the muscle.

muscle pull See **muscle strain**.

muscle pump A mechanism that returns venous blood towards the heart. Due to alternate contraction and relaxation of skeletal muscles, blood is squeezed through the veins towards the heart. Valves prevent backflow.

muscle pumping A temporary increase in muscle size during a single bout of exercise in which comparatively light weights are lifted many times in succession. The size increase results mainly from fluid accumulation in the interstitial and intracellular spaces of muscles. See also **hypertrophy**.

muscle rehabilitation Treatment of a muscle following an injury so that the muscle functions normally again. It is generally agreed that for muscle rehabilitation to be effective, muscle strengthening regimes should be combined with muscle flexibility exercises. See also **muscle scarring**.

muscle relaxant A drug that reduces the tension within a muscle.

muscle rupture Strictly speaking, an injury in which a muscle is completely torn in two; a third degree muscle strain (see **muscle strain**).

muscle scarring During healing of a muscle tear, the replacement of damaged contractile tissue with collagen tissue. The scar may result in pain which leads to immobility and loss of extensibility of the muscle. Scarring tends to cause the muscle to shorten as it heals. If this is not corrected by progressive mobilization of damaged tissue, the muscle will be susceptible to recurrence of the tear.

muscle selection A component of the motor program concerned with selecting the muscles to be used for the performance of a certain movement.

muscle soreness Pain and tenderness in a muscle which typically occurs after strenuous exercise, particularly if the exercise involved eccentric muscle actions. The underlying cause of muscle soreness is thought to be a change in the ultrastructure of muscle cells, with a rupture of the Z-line. Metabolic waste products, such as lactic acid, have also been implicated because they can stimulate pain receptors in the cell. Muscle soreness may occur during and immediately after exercise (see **acute muscle soreness**) or some time after exercise has ceased (see **delayed onset muscle soreness**).

muscle spasm See **spasm**.

muscle spindle A small, complex spindle-shaped sensory receptor located in skeletal muscle that senses how much the muscle is being stretched. A muscle spindle consists of several modified muscle fibres, called intrafusal fibres. The ends of these fibres are contractile but the central portion is noncontractile and innervated by special neurones (gamma motor neurones). Muscle spindles are sensitive to both the rate at which a muscle stretches (phasic stretch) and the extent to which the muscle is stretched (tonic stretch). Stimulation of muscle spindles elicits a reflex in the stretched muscle (see stretch reflex) and inhibits the action of antagonistic muscles (see **reciprocal inhibition**).

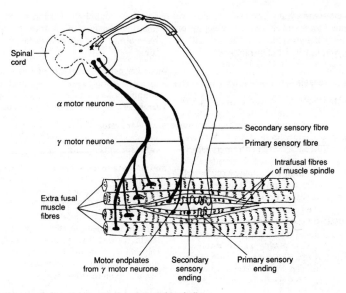

Spinal cord

α motor neurone

γ motor neurone

Secondary sensory fibre
Primary sensory fibre

Intrafusal fibres
of muscle spindle

Extra fusal
muscle
fibres

Motor endplates   Secondary   Primary sensory
from γ motor neurone   sensory   ending
                       ending

muscle spindle

muscle stiffness A measure of the resistance of a muscle to stretching. It is defined as the ratio of a change in muscle force divided by a change in muscle length. Muscle stiffness, therefore, increases as the muscle force associated with a given change in muscle length increases.

muscle strain (muscle pull) When unclassified, a muscle strain usually refers to a relatively minor injury in which muscle fibres are damaged but there is little if any rupture of blood capillaries. However, a strain is usually classified as a first, second, or third degree strain according to the severity of damage to the muscle. A first degree strain refers to tearing of less than 25 per cent of the muscle fibres; the muscle is tender but there is usually no impairment of muscle action. A second degree strain refers to tearing of between 25 to 75 per cent of the fibres, usually accompanied by swelling and bruising and some limitation of muscle mobility. A third degree strain refers to a complete rupture of the fibres with the muscle being completely torn in two; it is accompanied by

extreme tenderness, severe bruising (*see* **haematoma**) and impairment of movement. Rest, ice, compression, and elevation (*see* **RICE**) is the cornerstone of primary treatment. Ice should be applied immediately after the injury (*see* **ice treatment**). A doctor should be consulted if function is impaired. Mild and moderate strains often benefit from light stretching within the pain threshold. Strains, tears, and ruptures most commonly affect those muscles, such as the hamstrings, which span two joints (*see* **Lombard's paradox**). They occur most often in cold weather when joints are stiff and coordination is impaired by nerve conduction being slow. Wearing suitable clothes and warming-up adequately can reduce the risk of muscle strains. *See also* **muscle soreness**.

muscle strength Force or tension that a muscle or, more correctly, a muscle group can exert against a resistance in one maximal effort. Muscle strength can be measured using a dynamometer or a manumometer. *See also* **absolute strength**; and **relative strength**.

muscle tear When unclassified, usually refers to a relatively severe muscle injury in which muscle fibres and blood capillaries are ruptured and intramuscular bleeding occurs. *See also* **muscle strain**.

muscle tension *See* **muscle tone**.

muscle tone (tone; tonus) Tension in a relaxed resting muscle due to activity of some of the muscle fibres. Muscle tone is maintained involuntarily without fatigue through the activity of the nervous system, especially the reflex stimulation of the alpha-motor neurones by the muscle spindles in the muscle concerned. The natural elasticity or turgor of muscle and connective tissue may also contribute to muscle tone. Muscle tone is particularly evident in muscles which are opposing the effects of gravity and maintaining body posture. The degree of muscle tone can be judged by the ease with which joints can be passively stretched and flexed.

muscle tremor *See* **tremor**.

muscle twitch *See* **twitch**.

muscular 1 Pertaining to muscle. **2** Applied to a person with well-developed muscles.

muscular dystrophy A disease in which there is a progressive wasting of muscle.

muscular endurance The ability of a muscle to avoid fatigue. It is reflected by the length of time a muscle can perform repeated muscle actions against a submaximal resistance. It can be determined by the maximum number of repetitions performed at a given percentage of an individual's *one-repetition maximum.

muscular function test A test which evaluates the strength and stretching capacities of muscles that cooperate functionally, thus assessing the developmental level and the training state of intermuscular coordination.

muscular haematoma Bleeding caused by damage to a muscle. The extent of the bleeding is directly proportional to the muscle blood flow and is inversely proportional to muscle tension when the muscle is damaged. *See also* **intermuscular haematoma**; and **intramuscular haematoma**.

muscular power The ability of a muscle or muscle group to exert a maximum amount of force in the shortest period of time. *See also* **power**; and **sargent jump**.

muscular system The organ system consisting of skeletal muscles and their connective tissue attachments.

musculocutaneous nerve 1 A nerve arising from the brachial plexus, the network of nerves at the base of the neck which supplies the skin of the lateral forearm and some muscles of the arm, including the coracobrachialis and the biceps brachii. **2** A nerve which supplies the muscle on the fibular side of the lower leg, the dorsum (back) of the foot, and some areas of the skin on the lower leg.

musculoskeletal attachments Structures which attach muscle to bone and bone to bone. *See also* **ligament**; and **tendon**.

musculoskeletal system The body system comprising both the muscular system and skeletal system.

musculotendinous junction The connection between a muscle and its tendon. The junction contains muscle cells with *sarcomere membranes which are folded inwards in a complicated manner. The infolding reduces the ability of the muscle cells to generate stress on the junction during a muscle action, possibly reducing the risk of tears. If, however, a tear does occur (e.g. as a result of overtraining) the complex infolding of the terminal sarcomeres may not be repaired fully, increasing the risk of a 're-tear'.

MVV *See* **maximum voluntary ventilation**.

myelinated fibres *See* **myelin sheath**.

myelination The development of a *myelin sheath around motor neurones. Myelination improves the conduction speed of nerve impulses, enabling fast reactions and skilled movements to occur. Myelination of fibres in the cortex of the brain occurs most rapidly during childhood but continues until well after puberty. A motor skill can only become fully developed after maturity, when myelination of the nervous system is completed.

myelin sheath A whitish, fatty sheath covering many nerve fibres. The sheath is produced by *Schwann cells. Myelin consists of phospholipids and protein which protect and electrically insulate the fibres. Myelinated fibres (i.e. nerve fibres with myelin sheaths) transmit nerve impulses faster than fibres lacking a sheath. The velocity of nerve impulse transmission in a large myelinated fibre can reach about 120 metres per second (about 250 mph). See also saltatory conduction.

myelography A specialized X-ray technique, involving the injection of a radio-opaque substance, used to examine the spinal canal.

Myers–Briggs type indicator A *personality inventory indicating an individual's preferences for different types of activities. It consists of four basic dichotomous indices: extroversion/introversion, sensing/intuitive, thinking/feeling, and judgement/perception.

myocardial contractility The strength of ventricular contraction of the heart.

myocardial infarction (heart attack) A condition characterized by the formation of a dense wedge-shaped block of dead tissue in the *myocardium following an interruption to its blood supply. Heart tissue dies when deprived of oxygen and the patient has a 'heart attack'. If the interruption to the blood supply is towards the end of a coronary artery, the heart attack may be very mild. If it is towards the beginning of the artery, however, the amount of tissue affected may be large and the heart attack is severe. During a severe heart attack, the patient experiences sudden and very severe chest pains which may spread to the arms and throat. The risk of having a heart attack is increased during the period of vigorous exercise, but regular

aerobic exercise, if properly prescribed and supervised, significantly reduces the overall risk of heart attack. Exercise is often prescribed to post-myocardial infarction patients as an integral part of their rehabilitation programme. See also coronary heart disease risk factor.

myocarditis Inflammation of the muscular wall of the heart caused by a viral or bacterial infection. The risk of having myocarditis increases if the body is subjected to physical exertion when a viral infection is present. Physical activity should be resumed only after complete recovery from myocarditis, and even then exercise should be gradual and under medical supervision.

myocardium The middle region of the wall of the heart composed mainly of cardiac muscle. Compare endocardium; and epicardium.

myoclonus (jerk; muscle jerk) A sudden vigorous contraction of muscle, usually in the limbs. A myoclonus sometimes occurs in healthy individuals as they are falling asleep. It is thought to be caused by temporary reactivation of the reticular activating system. Myoclonus is also a feature of some neurological diseases.

myoelectric activity The electrical activity (change in potential difference) produced by a muscle. The technique for recording myoelectric activity is called electromyography.

myofibril A rod-like bundle of *myofilaments running the length of a *muscle fibre. They are the contractile elements of muscles. Each myofibril consists of a series of *sarcomeres containing *actin and *myosin. Its striated appearance results from a regular alternation of dark *A-bands and light *I-bands.

myofibril splitting Longitudinal splitting of a myofibril into two or more daughter myofibrils. This increases the total number of myofibrils within a muscle fibre, enabling the fibre to increase its cross-sectional area. An increase in the total number of myofibrils within existing fibres occurs during growth, and during *hypertrophy in response to overload.

myofibrosis Condition characterized by the replacement of muscle tissue by fibrous tissue with a consequent reduction in muscle function.

myofilament A contractile protein filament, made of either *actin or *myosin, found in a sarcomere.

myogenic Originating in muscle.

myogenic contraction A contraction initiated in the muscle itself and not dependent on neural stimulation. The contractions of cardiac muscle cells in the heart are myogenic, although the rhythm of the heartbeat can be modified by neural and hormonal stimulation.

myogenic factor A factor inherent in, or derived from, the activity of a muscle. Muscle *hypertrophy is an example of a myogenic factor contributing to muscle strength. See also **neurogenic factor**.

myoglobin An iron-containing pigment present in muscle. It combines with oxygen to form oxymyoglobin. This acts as a store of oxygen which can be used during strenuous exercise. Each myoglobin molecule consists of a single polypeptide chain with a haem group which has an affinity for oxygen stronger than that of *haemoglobin.

myoglobinuria The presence of *myoglobin in the urine. It sometimes occurs following very heavy exercise when muscle cells break down (exercise myoglobinuria), and it is occasionally associated with *carbohydrate-loading. Myoglobinuria can lead to acute kidney failure if it persists. See also **haemoglobinuria**.

myomesin See **M-line**.

myoplasm The living part of a muscle fibre inside the cell surface membrane, excluding the nuclei.

myosin A contractile protein that forms the thicker of the two types of filaments in muscle fibres. Each myosin molecule is composed of two polypeptide chains

twisted together. One end of each is folded into a globular head called the myosin head or myosin cross-bridge. In the presence of calcium ions, the heads with specific sites on the thinner actin filaments interact. The cross-bridges contain ATPase and generate the tension developed by a muscle fibre when it contracts. See also **sliding-filament theory**.

myosin cross-bridge A distinctive structure consisting of two globular heads on each *myosin molecule which interact in the presence of calcium ions with specific sites on a thin actin filament. The cross-bridges contain ATPase and generate the tension developed by a muscle fibre during a muscle action. See also **sliding-filament theory**.

myositis ossificans A condition in which calcium, and eventually bone, become deposited in muscle (often the *quadriceps) after severe bruising or a fracture. It usually takes a few weeks after the injury for myositis ossificans to develop. The calcium deposits are usually reabsorbed with no long-term effects, but the reabsorption may take several months. During this time, it is best to avoid aggressive rehabilitation of the muscle as this may result in microinjuries and pain which delays return to sport. Sometimes calcium deposits, especially those near the muscle insertion or origin, are not reabsorbed. These deposits may be severely disabling and may need to be removed surgically. Recurrent myositis ossificans may be related to bleeding disorders and clotting deficiencies.

myositis Inflammation of a muscle.

myotatic reflex See **stretch reflex**.

myotonia The lack of normal muscle tone.

myotonometer An instrument that measures *muscle tone.

myotonometry A measurement of muscle tone in which the state of muscle action and relaxation is examined; the greater the difference between the two states, the better the muscle tone.

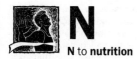

N to nutrition

N *See* Newton.

NAD *See* nicotinamide adenine dinucleotide.

naive falsification The notion that a theory or hypothesis can be decisively rejected on the basis of a single nonsupporting occurrence (the classical example is that the occurrence of one black swan would refute the hypothesis that all swans are white).

nanometre Unit of measurement equal to one thousandth of a micrometre.

naproxen A *nonsteroidal anti-inflammatory drug used to treat chronic inflammatory conditions, such as *arthritis. Its use for treating soft-tissue sports injuries has been advocated.

narcissism Self-love; an excessive preoccupation with oneself and one's self-importance. It is a normal stage of infant development and common in small degrees in sportspeople, but extreme narcissism may be a symptom of a mental disorder in adults.

narcosis An unconscious state induced by a *narcotic analgesic.

narcotic A substance which when swallowed, inhaled, or injected induces stupor, sleep, and insensibility. Substances classified legally into narcotics are divided into five groups: group I consists of substances such as cannabis, heroin, LSD, and mescaline which have no medical applications; group II includes habit forming drugs, such as amphetamines, cocaine, and morphine, which have some medical applications; and groups III, IV, and V, includes substances such as codeine and barbiturates which have greater medical use and less addictive properties.

narcotic analgesics A pharmacological class of agents, represented by morphine and its analogues, which are banned by the International Olympic Committee. Narcotic analgesics induce a state of reversible depression on the central nervous system (narcosis) and are administered to relieve pain. However, the use of these drugs carries a high risk of psychological and physiological dependence and side-effects include dose-related respiratory depression.

narrow focus An attentional style in which an individual has the ability to concentrate on relevant stimuli and ignore other stimuli. *See also* **attention**; *compare* **reduced focus**.

narrowing (focal narrowing; perceptual narrowing) The process whereby *attention is focused on a smaller area of interest so that specific sources of information are more likely to be perceived but rare events are more likely to be missed. It is sometimes referred to as tunnel vision because of its tendency to cause peripheral stimuli to be ignored. Narrowing tends to increase under stress. *See also* **selective attention**. *Compare* **scanning**.

nasal Pertaining to the nose.

nasal dilator (nose strip) A thin strip of plastic attached onto the bridge of the nose to dilate the nasal openings. It is claimed that dilators improve athletic performance by enabling athletes to breathe more easily, making more oxygen available during heavy exercise and recovery. Preliminary tests on athletes performing high intensity exercise and maximal cycling suggest that dilators have no significant physiological effect. However, they do make some athletes feel that they are breathing more easily, reducing their *perceived exertion.

nasal fracture *See* **nose injuries**.

nativism A theoretical perspective which emphasizes the importance of *natural endowment as forming the basis of human behaviour, rather than the effect of environment.

natural athlete *See* **born athlete**.

natural endowment A person's qualities and talents which are dependent on genetic factors (*see* **genetic endowment**).

natural frequency The frequency of free oscillations of any body in a system. *See also* **resonance**.

naturalism In sociology, a theoretical stance which adopts the *naturalistic approach.

naturalistic approach An approach to sociological research which assumes that there are multiple views of reality influenced by the social context and environment in which a situation is viewed. Therefore a question concerning a situation may have a number of valid answers dependent on the perspective of the viewers. *See also* **naturalistic research method**.

naturalistic research method In sport sociology, a method of conducting research which emphasizes the importance of studying social interactions of a sport in natural settings.

natural killer cells (NK cells) A class of large granular *lymphocytes that recognize and kill a variety of cancer cells and virus-infected cells. NK cells are an important part of the innate immune system, providing a major first-line defence against viral infection. NK cell activity is decreased in a number of conditions associated with reduced immune competence, including physiological stress. The total number of natural killer cells decreases for up to 24 hours after severe exercise. Although this may reduce the total activity of natural killer cells and make athletes more vulnerable to infection for a brief period following exercise, the activity of individual natural killer cells actually increases.

natural science model An approach to psychology based on the view that psychological events are physically based, observable processes. *Compare* **human science model**.

nature–nurture issue An issue concerned with the relative importance of heredity (nature) and environment (nurture) in various aspects of an individual's development and behaviour, including the ability to perform at sport. At one time there were two diametrically opposed viewpoints, but now it is generally realized that a person's behaviour and ability are determined by a variable mixture of the two factors. *See also* **genetic endowment**.

nausea A feeling of impending vomiting due to a change in the tone of muscles in the stomach and intestinal wall. The autonomic nervous system controls the vomiting response and nausea can be brought about by some irritant or heightened emotional state, such as that of an athlete prior to competition. As nausea can also be an early symptom of some acute illnesses, it is generally advisable to seek medical advice if it persists and the cause is not known.

navicular bone The boat-shaped ankle-bone of the *tarsus. It lies between the three cuneiform bones and the talus.

N-band A region within the light-band of a *sarcomere of a muscle fibre. It may be the site at which intracellular calcium is concentrated.

nearpoint vision The ability to focus and see clearly objects which are close to the eye.

nebulin A muscle protein associated with thin muscle filaments. It is thought to control the number of *actin monomers joined to each other in a thin filament.

nebulizer therapy A method of administering a drug in which the drug is dissolved in a solution, vaporized, and the vapour inhaled. It is used for the application of *bronchodilator drugs in the treatment of asthma.

neck Region of the body connecting the head to the trunk. The bony structure of the neck consists of seven vertebrae. These, with their associated ligaments and muscles, form joints which hold the head up when the body is upright. They are also responsible for head and neck movements. The head can move independently or with the neck. Other important structures in the neck include the oesophagus, trachea, larynx, thyroid gland, parathyroid gland, major blood vessels, and nerves. 2 Any narrow region of an organ or body part. For example, the neck of the *femur is a short bony connection between the head and the shaft, and is the weakest point of the bone.

neck girth In anthropometry, the circumference of the neck taken immediately above the larynx.

neck injuries Damage to the tissues and structure of the neck. Most neck injuries are sustained as a result of a fall, direct blow, or a twisting movement. These acute neck injuries include strains, sprains, contusions, fractures, and dislocations. All the vital nervous and circulatory connections between the head and the body pass through the neck, therefore some neck injuries can lead to permanent disability. However, it is difficult to differentiate between injuries which are potentially disabling and those which have minor effects. Therefore, all athletes with acute neck injuries should be treated the same. It should be assumed that the injury is serious and emergency medical assistance sought urgently. Patients with suspected neck injuries should not be moved unless they are in danger of further injury. Most neck injuries occur in collision sports such as American football and rugby. If a helmet is worn by a patient with a neck injury, it should not be removed on the field unless there is a danger of respiratory distress coupled with an inability to access the airway. If removal is essential, it should be performed only by trained personnel. Neck strengthening, acquisition of appropriate skills, and good refereeing can reduce the risk of serious neck injuries occurring in collision sports.

necrosis Death or disintegration of a cell or tissue due to disease, physical injury, or chemical injury.

need achievement theory A theory used in sport psychology to predict task preferences and performance outcomes. The theory adopts an *interactional model and considers that *achievement motivation results from the interaction of five components: personality factors, situational factors; resultant or behavioural tendencies, emotional reactions, and achievement related behaviour. Achievement related behaviour results from the interaction of the other four components (high achievers tend to perform better when evaluated and select challenging tasks with intermediate risks; low achievers tend to avoid risky and challenging tasks, and perform less well when evaluated).

need for achievement *See* **achievement motivation**.

needs The basic requirements for survival or for optimal adjustment to the environment, such as needs for food or water, and higher needs such as the need for self-actualization. Often the term is not applied with precision. *See also* **motivational hierarchy**.

needs analysis An assessment of which factors should be included in a training programme to make it suitable for a particular individual.

need to avoid failure A *personality factor which contributes to *achievement motivation. Those with a high need to avoid failure tend to avoid situations where they might be seen to fail and they tend to have a low need to achieve success.

negative acceleration (deceleration) The decrease of velocity over a given period of time.

negative energy balance Condition in which less energy (food) is taken in than is expended in metabolism, resulting in a decrease in body weight.

negative feedback A term used in cybernetics (the study of control and communications mechanisms in humans, other organisms, and machines) to describe how deviations in the output of a system switch on correcting mechanisms that bring the output back to normal. Negative feedback tends to maintain the output at a relatively constant level. It is the basis of the *homeostasis of many physiological systems.

negative motivation In sport, a source of either *primary motivation or *secondary motivation which has a detrimental effect on athletic performance. A series of bad performances may act as primary negative motivation; an audience heckling an athlete can act as a source of secondary negative motivation.

negative nitrogen balance A condition in which protein catabolism (breakdown) exceeds protein anabolism (synthesis) resulting in tissues losing protein faster than it can be replaced. A negative nitrogen balance may occur during physical or emotional stress, starvation, when an individual is on a very low calorie diet, or when the quality of protein is poor (e.g. when the diet is lacking essential amino acids). Adrenal cortical hormones, such as cortisone, released during stress enhance protein breakdown and the conversion of amino acids to glucose.

negative reinforcement A form of *reinforcement in which the removal of a negative or aversive stimulus, such as a loud noise or an unpleasant event, results in an increased probability that a particular behavioural response will occur in the future. *Compare* punishment; and positive reinforcement.

negative resistance training Strength-training which uses eccentric muscle actions. Lowering a barbell, bending down, running downhill, are all examples of negative resistance training. Many bodybuilders use this type of training because it is reputed to increase muscle size quickly. Typically, a training partner lifts the weight into position so that the subject can concentrate on lowering the weights.

negative transfer A form of *transfer of training in which a previously learned task makes it more difficult to learn a new task. *Compare* **positive transfer**.

negative work The absorption of mechanical work when an active muscle is stretched during an *eccentric action. A muscle stretched a distance D while exerting a force F, is said to do an amount FD of negative work. Running downhill, lowering a weight, bending down, and walking downstairs, are all examples of negative work.

neoglycogenesis *See* **glyconeogenesis**.

neopallium Part of the cerebral cortex of the brain associated with intelligence and muscular coordination.

neoplasm Any new and abnormal growth. Neoplasms include benign and malignant tumours. There is no clear relation between the incidence of neoplasms and exercise. Some sports activities may increase the risk of neoplasms (e.g. golf is associated with a high exposure to ultraviolet radiation and an above-average risk of skin tumours), but regular vigorous activity may decrease the incidence of certain cancers (e.g. colonic cancer). The overall risk of neoplasms among athletes is probably not significantly different from that of the general population.

nephritis Inflammation of the kidneys Nephritis has a number of causes. It can, for example, result from taking too much protein in the diet. Many athletes routinely consume more than 2 $gkg^{-1}day^{-1}$ to increase muscle bulk and to provide extra energy during endurance activities. However, this high protein intake provides no advantage, and could be hazardous. The recommended daily intake for protein is about 0.8 $gkg^{-1}day^{-1}$. Studies show that even professional soccer players who regularly engage in very strenuous activities need no more than 1.4–1.7 $gkg^{-1}day^{-1}$. *See also* **athletic pseudonephritis**.

nerve A bundle of *nerve fibres together with associated connective tissue and blood vessels. Nerves provide the wiring through which electrical messages (*see* **nerve impulse**) are transmitted to and from virtually all parts of the body. A nerve containing fibres from both sensory (afferent) and motor (efferent) neurones is known as a mixed nerve.

nerve axon conduction velocity The velocity at which a *nerve impulse is propagated along a neurone. It is affected by the diameter of the neurone, temperature, and the presence or absence of a *myelin sheath. Myelinated fibres have a conduction velocity of 12–20 ms^{-1}, while unmyelinated fibres conduct impulses at between 0.2–2 ms^{-1}. The slow conduction velocity of nerves during cold weather may contribute to the risk of sports injuries because coordination is likely to be impaired. A proper warm-up would overcome this problem.

nerve block A method of producing anaesthesia by blocking the passage of pain impulses along sensory neurones using a local anaesthetic.

nerve cell *See* neurone.

nerve fibre A long, slender process extending from a cell body and conveying *nerve impulses.

nerve growth factor (NGF) A protein produced by some tissues (e.g., smooth muscle) which is needed for the maintenance of some types of sympathetic and sensory neurones. NGF also stimulates the growth of nerve cell processes. When an athlete is injured, ideomotor training may stimulate nerve growth factors and accelerate recovery.

nerve impulse The electrical signal conducted along a *neurone. It is the means by which information is transmitted in the nervous system from one neurone to another, or from a neurone to an effector organ (e.g., a group of muscle fibres). A nerve impulse takes the form of a wave of *depolarization which passes along a nerve fibre. During its passage, the resting potential of the neurone is reversed and becomes an *action potential. A nerve impulse in a single neurone obeys the *all-or-none law.

nerve injury Damage to a nerve. In sport, nerve injuries are most commonly associated with overtraining or poor technique when the nerves are compressed repeatedly against a bone. Serious nerve injuries are sometimes sustained during collision and contact sports. Nerve injuries can be classified according to their severity as grade 1 (*see* **neurapraxia**), grade 2 (*see* **axonotmesis**), and grade 3 (*see* **neurotmesis**).

nervous system A body system consisting of the brain, spinal cord, and nerves. It works in conjunction with the *endocrine system to coordinate and direct all the activities of the body. It has a complex system of neurones which carry information in the form of nerve impulses. The nervous system provides a fast communication and coordination system between different parts of the body as well as with the outside world. *See also* **autonomic nervous system**; **central nervous system**; and **peripheral nervous system**.

net cost of exercise *See* net oxygen cost.

net force The single resultant force derived from the combination of two or more forces. The net force acting on a static body is zero.

net oxygen cost (net cost of exercise) The amount of oxygen above resting values required to perform a given amount of work. It includes both the extra oxygen consumed during the exercise and during the recovery period. The net oxygen cost can be used to estimate the energy required for the exercise.

neural adaptation Adaptive changes in the nervous system in response to training. Neural adaptations are concerned with the ability of the nervous system to activate and coordinate the appropriate muscles for a task. The adaptations may include increased activation and selective activation of agonists within a muscle group, and inhibition or co-contraction of antagonists (*see* **antagonist co-contraction**). Neural adaptations predominate in the first weeks of a new training programme, preceding morphological adaptations. In strength training, for example, improvements due to neural adaptations precede those due to muscle hypertrophy.

neural arch *See* vertebra.

neuralgia An acute pain without inflammation along the course of a sensory nerve. In sport, neuralgia is often the result of pressure from ill-fitting kit, but it may be due to fatigue or illness.

neural pathway The route, such as a *reflex arc, along which a connected sequence of nerve impulses is conveyed from one neurone to another.

neural processing The processing of information, conveyed in the nervous system as *nerve impulses, in order to obtain the appropriate responses. See also **parallel processing**; and **serial processing**.

neural spine See **vertebra**.

neurapraxia A relatively mild form of nerve injury (grade 1 neuropathy) caused by compression of a nerve. It involves no structural damage to the nerve axon although the *myelin sheath may be temporarily disrupted. It is characterized by temporary loss of nerve function, tingling, numbness, and weakness. It usually heals quickly.

neuritis An inflammation of a nerve characterized by pain, tenderness, and loss of function. It is not common in athletes but it can occur as a result of a physical injury to a nerve. This is known as traumatic neuritis. It may be due to a blow, pressure from ill-fitting sports gear, or pressure from a bony exostosis.

neurogenic Derived from, or produced by nerve stimulation. *Compare* **myogenic**.

neurogenic factor A factor related to the activity of nerves. For example, the nervous coordination of the muscles is a neurogenic factor affecting muscle strength.

neuroglia (glia) Cells in the nervous system which are nonconducting. They support and protect delicate *neurones.

neurohypophysis The posterior portion of the *pituitary gland.

neuroma A benign tumour growing from the fibrous tissue around a peripheral nerve. See also **Morton's syndrome**.

neuromuscular Pertaining or involving both nerves and muscles.

neuromuscular electrodiagnosis An examination of the excitability of a nerve or muscle which involves measuring the time taken for a nerve or muscle to respond to a stimulus. Its use to monitor the recovery of a muscle after injury has been largely superseded by *electromyography.

neuromuscular feedback theory See **psychoneuromuscular feedback theory**.

neuromuscular functional test An evaluation of the coordinated functioning of nerves and muscles.

neuromuscular hypertension A condition characterized by an exaggerated *muscle tone and the production of excess tension during muscle actions, far beyond that needed to perform a given task.

neuromuscular junction The site at which a *motor neurone meets and communicates with a muscle fibre. At the junction, a small gap (the synaptic cleft) separates the neurone from the muscle fibre. This gap is bridged by the release of a *neurotransmitter, such as *acetylcholine.

neuromuscular spindle See **muscle spindle**.

neuromuscular stimulation A physical therapy used to treat athletes with muscle atrophy associated with nonuse, postsurgery, or after an incomplete spinal injury. Motor nerves supplying the affected muscle are stimulated with electric pads applied directly on the skin. This causes the muscles to contract, improving their strength and range of movement. The muscle contractions also reduce oedema (swelling) by helping to pump blood through the tissue. Neuromuscular stimulation can also be used for muscle re-education after a cerebrovascular accident (e.g. a stroke).

neuromuscular system Body system that depends on the coordinated activities of nerves and muscles.

neuron See **neurone**.

neuronal pools Functional groups of *neurones occurring in the *grey matter of the brain and spinal cord which process and integrate incoming information received from other sources, such as the sense organs, and transmit the processed information to other destinations.

neurone (nerve cell; neuron) A highly specialized cell that generates and conducts a *nerve impulse. Typically, a neurone is very long and branching, and consists of a *cell body, dendrites, and an *axon.

neuropathy A disorder of the peripheral nervous system, usually presented as a weakness and numbness of the muscles supplied by the affected nerve or nerves.

neuropeptides Chains of amino acids which can function as *neurotransmitters. They include *endorphins and *enkephalins.

neurophysiology The study of the chemical and physical changes which take place in the nervous system.

neuroprobe An instrument for locating and stimulating *trigger points to relieve pain. *See also* **Transcutaneous Nerve Stimulation**.

neurosis A functional behaviour disorder with no apparent underlying physical cause for the feelings of ill-health it engenders. Neuroses include a number of affective disorders, such as anxiety, depression, and obsessive states.

neurotic A loosely applied term to describe a person who suffers from a *neurosis or who has a *personality trait tending towards the unstable end of the neuroticism-stability continuum. *See also* **neuroticism**.

neuroticism A personality trait which is usually described by a continuum from complete instability to complete stability (the neuroticism-stability continuum). Generally, neurotics tend to be more easily aroused than stable individuals and may become over-aroused in stressful situations such as a competition. The degree of neuroticism a person exhibits is complex and is dependent on factors peculiar to each situation.

neuroticism-stability continuum *See* **neuroticism**.

neurotmesis A severe nerve injury that disrupts the entire nerve and usually results in a permanent neurological impairment.

neurotransmitter A chemical released across a *synapse of a neurone which affects the activity of another neurone or a muscle fibre. More than 40 neurotransmitters have been identified. They are classified as either (a) small-molecule rapid-acting neurotransmitters (e.g., acetylcholine and norcadrenaline), or (b) large, slow-acting neuropeptides (e.g., endorphins). Neurotransmitters may be excitatory or inhibitory. They include *adrenaline, *acetylcholine, and *dopamine.

neutral equilibrium Position of a body which, when subjected to a slight displacement has no tendency either to return to its original position or to move further away from its original position. *Compare* **stable equilibrium**; and **unstable equilibrium**.

neutral fat *See* **triacylglycerol**.

neutral hypnosis A state of *hypnosis in which the subject's physiological responses are the same as during complete relaxation.

neutralizer During a particular movement, the role of a muscle which acts to neutralize undesirable actions of another muscle including unwanted accessory actions of the *agonist.

neutral position *See* **anatomical position**.

neutral stimulus A stimulus that does not evoke a response.

neutropenia A decrease in the number of *neutrophils in the blood. It is associated with an increased risk of infection caused by a number of diseases.

neurophil A white blood cell which has a neutral reaction to acid and alkaline stains. It is the most abundant type of white blood cell, and can kill and ingest bacteria.

newton (N) The SI unit of *force. One newton is equal to the force required to give a mass of 1 kg an acceleration of 1 ms^{-2}.

Newton's laws of motion The fundamental laws of motion, first described by Sir Isaac Newton (1642–1727) which form the basis of classical mechanics (*see* **acceleration, law of; inertia, law of; reaction, law of; and gravitation, law of**)

new vegetarian An individual who has a diet of plants supplemented by animal products, but who prefers to eat natural, unprocessed foods. *See also* **vegetarian diet**.

NGF *See* **nerve growth factor**.

niacin (nicotinic acid; vitamin B_3) A water-soluble *vitamin belonging to the B-complex. It is a component of *nicotinamide adenine dinucleotide (NAD and plays an important role in respiratory metabolism. When niacin is present in the blood in high concentrations, it has insulin-like effects and inhibits fat mobilization. Enteric bacteria may produce some niacin in the intestine. Meat and yeast products are rich sources of niacin. Deficiency causes pellagra, characterized by diarrhoea, dermatitis, and mental disturbance. In the UK, the daily Reference Nutrient Intake is 13 mg for females and 17 mg for males; in the USA the Recommended Dietary Allowance is 19 mg for males and 15 mg for females.

nicotinamide adenine dinucleotide (NAD) A coenzyme which readily accepts or gives up hydrogen. It acts as a hydrogen carrier in cells and plays an important role in *glycolysis, when its reduction is coupled with the formation of ATP.

nicotine A poisonous alkaloid obtained from the tobacco plant, *Nicotiana tobacum*. The psychological and addictive effects of smoking cigarettes and chewing tobacco are attributed to nicotine. It is a cholinergic agonist, stimulating the central nervous system and enhancing *arousal. Paradoxically, users also believe it has relaxing properties. Nicotine is generally detrimental on physical performance because of the adverse effects it can have on the cardiovascular, respiratory, and endocrine systems.

nicotinic acid *See* **niacin**.

Nideffer's attentional model A model which proposes that *attentional style exists along two dimensions: width and direction. Width ranges from broad to narrow. Those with broad attention can focus on a large range of things, while those with narrow attention tend to focus on a limited range of cues. The direction of attentional style varies on a continuum from an internal focus to an external focus.

ninety-five per cent rule The rule that an athlete recovering from an injury should not return to full activity until he or she has regained at least 95 per cent of the function in the injured part. Assessment of function is usually based on a comparison of the injured part (e.g. right ankle) with its opposing uninjured part (e.g. left ankle). This assumes that the two parts had equivalent pre-injury functions.

NIPED A mnemonic for remembering the secondary therapies for soft tissue injuries. N represents nonsteroidal anti-inflammatory drugs; I, injections, such as corticosteroids, if appropriate; P, physical therapies including cryotherapy, heat treatment, massage, and ultrasound; E, exercise and stretching; D, devices and braces.

nitrogen balance A condition which occurs when a person's nitrogen intake, in the form of *protein ingested, is equal to the nitrogen utilized in protein synthesis and excreted in the urine and faeces. Estimates are based on the assumption that the nitrogen content of protein averages 16 per cent.

nitrogen narcosis (raptures of the deep) A condition caused by breathing air at high atmospheric pressure. Nitrogen is forced into solution and has a narcotic-like affect on the nervous system, causing dizziness, slowing of mental processes, euphoria, and fixation of ideas.

nitrogen waste The by-product of nitrogen metabolism in the body involving amino acids and *protein. Nitrogen waste is eliminated mainly as urea.

NK cells *See* **natural killer cells**.

NMR *See* **nuclear magnetic resonance**.

Noble test A diagnostic test for *iliotibial band syndrome. The examiner applies pressure on the lateral side of the injured knee directly over the femoral epicondyle. The knee is slowly straightened from a 90° position. Pain is felt by the patient when the knee reaches about 30° flexion, as the band slips over the femoral condyle directly underneath the examiner's finger.

nociceptor A sensory receptor that responds selectively to potentially damaging stimuli. Its stimulation results in *pain. Nearly every type of sensory receptor can function as a nociceptor if the stimulus strength is high enough.

node A swelling or protuberance.

nodes of Ranvier Regularly spaced constrictions of the *myelin sheath on medullated nerve fibers. The nodes allow *saltatory conduction to take place. A *nerve impulse appears to leap from one node to the next.

nodule A small swelling or aggregation of cells.

noise 1 A term used in information theory to indicate a disturbance that does not represent any part of a message from a specified source. **2** Background stimuli (or information) which a person might or might not be aware of, but which is not directly relevant to the task in hand. **3** In signal detection theory, the random firing of the *nervous system; that is background neural activity.

nominal analysis The identification and naming of components of a system. Nominal analysis forms one of the first stages in the development of any scientific study.

nominal measurement The designation of an observation with a value which is merely a name or label such as, big or small. Sometimes numerical values are given to the categories, but these nominal numerical values are without reference to the ordering or distance between categories. Consequently, many statistical applications are not valid with nominal measurements. *Compare* **ordinal measurements**.

nominal variable A variable for which values represent the names of things, with no order implied.

nomogram (nomograph) A chart with three or more scales so aligned that the value of an unknown variable can be found without calculation. A straight line is drawn between known values of two variables to give the related value of another variable. For example, the Lewis nomogram consists of three scales (jump-height, power, and body weight) for determining anaerobic power from a Sargent jump. A line connecting the appropriate points on the jump height and body weight scales intersects the power scale, giving the subject's power output.

nomograph *See* nomogram.

nonaxial joints Joints such as the intertarsal joints, which allow only a very limited movement (e.g., side to side, or back and forth).

nonconscious motor control The control of muscle movements made unconsciously, such as the peripheral corrections which occur in ballistic responses via the muscle spindle reflex and which take only 20–30 ms to complete.

nonconsequential injuries Injuries which are not sustained during a sport but which interfere with athletic performance.

nonessential amino acid An amino acid that can be synthesized in the body and which does not have to be obtained from the diet.

nonfreezing cold injury Tissue damage caused by cold without freezing. Nonfreezing cold injuries (NFCIs) tend to affect areas of a limb more proximal than those affected by frostbite. NFCIs to the feet, known as trench feet, were frequent among soldiers living in wet trenches. Prolonged standing in seawater or walking through wet terrain in a cold environment can also result in NCFIs. These injuries are more likely if the limb is wet, and if the subject is dehydrated, malnourished, ill, or in poor physical condition. Primary treatment consists of removing the patient from the hostile environment, administering analgesics to relieve the pain, and bed rest. Unfortunately there is no satisfactory treatment for the long-term effects of NFCI. These may include chronic damage to muscles, nerves, cartilage, and bone. Preventative measures include limiting exposure to the cold (NFCI takes longer to develop than frost bite);

taking hot drinks whenever possible; taking extreme care to keep feet as dry as possible; and awareness of early signs of injury (e.g., cold, swollen, and blotchy pink-purple or blanched feet that feel heavy and numb). *See also* **frost bite**.

nonhaem iron Iron not contained within the prosthetic haem group of respiratory pigments (primarily, haemoglobin). Nonhaem iron makes up all of the iron in eggs, plants, and dairy products, and up to 60 per cent of the iron in animal tissue. Nonhaem iron is not as readily absorbed as haem iron from the digestive tract.

noninsulin dependent diabetes *See* **diabetes mellitus**.

noninteractive audience A passive audience that does not interact verbally or emotionally with performers.

noninvolvement A lack of involvement in sport exhibited by individuals who have never been involved in sport and who abhor any association with sport, and those who have been active participants but who have lost interest in sport.

non-narcotic analgesic A drug, such as *acetylsalicylic acid (aspirin), which relieves pain but which does not have narcotic effects. *Compare* **narcotic analgesic**.

nonparametric statistics Methods of statistical analysis which can be applied to both ordinal and nominal measurements. They are sometimes referred to as distribution-free statistics because they can be applied to samples from populations without regard to the shapes of their population distribution. Although the tests are robust, they are not as powerful as *parametric statistics.

nonresponders Individuals who do not improve or who improve only slightly compared with others who complete the same training programme. *Compare* **responders**.

nonresponse The incompletion of questionnaires. Nonresponse may produce a bias in a sample.

nonscreeners Individuals with low *selective attention, who have difficulty shifting attention from one stimulus to another.

Nonscreeners generally have higher levels of *anxiety and show higher empathy than screeners.

nonshivering thermogenesis *See* **thermogenesis**.

nonsteroid hormones Hormones derived from amino acids, or proteins and peptides. They are not lipid-soluble, so they cannot pass across cell membranes easily.

nonsteroidal anti-inflammatory drug (NSAID) A drug, not related to steroids, which has anti-inflammatory and pain-reducing properties. Commonly used NSAIDs include naproxen and acetylsalicylic acid (aspirin). NSAIDs are widely used in the treatment of acute soft tissue injuries, but less so for chronic injuries such as tendinitis. The exact mechanism of action of NSAIDs is not known, but they are thought to reduce the synthesis and release of prostaglandins. NSAIDs are permitted by the International Olympic Committee for use by athletes.

nonuniform speed The speed of an object which varies over a certain period of time.

nonverbal communication Forms of communication, such as smiling and frowning, patting on the back and blowing on a whistle, which convey ideas, feelings, and attitudes without using words. Experimental evidence shows that nonverbal communication can be a very important source of motivation. *See also* **kinesics**; and **paralanguage**.

nonzero-sum competition Competition in which all the participants may achieve some if not all of their goals. For example, in a marathon, all participants can share the achievement of completing the course or obtaining a personal best time, even though there is only one winner.

'no pain, no gain' concept The concept that an athlete can improve only by working hard enough to feel discomfort. In order to benefit from training, the effort exerted during exercise must be greater than that used during normal daily activities (*see* principle of progressive overload). However, if athletes exercise beyond their normal limits of tolerance and suffer real pain, they are likely to succumb to new injuries and aggravate pre-existing ones.

noradrenaline (norepinephrine) A drug belonging to the stimulants which are on the International Olympic committee list of *banned substances. Noradrenaline is an endogenous hormone secreted by the adrenal medulla and released as a *metabotropic neurotransmitter from nerve-endings in the sympathetic nervous system and some areas of the cerebral cortex. Its effects may be excitatory or inhibitory. Low levels of noradrenaline are associated with depression. Its release is enhanced by *amphetamines and its removal from synapses is blocked by *cocaine. Noradrenaline is closely related to *adrenaline and has similar actions. *See also* **biogenic amine**.

noradrenaline

norepinephrine *See* noradrenaline.

norm 1 The set point or reference point in a system which has its output maintained at a constant level. For example, the norm for body core temperature is approximately 37 °C. *See also* **homeostasis**. **2** An empirically established standard. Sometimes the norm refers to the normal or average value. **3** A social rule, regulation, law, or informal agreement which prescribes and regulates behaviour in a particular situation; violations of norms are subject to sanctions. Many sports sociologists consider that harmonious social interactions within teams are dependent on these shared expectations and obligations. *Compare* **values**.

normal A line perpendicular to the surface at the point of contact of a body.

normal active range Range of motion of a joint during activities which are a normal part of everyday life. *Compare* **maximum active range**.

normal distribution (Gaussian distribution) In statistics, a continuous distribution of a random variable with its mean, median, and mode equal. The normal distribution is depicted graphically by a symmetrical, bell-shaped curve.

normal force *See* normal reaction force.

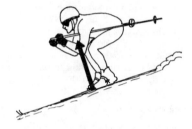

normal force

normal involvement A pattern of sport involvement in which individuals participate regularly in sport and the participation has become integrated into their lifestyles.

normal reaction force A force acting perpendicular to two surfaces in contact with each other. It is a measure of the force holding the two surfaces together. The larger the normal reaction force, the larger the value of *limiting friction. If weight is the only vertical force acting on an object lying or moving on a horizontal surface, the normal reaction force is equal in magnitude but opposite in direction to the weight. Friction, therefore, is increased by increasing the weight.

normative Pertaining to a *norm or norms.

normative approach A theoretical, prescriptive approach to sociological studies which has the aim of appraising or establishing the values and norms which best fit the overall needs and expectations of society. *Compare* **value-free approach**.

normative theory Any theory which adopts a *normative approach.

normative theory of leadership A theory which suggests that one of the primary functions of a leader, such as a coach, is to make decisions. When making the decision, the coach should consider the relative importance of the quality of the decision, and the acceptance of the decision by his or her athletes. According to the theory, in some circumstances the quality of the decision is of prime importance, in other circumstances acceptance is of greater importance. Depending on the particular circumstances, the coach should use one of three decision-making coaching styles: autocratic, in which the coach makes decisions with little consultation; delegative, in which the coach delegates decision-making to others; or participative, in which the coach makes decisions jointly with the athletes.

norming See team.

normotensive Applied to a condition in which blood pressure is within the normal range.

norm-referenced test A test in which an individual's scores are evaluated in the context of the performance of others. In sport, such norm-referencing is often used for purposes of team selection and for identifying individual differences. Compare criterion referenced tests.

nosebleed (epistaxis) Loss of blood through the nose due to changes in the continuity of the blood vessels of the nasal septum and surrounding mucosa. A nosebleed may be caused by a blow to the head, fever, high blood pressure, barotrauma, or blood disorders. Most nosebleeds in sports are caused by physical trauma. An athlete with a bleeding nose should sit with the head tilted forward, pinch the nostrils with the thumb and forefinger, and apply ice to the bridge of the nose (see ice treatment). If bleeding does not stop or if the nose is put out of shape by the injury, medical advice should be sought.

nose fracture See nose injuries.

nose injuries Damage to the cartilage, bone, or soft tissues in the nose. Nose fractures are the most common facial injuries sustained in sport. Although they are not normally dangerous, they can be disfiguring and athletes should seek medical advice. Nosebleeding, nasal airway obstruction, and a nasal deformity are the most common symptoms of a nasal fracture. The most important concern in primary treatment is to ensure an airway is open and breathing is not restricted. Then, the bleeding should be controlled (see **nosebleed**), and the nose protected from further injury while medical assistance is acquired. See also **pugilist's nose**.

nose strip See nasal dilator.

notch A depression in a bone.

novelty problem A problem encountered with early definitions of *motor programs as structures that carry out movements in the absence of *feedback. Such programs would prevent the generation of movements that had not been produced previously.

NSAID See nonsteroidal anti-inflammatory drug.

nuclear cardiology See cardiac imaging.

nuclear magnetic resonance (magnetic resonance imaging; MRI: NMR) A technique that produces images of internal soft structures, such as muscles and tendons. The images are much clearer than those produced by X-radiography or even computerized tomography, and without known risk to the patient. NMR is used to diagnose joint injuries, prolapsed intervertebral discs, and muscle injuries. It is especially useful in investigating the cause of exertional or postconcussive headaches. The technique depends on atomic nuclei behaving like small magnets. When in a magnetic field, these nuclei arrange themselves nonrandomly, producing signals which can produce an image.

nucleus pulposus The spongy, semifluid inner contents of an intervertebral disc. The nucleus pulposus of a young, healthy disc is approximately 90 per cent water making the disc highly resistant to compression. *See also* **annulosus fibrosus**.

null hypothesis A hypothesis used in experimental analysis which postulates that there will be no statistical difference between two or more sets of results. For example, if two groups of people are tested for physical fitness, the null hypothesis would state there is no significant difference between the two groups and that any differences that do occur are due to random chance. A significance test, such as the t-test, would then confirm whether the null hypothesis should be accepted or rejected.

nutation 1 Wobbling; tilting of a body's axis of rotation from its original position. See also twisting. **2** The act of uncontrollably nodding the head.

nutrient A substance present in food that is used by the body to promote normal growth, maintenance, and repair. The major nutrients needed to maintain health are *carbohydrates, *lipids, *proteins, *minerals, *vitamins, and *water. Roughage (*fibre) although never assimilated into the body and therefore not a nutrient, is also regarded as an essential component of a balanced diet.

nutrient artery (medullary artery) A large artery which supplies the central medullary cavity of a long bone with nutrients and oxygen.

nutrient density A measure of the amount of nutrients per unit energy of food. Nutrient density usually relates to the amount of vitamins and minerals (and sometimes proteins) per 100 kilocalories of food.

nutrition 1 The process of taking in and assimilating nutrients. **2** The study of food in relation to the physiological processes used to acquire sufficient nutrients to maintain good health.

O

Ober's test to ozone

Ober's test A diagnostic test which assesses the degree of tautness in the *iliotibial band. The patient adopts a side-lying position with hips at 0° flexion and the examiner passively adducts the leg. Pain or tightness is a sign of *iliotibial band syndrome. Tenderness localized on the supralateral aspect of the greater tuberosity indicates a *bursitis.

obesity The storage of excessive amounts of fat, particularly under the skin and around certain internal organs. Obesity usually results from a positive energy balance and not having a balanced diet. Obesity is a well-recognized predisposing factor for a number of diseases, including *diabetes mellitus, *hypertension, and other cardiovascular diseases. Some medical experts estimate that life expectancy decreases by approximately 1 per cent for each pound (about 450 g) of excess fat fat carried by an person of forty-five to fifty years of age. Obesity is difficult to define quantitatively, but it is generally accepted that anyone who has a *body mass index (BMI) greater than 30 is obese. According to this definition, it is possible to be obese without being overweight. Conversely, muscular athletes may be overweight without being obese.

object In biomechanics, anything which has mass and occupies space.

object cueing An exercise that improves *attention. The subject, assuming a relaxed position in a distraction-free environment, holds an object and looks at it while repeating a meaningful cue word related to the object. When the object is taken away, the subject is instructed to repeat the cue word and visualize the object. Athletes often use a sport-related object, and use the appropriate cue word during an actual performance to block out irrelevant thoughts, and when concentration is waning.

objective **1** Applied to a material object or phenomenon which exists independently of perception. **2** Applied to studies and opinions which are free from distorting, subjective, personal, or emotional bias. *See also* **objectivity**. **3** In medicine, applied to symptoms of a disease which can be perceived by persons other than the sufferer. **4** The object of one's efforts; sometimes used synonymously with *goal.

objective competitive situation Competitive situation that an athlete is placed in. It usually incorporates the following: a standard evaluation of the quality of performance; an evaluator who is familiar with the standard; and a comparison of the performance outcome against the standard.

objective danger A risk, such as an avalanche, flood, or storm, over which a person has little or no control, and which is not merely a figment of his or her imagination. *Compare* **subjective danger**.

objective demand An environmental situation or stimulus which contributes to *stress.

objective descriptive feedback A nonjudgemental type of *augmented feedback which describes as clearly as possible the behaviour observed. For example, a coach stating that 'Your knees were bent when you were leaning out over your skis.'

objectivism The view that it is possible to describe the real physical and social world in purely objective terms, free from personal bias. *See also* **objectivity**.

objectivity The quality of being free from personal bias. Objectivity is the aspect of measuring and testing related to the extent to which two observers achieve the same results independently. An experimental procedure is said to have objectivity if it is not influenced by the views and perceptions of the experimenter, and is a true reflection of reality. Knowledge gained from such procedures should have validity, reliability, and be free from bias. The subdisciplines of sports science all have working criteria of objectivity which they aim to fulfil. Many philosophers, however, maintain that strict objectivity is an unattainable goal and that all views of reality are to some extent influenced by the perceptions of the observer.

OBLA *See* **lactate threshold**.

obligatory activities Physiological activities, such as eating and sleeping, which a person is compelled to perform to satisfy the demands of the body.

oblique impact The collision of two objects not moving along the same straight line before impact, or the collision of a stationary object with another object travelling at an angle other than 90° to the surface on which the impact occurs. *Compare* **direct impact**.

O'Brien technique Technique demonstrated in the 1952 Olympic Games by Parry O'Brien of the USA, for putting the shot. He moved across the circle to apply force to the shot for a longer period than was possible from a standing putt, thereby increasing the *impulse.

observation The deliberate act of an observer who studies events using his or her sensory processes. Observation is usually the first step taken in a scientific investigation.

observational learning **1** Learning (for example, a skill) by observing the behaviour of someone else rather than by direct experience. It may involve learning about the consequences of another individual's actions with or without copying the actions. **2** A term sometimes used as synonym for cognitive learning.

obsession A thought which persistently recurs despite attempts to resist it. An obsession provokes *anxiety and dominates a person although the person regards it as being senseless.

obturator externus A flat triangular muscle deep in the medial aspect of the thigh. It has its origins on the outersurface of the obturator membrane on the pubis and ischium and the margins of the obturator foramen; its insertion is via a tendon into the trochanteric fossa on the posterior aspect of the femur. Its primary action is lateral (outward) rotation of the femur. It also helps to stabilize the hip.

obturator foramen An opening through which blood vessels and nerves pass in the hip bone, slightly in front of and below the *acetabulum. The obturator foramen is formed from a fusion of the pubic bone and the ischium, and is nearly closed by a fibrous membrane.

obturator internus A muscle which surrounds the *obturator foramen in the pelvis. It has its origins on the inner surface of the membrane around the obturator foramen, on the greater sciatic notch and the margins of the obturator foramen. It leaves the pelvis via the sciatic notch and then turns acutely forward to insert on the greater trochanter of the femur, in front of the *piriformis muscle. Its primary action is lateral (outward) rotation of the femur. It also helps to stabilize the hip joint.

obturators Either of two muscles covering the outer anterior wall of the pelvis (*see* **obturator externus** and **obturator internus**).

occipital Pertaining to the area at the back of the head or at the base of the skull.

occipital bone Bone which forms part of the back and base of the cranium, and encloses the foramen magnum.

occipito-atlantal joint The joint between the two condyles at the base of the *occipital bone and the *atlas vertebra.

occipito-axial joint The joint formed between the *occipital bone of the cranium and the *axis.

occluded circulation The closure or obstruction of a blood vessel.

occlusion Closure or obstruction of a hollow body structure.

occupational sport subculture A group of people, including athletes and all types of producers, who earn a livelihood from a particular sport. *Compare* **avocational sport subculture; deviant sport subculture**.

octacosanol A 28-carbon alcohol found in wheatgerm oil. It has been taken as an *ergogenic aid in the belief that it enhances endurance. However, there is no clear, scientific evidence that it acts as a performance enhancer.

ocular Pertaining to movements of the eye.

ocular injuries *See* **eye injury**.

oculomotor Pertaining to movements of the eye.

odontoid process Toothlike process on the superior surface of the *axis which acts as a pivot for the rotation of the *atlas.

oedema An atypical accumulation of fluid in the interstitial space leading to a swelling. An oedema may be caused by any event that increases fluid flow out of the bloodstream or hinders its return. Many sports injuries are associated with oedema. *See also* **high altitude pulmonary oedema**.

oestrogen A group of steroid hormones (including oestradiol, oestriol, and oestrone) produced by the ovary, the placenta, and, in small amounts, by the male testis and adrenal cortex. In females, it maintains the secondary sexual characteristics and is involved in the repair of the uterine wall after menstruation. Synthetic oestrogens are major constituents of contraceptive pills. Side-effects of oestrogen administration include nausea and vomiting, irregular vaginal bleeding in females, and feminization in males.

old age The final stage in the life course of an individual. Old age is usually associated with declining faculties, both mental and physical, and a reduction in social commitments (including sport participation). The precise onset of old age varies culturally and historically. It is a social construct rather than a biological stage.

olecranal Pertaining to the back of the elbow.

olecranon bursa A superficial *bursa underneath the skin at the point of the elbow which, because of its position, is particularly vulnerable to direct trauma and bursitis.

olecranon bursitis Inflammation of the olecranon bursa. It is caused by a single blow or repeated blows to the elbow (for example, in kareteka who break objects with the elbow). It is characterized in the acute phase by an egg-shaped-swelling, pain, and tenderness. A redness around the bursa may indicate an infection. This requires medical evaluation which usually takes the form of microscopical analysis of bursal fluid withdrawn by aspiration. An infection is treated with antibiotics. Immediate treatment of olecranon bursitis includes rest, ice, compression, and elevation (*see* **RICE**), and anti-inflammatories. An athlete experiencing persistent pain and loss of mobility of the elbow should consult a doctor. An uninfected olecranon bursitis in which the swelling persists after the acute stage can be treated effectively with a localized steroid injection. Chronic, or recurrent bursitis may warrant surgical excision of the bursa.

olecranon fossa Depression on the posterior surface of the *humerus which allows free movement of the ulna during flexion and extension.

olecranon fracture Fracture of the ulna at the point of the elbow joint. It is usually caused by a fall onto the arm or elbow. Olecranon fractures occur most commonly in contact sports and in sports, such as horse-racing, in which falls are frequent. Primary treatment includes protecting the arm by securing it to the body, gently applying ice over the injured area for twenty minutes, and obtaining medical assistance. X-radiography will determine the nature of the injury. Fractures should be dealt with by an orthopaedic surgeon as surgical fixation may be required. However, if no displacement has occurred, the injury may be managed by splinting the arm at 90 degrees in a sling for a few weeks. If displacement has occurred, it is important that the bones are realigned exactly to ensure no long-term loss of joint function.

olecranon process Prominent projection at the proximal end of the elbow. It forms the point of the elbow and forms the attachment point for the *triceps brachii muscle.

oligomenorrhoea Reduced frequency of menses (menstruation). Menstrual dysfunctions are common in female athletes but their classification is confused. A woman who has not experienced menses for five months may be classified as oligomenorrhoeic in one study and amenorrhoeic in another. *See also* **amenorrhoea**.

omega-3 fatty acids A group of unsaturated fatty acids found in some fish oils and linseed oil. They appear to change blood chemistry, reducing blood clotting and may lessen the risk of heart disease.

omnidirectional information transmission Transmission of information in a group in which each member can use and benefit from the information given by any other member of the group, and can in turn ask questions and exchange information with other members. *See also* **social facilitation**. *Compare* **unidirectional information transmission**.

one-area-target-type procedure A procedure for testing the accuracy of an individual attempting to hit a single target. The successful attempts gain points and the misses count as errors. There are a number of variations: for example in basketball, a basket made can score one point and a basket missed no points; or a clean shot may score four points, a rim shot that goes in 3 points, a rim shot that goes out 2 points, and a shot that touches the basket 1 point, and a complete miss scores no points.

one-leg study A physiological study in which one leg of each subject is treated differently to the other leg; for example, a group of subjects may perform one-leg endurance training on a cycle ergometer for several weeks. During such a study, physiological parameters of aerobic fitness (e.g., succinic dehydrogenase levels) can be compared in the trained and untrained leg. After the training period when one leg is well-trained, the subjects can perform a two-leg endurance exercise in which both legs perform identically. The effects of this exercise on the trained and untrained leg can be compared by means of arterial and venous catheterization and muscle biopsy analysis.

one-repetition maximum (1–RM) In weight-training, the maximum weight an individual can lift just once.

onset of blood lactate accumulation (OBLA) See **lactate threshold**.

ontogenesis The development of a particular individual.

ontogeny The general development of a race or other group of people.

ontology A branch of philosophy which deals with the nature of the fundamental things which exist in society.

onychia Inflammation of the bed of a nail in which pus forms. This is followed by the nail becoming loose and eventually falling off. See also **black nail**.

open-circuit spirometry A method of *indirect calorimetry in which the subject breathes air from the atmosphere. The composition of the air flowing in and out of the lungs is measured to estimate oxygen consumption. Compare **direct calorimetry**.

open-closed continuum A continuum extending from an open situation to a closed situation which describes the extent to which environmental conditions affect performance.

open-ended attribution An *attribution freely made by an athlete who can identify his or her own cause for a particular outcome without any suggestion or constraints of a questioner. Sometimes open-ended attributions are difficult to categorize. See also **structural rating scale**.

open-ended question A question, for instance in a questionnaire, in which the respondent does not have to choose from a number of pre-structured answers but is left to answer entirely free from any constraints. Compare **fixed-choice question**.

open fracture See **compound fracture**.

open-loop system A control system with a preprogrammed set of instructions to an effector which has no feedback or error-detection process; consequently, the system is unable to make compensatory adjustments. It has been suggested that open-loop systems control certain movements which are executed without any alterations due to sensory feedback. However, the performance of complex, skilled movements probably involves the use of many mechanisms, including both open-loop systems and *closed-loop systems.

open situation An environmental situation which is unpredictable and changing.

open skill A *motor skill performed in an unpredictable, changing environment which dictates how and when the skill is performed. Compare **closed-skill**.

operant conditioning (instrumental conditioning) A form of learning where an individual forms an association between a particular behavioural response and a particular reinforcement. The process may be positive, for example when a player learns to associate a particular activity with a pleasant result, or negative, for example when a player associates an activity with an unpleasant result. Compare **classical conditioning**.

operant technique Learning method in which certain behaviours are reinforced or rewarded, leading to an increase in the probability that the behaviours will be repeated. See also **operant conditioning**.

operational hypothesis See also **working hypothesis**.

ophthalmic Pertaining to the eye.

opiate Any drug containing or derived from opium. Opiates include codeine and morphine. All opiates are *narcotic analgesics on the IOC list of *banned substances.

opium The dried latex from unripe seed-heads of the oriental poppy Papaver *somniferum*, from which morphine is extracted. Opium is a highly addictive drug belonging to the *narcotic analgesics which are on the IOC list of *banned substances.

opponens digiti minimi An intrinsic muscle of the hand. Its origin is on the hamate and its insertion is on the fifth metacarpal. Its primary action is on the fifth (little) finger, enabling opposition with the thumb.

opponens pollicis A muscle in the hand that has its origin on the *trapezium and its insertion on the radial side of the first metacarpal. Its primary action is opposition at the carpometacarpal joint of the thumb.

opportunity cost The cost of taking part in one activity in terms of the lost opportunities which could have been pursued using the same resources of time and money. Opportunity cost is mainly an economic concept, but it is also applied to sport where success commonly depends on the athlete devoting his or her youth to the pursuit of success, often at the expense of career opportunities.

opposition The muscle action which enables the pad of the thumb to make contact with the pad of the other fingers and so provide a firm and sensitive grip. It is a unique action involving a combination of abduction, circumduction, and rotation.

optic Pertaining to vision or the eye.

optimal angle of release The angle at which a projectile leaves the ground and gains maximum horizontal displacement. When the height of release and landing are the same, assuming no air resistance, the theoretical optimal angle of release is 45°. However, the actual optimal angle is usually 35–45° to compensate for the effects of air resistance. When the height of release is greater than the height of landing, as in shot-putting, the optimum angle is always less than 45°. When the height of release is less than the height of landing, for example when playing a bunker shot in golf, the optimal angle is more than 45°.

optimal arousal *See* **zone of optimal functioning**.

optimal arousal theory A theory which postulates that each athlete has his or her own *zone of optimal functioning* (ZOF), and that the athlete performs best when his or her level of arousal falls within the ZOF. *See also* **catastrophe theory**.

oral Pertaining to the mouth.

oral contraceptives *See* **contraceptive pill**.

orbit 1 The bony cavity containing the eye. **2** The curved path of a body moving around another body.

orbital blow-out fracture A dramatic eye injury in which the globe of the eye is forced posteriorly, fracturing the floor of the orbit and trapping the inferior rectus muscle (one of the oculomotor muscles that move the eye). Classically, the rim of the orbit remains intact so that the fracture is not palpable. A blow-out fracture is indicated by the eye appearing abnormally sunken (enophthalmus), double vision (diplopia), and, if the infraorbital nerve is trapped, lack of feeling underneath the eye. Typically, a blow-out fracture is caused by a knee, elbow, or fist hitting the eye during a contact or collision sport.

ordinal measurement The designation of values into rank order so that if 'A' is greater than 'B', then 'B' is greater than 'C'. Often numbers are used to identify the rank, but it does not indicate relative distances between the ranks. Thus a group of footballers may be arranged in rank order of aggressiveness and although it might be possible to say that one player is more aggressive than another, it is not possible to state precisely by how much the relationship differs. *Compare* **interval measurement**; **nominal measurement**; and **ratio**.

ordinal variable A variable for which values imply rank-order relations only. *See also* **ordinal measurement**.

organ A multicellular structure containing different types of tissue and which carries out a specific role.

organelle A discrete structure within a cell that carries out a specific function (e.g. *mitochondrion and nucleus).

organic 1 In biochemistry, pertaining to carbon-containing substances other than carbon dioxide and carbon monoxide. **2** Pertaining to an organ or organs of the body.

organic fitness The fitness of the body and its physiological systems in terms of functional efficiency and state of repair. Organic fitness is regarded as an integral part of health.

organismic theories of personality Clinically oriented theories which view *personality as being shaped by the overall field of forces acting on individuals, and posit self-change or growth as central features.

organization A social, administrative structure formed to pursue certain goals. An organization is characterized by having a formal set of rules and having a limited membership which is often hierarchical with a well-defined division of labour.

organization theory Knowledge concerned with the structure and functioning of an organization, particularly with regards to the dynamics of the social relationships. Organization theory includes topics such as rewards and motivation, decision-making and leadership, all of which have particular relevance to sports organizations.

organ system A group of organs in the human body that work together to carry out a vital body-function.

orientation The ability of a person to be aware of his or her position with respect to both time, place, and circumstantial situation.

orienting response An autonomic mechanism which directs *attention to anything unusual or different. Its function is to alert a person to potential danger. It is possible, with training, to override this response. It is often useful for athletes to be able to override the orienting response during competition.

origin 1 The attachment point of a muscle that remains relatively fixed during the action of the main muscle; it is usually proximal to the *insertion. **2** A point at which a blood vessel or nerve branches from a vessel or nerve.

origin–pawn relationship A term based on the observation that some people like to control their own destiny, while others feel powerless to control their destiny: the former have been called origins and the latter pawns. *See also* **locus of control**.

origins *See* origin–pawn relationship.

ornithine An amino acid produced in the liver during the formation of urea from ammonia.

ornithine cycle A series of reactions which take place in the liver in which ammonia, produced from the breakdown of excess amino acids, is combined with carbon dioxide to form urea.

orthopaedics A branch of medicine dealing with skeletal deformities and disorders caused by disease or injury.

orthoses (orthotics) Moulded foot-supports (ideally, custom-made) that fit in a shoe to make foot motion more efficient, reduce the risk of foot injuries, and to correct certain structural imbalances (e.g. flat feet and high arches) which may lead to pain in the back, hips, knees, lower legs, or feet. Soft orthoses provide extra cushioning for those with very inflexible feet (e.g. those with high arches). Rigid orthoses provide extra stability to those who have flat feet or who overpronate. Many élite athletes, including runners, cyclists, and skiers, benefit from using orthoses during training and competition.

orthostatic Pertaining to, or caused by, standing erect.

orthostatic hypotension (postural hypotension) A fall in blood pressure that occurs on standing up after lying down.

orthostatic proteinuria (postural proteinuria) Occurrence of *protein in the urine as a result of prolonged standing. It disappears after bed-rest. Orthostatic proteinuria has been linked to the peripheral sequestration of blood during exercise, especially in young adults.

orthotics *See* orthoses.

os (pl. ossa) A bone.

os (pl. ora) The mouth or any mouth-like opening.

O-scale A system of assessing physique based on a scale constructed from anthropometric data, including measurements of skinfold, body-height, body-girth, and body-weight.

oscillatory motion A motion which recurs back and forth over the same pattern. An example of an oscillatory motion is that of the legs during running when the same cycle of movements is repeated.

Osgood's semantic differential scales Measures of *attitude which require that individuals rate the attitude object on a set of semantic scales which are bipolar adjectives generally seven steps apart. For example, a scale for rating how a person feels about doing aerobics may include the following: FOOLISH: −3 −2 −1 0 +1 +2 +3 :WISE PLEASANT: −3 −2 −1 0 +1 +2 +3 :UNPLEASANT etc.

Osgood–Schlatter disease An injury in growing children in which the attachment of the *patellar tendon on the tubercle at the top of the tibia is damaged through overuse. Osgood–Schlatter disease is a form of *apophysitis in which the tibial apophysis and the growth centres of the bones of the tubercle of the tibia become inflamed. It is usually presented as pain over the tibial tubercle, and pain when extending the knee against a resistance. It commonly occurs in children aged 9 to 14 years who take part in sports that involve repetitive knee-bending, such as football, skating, and jumping. Knee-bending imposes great tensile stress at the attachment point of the patellar tendon which, in young athletes, is still soft. Repeated, excessive stress may cause an *epiphyseal avulsion. Osgood–Schlatter's disease usually heals spontaneously as the athlete matures and the cartilage in the epiphysis is replaced by bone. Some doctors believe that the knee should be immobilized and all activity restricted for a period from a few weeks to three years. Other doctors believe that athletes with this condition can continue exercising with slight discomfort, but they should avoid activities that cause pain sufficiently severe to limit movement. Sometimes a piece of bone (a fragment of the tubercle) develops in the tendon. This bone may have to be removed surgically. Removal is best delayed until growth has been completed to avoid growth plate arrest and structural abnormalities such as valgus of the knees.

osmolality The ratio of solutes (such as electrolytes) to fluid. It is measured in osmoles per kilogram of fluid. One osmole is equal to the molecular weight of the substance in grams divided by the number of ions or other particles the substance dissociates into when in solution.

osmoles *See* osmolality.

osmoreceptor A cell which is sensitive to changes in solute concentration of the blood. A group of osmoreceptors occur in the *hypothalamus and monitor changes in the osmotic pressure of the blood.

osmoregulation The homeostatic control (*see* homeostasis) of osmotic potential or water potential, resulting in the maintenance of a constant volume of body fluids.

osmosis The net movement of water (or another solvent) from a high *water potential (or low solute concentration) to a low water potential (or high solute concentration) through a semi-permeable membrane.

osmotic potential *See* solute potential.

osmotic pressure The pressure needed to prevent the osmotic movement of water or another solvent though a semipermeable membrane (*see* osmosis).

os pubis *See* pubis.

ossa coxae *See* coxal bone.

osseous tissue Bone.

osseous Applied to tissue which is bony.

ossicle A small bone, such as the auditory ossicles in the middle ear.

ossification (osteogenesis) The transformation of fibrous tissue or cartilage into bone. In long bones, special cells (osteoblasts) carry out the process in three main stages: first, a framework of collagen fibres is laid down; then a cementing polysaccharide is produced; finally, calcium salts are deposited in the cement. A bone is unable to elongate any further after ossification is completed. Exercise and an adequate diet (especially with respect to calcium and vitamin D) are essential for proper ossification. Weight-bearing exercise can increase the width, density, and strength of bone, but not its final length. *See also* **intramembranous ossification**.

osteitis Inflammation of bone due to disease or injury.

osteitis pubis Inflammation of the cartilaginous disc in the pubic bone (the *symphysis), causing groin pain.

osteoarthritis Degeneration of articular cartilage which may also affect the underlying bone of a joint, causing pain and stiffness. Osteoarthritis may result from trauma, incorrect loading of a joint, ligament injuries, or recurrent dislocations. It is often associated with *obesity, low bone density, repeated mechanical stress, and structural abnormalities of the joint. Although it may affect any joint, it most commonly affects the hips, knees, and thumbs. The relationship between osteoarthritis and exercise is complex: in some cases it may exacerbate the condition, in others it may delay its progress. Athletes with osteoarthritis of the hips or knees are often advised not to participate in activities, such as running, which impose high impact forces on the joints. However, there is no scientific evidence that running causes arthritis in athletes whose joints were normal before they started running. Nonweight bearing activities, especially swimming, are recommended for those with mild forms of arthritis. Although children can have osteoarthrits, it tends to be an age-related disease, but it is not an inevitable consequence of ageing. Once it has started to develop, osteoarthritis can usually be kept under control for many years by using anti-inflammatories and analgesics.

osteoblasts Specialized bone cells that build new bone tissue (*see* **ossification**).

osteochondritis *See* osteochondrosis.

osteochondritis dissecans A disease process by which subchondral bone (bone just below the articular cartilage of a joint) loses its blood supply. The bone and its overlying cartilage become damaged, and a fragment of bone may separate from contiguous bone to form *loose bodies in the joint; the articular cartilage may or may not remain intact. The process occurs particularly in the femoral condyles of the knee, and also in the ankle and hip joints. The condition may be due to inherited anatomical abnormalities, obstruction of the blood supply to subchondral bone, or physical trauma to the joint. In young people, osteochondritis dissecans is most likely to be due to cumulative stresses on the subchondral bone. Treatment varies from observation to surgical intervention, depending on the age of the patient and severity of the condition. Observation and conservative treatments (e.g., physiotherapy, orthotics, and immobilization) are the usual option for younger patients.

osteochondrosis An assorted group of conditions affecting the growing epiphysis. Osteochondroses often occur in young athletes who subject the growth regions of their bones (epiphyses) and their *apophyses to repeated mechanical stress. It is characterized by inflammation of bone and cartilage (osteochondritis) that can cause pain. The conditions, although appearing similar in radiographs, differ in their pathology. They may involve fragmentation, distortion, and collapse of the affected cartilage and bone which, after a time, becomes ossified into an irregular shape. *See also* **Freiberg's disease, Kohler's disease, Osgood–Schlatter disease**; **Perthe's disease**; and **Sever–Haglund disease**.

osteoclast A large multinucleated cell of uncertain origin which destroys bone cells and reabsorbs calcium. Osteoclasts play a key role in bone-remodelling.

osteocyte A spider-shaped, mature bone cell derived from an osteoblast. Osteocytes lie in a small cavities (the lacunae) in bone.

osteogenesis *See* ossification.

osteolysis The breakdown of bone through disease. It is usually associated with a restriction or loss of the blood supply to the bone.

osteomalacia A term applied to a number of conditions in which the bones are inadequately mineralized and are abnormally soft. It may occur as a result of vitamin D deficiency.

osteomyelitis Inflammation of bone resulting from an infection of bone marrow.

osteon The structural and functional unit of compact bone, also called an *Haversian system.

osteopenia A progressive condition characterized by reduced bone mineral density without the presence of a fracture, but which predisposes the individual to *osteoporosis.

osteoperiostitis Inflammation of bone and the periosteum. *See also* **periostitis**.

osteophyte A bony deposit or outgrowth which often develops at the site of cartilage degeneration near a joint.

osteoporosis (brittle bone disease) A group of diseases characterized by decreased bone mineral content that increases bone porosity and causes them to become more brittle and more inclined to fracture. Osteoporosis is an age-related disease which primarily affects postmenopausal women. Physical exercise when young can reduce the risk of developing the disease in later life. Moderate weight-bearing exercise (e.g. dancing, walking, and tennis) stimulates the deposition of calcium, strengthening bones. Women with osteoporosis should avoid contact sports and high-impact exercise which puts undue stress on bones and joints. Sit-ups are also harmful because of the stress they impose on vertebrae. A premenopausal diet rich

in calcium and vitamin D also reduces the risk of osteoporosis.

osteosclerosis An increase in the density of bone.

osteotomy Surgical bisection of bone. The operation may be performed so that the two parts can be realigned to facilitate healing, or to reduce pain and disability of an arthritic joint.

os trigonum A small bone behind the ankle. It is present in only about 7 per cent of the population. The bone develops as an extension of the ankle bone and then becomes detached. It usually causes no problems except during certain activities, such as repeated, energetic bounding movements, commonly performed by gymnasts, basketball players, and jumpers. The bone may become squeezed between the ankle bone and the shin bone, causing pain and damaging surrounding tissue. Surgical removal may then be necessary.

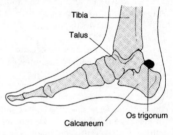

os trigonum

otitis externa (surfer's ear; swimmer's ear) Inflammation of the outer ear characterized by an itchy irritation and watery discharge. It commonly affects swimmers and surfers who neglect to dry the outer ear canal adequately after long periods of immersion. Ear plugs may exacerbate the condition. Water trapped in the ear canal breaks down the lining of the canal, providing an opportunity for infection with bacteria or fungi. Initial treatment includes gentle cleaning of the canal. Ear drops containing acetic acid are often used for mild cases. Overzealous use of ear cotton buds may abrade the canal and perpetuate the problem. For severe cases, solutions containing antibiotics with or without hydrocortisone may be used. Cases which are resistant to simple treatments should be referred to an ear specialist. Otitis externa need not interfere with physical activity except in the acute infective stage, as long as appropriate precautions are taken (e.g., application of alcohol drops to help dry the ear and restore the correct pH).

otitis interna Inflammation of the inner ear (labyrinthitis) causing vomiting, vertigo, and loss of balance.

otitis media Inflammation of the middle ear usually resulting from blockage of the Eustachian tube and subsequent invasion by bacteria. Pus accumulates in the middle ear, creating pressure against the eardrum which leads to pain and impairment of hearing. The pain may be excruciating and the eardrum may perforate. Physical exertion should be avoided during the infective stage. This applies especially to swimmers since water entering the middle ear may seriously damage the auditory ossicles. Treatment is usually with oral (and rarely intravenous) antibiotics; antibiotic eardrops are rarely useful.

otolith 1 A calcareous granule of which there are several in the inner ear. An otolith is attached to sensitive cells which enable body position to be assessed. **2** A bony secretion in the middle ear.

outcome The result or consequence of a performance in terms of success and failure. The outcome may be absolute, as with a team winning by scoring more goals than opponents, or dependent on the perception of particular individuals (*see* **perceived importance**).

outcome goal A *goal which depends on the result or outcome of a competition. Such goals are only partly under the control of any one individual and are partly dependent on others, including team mates, opponents, and officials. *See also* **goal setting**; **performance goal**.

outcome goal orientation (competitive goal orientation) The orientation of an athlete who tends to compare his or her performances with those of other athletes, and whose aim is to be better than them or to defeat them. Outcome goal orientation can have positive psychological effects when the athlete is winning (e.g., increasing perceived competence), but has negative effects when losing (e.g., lowering perceived competence and reducing effort during competitions).

outdoor education Education which takes place in the natural environment. It includes conventional field studies, outdoor pursuits, and any other educational activity which takes place in the open air.

outdoor pursuits Physical activities, such as sailing, canoeing, and rock-climbing, which take place in a natural setting where part of the activity involves the challenge of coping with the natural elements.

outdoor recreation Leisure activities, such as hill-walking, which take place in the open air, usually in the natural environment, and are more obviously recreative than competitive.

outer ear *See* **pinna**.

outer range That third of the range of movement of a joint at which the muscle is at its most elongated and the joint surface is at its greatest angle. *See also* **inner range**; and **midrange**.

output A term used in systems theory and systems models to describe the product of a particular device or physiological process, or the motor response of a person to a particular situation.

outsole Part of a *training shoe which comes into contact with the ground.

overall duration parameter A parameter of a generalized *motor program that helps to specify how a movement is to be expressed. The overall duration parameter defines the overall duration of the movement; it is sometimes called a 'speed' parameter.

overall force parameter A parameter of a generalized *motor program that defines overall force of the combined contractions of the participating muscles in an action.

overcompensation A mental process by which a person tries to overcome a disability by making greater efforts than are necessary. For example, a person may compensate for feelings of emotional insecurity by being over-aggressive or by showing off.

overcorrection An overcompensation of a mechanical fault during the performance of a motor skill. For example a canoeist falling over towards the water on one side may adjust by going over too far on the other side. Overcorrection often occurs during the early stages of skill learning.

overdetermination In psychology, a process in which several factors act simultaneously to produce a single mental phenomenon, such as an image in a dream or a neurotic symptom, but in which any one of the several factors on its own can produce the same phenomenon.

overdistance training Training over a distance greater than the competition distance, but at a slower than race pace. Overdistance training is thought to improve fat metabolism, enabling a competitor to use fat stores more efficiently during competition. This would spare *muscle glycogen and delay the onset of fatigue.

overjustification hypothesis A hypothesis which posits that an individual's intrinsic interest in an activity may be decreased by inducing him or her with *extrinsic rewards to take part in the activity. If the reward is perceived to be too great, the individual infers that the behaviour is motivated by extrinsic rewards rather than intrinsic motivation. Consequently, the individual tends to become less interested in the activity. See also **discounting principle**.

overlearning Repeating a technique or skill after it has been learnt sufficiently well to be performed in training, so that it can be reliably performed during the stress of competition. It is generally assumed that it takes longer to learn a skill for a competition than for a noncompetitive situation.

overload See **principle of progressive overload**.

overload theory The theory that some *stress fractures develop because certain muscle groups contract in such a way as to bend the bones to which they are attached. Repeated bending produces microscopic stress fractures in the bone. Compare **fatigue theory**.

overpractice Practising a skill which has already been learned. See also **overlearning**.

overpronation Movement of a runner whose foot rolls too far inwards and puts a strain on the muscles, tendons, and joints of the lower leg. Overpronation may be due to anatomical abnormalities or it may be caused by shoes which tilt the foot inwards. Overpronation can be diagnosed by looking at the wear-pattern of well-used shoes; it increases the wear along the inside edge of the shoe. In normal runners, wear is greatest on the outer edge of the heel, under the ball of the foot, and at the front of the sole.

overreaching The process of hard training which forms part of an athlete's planned training programme to stimulate physiological adaptation. When combined with adequate rest, overreaching is normal and beneficial. Signs of overreaching include high serum creatine kinase concentration, low serum testosterone to cortisol concentration, a fall in muscle glycogen, and raised heart rate and feelings of fatigue, but these return quickly to normal after rest.

overstrain A form of *rundown which develops in those training beyond the adaptation capacity of the body. Overstrain occurs commonly in those taking part in sports which require excessive energy outputs, such as long-distance running and cross-country skiing. Unlike overtraining, it includes physiological fatigue which causes both nervous and hormonal disturbances. These are indicated by a decrease in activity of the *sympathetic nervous system with a reduction in adrenal function, and greater activity of the parasympathetic nervous system.

oversupination An excessive outward rolling of the foot during running. Oversupination can be diagnosed by looking at the wear-pattern of well-used shoes; it increases the wear along the whole outer edge of the shoe, especially the outer edge of the heel. *Compare* **overpronation**.

overt behaviour Behaviour which can be observed by others.

overtraining Training at a work level beyond physical tolerance limits so that the body is unable to recover completely during rest periods. Overtraining is associated with *rundown and *burnout. It commonly causes physical and mental fatigue resulting in a decrease in the quality of performance. Overtrained athletes typically complain of feeling tired and having difficulty sleeping. *See also* **overtraining syndrome**; **overuse injury**; and **overuse syndrome**.

overtraining syndrome A combination of signs and symptoms resulting from overtraining which typically causes the overtrained athlete to feel mentally fatigued and unable to perform maximally. The symptoms of overtraining are highly individualized but many overtrained athletes have an increased *basal metabolic rate and elevated resting heart rate; they suffer from insomnia, decreased appetite, and nausea; they lose body weight because of a negative *nitrogen balance; and the rate of return of their exercise pulse rate to resting pulse rate is delayed. The presence of any one or more of these symptoms should alert a coach or athlete to the possibility of overtraining. Overtraining syndrome is thought to involve changes in the nervous system and endocrine system, particularly the hypothalamus. Overtraining appears to be associated with depressed immunity, increasing the risk of infection.

overuse injury An injury caused by over-exerting the body with excessive workloads at a normal frequency of movement, with normal workloads at an increased frequency of movement, or with low workloads at an excessively rapid frequency of movement. Overuse injuries often occur at the microscopic level and are caused by repeated microtrauma.

overuse syndrome The pathological signs and symptoms created by repeated use of the body in physically stressful conditions. *See also* **overstrain**; and **overtraining syndrome**.

overweight A body weight that exceeds a normal or standard weight for a person of a particular sex, height, and frame size. Although there is no universally agreed system, a person is generally regarded as overweight if he or she is 15 to 20 per cent heavier than the appropriate weight as determined by standard tables. Although there is no universally agreed set of tables, those prepared by the Metropolitan Life Insurance Company are often used. These are based on population averages. Those who are overweight are assumed to be a greater health risk because excess weight is often in the form of fatty tissue which increases the risk of cardiovascular diseases. Excess weight can also overload the joints. However, the standard tables are based on population averages which do not necessarily apply to athletes. According to the tables, many American Footballers are overweight, yet they are much fitter and leaner than people of a comparable age and body build in the general population. *See also* **obesity**.

oxalic acid Chemical found in vegetables such as spinach and rhubarb that combines with calcium in the body to form insoluble salts which impede the absorption of some nutrients.

Oxendine's taxonomy of sport A classification system, not yet fully tested, which matches sport skills with optimum levels arousal. The system is based on the assumption that gross motor skills (e.g., shot putting) are improved by high levels of *arousal, whereas fine motor skills (e.g., pistol shooting) are improved by low levels.

oxaloacteric acid A four-carbon organic acid involved in the *Krebs cycle in which it combines with acetyl coenzyme A to form citric acid.

oxidase Any enzyme such as cytochrome oxidase, involved in oxidation reactions. These enzymes are also known as oxidoreductases.

oxidation A chemical reaction involving the addition of oxygen, the removal of hydrogen, or the removal of an electron from a substance.

oxidative capacity (QO2) A measure of a muscle's maximal capacity to use oxygen in microlitres of oxygen consumed per gram of muscle per hour. Factors which affect the oxidative capacity of muscles include the activity of oxidative enzymes (e.g. succinic dehydrogenase), fibre-type composition (*see* **muscle fibres**), and availability of oxygen.

oxidative decarboxylation The catabolic process which takes place in the *Krebs cycle in the mitochondria, in which both hydrogen and carbon dioxide are released during the conversion of citric acid to oxaloacetic acid. The hydrogen is passed on to the respiratory chain; the carbon dioxide is eventually exhaled from the lungs.

oxidative phosphorylation The process by which ATP is synthesized during aerobic metabolism in the mitochondria.

oxidative system *See* **aerobic energy system**.

oxidoreductase A member of a group of enzymes involved in redox reactions. Oxidoreductases were formerly known as oxidases or dehyrdogenases.

oxygen An odourless, colourless gas that makes up about one fifth of the atmosphere. It is essential for human survival. Attempts have been made to use oxygen as an ergogenic aid, but there is no evidence that it is beneficial before or after exercise. Oxygen taken *during* exhaustive exercise may boost performance, but it is of little practical use because of the problems of administering the gas to an active athlete.

oxygenation The addition of a molecule of oxygen to another molecule. The term is used in particular to describe the process whereby *haemoglobin becomes loaded with oxygen to become oxyhaemoglobin. Molecules of oxygen are carried by the haem groups, but the iron in haem remains in the ferrous state and does not become oxidized.

oxygen capacity The maximum volume of oxygen which can be carried by *haemoglobin in the blood. It is usually expressed as ml of oxygen per 100 ml of blood. Since each g of haemoglobin can carry 1.3 ml of oxygen, the total oxygen capacity of haemoglobin equals the haemoglobin concentration (in g of haemoglobin per 100 ml of blood) multiplied by 1.3.

oxygen cost (oxygen requirement) The volume of oxygen used by body tissues during an activity. It is directly related to the energy demands of the activity, but it is also affected by the nature of the substrate respired.

oxygen debt *See* **excess post-exercise oxygen consumption**.

oxygen deficit The difference between the oxygen required for a given rate of work and the oxygen actually consumed. During intensive exercise, muscles expend more energy than can be supplied by the aerobic system, consequently the muscles have to respire anaerobically to satisfy their energy needs.

oxygen diffusion capacity The rate at which oxygen diffuses from one place to another. In the lungs, oxygen diffusion capacity increases from rest to exercise and tends to be higher in trained endurance athletes.

oxygen–haemoglobin dissociation curve (oxyhaemoglobin dissociation curve) A graph of the relationship between the percentage oxygen saturation of blood and the partial pressure (or tension) of oxygen. The curve is S-shaped and indicates that haemoglobin has a high affinity for oxygen. The blood becomes highly saturated at relatively low oxygen partial pressures but, within respiring tissues, a small drop in oxygen partial pressure results in a big

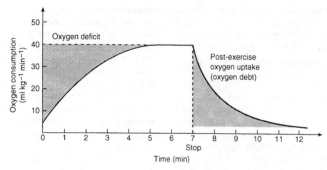

oxygen debt

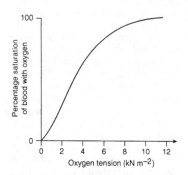

oxygen–haemoglobin dissociation curve

fall in oxygen saturation of the blood. During exercise, increased temperature and hydrogen ion concentration affect the oxygen–haemoglobin dissociation curve in such a way that more oxygen can be unloaded to supply the active muscles (*see* **Bohr shift**).

oxygen-independent glycolysis *See* **anaerobic glycolysis**.

oxygen plateau A condition reached by an athlete exercising at increasing workloads whose oxygen consumption no longer increases with further increments of workload. The oxygen plateau is most easily studied under controlled conditions using a treadmill, bicycle ergometer, etc. Results vary according to the type of exercise equipment and type of workload increment (for example, increases in speed or gradient). The plateau does not occur in all

subjects; the oxygen consumption of some subjects increases steadily with increasing workloads until exhaustion.

oxygen poisoning Condition caused by breathing pure oxygen under high atmospheric pressure. Symptoms include tingling of the fingers and toes, visual and auditory hallucinations, mental confusion, muscle-twitching, vertigo, and convulsions.

oxygen pulse The oxygen uptake per heartbeat. The oxygen pulse can be used as an indirect measure of stroke volume, and is closely related to body-weight.

oxygen pump theory The theory that regular exercise increases the ability of heart muscle to pump blood and thereby improve oxygen transport.

oxygen requirement *See* **oxygen cost**.

oxygen supplementation The administration of oxygen as an ergogenic aid. Extra oxygen enhances performance only slightly if taken immediately (i.e. a few seconds) before a short-duration activity, but it can improve endurance significantly if taken during an activity. However, this is of little practical use because administration of the gas is too cumbersome. Despite its almost routine use after a burst of activity in some sports, oxygen supplementation does not seem to accelerate the recovery process.

oxygen system *See* **aerobic energy system**.

oxygen transport Transport of oxygen in the blood. More than 98 per cent is transported as oxyhaemoglobin, with the rest carried in solution in the plasma.

oxygen transport system The body system which transports oxygen from the lungs to respiring tissue. It depends on the ability of the heart to pump blood around the body and the ability of tissues to extract oxygen from the blood. Thus the functioning of the oxygen transport system is determined by the stroke volume, heart rate, and the arterial–venous oxygen difference. The product of these values equals the rate at which oxygen is being consumed by the body tissues. Endurance training enables the oxygen transport system to function more effectively.

oxygen uptake The volume of oxygen extracted from inspired air at STPD in a given time. If the oxygen content of the body remains constant, the oxygen uptake equals the volume of oxygen utilized in the metabolic oxidation of foodstuffs, with one litre of oxygen corresponding to 19.7 to 21.2 kJ (4.7–5.9 kcal). The oxygen uptake reflects the ability of the heart to pump oxygenated blood to the tissues, and the ability of the tissues to extract oxygen from the blood. Therefore, oxygen uptake of a particular tissue is a product of cardiac output and arterial–venous oxygen difference. The oxygen uptake of the whole body is a product of cardiac output and the arterial mixed-venous oxygen difference.

oxyhaemoglobin Haemoglobin which has combined reversibly with oxygen, Oxyhaemoglobin is a relatively unstable, bright red substance and is the means by which most of the oxygen is transported in the bloodstream from the lungs to the tissues. Each molecule of haemoglobin can carry four molecules of oxygen.

oxyhaemoglobin dissociation curve *See* oxygen–haemoglobin dissociation curve.

oxymyoglobin A combination of oxygen and myoglobin. Each molecule of myoglobin can carry one molecule of oxygen. Oxymyoglobin acts as a store of oxygen in muscles (with an average of 11.2 ml of oxygen per kg of muscle mass), and is important during intermittent exercise. Oxygen is released during the work intervals and oxymyoglobin restored during the recovery periods. It is also thought to be functionally important in transporting oxygen from the blood to muscle mitochondria.

ozone A gas containing three atoms of oxygen per molecule. Ozone occurs naturally at about 0.01 parts per million (ppm). When it reaches concentrations above 0.1 ppm, it is regarded as toxic and can be a potent eye and airway irritant causing chest tightness, breathlessness, and coughing. Exposures to concentrations above 0.775 ppm for longer than 2 hours, significantly reduce oxygen uptake. High ozone levels in cities hosting marathon races have been the cause of respiratory distress in some athletes.

P

Pa to **Pythagorean theorem**

Pa *See* Pascal.

PABA (para-aminobutyric acid) A member of the vitamin B group of chemicals, PABA is one of the most common ingredients of lotions and creams used to prevent sunburns. The derivatives made from it effectively screen out the ultraviolet rays responsible for sunburn, but do not offer protection against the full spectrum of ultraviolet rays, including those linked with skin cancer.

pace The rate of movement, especially of walking, running, and swimming.

pace clock Clock used in swimming pool training so that swimmers can learn pace judgement by self-timing. The clock is positioned at the side of the pool where the swimmer can observe it easily at the end of a length; ideally, two clocks are used, one at each end of the pool.

pace judgement An inherent awareness of rate of movement without the use of external timing devices. Pace judgement is an important ability for racing and can be learned.

pacemaker 1 A small region of cardiac tissue in the right atrium of the heart (*see* **sinoatrial node**) which controls the rate of contraction of the heart as a whole. **2** A device which controls the heart rate of a patient who has heart block.

pacing continuum A continuum, extending from *self-paced tasks to externally paced tasks, concerned with the extent to which the performer has control over his or her actions.

Pacinian corpuscle A specialized sense receptor in the skin which responds to firm pressure; named after F. Pacini (1812– 1883), an Italian anatomist.

pack A pad of folded material moistened, or containing hot or cold material, which can be applied to the surface of the body. *See also* **ice treatment**.

paddler's wrist *See* **de Quervain's disease**.

paediatrics Branch of medicine dealing with the treatment of children.

PAI *See* **Physical Activity Index**.

pain A feeling of distress, suffering, or agony usually caused by the stimulation of specialized nerve endings. Pain has a protective function, acting as a warning sign and preventing further injury. However, even mild pain can have a detrimental effect on performance, and severe pain will limit movement. Pain can be classified functionally into five levels: at level 1, pain occurs only after a specific activity; at level 2, pain occurs during and after specific activities, but it does not affect performance; at level 3, pain occurs during and after specific activity, and affects the performance of the activity; at level 4, pain occurs with activities of daily living; at level 5, pain occurs at rest. This classification enables an athlete to describe their pain to a physician. Also, during rehabilitation from a sports injury, the functional level of pain can be used as a guide to how recovery is progressing. Pain can be relieved by *acupuncture, *ice treatment, *heat treatment, *anaesthetics, *anti-inflammatory medicines, *analgesics, *NSAIDs, *opiates, and *transcutaneous nerve stimulation therapy. Substances which increase sensitivity to pain include bradykinins, free radicals, histamine, potassium, and serotonin. Some of these substances evoke pain by affecting nerves directly, others cause an inflammatory reaction.

pain cycle A vicious cycle resulting from training when in pain. Initially, pain may occur only after intensive activity. Instead of taking this as a warning sign, an athlete may attempt to train through it. The pain may disappear during warm-ups, allowing the athlete to continue training which may aggravate the injury, worsening the pain. The pain cycle continues until the

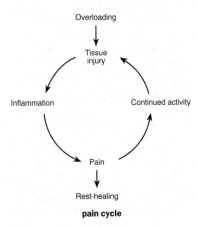

pain cycle

athlete suffers a chronic injury which prevents training, or until the cycle is broken by rest and treatment of the injury. Generally, the earlier the escape from the pain cycle, the less rest is required, and the easier the treatment.

pain-killer *See* analgesic.

pain receptor *See* nociceptor.

pain threshold The lowest stimulus intensity which results in the perception of pain. Pain threshold may be influenced by genetic factors beyond an individual's control. *Compare* **pain tolerance**.

pain tolerance An individual's reaction to pain. The ability to continue an activity despite the perception of pain indicates a high pain tolerance. Pain tolerance varies widely and is strongly affected by genetic, psychological, and cultural influences. Training which is painful, but not damaging, may improve the ability of some athletes to tolerate pain.

PAL *See* Physical Activity Level.

palliative A medicine which provides temporary relief, alleviating symptoms, but which does not provide a cure for a disease.

palmar Pertaining to the palm of the hand.

palmar interossei Three muscles with origins on the second, fourth, and fifth intercarpals, and insertions on the base of the proximal phalanx of digits 2, 4, and 5. The primary action of the palmar interossei are abduction and flexion of the metacarpophalangeal joints of digits 2, 4, and 5.

palpation Examination of an area of the body by the sense of touch. Palpation is often used by physiotherapists to examine the condition of superficial muscles, tendons, and ligaments.

palpitation Condition in which the heart beats forcibly or irregularly, and an individual becomes conscious of its action. Palpitations may be precipitated by a number of factors including undue excitement, dyspepsia, drinking alcohol, frequent coffee- or tea-drinking, or smoking. Although unpleasant and worrying, palpitations are not usually caused by heart disease. Moderate exercise is often useful in alleviating palpitations not associated with disease.

pancreas A mixed gland located behind and slightly below the stomach. It produces hormones (*insulin and *glucagon) from the Islets of Langerhans, and digestive juices from small sacs known as acini. The digestive juices (also known as pancreatic juices) are released the into duodenum. They contain amylase, lipase, nucleases, peptidases, and other proteases (e.g. trypsin). Production of pancreatic juices are stimulated by hormones secreted by the duodenum (e.g. secretin).

pancreatic juices *See* pancreas.

panel study A form of longitudinal study used in sociology which involves the questioning of the same sample at regular intervals to observe trends of opinion. It is usually of shorter duration and more focused than other forms of longitudinal studies.

pangamic acid (vitamin B15) A member of the B-complex. Although it is not a true vitamin, it is marketed in the form of sodium or calcium pangamate as one of the 'super-vitamins' which improves physical performance. There is little scientific evidence to support this claim.

panic A sudden unreasoning and overwhelming fear or terror, often affecting a group. It may occur in a state of high anxiety.

Panner's disease An overuse injury of the *capitellum in the elbow. It tends to occur in young athletes as a result of lateral compression forces in throwing activities. It involves the ossification centre of the capitellum but, unlike osteochondritis dissecans, it is associated with no loose bodies and recovery is usually complete, albeit slow.

pannus 1 The growth of vascular tissue in the cornea of the eye which may occur after inflammation of the cornea; it impairs vision. **2** Extension of thickened synovial membrane onto the cartilage of a joint surface.

panting Breathing with noisy, deep gasps, as occurs during or after strenuous exercise. The uncontrollable desire to pant indicates lack of oxygen supply to tissues. *See also* **hyperventilation**.

pantothenic acid (vitamin B₅) A water-soluble vitamin that plays a part in carbohydrate and fat metabolism. It is a constituent of coenzyme A. Deficiency causes neuromuscular dysfunction and fatigue. Pantothenic acid is found in liver, yeast, peas, and other legumes. No Reference Nutrient Intake is set in the UK because of insufficient information. In the USA, the Recommended Dietary Allowance is 4–7 mg.

papillary muscles Nipple-shaped projections of ventricular muscle to which the tendinous cords (*see* **chordae tendinae**) of the atrioventricular valves are attached. Contractions of the papillary muscles assist the tendinous cords in preventing the valves from being thrust out into the atrial cavity during ventricular systole.

papular Applied to a rash which appears as small raised spots on the skin.

para-aminobutyric acid *See* **PABA**.

parabola A curve traced out by a point moving so that its distance from a fixed point (its focus) is equal to its distance from a fixed straight line, the directrix. In the absence of air resistance the flight path of a projectile, such as a long-jumper's body, is parabolic.

paracetamol (actaminophen) An *analgesic which has very little anti-inflammatory effects and, unlike acetylsalicylic acid (aspirin), it does not increase the tendency to bleed. The use of paracetamol in sport is permitted by the IOC.

paracrine Applied to cellular secretions that act on cells a short-distance from their site of secretion. For example, *insulin-like growth factors secreted by a muscle cell may promote the growth of neighbouring muscle cells and connective tissues.

paradigm Any generalized example or representative instance of a concept or a theoretical approach which provides a means by which the real world can be studied.

paradox A person or thing exhibiting apparently contradictory features, as in *Lombard's paradox; or a phenomenon, such as a medical symptom, in conflict with what is expected.

paraesthesia An abnormal tingling sensation, often described as 'pins and needles'. It is a symptom of partial damage of a peripheral nerve (e.g. from a head or spinal injury) or lack of blood supply to a nerve. It can be caused by an external pressure of a bone on a nerve, for example as a result of a dislocation.

paraffin bath A form of *heat treatment for joint injuries, particularly those of the hand and foot. The limb is dipped into warm paraffin (52–58 °C) or the warm

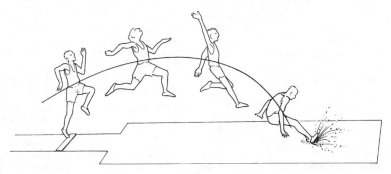

parabola

paraffin is applied with a paintbrush to the injured part.

paralanguage Communication conveyed by the intonation of the voice and other vocal components of speech which do not depend on the actual words spoken. Paralanguage refers not to what people say, but to how they say it. Many sportspeople are unaware of the powerful effects, beneficial or detrimental, of paralanguage on the behaviour of their team mates and officials.

parallax An optical effect which contributes to the perception of relative distances. Parallax occurs when movement at right angles to the line of vision alters the relative position of two unequally distant objects. The same effect is achieved by the difference in view point of the two eyes when the distance between the eyes relative to the distance of the objects is significant.

parallel axes theorem A theorem relating the *moment of inertia about an axis through a body segment's centre of gravity to the body's movement about any other parallel axis. The theorem is stated in algebraic form in the following equation: $I_a = I_{cg} + md^2$, where I_a = the moment of the body about an axis through the point a, I_{cg} = the moment of inertia of the body about a parallel axis through its centre of gravity, m = the mass of the body, and d = the distance between the parallel axis.

parallel competition A competition in which contestants compete with each other indirectly by taking turns contesting in separate areas. *See also* **indirect competition**.

parallel elastic component The component of a muscle that provides resistive tension when a muscle is passively stretched. The parallel elastic component is noncontractile and consists of the muscle membranes which lie parallel to the muscle fibres. Along with the *series elastic component, this component enables muscle to stretch and recoil in a time-dependent fashion.

parallel fibre arrangement Pattern of fibres within a muscle in which the fibres are roughly parallel to the longitudinal axis of the muscle. Muscles, such as the *biceps brachii, with a parallel fibre arrangement are able to shorten greatly, moving body segments through large ranges of motion, but they are not as powerful as muscles with a pennate fibre arrangement (*see* **pennate muscle**). *See also* **fusiform muscle**.

parallelogram A plane four-sided rectilinear figure with opposite sides parallel. The opposite sides and angles of a parallelogram are equal; the diagonals bisect each other and the parallelogram itself.

parallelogram of forces A method of calculating the resultant of two forces acting on a body. The two forces are represented in direction and magnitude by the two sides of a parallelogram drawn from a common point, and the resultant of the two forces is represented by the diagonal of the parallelogram drawn from that point.

parallelogram of vectors A method of obtaining a resultant vector from two or more component vectors. The two component vectors form the adjacent sides of a parallelogram drawn to scale. The resultant vector is given by the direction and length of the diagonal of the parallelogram. If necessary, the resultant vector can be used as a component vector in another parallelogram. The process is then repeated until one resultant vector remains.

parallelogram of velocities A method of calculating the resultant of two velocities acting on a body. The two component velocities are represented in magnitude and direction by two adjacent sides of a parallelogram drawn from a common point, and the resultant velocity of the body is represented by the diagonal of the parallelogram drawn from that point.

parallel processing A type of information processing in which at least two processes can occur simultaneously. In the human body, parallel processing is a form of neural integration which underlies complex mental processes. Nerve impulses are conveyed simultaneously along several

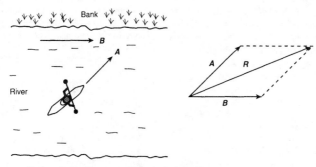

A is the velocity of the canoe with respect to the water;
B is the velocity of the water with respect to the bank;
R is the resultant velocity of the canoe with respect to the bank.

parallelogram of vectors

pathways to different centres of integration. *Compare* serial processing.

paralysis A loss or impairment of motor function due to a disorder in some part of the neuromuscular system. The extent of the paralysis will vary according to the location and extent of the disorder. The term is also applied to concomitant loss of sensory function. Paralysis is a symptom rather than a disease.

paralysis by analysis The idea that, once a skill has become automated, thinking too much about its execution can disrupt performance. For example, if an experienced golfer at the tee thinks too much about the position of his or her hands, feet etc., he or she is likely to become tense and miss hit the drive.

paramedical 1 Pertaining to a person, such as a physiotherapist, associated with the medical profession in providing health care. **2** Refers to a person known as a paramedic, usually an ambulance crew member, who has advanced training in resuscitation.

parameter 1 An arbitrary constant or variable in a mathematical expression which gives rise to various cases of a particular phenomenon. **2** A quantity which is constant under a particular set of conditions but which differs with changing conditions.

parametric statistic Statistic which assumes that the sample has been drawn from a population which has a particular distribution (for example, a normal distribution) and shares certain parameters (for example, equal variance).

paranoia A mental disorder characterized by persistent delusions. The sufferer may show no symptoms of mental illness and apparently has an intact *personality. The term is commonly applied more loosely to a person who feels unduly persecuted.

parasympathetic nervous system Part of the autonomic nervous system which has cholinergic nerve-endings (i.e., it uses *acetylcholine as a neurotransmitter). The parasympathetic nervous system typically affects the body in an opposite way to the *sympathetic nervous system. Whereas the parasympathetic nervous system helps to create the internal body conditions found during rest, sleep, and digestion, the sympathetic nervous system prepares the body for physical activity. The parasympathetic nervous system causes constriction of the bronchioles, decreased heart rate, and constriction of coronary blood vessels.

paratelic Applied to the mental orientation of a person who has a fun loving attitude to a situation and seeks excitement. A paratelic state of mind is activity oriented and pleasure seeking. *Compare* **telic**.

paratenon Tissue between a tendon sheath and its tendon. The paratenon surrounds and nourishes the tendon.

parathormone *See* **parathyroid gland**.

parathyroid gland One of four small endocrine glands on the back of the thyroid gland. It secretes parathormone (PTH or parathyroid hormone) which affects calcium and phosphate levels in extracellular fluid. High levels of PTH cause calcium to be transferred from bones to blood; abnormally low levels result in a lowering of blood calcium levels which can lead to *tetany. An overproduction of PTH has been linked to the development of fragile bones in a group of female long-distance runners.

parathyroid hormone *See* **parathyroid gland**.

parenteral administration The application of a medicine or other substance by routes other than the rectum or mouth. The medicine is usually injected directly into a blood vessel.

parietal Pertaining to the walls of a cavity.

parietal pleura Thin membrane lining the inner surface of the thoracic wall. It secretes serous fluid. *See also* **pleura**.

parking thoughts A technique for coping with intrusive thoughts during an athletic performance, by putting the thoughts aside to be dealt with later. Typically, the athlete imagines recording the intrusive thought on a piece of paper and putting it in some other place until after the performance.

PARQ *See* **Physical Activity Readiness Questionnaire**.

pars A specific part of an organ or structure.

pars interarticularis The weakest portion of the neural arch of a vertebra, between the superior and inferior articular facets. A fracture of the pars interarticularis is called a *spondylolysis.

part-method of learning A method of learning a skill which can be subdivided into parts forming a natural and meaningful sequence. Each part is learned separately to a criterion and then an attempt made to join the parts together sequentially until

they are combined to form the whole skill. The order in which they are learned and combined together usually follows the natural order in which they occur in the skill. *Compare* **part-whole method of learning**.

part-whole method of learning *Learning technique in which the task to be learned is broken down into its parts for separate practices. The part-whole method is commonly used when parts do not form a natural and meaningful sequence of actions and do not need to be practised together. They can be learned in any order, practised separately, and, once mastered, can be incorporated together in, for example, a game. *Compare* **part-method learning**.

partial dislocation *See* **subluxation**.

partial muscle tear *See* **muscle strain**.

partial pressure The pressure exerted by a single gas in a mixture of gases. It can be calculated by multiplying the total pressure of the mixture of gases within which the particular gas occurs, by the total volume the gas occupies. Thus, if the normal pressure of atmospheric gases is 760 mmHg and there is 21 per cent oxygen, the partial pressure of oxygen is $760 \times 0.21 = 160$ mmHg.

participant observation A method of research in which the researcher becomes a participant in the activity being investigated.

participatory modelling A coaching technique in which a *model helps an athlete to perform a skill successfully. The athlete first observes the model perform the task. Then the model assists the athlete to perform the task successfully, not allowing the athlete to fail. Participatory modelling is used to promote strong feelings of *self-efficacy.

Pascal (Pa) The SI unit of pressure which is equivalent to 1 Nm^{-2}.

passive immunity Short-lived immunity resulting from the introduction of *antibodies obtained from an animal or human donor.

Physical Activity Readiness Questionnaire (PAR-Q)*

NAME OF PARTICIPANT ______________________

DATE ______________________

PAR Q & YOU

PAR-Q is designed to help you help yourself. Many health benefits are associated with regular exercise, and completion of PAR-Q is a sensible first step to take if you are planning to increase the amount of physical activity in your life.

For most people, physical activity should not pose any problem or hazard. PAR-Q has been designed to identify the small number of adults for whom physical activity might be inappropriate or those who should have medical advice concerning the type of activity most suitable for them.

Common sense is your best guide in answering these few questions. Please read them carefully and check (✓) the ☐ YES or ☐ NO opposite the question if it applies to you.

YES	NO	
☐	☐	1 Has your doctor ever said you have heart trouble?
☐	☐	2 Do you frequently have pains in your heart and chest?
☐	☐	3 Do you often feel faint or have spells of severe dizziness?
☐	☐	4 Has a doctor ever said your blood pressure was too high?
☐	☐	5 Has your doctor ever told you that you have a bone or joint problem such as arthritis that has been aggravated by exercise, or might be made worse with exercise?
☐	☐	6 Is there a good physical reason not mentioned here why you should not follow an activity program even if you wanted to?
☐	☐	7 Are you over the age of 65 and not accustomed to vigorous exercise?

If You Answered

YES to one or more questions

If you have not recently done so, consult with your personal physician by telephone or in person BEFORE increasing your physical activity and/or taking a fitness appraisal. Tell your physician what questions you answered YES to on PAR-Q or present your PAR-Q copy.

programs

After medical evaluation, seek advice from your physician as to your suitability for:

- unrestricted physical activity starting off easily and progressing gradually.
- restricted or supervised activity to meet your specific needs, at least on an initial basis. Check in your community for special programs or services.

NO to all questions

If you answered PAR-Q accurately, you have reasonable assurance of your present suitability for:

- A GRADUATED EXERCISE PROGRAM – a gradual increase in proper exercise promotes good fitness development while minimizing or eliminating discomfort.
- A FITNESS APPRAISAL – the Canadian Standardized Test of Fitness (CSTF)

postpone

If you have a temporary minor illness, such as a common cold.

• Developed by the British Columbia Ministry of Health. Conceptualized and critiqued by the Multidisciplinary Advisory Board on Exercise (MABE).

Reference PAR-Q Validation Report, British Columbia Ministry of Health, May, 1978.

• Produced by the British Columbia Ministry of Health and the Department of National Health & Welfare.

par Q & you

passive insufficiency The inability of a muscle that spans two or more joints to be stretched sufficiently to produce a full range of motion in all the joints simultaneously.

passive learning *See* incidental learning.

passive mobility exercise An exercise performed on a subject by a partner who exerts an external force not only to produce a passive movement, but also to increase the range of movement of a joint. The partner presses the joint into its end-position (i.e. end of range) while the subject's muscles which normally carry out the movements are completely relaxed. There is a danger of over-extension beyond the range of movement and damage to the joint if the exercise is not carried out carefully.

passive movement Any movement produced by a force which is external to the muscle or muscle group normally responsible for the movement. Passive movements are used in the diagnosis of some sports injuries to distinguish between injuries of the muscle and the ligaments of a joint.

passive stability Joint stability provided by passive forces, mainly from the ligaments. *Compare* active stability.

passive stretching Stretching of muscles, tendons, and ligaments produced by a stretching force other than that of the subject's own muscle actions (e.g., gravity or a force applied by a partner). Passive stretching can carry a movement beyond the normal active range, but there is an increased risk of tissue injury. *Compare* active stretching.

patella A small lens-shaped sesamoid bone encased in the patellar tendon at the front of the knee. The patella protects the knee-joint anteriorly and improves the leverage of the knee extensor muscles by as much as 50 per cent. It also increases the area of contact between the patellar tendon and the femur decreasing mechanical stress on the patellofemoral joint. The patella is poorly nourished and poorly protected, consequently it is susceptible to injury.

patella alta High-riding kneecaps. Patella alta is a structural abnormality occurring especially in tall, thin, people, predisposing them to anterior knee pain caused, for example, by quadriceps tendinitis and *patellofemoral pain syndrome.

patellar Pertaining to the front of the knee. *Compare* popliteal.

patellar ligament A strong flat band which connects the apex of the patella to the tibia. Its central, superficial fibres are continuous with the *quadriceps tendon.

patellar tendinitis *See* jumper's knee.

patellar tendon That part of the *quadriceps tendon which attaches onto the patella. Its superficial fibres are continuous with the fibres of the patellar ligament which attach onto the tibia.

patellectomy Surgical removal of the patella, for example, to treat recalcitrant cases of *chondromalacia patella. The patellectomy often alleviates symptoms, but increases knee instability due to a reduction in leverage of the extensor muscles.

patellitis Inflammation of the patella commonly caused by a strain on its inferior border causing tenderness and swelling. *See also* chondromalacia patellae; and jumper's knee.

patellofemoral Pertaining to the area of the femur adjacent to the patella.

patellofemoral joint The joint in the knee between the patella and femur.

patellofemoral pain syndrome An overuse injury characterized by a dull pain felt at the kneecap. Patellofemoral pain syndrome is most common among runners who overtrain, and who continue to train through injuries (*see also* pain cycle). The pain tends to worsen when ascending or descending stairs, and when running downhill. Typically, the knee stiffens when trying to straighten it after sitting for prolonged periods (the so-called theatre sign). The pain is thought to arise from nerve fibres in the subchondral bone of the patella or from inflammation of the synovial membrane. Patellofemoral pain syndrome is often confused with chondromalacia patella, but in the syndrome there is no softening of the articular cartilage. Flat feet, hyperpronation, femoral anteversion, high Q-angle, and weakness and tightness in the *quadriceps, *hamstrings, and calves are often associated with the syndrome. Treatment of patellofemoral pain syndrome varies. It includes rest from running, ice-treatment, anti-inflammatories, correction of anatomical defects, exercises which strengthen the muscles around the knee, and stabilization of the kneecap with a knee brace. Sometimes knee surgery is required to relieve the pain. A key feature of rehabilitation is strengthening the vastus medialis (obliquus) muscle by suitable static muscle actions (isometric contractions).

paternalism A system by which an organization deals with its members in a manner similar to that of a benevolent father dealing with a child. Paternalism is used widely in personal relationships such as those between a coach and athletes.

path analysis A method of quantifying the relationship between *variables. A diagram, called a path diagram, is constructed using regression to show how the variables are assumed to affect each other. The assumptions can be tested by seeing if the relationships depicted in the diagram are compatible with observed data.

path–goal theory of leadership A theory of *leadership which can be applied to a coach–athlete relationship. The basic proposition of the path–goal theory is that the function of the coach is to assist athletes to achieve their own goals. It hypothesizes an interaction between the coach and any situation (including the *personality of the athlete and the environmental demands of the task), in which the emphasis is on the needs and goals of the athlete. The coach is viewed as a facilitator helping an athlete to select worthwhile goals, and by pointing out the 'path' to follow in order to reach the goals successfully. To be successful, the coach's behaviour needs to vary according to the situation.

pathogenic Applied to microorganisms which are capable of producing illness.

pathognomic Applied to a symptom or sign which is characteristic of a specific disease.

pathological condition A condition associated with disease.

pathology A study of the nature of diseases, especially how they affect the human body and what causes them.

pattern generator See **central pattern generator**.

Pavlovian conditioning See **classical conditioning**.

PCr See **phosphocreatine**.

PCR See **polymerase chain reaction**.

PCSA See **physiological cross-sectional area**.

peak aerobic power See **maximal oxygen uptake**.

peak experience Rare moments of extreme happiness and fulfilment which are accompanied by loss of fears, inhibitions, and insecurities. Peak experiences occur during optimal performances and are marked by a heightened sense of awareness. Athletes generally report the experience as temporary, unique, and beyond their own control, but when it does happen it stands apart from normal happenings and experiences. The physiological basis of the experience has not been fully analysed although it may be associated with increased levels of *endorphins in the brain. See also **flow**; **runner's high**.

peak force (peak torque) The maximum force (in newtons) of *torque (newton metres) developed during a muscle action.

peak heart rate The highest heart rate during a specific activity.

peaking The process of achieving an optimal performance on a specific occasion. Ideally, peaking will occur on the very day, even the very minute, of an important competition. Peaking requires a thorough knowledge of training and its effects on an individual athlete so that the training programme will produce the required response.

peak performance *See* **ideal performance**.

peak torque *See* **peak force**.

Pearson product moment correlation coefficient A correlation coefficient (r) for use with continuous variables with a *normal distribution.

pecs *See* **pectoralis muscles**.

pectineus A short flat muscle in the medial compartment of the thigh. It has its origin on the pubic bone and insertion on the proximal medial surface of the femur. It is one of the *adductor muscles, causing adduction, flexion, and lateral rotation of the femur.

pectoral Pertaining to the chest.

pectoral girdle (shoulder girdle) Bony structure which attaches the arms to the axial skeleton. The pectoral girdle consists of the right and left shoulder blades (*see* **scapula**) and collar bones.

pectoralis major Large, fan-shaped muscle covering the upper part of the chest and forming the anterior axillary fold (front part of the armpit). The pectoralis has two origins: the clavicular pectoralis major originates from the median half of the clavicle; and the sternal pectoralis major originates from the anterior sternum and the cartilage of the first six ribs. The fibres of the muscle converge to insert onto the lateral aspect of the humerus, just below its head. The primary actions of the clavicular pectoralis major are flexion and horizontal adduction about the shoulder; those of the sternal pectoralis major are extension, adduction, and horizontal adduction. The pectoralis major plays an important role in climbing and throwing. When the scapula and arm are fixed, the pectoralis major pulls the ribcage upwards, contributing to inspiratory movements.

pectoralis minor A flat, thin chest muscle which has its origin on the anterior surface of ribs 3–5, and its insertion on the *coracoid process of the scapula. When

the ribs are fixed the pectoralis minor draws the scapula forward and downward; when the scapula is fixed, it draws the ribcage superiorly.

pectoral muscles (pecs) Two pairs of chest muscles which contribute to movements of the upper arm and shoulder (*see* **pectoralis major** and **pectoralis minor**).

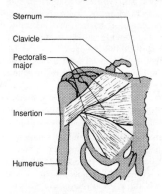

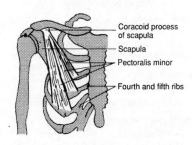

pectorals

peer group A group of individuals sharing the same *status.

peer group interaction The social exchanges which occur between individuals with the same *status. Peer group interaction usually refers to the interactions of children and adolescents within groups of their own age.

pellagra A disease due to a deficiency of *niacin. Early signs of the disease include listlessness, headache, and weight loss, which progresses to tongue soreness, nausea, vomiting, and photosensitive dermatitis. The symptoms of pellagra are sometimes referred to as the 'four Ds': dermatitis, dementia, diarrhoea, and death.

pelvic girdle The paired coxal (hip) bones plus the sacrum that attach the lower limbs to the axial skeleton. The pelvic girdle can move in all three planes to optimize the positioning of the hip joint. Movements of the girdle also coordinate with certain movements of the spine.

pelvis A deep basin-like bony structure formed by the two coxal bones, the sacrum, and coccyx. The pelvis forms the lower portion of the trunk.

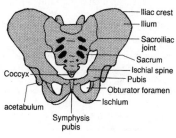

- Iliac crest
- Ilium
- Sacroiliac joint
- Sacrum
- Ischial spine
- Pubis
- Obturator foramen
- Ischium

Coccyx

acetabulum

Symphysis pubis

pelvis

pendular model A model of *group cohesion which suggests that the amount of cohesion oscillates in a pendular fashion throughout a group's existence. For example, an American football team may have high cohesion when it first meets; the cohesion is reduced due to competition among players for selection to the final cut; and then cohesion rises again after the selection has been made prior to the first match.

pendular motion The regular swinging or oscillating movements of a body suspended from a fixed point. A form of pendular motion is exhibited in running. It is very complex, not only because it consists of three links in simultaneous rotation and translation, but also because it depends on the speed of other links in the kinetic chain, and on external forces and their torques.

pendular period (period) The time taken for one complete to and fro movement of a vibration or oscillation.

pendulous abdomen The hanging downwards of the abdomen over the pelvis, usually due to weakness and lack of firmness of the abdominal muscles.

pendulum A body suspended from a fixed point so that it is free to swing or oscillate with a known pendular period. *See also* **double pendulum**.

pennate muscle (penniform muscle) Flat muscle with fibres arranged around one or more central tendons like the barbs of a feather. Pennate muscles shorten only to a limited extent, but they can produce very powerful actions. Pennate muscle may be unipennate, when the fibres insert onto only one side of a tendon (e.g. extensor digitorum longus); bipennate, when fibres insert onto opposite sides of a tendon so that the muscle resembles a feather (e.g. rectus femoris); or multipennate, when fibres converge onto several tendons, giving a herringbone appearance (e.g. deltoid muscle). *Compare* **fusiform muscle**.

penicillin Antibiotic used to treat a wide range of bacterial infections. Some people are allergic to penicillin and may develop painful rashes, swelling of the throat, and fever.

penniform muscle *See* **pennate muscle**.

pentose-phosphate cycle *See* **hexose monophosphate shunt**.

pep pills Artificial stimulants taken orally to improve physical and mental performance. Drugs used as pep pills include *amphetamines, *caffeine, and *epinephrine.

pep talk A motivational strategy aimed at heightening *arousal. Pep talks are usually given prior to competition or during an interval in play. They are a characteristic feature of managerial talks to football teams before a game and at half-time. Exhortations to try harder may help some athletes to reach an optimal level of arousal, but may cause others to become overaroused.

peptide hormones and analogues A pharmacological class of agents banned by the IOC (*see* **doping class**). The class includes *human chorionic gonadotrophin, *adrenocorticotrophic hormone (ACTH), *erythropoietin, and *human growth hormone (hGH). All the respective releasing factors which stimulate the secretion of these hormones are also banned. Most peptide hormones are produced endogenously, and several are now produced synthetically by recombinant DNA technology. The synthetic forms are identical to the endogenous forms, making drug detection difficult.

perceived ability An individual's assessment of his or her own ability. In sport, it is regarded as a major construct of achievement behaviour and an important determinant of *motivation. Individuals who perceive themselves as having high ability, tend to be more motivated than those who perceive themselves as having low ability.

perceived competence scale for children (PCSC) A scale which assesses a child's competence in three domains: cognitive (school competence), social (peer-related competence), and physical (skill at sport). Results from several sport-related studies using the scale have provided support for *Harter's competence motivation theory.

perceived contingency Situation in which a person feels that success at a future activity depends on success at a present activity: i.e. present performance affects future opportunities.

perceived exertion *See* **Ratings of Perceived Exertion**.

perceived fatigue *See* **subjective fatigue**.

perceived importance The importance an athlete assigns to the outcome of a performance. It is strongly affected by the presence of significant others and their perception of the importance of the event. Perceived importance has an important affect on *anxiety levels. Several stress management techniques are aimed at reducing the perceived importance of an event.

perceived success A performer's own assessment of whether he or she has achieved goals. *See also* **perceived ability**.

percentage change in maximal aerobic power A measure of the effect of ageing on aerobic fitness. The percentage change in maximal aerobic power (VO_2 max) = VO_2 max at age × years–VO_2 max at age × + y years/ VO_2 max at × years × 100. Maximal aerobic power usually decreases by about 10 per cent per decade with ageing, starting in the mid-20s for men and in the late teens for women. The decrease is associated with a decrease in cardiorespiratory efficiency (e.g., the stroke volume decreases with age). Endurance athletes who maintain high-intensity training as they age exhibit a smaller decrease in maximal aerobic power than those who stop training.

perception The mental process by which the *brain interprets and gives meaning to *information it receives from sense organs. Perception depends on both the psychological and physiological characteristics of the perceiver, in addition to the nature of the stimuli.

perceptual ability The ability to be able to deal with and give meaning to sensory stimuli.

perceptual anticipation A form of *anticipation in which temporal predictions are made when the subject cannot measure the true passage of time with an external timing device. Perceptual anticipation is thought to depend on an internal biological clock. An athlete able to run at a regular pace may use internal feedback from his or her limbs to keep track of the time (*see* **pace judgement**).

perceptual motor *See* **motor**.

perceptual motor skill learning Acquisition of skill in which movement is an important part. The term emphasizes that the process depends on perceptual mechanisms which deal with the sensory input, mental processes which select and control the movement, and on muscle effectors which carry out the movements.

perceptual narrowing *See* narrowing.

perceptual skill A motor skill which is dependent on high *perceptual ability. Perceptual skills are particularly important in sports, such as tennis and basketball, in which the performer has to be able to adapt his or her skills to a changing environment. There are strong similarities between a perceptual skill, an *externally paced skill, and an *open skill. *See* habitual skill.

perceptual trace *See* closed loop theory.

percussion The tapping of a body-part with a hammer or fingers to gain information about the condition of underlying structures.

perforation Formation of a hole in an organ or tissue, as in a burst eardrum. Causes include disease and physical trauma, such as a deep penetrating wound.

performance 1 The observable act of carrying out a process, such as a *motor skill, which may vary according to circumstances, mood, etc. **2** The manner or quality of carrying out an activity, including a sporting activity. *Compare* learning. *See also* performance curve.

performance curve A plot of the average level of performance of a group of subjects for each of a number of practice trials or blocks of trials. Graphs of changes in performance plotted against time are often used to estimate changes in *learning, but the level of performance will fluctuate from time to time due to performance variables such as fatigue, motivation, and boredom, even when no change in learning has taken place.

performance dependence A situation in which a person is dependent on the performance of another person to reach a particular goal. For example, in netball, a shooter relies on team mates to provide a pass before being able to score a net.

performance goal A desire or objective to improve the level of personal performance at a task (as opposed to an outcome relative to others) which is observable, measurable, and relatively independent of the actions of others. *See also* goal; goal setting; and outcome.

performance plateau *See* plateau; and arrested progress.

performance ratio The level of a performance of one group expressed as a ratio of the level of performance of another group for the same observable, measurable activity. Such performance ratios have been used to examine the effect of gender on performances in each event of athletics by dividing the women's world record by the men's world record.

performance variable An independent variable that affects performance only temporarily and does not affect learning of the task.

performing A stage in the formation of a team (*see* team).

perfusion The flow of fluid, usually blood through the vessels of an organ.

pericarditis Inflammation of the membrane surrounding the heart. It is usually caused by bacterial or virus infections, but it may also be linked with rheumatic fever. The pericardial cavity swells with fluid, constricting the heart. Symptoms include chest pains, anxiety, and fear. Physical activity should be avoided until the inflammation is completely resolved, and then activity should be resumed only with medical guidance. *See also* myocarditis.

pericardium The double-layered envelope surrounding the heart which prevents overextension during heart beats.

perichondrium Dense, fibrous connective tissue membrane covering the external surface of cartilaginous structures.

perimysium *See* fasciculus.

perineal Pertaining to the region between the anus and the external genitalia.

perineum Region of the body between the muscular floor of the pelvis and the thighs, containing the anal canal and external genitalia.

period *See* pendular period.

periodic load test An *aerobic endurance test in which the subject performs successive phases of activity at one intensity level with rest periods between each phase. *See also* **interval training**.

periodic motion A motion that repeats itself. *See also* **harmonic motion**; and **oscillatory motion**.

periodization (cycling of training) A planned training programme in which the year is divided into periods or cycles often of different duration. Each period has a different purpose. A typical example consists of four periods: a preparation period, a pre-competition period, a maintenance or competition period, and finally a transition or recovery period. During the first two periods, training gradually changes from nonspecific, general conditioning activities of long duration and short intensity, to more specific, special training of high intensity and short duration. The programme is designed so that athletes peak during the maintenance period; this peak is timed to coincide with major competitions. Periodization also helps to prevent overtraining by varying the training stimulus. The main periods of training are called macrocycles and the phases of training within the macrocycles are called mesocycles. Thus within the pre-competition period there might be a mesocycle for general conditioning, another for strength training, and a third for speed work. Daily and weekly training sessions are called microcycles and are described in terms of the type of exercise, its intensity and duration. The precise duration of the periods and the total length of the complete cycle depends on when the athlete wants to peak. Most training programmes adopt a single periodization per year; some adopt a double periodization in one year so that the athlete can peak twice; and others have a periodization lasting 2 to 4 years (for example when preparing for the Olympic Games) or even longer. *See also* **Matveyev's six phases**.

periorbital haematoma *See* **black eye**.

periosteal Pertaining to the perisoteum.

periosteum A glistening-white, double-layered membrane of connective tissue covering the outer surface of bone. It is composed of an outer fibrous layer of dense, irregular connective tissue, and an inner layer of bone-forming cells called osteoblasts. The periosteum is richly supplied with nerve fibres, lymph vessels, and blood vessels. It is secured to the underlying bone by strong fibres (Sharpey's fibres) which are exceptionally dense where the periosteum provides anchoring points for tendons and ligaments.

periostitis Inflammation of the periosteum of any bone. It is usually an *overuse injury due to severe strain at the tendon insertions where the muscle fibres or muscle tendons pull, stretch, or tear. Periostitis of the lower leg is particularly common among athletes who change from one playing surface to another, or who change techniques or equipment. Treatment includes rest, anti-inflammatories, and correction of technical or training faults. *See also* **shin splints**.

peripheral blood flow Blood flow to the skin and extremities.

peripheral nervous system That part of the nervous system derived from the cranial nerves, the spinal nerves, and the autonomic nervous system. *Compare* **central nervous system**.

peripheral resistance A measure of the opposition encountered by the blood as it flows through blood vessels. It is the sum of all the regional individual resistances to arterial blood as it passes through the many and varied circuits to body organs and tissues. Peripheral resistance is caused by friction between the blood and the walls of blood vessels. It varies inversely to the fourth power of the radius of the vessel. Thus, if the radius is halved, resistance increases sixteenfold enabling substantial blood flow changes to be effected by relatively small adjustments to the radius of the vessels (*see* **shunting**). Peripheral resistance is an important indicator of *cardiovascular fitness. Physical training can favourably and significantly lower total peripheral resistance, reducing the load on the heart.

peripheral vascular disease A disease of blood vessels in the body extremities that impedes blood flow.

peritendinitis *See* **tenosynovitis**.

peritendinitis crepitans Inflammation of the sheath around a tendon, which has been caused by friction or overuse, not by a trauma.

peritoneum A membrane lining the interior of the abdominal cavity and surrounding its organs.

pernicious anaemia A progressive decrease in the number, but an increase in the size, of red blood cells. Pernicious anaemia is due to lack of vitamin B_{12}. In addition to the symptoms of other forms of anaemia, those with pernicious anaemia often have a sore tongue, fever, and abdominal pain.

peroneal Pertaining to the outer (fibular) side of the lower leg.

peroneus brevis Muscle in the lateral compartment of the lower leg, lying deep to the peroneus longus. It has its origin on the distal fibula shaft and its insertion on the peroneal tendon which runs behind the *lateral malleolus to insert on the proximal fifth metatarsal. Its primary actions are *plantar flexion and *eversion.

peroneus longus A superficial muscle in the lateral compartment of the lower leg. It has its origin on the lateral upper two-thirds of the fibula and its insertion on the lateral surface of the first *cuneiform and first metatarsal. Its primary actions are *plantar flexion and *eversion.

peroneus tertius A small muscle, not always present, in the anterior compartment of the lower leg. It is usually fused with and continuous with the distal part of the extensor digitorum longus. It has its origin on the distal anterior surface of the fibula and the interosseus membrane, and its insertion on the dorsal surface of the first metatarsal. Its primary actions are dorsiflexion and eversion.

peroral By mouth.

personal attribute Physical and psychological characteristics of an individual.

personal attribute questionnaire (PAQ) A questionnaire which measures a person's perceived sex role, that is, the person's perception of his or her masculinity or femininity. The results of the questionnaire suggest that athletes differ in achievement motivation consistent with differences in perceived sex role.

personality The relatively stable organization of a person's character, temperament, intellect, and physique which predisposes him or her to behave and act in particular ways in given situations, and which differentiates one individual from another. There are many different theories about the nature of personality and how it develops. Sheldon's *constitutional theory and trait theories are two which have often been used in trying to explain behaviour in sport. Personality is sometimes viewed as consisting of three levels: the psychological core, typical responses, and role related behaviour. *See also* **personality trait**; and **personality structure**.

personality development An area of sport psychology which includes the study of the genetics and environmental processes that influence *personality.

personality dynamics The study of how an individual's various characteristics interact and operate to influence behaviour. Sport psychologists have been particularly interested in how *anxiety levels interact with *achievement motivation to influence behaviour or performance.

personality profile *See* **psychological profile**.

personality structure The basic psychological components or traits of an individual's *personality and how they combine together to produce that individual's particular behavioural tendencies in certain situations. *See also* **personality traits**.

personality trait Relatively general and enduring personal characteristics which predispose a person to think and behave in certain ways in given situations.

personology The study of *personality.

perspiration *See* **sweating**.

Perthe's disease (pseudocoxalgia) Deformity of the head of the femur in the hip joint, causing aching and limping. It may be due to an injury disturbing the blood supply. Perthe's disease occurs mostly in children between the ages of 3 and 10 years, with a peak occurrence between 6 and 8; it is more common in boys than girls. Young athletes with Perthe's disease may lose the rotatory function of their knee and may develop secondary *overuse injuries. *See also* **osteochondrosis**.

pertinence model A model of selective attention which suggests that all stimuli are analysed but only the most relevant are attended to. *Compare* **Triesman model**.

pes Pertaining to the foot or a structure resembling a foot.

pes anserine A division of the facial nerve which has the appearance of a bird's claw.

pes anserinus An area of the proximal tibia onto which tendons of the *sartorius, *gracilus, and *tendinosus muscles are attached.

pes anserinus bursitis Inflammation of the bursa located between the medial ligament of the knee and the pes tendon approximately 2 cm distal to the anteromedial line of the knee joint.

pes cavus *See* **cavus foot**.

pes malleus valgus *See* **hammer toe**.

pes planus *See* **flat feet**.

PET *See* **positron emission tomography**.

petrissage A form of *massage in which the masseur kneads muscles by applying pressure into a muscle rather than along it. The massage is applied by grasping or picking up the muscle tissue then compressing, pinching, and rolling it.

PFK *See* **phosphofructokinase**.

pH A measure of the relative acidity or alkalinity of a solution expressed in terms of the reciprocal of its hydrogen ion concentration. $pH=\log_{10}(1/H)$, where H is the hydrogen ion concentration in mol l^{-1}. A pH of 7 indicates neutrality, values above 7 indicate alkalinity, and those below 7 indicate acidity.

phagocyte A cell capable of engulfing and digesting foreign particles or other cells.

phagocytosis The act of engulfing foreign solids by cells.

phalanges (sing. phalanx) The bones of the fingers and toes. Each toe and finger contains three bones, except the great toe (hallux) and thumb (pollex) which have two bones each. The phalanges of the toes are smaller than those of the fingers, and less mobile.

phantom (reference human; unisex reference human) A hypothetical human used as a model for assessing human proportionality, particularly among élite athletes. The unisex phantom is defined by designated body length, body girth, body breadth, and skinfold measurements, and has an arbitrary stature of 1.7018 m and body mass of 64.58 kg.

pharmacological agent A drug thought to enhance physical performance.

pharmocopoeia A book containing an official list of the drugs used in medicine together with information about their purity, and physical and chemical properties.

pharmokinetics The mathematical study of the time courses and absorption, distribution, and excretion of drugs in the human body.

phase Period of the year during which there is a particular training emphasis dependent on the specific requirements of a sport. Commonly used phases include preparatory phase, competition phase, and transition phase. *See also* **periodization**.

phasic stretch A type of stretch imposed on a muscle by a load which affects the velocity or rate of change in muscle fibre length. *Compare* **tonic stretch**.

phasing The temporal structure (timing) of a sequence of muscle actions needed to perform a skill. Phasing is usually measured by the ratios of the duration of the component elements of a movement to the overall duration of the movement.

phenomenalism The doctrine advanced by J. S. Mill that only things capable of being permanently perceived as an occurrence or fact by the human senses are real.

phenomenology A philosophical approach which concentrates on the detailed description of conscious experiences. Supporters of this approach do not deny objective reality but emphasize the importance of each person's unique subjective experience of events on the way he or she reacts to the events.

phenomenon Anything capable of being perceived by human senses.

phenotype The observable characteristics of an individual, determined by both the genotype and environment.

phenylalanine One of 20 amino acids commonly found in proteins.

phobia A strong but apparently irrational fear, such as a fear of open spaces, or a fear to stand in a high place even though there is no danger of falling.

phonocardiogram Recording of the sounds made by the heart during a *cardiac cycle. The sounds are thought to result from vibrations created by closure of the heart valves. There are at least two: the first when the atrioventricular valves close at the beginning of systole, and the second when the aortic valve closes at the end of systole.

phonophoresis A technique which uses ultrasound to drive molecules of a medication through the skin into underlying tissue.

phosphagen A member of a group of energy-rich phosphate compounds, e.g. phosphocreatine.

phosphagen system See ATP–PCr system.

phosphate loading Ingestion of sodium phosphate as an *ergogenic aid. It is claimed that phosphate loading increases the availability of phosphates for oxidative phosphorylation (production of ATP). These, and other effects, are thought to improve energy capacity and endurance. Although some scientific studies show significant improvements in VO_2 max, other studies show no such effect.

phosphocreatine (PCr) An energy-rich compound used in the production of ATP from ADP in muscle cells The breakdown of phosphocreatine to creatine and inorganic phosphate is an exergonic reaction coupled to the synthesis of ATP. PCr plays a critical role in providing energy for muscle actions by maintaining ATP concentration. See also **ATP–PCr system**.

phosphocreatine

phosphofructokinase (PFK) An enzyme which plays a key part in *glycolysis, accelerating the conversion of a phosphate of glucose to a phosphate of fructose. PFK activity is particularly important in power events, such as sprinting, during which glycolysis must take place several hundred times faster than at rest. The concentration of PFK is higher in muscle fibres of sprinters than those of endurance athletes. The limited ability of children to perform anaerobic activities may be due to their relatively low concentration of PFK. Those with McArdle's disease (a deficiency in phosphofructokinase or phosphorylase) have an impaired ability to utilize intramuscular glycogen as an energy substrate.

phospholipid An organic compound consisting of a hydrophobic tail of two chains of fatty acid and a hydrophilic head of glycerol and phosphate. Phospholipid is a major component of all cell membranes, and is involved in fat transport in blood and lymph. Phospholipids are also involved in many metabolic reactions.

phosphorus An essential *macronutrient that constitutes approximately 22 per cent of the body's total mineral content. Most of the phosphorus is combined with calcium in bones. Phosphorus is a constituent of many vital compounds including DNA, ATP, and phospholipids. Dietary deficiency is rare. In the UK, the daily adult Reference Nutrient Intake is 550 mg; in the

USA, the Recommended Dietary Allowance is 1200 mg. Phosphorus is required in greater amounts by lactating women.

phosphorylase An enzyme which plays a key part in regulating *glycolysis in muscle cells. It catalyses the conversion of glycogen to a phosphate of glucose. Phosphorylase is activated during exercise by increased amounts of AMP, calcium, and epinephrine. Those with McArdle's disease (a deficiency in phosphorylase or phosphofructokinase) have an impaired ability to utilize intramuscular glycogen as an energy substrate.

phosphorylation Addition of one or more phosphate groups to a molecule.

photophobia Intolerance of the eyes to light due to systemic or environmental causes. An athlete suffering from photophobia is often helpless under stadium lights or in bright sunlight. *See also* **snow-blindness**.

photosensitivity A heightened sensitivity to light which can be caused by certain medications, drugs, or other chemicals. It may lead to phototoxicity.

phototoxicity A toxic reaction provoked by light and often linked to photosensitivity. It usually takes the form of a sunburn reaction (e.g., blistering and peeling of the skin).

phrenic 1 Pertaining to the mind. **2** Pertaining to the diaphragm.

phrenic nerve One of a pair of nerves supplying the diaphragm.

physical Pertaining to the body rather than the mind.

Physical Activity Index *See* **Physical Activity Level**.

physical activity Any form of body movement that has a significant metabolic demand. Thus physical activities include training for and participation in athletic competitions, the performance of strenuous occupations, doing household chores, and nonsporting leisure activities that involve physical effort.

Physical Activity Level (PAL; Physical Activity Index; PAI) Daily physical activity; the sum of the cost of all the physical activities over a 24 hour period. PAL = total energy required over 24 hours/ BMR over 24 hours. According to World Heath Organization statistics, the desirable PAL for cardiovascular health is 1.7; the average PAL in the UK is 1.4, with only 13 per cent of women and 22 per cent of men achieving a PAL of 1.7. For those engaged in hard physical activity, the PAL is 2.14. In a group of novice athletes training for the half marathon, the average PAL at the start of training was 1.66, and after 10 weeks of training it was 2.03.

Physical Activity Ratio (PAR) The energy used for a particular activity calculated by multiplying the *basal metabolic rate (BMR) by a factor appropriate to that activity: PAR = energy cost of an activity per minute/energy cost of BMR per minute. Thus the energy cost of sitting at rest is 1.2; for walking at a normal pace, 4; and for jogging, 7.

Physical Activity Readiness Questionnaire (PARQ) A questionnaire developed by the British Columbia Ministry of Health and the Multidisciplinary Board on Exercise. The questionnaire requires a yes/no response to a series of questions concerning the health risks of the subject, such as 'Are you over 60 years of age?', and 'Do you suffer from chest pains?' It is designed for self-screening by anyone who is planning to start an exercise programme that includes moderate to strenuous activities, such as aerobics, jogging, cycling, power walking, and swimming. Trials of the questionnaire in Canada show that it detects at least half of those in whom an increase in physical activity would cause an increase in the risk of a heart disorder.

physical conditioning *See* **conditioning**.

physical culture The sum total of a society's activities and attitudes connected with physical development and education.

physical dependence A state in which an abrupt termination of the administration of a drug produces a series of unpleasant symptoms known as the abstinence syndrome. The symptoms are reversed rapidly after readministration of the drug. *See also* **drug dependence**.

physical education 1 Any planned programme of motor activities that helps individuals to develop and control their bodies. Physical education is a process through which favourable adaptation and learning (organic, neuromuscular, intellectual, social, cultural, emotional, and aesthetic) result from and proceed through, fairly vigorous activity. **2** A formal area of educational activity in which the main concern is with bodily movements and which takes place in an educational establishment. *See also* **physical recreation**; **play**; and **sport**.

physical fitness The ability to function efficiently and effectively, to enjoy leisure, to be healthy, to resist disease, and to cope with emergency situations. Health-related components of physical fitness include body-composition, cardiovascular fitness, *flexibility, *muscular endurance, and *strength. Skill-related components include *agility, *balance, *coordination, *power, *reaction time, and *speed. The relative importance of each of the components varies for each sport. Physical fitness is not only sport specific, it may also be position specific.

physical recreation Physical activity pursued for enjoyment and to refresh health or spirits. Physical recreation is usually more purposeful and planned than play, but it tends to have a limited organizational structure. Some highly competitive and organized sports are pursued as recreation, but the main purpose of participation is to gain refreshment, not to compete. *See also* **leisure**; and **sport**.

physical sign A sign that can be detected by a physician during observation or examination of a patient.

physical work capacity The maximum amount of work a person can perform. Physical work capacity is usually related to a specific heart rate and is used as a measure of aerobic fitness. The most common test of physical work capacity is called the PWC$_{170}$, which relates to the maximum amount of work that can be done at a heart rate of 170 beats/minute. This value is chosen because, for most people, it is a high but well-tolerated work level. However, an extrapolation taken at maximum heart rate (assuming HR=220−age) is sometimes used for athletes.

physician A registered practitioner of medicine who diagnoses and treats physical diseases and injuries.

physics The study of the properties of matter and energy.

physiological Pertaining to functions in a normal, healthy person.

physiological age *See* **age**.

physiological agent An agent normally present in the body, supplements of which are thought to enhance performance. *See also* **blood doping**; **erythropoietin**; and **oxygen supplementation**.

physiological arousal Unconscious *anxiety which manifests itself in physiological changes. For example, increases in physiological arousal are accompanied by increases in heart rate and sweating. *See also* **cognitive anxiety**.

physiological cross-sectional area (PCSA) The area of a transverse section of muscle. When a muscle is tested physiologically in situ and then removed: PCSA= (muscle mass) (cosine theta)/ (fibre length) (muscle density), where muscle mass is the wet weight of the muscle; theta is the angle of fibre pinnation; fibre length is the mean fibre length within the muscle; and muscle density is assumed to be a constant (1.067 gcm^{-3}). The PCSA of a muscle or muscle group can be estimated *in vivo* from the following equation: PCSA = muscle volume/fibre length, where muscle volume is determined, for example, noninvasively by *nuclear magnetic resonance imaging; and fibre length is estimated from the relatively consistent fibre length to muscle length ratios reported for dissected muscles. PCSA is an important anatomical parameter because the maximum force that a muscle can generate is directly related to its physiological cross-sectional area, with maximum force being approximately 80 Ncm^{-2}.

physiological dead space The volume of alveolar space which is underventilated. *Compare* **anatomical dead space**. *See also* **lung volumes**.

physiological drive A state of *arousal which stems from biological needs such as the need for food and sleep.

physiological fatigue Reduction in the capacity of the neuromuscular system to carry out its functions as a result of physiological overwork and strain. *Compare* **subjective fatigue**. *See also* **fatigue**.

physiological functions Processes carried out by organs, tissues, and cells to maintain health. Major physiological functions include respiration, coordination, excretion, circulation, and reproduction.

physiological limit Level of performance beyond which, by reason of physiological limitations, an individual cannot go. In ordinary circumstances athletes do not reach their physiological limit although it might be approached in the heat of competition when *motivation is high. Improvements gained from training usually often occur when athletes think they have reached their limit; this may be well short of their actual physiological limit (*see* **arrested progress**).

physiological response The reaction of the physiological system to a stressor.

physiological testing Tests designed to measure a specific physiological function thought to be a primary determinant in the performance outcome of a sport. Physiological testing is used to monitor progress of athletes and provide *feedback; to compare different groups of individuals; and to compare different training procedures. Physiological testing is generally a poor predictor of future performance since this will be determined by a complex mixture of factors of which physiological function is only one.

physiology In humans, the study of the functioning of normal, healthy people and their body structures. *Compare* **pathology**.

physiotherapist A practitioner of physiotherapy. In addition to using physical therapies to treat sports injuries, sports physiotherapists also help prevent injury by giving athletes of every standard advice on training, body conditioning, and protective exercises. They also provide prophylactic treatment to help minimize the occurrence of an injury, or prevent the recurrence of an old injury.

physiotherapy Use of physical methods, including manipulation, massage, electrotherapy (e.g. electrical muscle stimulation), hydrotherapy, and exercise therapy, to assist recovery of damaged tissues. Physiotherapy is also used as a prophylactic treatment of athletes, reducing their risk of sustaining sports injuries during strenuous training or competition.

physique The characteristic appearance or physical power of an individual. *See also* **somatotype**.

Piagetian Applied to theories, particularly of cognitive development, proposed by the psychologist Jean Piaget (1896–1980). Although he did not deny the effects of environment in cognitive development of the child, he emphasized the role of innate mechanisms. He suggested that development took place in a series of stages with each stage being the foundation of the next.

pick-up sprint training A form of incremental training that begins with walking, moving on to jogging, then striding and sprinting, and ending with walking. The sequence is repeated as often as possible. Pick-up sprint training improves both aerobic and anaerobic fitness, and trains athletes to cope with changes of pace.

pie chart (pie graph) A diagrammatic representation of the proportions of an identifiable whole in which a circle is divided into sections proportional to the magnitude of the quantities represented.

pie graph *See* **pie chart**.

pigeon toed An abnormal inward turning of the feet so that the toes of one foot point towards the toes of the other foot. It is often associated with *genu valgum (knock-knees), and causes biomechanical ineffi-ciencies during walking and running, increasing the risk of injury.

pilot-study A small-scale version of a planned investigation used to test its feas-ibility and design, and to identify prob-lems.

pinna (auricle) The flap of tissue projecting from the external ear.

piriformis A pear-shaped muscle in the pos-terior aspect of the thigh, inferior to the *gluteus minimus. Its origin is on the anterolateral surface of the sacrum, and its insertion is on the superior border of the greater trochanter of the femur. Its pri-mary action is lateral (outward) rotation of the femur. Its also assists in abduction when the hip is flexed, and helps to stabil-ize the hip joint.

pirformis syndrome A condition character-ized by a dull ache in the mid-buttock region, night pain, and pain when walk-ing upstairs. Symptoms increase when sit-ting, walking, or running, and decrease when supine. It is due to entrapment of the sciatic nerve within the piriformis muscle and may be related to any irrita-tion which causes the muscle to spasm and constrict the nerve. The sciatic nerve passes directly through the piriformis of about 20 per cent of the population making them susceptible to this form of nerve entrapment. Appropriate stretch-ing exercises, nonsteroidal anti-inflamma-tories, ultrasound, aggressive massage, and, occasionally, steroid injections, have been used to treat the syndrome. Surgical release of the piriformis was common in the past but conservative treatments are now generally preferred.

piroxicam A nonsteroidal anti-inflammatory drug (NSAID) used to treat musculoskel-etal injuries. Side-effects are similar to those of aspirin.

pisiform bone A small pea-shaped bone in the wrist which articulates directly with the triquetral bone and indirectly via cartilage with the ulna.

pisiform-hamate tunnel *See* tunnel of Guyon.

pitcher's elbow *See* golfer's elbow.

pitching moment *See* centre of pressure.

pituitary gland An *endocrine gland which coordinates the activities of many other endocrine glands. The pituitary gland is derived from, and attached to, the base of the brain. The activity of the pituitary gland is largely controlled by inhibiting and releasing factors secreted by the *hypothalamus. *Hormones produced by the pituitary include adrenocorticotropin (ACTH), follicle stimulating hormone (FSH), growth hormone (GH), and thyroid-stimulating hormone (TSH).

pivot A short shaft or pin supporting some-thing that turns a fulcrum.

pivot joint (trochoides; trochoid joint) A ring-shaped joint which permits rotation around one axis only; for example, the atlantoaxial joint and the radioulnar joint.

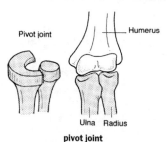

pivot joint

placebo An inactive substance or situation that should not have any effect on a person but which may do so, possibly as a result of suggestion, but for no other biochemical or physical reason. Placebos are used in drug tests as a control to distinguish be-tween effects caused specifically by the drug and effects caused by suggestion. In such tests, neither the investigator or sub-ject should know which is the placebo and which is the genuine drug (a double-blind trial).

placebo effect A positive response to a placebo, similar to that of an active sub-stance, brought about by a person's expectations of the placebo. The placebo effect is well established in sport and is often used as an ergogenic aid. Placebo salves with no pharmacologically active ingredients have been used to relieve muscle fatigue. This demonstrates that although a placebo may have a psychological origin, it can produce a real physical response.

plane A two-dimensional surface with an orientation defined by three distinct points not all contained in the same line. It can be thought of as an imaginary, flat, rectangular surface. *See* **cardinal planes**.

plane joint A nonaxial joint in which the articular surface is flat or only slightly curved. Theoretically, a plane joint allows slipping or gliding movements of one bone on another in all directions, including twisting. However, because such joints are bound tightly in a ligament, movement is limited (e.g., to back and forth or sliding movements). *See also* **intercarpal joint**; and **sternoclavicular joint**.

plane of motion A body plane in which movement occurs. Three planes of motion pass through the human body: the sagittal plane or anteroposterior plane, the frontal plane or coronal plane, and the horizontal or transverse plane. They are the basic references for describing motion. However, motion may also take place through an oblique plane.

plantar Pertaining to the sole of the foot.

plantar aponeurosis A thin, strong fibrous sheet running from the *calcaneus to the toes.

plantar arch The arch-shaped arrangement of interconnecting branches of the plantar arteries on the sole of the foot.

plantar eversion *See* **eversion**.

plantar fascia Thick, fibrous, interconnected bands of connective tissue extending over the sole of the foot. The plantar fascia help support the arches and joints which they cross.

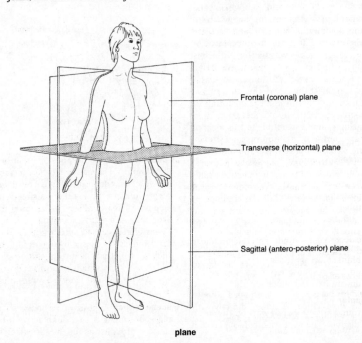

Frontal (coronal) plane

Transverse (horizontal) plane

Sagittal (antero-posterior) plane

plane

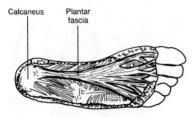

Calcaneus   Plantar
              fascia

plantar fascia

plantar fasciitis An inflammation of the plantar fascia at its attachment to the heel-bone. Plantar fasciitis is characterized by a gnawing pain or discomfort in the heel that radiates along the sole of the foot. It may also be caused by the partial tear of the fascia in the arch of the foot. Plantar fasciitis is most commonly associated with *flat feet. Treatment includes rest and ice in the first 72 hours; thereafter, heat before exercise and ice afterwards. A special programme of massage and exercise is also often recommended. *See also* **tarsal tunnel syndrome**.

plantar flexion A movement that points the toes downwards by extension (straightening) of the ankle. *Compare* **dorsiflexion**.

plantar flexors Muscles in the posterior and lateral compartments of the lower leg which effect *plantar flexion. The major plantar flexors are the *gastrocnemius and *soleus. They may be assisted by the tibialis posterior, flexor digitorum longus, flexor hallucis longus, peroneus longus, and peroneus brevis.

plantaris A small, weak muscle at the back of the lower leg. It varies in size and may even be absent. It has its origin on the distal, posterior femur and its insertion on the tuberosity of the *calcaneus via the *Achilles tendon. Its primary action is knee flexion and plantar flexion.

plantar reflex A reflex induced by running a blunt object along the sole of the foot. The normal response is for the toes to curl downwards and bunch together.

plantar wart (verruca; verruca plantaris) A round or oval-shaped wart on the sole of the foot. The wart usually has a crack or dark spot at its centre. It can be painful when pressed against underlying tissue. Plantar warts are caused by viruses. They are very contagious and are often transmitted by walking bare foot in changing rooms.

plaque Strands of fibrous tissue that attach to the inside of blood vessels. Plaque formation contributes to the development of *atherosclerosis which may lead to a heart attack or a stroke. Its rate of development depends on heredity, diet, and other aspects of lifestyle; regular aerobic exercise may reduce plaque formation.

plasma (blood plasma) The fluid, noncellular component of the blood within which formed elements and various solutes are suspended and circulated. *Compare* **serum**.

plasma membrane A boundary membrane surrounding and enclosing the cytoplasm of a cell.

plasma proteins Proteins, such as albumins and globulins, which circulate in the plasma of blood. Levels of plasma proteins tend to increase during training in relation to the strength and endurance effort.

plasma volume The volume of *plasma in the blood vessels. At the onset of a bout of intense strenuous exercise, the plasma volume decreases by as much as 20 per cent. The reduction is due to fluid moving from the blood vessels into the surrounding tissue fluid, probably as a result of the increase in hydrostatic pressure within blood vessels and an increase in metabolites in the tissue fluid. During prolonged, strenuous exercise, further decreases of plasma volume result from sweating. As the plasma volume becomes reduced, the concentration of red blood cells increases. This causes the blood viscosity to increase and the heart has to work much harder to pump the blood around the body. Consequently, a reduction of plasma volume is likely to impair athletic performance. One of the adaptations to regular endurance training is an increase of plasma volume.

plasmin An enzyme found in the blood which catalyses the breakdown of fibrin clots.

plaster An adhesive material which can be applied as a simple dressing to treat superficial skin-wounds. A few people have an allergic reaction to the adhesive.

plastic behaviour *See* plasticity.

plastic A material which can be distorted permanently when a force is applied to it. *Compare* **elastic**.

plasticity (plastic behaviour) **1** Property of a body that causes it to be deformed permanently when a force is applied. *Compare* **elasticity**. **2** In sociology and psychology, applied to the modifiability of human behaviour; plastic behaviour.

plastic surgery Surgery which revises or reconstructs tissue of superficial organs (i.e. those which can be seen) in a damaged area.

plateau *See* **arrested progress**.

platelet *See* **blood platelet**.

play Spontaneous, childlike, physical activity from which pleasure can be derived immediately. Play is a voluntary activity which has no goal other than enjoyment. It is an activity which takes place within certain limits of time and space, with components having an observable order determined by rules freely accepted. Play is conducted outside the sphere of necessity or material utility. The play mood is one of rapture and enthusiasm, and is sacred or festive, according to the occasion. A feeling of exhilaration and tension often accompanies the action, with mirth and relaxation following. Play among children is believed to be necessary for physical development, learning, social behaviour, and personality development. Among adults, it is conducive to good mental and spiritual health.

plethysmography The process of recording changes in the volume of a limb which reflect changes in blood pressure.

pleura A thin two-layered membrane that secretes fluid, and lines the thoracic wall (parietal pleura), the diaphragm (diaphragmatic pleura), and the lungs (visceral pleura).

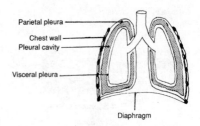

pleura

pleural cavity A fluid-filled cavity between the parietal and visceral pleura surrounding the lungs.

plexus A network of blood vessels or nerve fibres. There are five major nerve plexuses: the brachial, cervical, coccygeal, lumbar, and sacral plexuses. Some of their fibres carry sensory messages to the central nervous system (CNS), and others carry motor impulses away from the CNS to the effector organs, such as muscles.

plica A fold of tissue or fold-like structure. *See also* **knee plica**.

plyometrics A form of training that develops explosive power. It consists of performing of hops, bounds, and jumps so that maximum effort is expended while a muscle group is lengthening. During plyometrics, a concentric muscle action (shortening) is immediately followed by an eccentric action (lengthening). This combination of dynamic muscle action is believed to use the stretch reflex in such a way that more than the usual number of *motor units are recruited. Plyometrics forms part of the training programmes for most sprinters, jumpers, and throwers. However, there is a high risk of injury for those who are not well-conditioned.

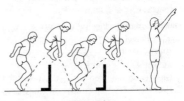

plyometrics

PMS *See* **premenstrual syndrome**.

PMT Premenstrual tension. *See* **premenstrual syndrome**.

pneumotachograph A meter for measuring gas flow rates during breathing by recording pressure differences across a device of fixed-flow resistance that has known pressure flow characteristics. Pneumotachographs are often used in conjunction with computers to give *minute ventilation and breath-by-breath measurements of ventilation.

pneumotaxic centre One of the *respiratory centres in the upper part of the pons of the brain; it controls the frequency and rhythm of breathing.

pneumothorax The entrance of air into the pleural cavity which may lead to lung collapse. It may result from a perforation of the chest wall, but a spontaneous pneumothorax has an internal cause, such as the rupture of the alveoli which can occur if a diver ascends too rapidly with air trapped in the lungs.

PNF *See* **proprioceptive neuromuscular facilitation**.

pO₂ Partial pressure of oxygen.

pocket valve *See* **semi-lunar valve**.

podiatrist A practitioner of podiatry; commonly called a 'foot doctor'. One of their functions is to correct foot defects by making shoe inserts (*see* **orthoses**).

podiatry A branch of the paramedical profession dealing with biomechanical disorders of the feet, the relationship between foot disorders and malalignments of the legs, and how foot disorders affect leg movements.

point of application The precise point at which a force is applied on the body or system receiving the force.

point of release *See* **release point**.

point of resistance In a lever, the point at which the load acts. In human skeletal movements, it is the centre of gravity of the segment of the body being moved plus the centre of gravity of the external resistance or load. *See also* **moment arm**.

poise The CGS unit of *viscosity; it is the tangential force per unit area (measured in dynes per square centimetre) required to maintain unit difference in velocity between two parallel planes separated by one centimetre of fluid.

Poiseuille flow *Laminar flow of a fluid, such as blood, through a long tube with a circular cross-section.

pollex The thumb, the first digit of the hand. It consists of two phalanges.

polycythaemia (erythrocytaemia) An abnormal increase in the number of red blood cells per mm³ of blood. The number of these cell varies considerably among healthy people, but there are normally about 5 million per mm³. A figure above 6 million per mm³ indicates polycythaemia. Relative polycythaemia occurs when the total number of red blood cells in the circulation is normal but the volume of circulating fluids has decreased due to dehydration, injury, or disease. Absolute polycythaemia occurs in response to an oxygen deficiency, for example, as a part of *altitude acclimatization and in those suffering from cardiorespiratory disease. *Compare* **anaemia**. *See also* **blood doping**.

polymer A large molecule formed by the linkage between a large number of smaller molecules. For example, proteins are polymers made from amino acid molecules, and glycogen is a polymer made from glucose molecules.

polymerase chain reaction (PCR) A technique used to replicate specific sequences of DNA (the chemical containing hereditary information) in cells. In the 1992 winter Olympic Games at Albertville, PCR was used to verify the gender of 557 women athletes. PCR can replicate the male-determining SRY gene on the Y-chromosome, enabling it to be detected. The majority of tests can be completed in 24 hours and are highly, but not completely, reliable. *See also* **gender verification**.

polyneuritis Simultaneous inflammation of nerves in many parts of the body.

polyp A growth, usually benign, on a stalk from the skin or mucous membrane.

polypeptide chain A chain of amino acids linked together by peptide bonds.

polysaccharide A *carbohydrate formed of long chains of *monosaccharide units linked together. Polysaccharides may form linear or branched chains. They include the storage substances, *glycogen and *starch, and the structural substance cellulose (*fibre or roughage). They are relatively insoluble, not sweet, and have a low osmotic effect.

polyunsaturated fatty acid See **unsaturated fatty acid**.

POMS See Profile Of Mood States.

ponderal index See body size.

pons Any bridge-like structure that joins two parts of an organ.

pons Varolli A short segment of the brainstem connecting the medulla with the midbrain. It is composed of conduction tracts of nerve fibres linking the upper and lower leaves of the central nervous system. It also contains the *respiratory centres which help maintain the rhythm of breathing.

pooling The accumulation of blood in the lower limbs due to gravity. See also **orthostatic hypotension**.

poor motivation An element of *subjective fatigue characterized by feelings of reduced drive, and lack of determination and vigour.

popliteal Pertaining to the back of the knee.

popliteal artery entrapment syndrome Pain in the lower leg due to entrapment of the popliteal artery in the popliteal fossa behind the knee. The artery may become temporarily occluded when the knee is flexed during exercise producing a pain that may be confused with the pain of shinsplints. Popliteal artery entrapment can be differentially diagnosed by palpating the dorsalis pedis pulse (the pulse on the top of the foot). Entrapment is indicated by the pulse disappearing when the knee is flexed (however, transmission of a pedal pulse does not always mean there is no arterial injury). It can be confirmed by arteriography.

popliteus A thin, triangular muscle deep in the back of the knee. It has its origin on the lateral condyle of the knee and its insertion on the medial, posterior tibia. Its primary action is medial rotation and flexion of the lower leg. It is also known as the unlocker of the knee because it can bring about lateral rotation of the femur with respect to the tibia when the knee is fully extended.

Poppelreuter's law A law which states that when teaching a skill where both speed and accuracy are required, it is better to retard the speed of movement in the early stages of practice until a high degree of accuracy is reached, and then gradually to increase the speed. The law is based on the assumption that it is easier to speed-up accurate movements than to correct fast, inaccurate ones. However, it has also been argued that the law has not got universal application, and that, where speed is a vital component of the performance and influences technique, speed should be emphasized from the beginning.

popular culture Cultural and recreational activities, including many sports, shared by many people in society. Popular culture originates and evolves from the general population itself in contrast with activities which have been created by the *mass media. Compare high culture, mass culture. See also **taste culture**.

population In statistics, the aggregate of individuals or items from which a sample is taken.

population code A means of conveying information in the nervous system by the number of nerve cells involved in transmitting nerve impulses. Compare **frequency code**.

porphyrin A class of pigments containing *pyrolle rings and a metal. Porphyrins include the iron-containing *haemoglobin, *myoglobin, and *cytochromes, and the magnesium-containing chlorophyll.

position The attitude of a body or the posture of a person.

positional segregation *See* stacking.

positive acceleration An increase in the velocity of an object during a given period of time.

positive energy balance A condition in which more energy is taken in as food than is expended during metabolism; body weight increases as a result.

positive feedback A form of *feedback in a *closed loop system in which small changes in the level of output tend to be exaggerated so that deviations from the *norm are increased. *Compare* **negative feedback**.

positive motivation In sport, a source of *primary motivation or *secondary motivation which has a beneficial effect on athletic performance. A series of consistently good performances can act as a source of primary positive motivation. A supportive audience can act as a source of secondary positive motivation.

positive nitrogen balance A condition in which the rate of protein synthesis is greater than protein breakdown or loss, resulting in tissue growth. A positive nitrogen balance is the normal situation for children and expectant mothers. Anabolic steroids accelerate protein synthesis and tend to create a positive nitrogen balance.

positive reinforcement *Reinforcement with pleasant properties which an *athlete will pursue if at all possible. If such a reinforcement is to be effective, it must follow the response, preferably immediately, and increase the likelihood that the response will occur in the future under the same or similar conditions.

positive transfer Transfer of training is positive when previous learning accelerates the learning of a new task. For example, there is positive transfer when an individual who has learned to roller skate can acquire ice skating skills more quickly than he or she would otherwise have done. *See also* **transfer of training**.

positive work Work done by muscles when both the net muscle *torque and the direction of angular motion at the joint are in the same direction. During positive work (e.g. when lifting a barbell) concentric muscle action predominates. *Compare* **negative work**.

positivism (positivistic approach) A philosophical approach which argues that the one true knowledge is scientific knowledge (that is, knowledge which can be gained from observed facts and experiences). Supporters of this approach assume that there is one reality which everyone can view in the same way, or that there is a single answer to a posed question although the answer may be composed of different variables. Positivistic research methods tend to be quantitative.

positron emission tomography (PET) A technique in which extremely short-lived isotopes are injected into the blood stream and their behaviour in specific tissues monitored with an external camera. PET can be used to study muscle metabolism and the activity of brain tissue.

post-calcaneal bursitis *See* Achilles bursitis.

post-concusssion syndrome A combination of signs and symptoms which follow *concussion. They include headaches, irritability, giddiness, and mental fatigue. Athletes exhibiting postconcussive syndrome should not be allowed to return to participation in sports (especially contact or collision sports) until it has resolved completely because they are particularly susceptible to a serious injury at this time (*see* **second impact syndrome**).

posterior (dorsal) Toward the back of the body. *See also* **directional terms**.

posterior cruciate ligament A knee ligament attached to the posterior surface of the tibia from which it passes anteriorly, medially, and upward to attach to the anterolateral surface of the medial femoral condyle. The posterior cruciate ligament is very strong and prevents the femur from sliding anteriorly, the tibia from backward displacement, and the knee from overflexion.

posterior deep compartment syndrome An *overuse injury affecting the posterior deep compartment containing the tibialis posterior, flexor hallucis longus, and the flexor digitorum longus muscles in the lower leg. The condition may be either acute or chronic. *See also* **compartment syndrome**.

posterior superficial compartment syndrome A *compartment syndrome affecting a muscle compartment containing the *gastrocnemius and *soleus muscles at the back of the lower leg.

postganglionic neurone A *motor neurone of the *autonomic nervous system; it has its cell body in a peripheral ganglion and projects its axon to an effector (a muscle or gland).

posthypnotic suggestion A suggestion given during the alert hypnotic trance that is to be carried out when the subject is awake.

post-knowledge of results delay Interval of time from delivery of *knowledge of results to production of the next response. If the interval is too short, performers have difficulty generating a new and different movement at the next response.

post-lunch dip The observation that the level of some physical performances show a slight decrease in the early afternoon. It occurs in some tasks even when no lunch is taken, suggesting that it may be a regular component of *circadian rhythms. Some athletes take an afternoon nap to coincide with this dip, and train later in the afternoon when they are able to perform better.

postsynaptic membrane A cell membrane of a neurone or muscle fibre which conducts impulses away from a synapse.

postsynaptic neurone A *neurone that carries *nerve impulses away from a synapse.

postsynaptic potential A *graded potential in a postsynaptic membrane resulting from the release of neurotransmitter across a synapse.

post-traumatic amnesia *See* **amnesia**.

postulate A statement in a theory that describes the relationship of the hypothetical constructs.

postulate of adequacy The sociological doctrine that descriptions or explanations of social situations must be comprehensible to those involved.

postulate of functional indispensability (universal functionalism) The sociological doctrine that every aspect of culture fulfills an important function for the society in which it occurs.

postural discrimination The ability to respond to changes in posture and make precise compensatory movements in the absence of visual cues (e.g., when walking in the dark). Postural discrimination depends on postural cues from *proprioceptors.

postural hypotension *See* orthostatic hypotension.

postural hypotension drop The amount by which *blood pressure is reduced when a person moves from a lying position to a standing position. A low postural hypotension drop is an indication of good physical fitness.

postural muscle A muscle or group of muscles which play an important part in maintaining body *posture.

postural sway *See* body sway.

posture The position or attitude of the body as a whole.

posture plate *See* arch support.

posturography A technique for assessing body balance by measuring deviations from an erect posture of a subject attempting to balance on a platform. The subject carries out the test once with the eyes open and once with eyes closed while making movements in the vertical, frontal, and transverse axes. Movements of the platform are recorded on a computer and may be converted to graphs for analysis.

potassium An essential mineral which forms the main cations (negative ions) in intracellular fluid. Potassium plays an important role in muscle and nerve function. Although deficiencies are rare, they can lead to muscle weakness, irregularities of heart rate, and nausea. Severe deficiencies may lead to heart failure. Toxicity due to an excessive intake of potassium is also rare, but it can lead to muscle weakness, and heart and kidney disorders. The daily potassium requirement is about 2–4 g (the UK recommended daily adult level is 3.5 g). The best dietary sources of potassium are fruit (especially bananas) and vegetables because they are high in potassium but relatively low in sodium.

potential energy The capacity to do mechanical work by virtue of a body's position. A stretched elastic band and a bicycle at the top of a hill both have potential energy. Potential energy is measured by the amount of work the body performs in passing from a high position to a standard position (usually the ground) in which the potential energy is considered to be zero. A mass raised through a height has a potential energy given by the equation: $U = mgh$, where U is the potential energy in joules; m, is mass in kilograms; g is the acceleration of free fall; and h is height in metres.

Pott's fracture A fracture-dislocation of the ankle joint with the lower parts of the fibula and tibia (the malleoli) being broken. All such fractures require hospital treatment.

pound A unit of weight in the old UK system of weights and measure. It is equivalent to 0.45359237 kg; it is also used as a unit of *force and *mass.

poundal A unit of *force. One poundal acting on a mass of one pound will accelerate the body one foot per second per second. One poundal = 0.138 255 N.

Poupart's ligament *See* **inguinal ligament**.

power 1 Technically defined as 'the rate at which energy is expended or work is done', power is measured in watts (W) of work per unit time (power = work done/time taken). The amount of power generated by a person, therefore, depends on two important components: speed and strength. Power is the key component for most athletic activities. A powerful athlete has to be able to transform physical energy into force at a fast rate. This ability depends on the amount of *ATP he or she can produce per unit time. Sprinting, jumping, and throwing events are activities requiring great power and very high rates of ATP production. *Compare* **capacity**. **2** The ability of a person or group to control the behaviour of others even when actively opposed. **3** The capacity to intervene in a given set of circumstances to alter them in some way.

power stroke *See* **sliding-filament theory**.

power system A leadership approach in which influence and power tends to flow from the coach to the athlete in one direction only. The source of power in such systems includes coercion, reward, authority, expertise, and affection. *Compare* **influence system**.

practical knowledge The things a person knows in relation to his or her behaviour and situation but cannot necessarily express.

practical reasoning Thought which is directed to a practical outcome.

practice The repeated performance of techniques and skills, often taken out of the context of a whole game or event, so that they may be improved. As practice sessions increase, there is generally an improvement in performance (*see* **learning curves**). However, at high levels of performance, much of the time spent in practice is used to maintain the level of performance. Practice conditions which are most effective are those which are similar to those during actual competition. In addition, practice staggered over several short sessions is more effective than an equivalent amount of practice in one long session.

praise A motivational strategy in which a coach or some other person commends a good performance of an athlete. To be effective, praise must be warranted and not excessive. Too much unwarranted praise can be counter-productive. Praise should be given either during the performance or immediately following it. If applied properly, praise can encourage players to persist with their training and playing despite difficulties. *Compare* **criticism**.

precapillary sphincter A ring of muscle surrounding a blood vessel at the junction between an *arteriole and *capillary. It can effectively open and close the capillary and facilitates *shunting.

precession *See* twisting.

precision The number of significant figures to which data or readings are taken. The higher the number of significant figures, the greater the precision. *Compare* **accuracy**.

pre-competition meal (pre-game meal) The meal taken before an athletic competition. Sports nutritionists generally advise athletes to avoid protein-rich and fatty foods, such as steaks, for at least 12 hours before intensive exercise. These types of food take a long time to digest and the digestive system will compete with muscles for the blood supply. A meal taken two to three hours before strenuous activity (the optimum time will depend on the individual) should consist of familiar food containing complex carbohydrates with an energy content of between 200 to 500 kcal. Such a meal will ensure a normal blood glucose level and prevent hunger. Overeating should be avoided.

preconscious In Freudian theory a relatively minor part of the mind that can be readily recalled to the conscious.

predictive value 1 The extent to which a test predicts future performance accurately. **2** The ability of a test to measure what it claims to measure.

predictor variable A causal variable which when changed produces an effect on an event, and which can be used to predict the event. Usually a number of causal variables contribute to an event. For example, an athlete who is very nervous before competition may have many predictors of his or her *anxiety response. The athlete may have a high trait anxiety, may have had

bad experiences at other high level competitions, or may be focusing upon negative thoughts. These predictors must be accurately identified before a sport psychologist can help the athlete control his or her anxiety.

predisposition A tendency to be affected by a particular disease or injury. The predisposition may be inherited or acquired. Athletes who do not warm-up prior to training have a predisposition to joint and muscle injuries.

preferred leader behaviour A style of *leadership behaviour preferred by members of a group. For example, the athletes' preference for a particular style of leadership from their coach. *See also* multidimensional model of leadership.

prefrontal cortex Part of the brain located in the front of the *cerebral cortex and concerned with thought, intelligence, motivation, and personality.

pre-game meal *See* pre-competition meal.

preganglionic neurone A *motor neurone of the *autonomic nervous system with its cell body in the central nervous system and its axon extending to a peripheral ganglion.

pregnancy The period of time (about 280 days) between conception and birth. Although women with a history of poor health may be prescribed rest at various stages of pregnancy, many women exercise and even compete during pregnancy with no ill effects. It is generally agreed that as long as an exercise programme is properly designed, the benefits of exercise during pregnancy outweigh the potential risks. However, all pregnant women should obtain medical clearance before engaging in exercise and should acquire expert advice in designing an individualized programme. The best exercises are nonweight-bearing (e.g., cycling and swimming). Exertion levels should be individually determined. Contact sports, exercises in the supine position, and exercising in a warm, humid environment should be avoided. It is important that pregnant women drink plenty of liquids before and after exercise to avoid dehydration. Maximal physical exertion is generally not recommended after the fifth month of pregnancy.

prejudice Any *attitude held towards a person or group which is not justified by the facts. Prejudice includes negative and positive attitudes towards people solely on the basis of their race, ethnicity, gender, or sex.

premenstrual syndrome (premenstrual syndrome; premenstrual tension; PMS; PMT) Disruptive emotional and physical symptoms, including irritability and headaches, that appear to precede menstruation and may last two weeks or more. The symptoms tend to disappear with the onset of menstruation. PMS can affect adversely the athletic performance of some female athletes. It is generally recognized that the cause of PMS is an altered balance of sex hormones, progesterone becoming relatively dominant in the premenstrual phase of the menstrual cycle. PMS can be treated by hormonal adjustment or by *diuretic drugs. Female athletes who are prescribed mild diuretics to alleviate PMS should ensure they are in no danger of failing a drug test. *See also* **menstrual adjustment**.

premenstrual tension *See* **premenstrual syndrome**.

premotor area *See* **premotor cortex**.

premotor cortex (premotor area) Part of the brain, in front of the *primary motor cortex, which controls motor skills of a repetitious or patterned nature. The premotor cortex contains neurones which coordinate the movements of several muscles by sending impulses to the primary motor cortex and other motor centres in the brain, such as the *basal ganglia.

premotor reaction time The interval from the presentation of a stimulus to the initial changes in the electrical activity of a muscle.

preorbital haematoma *See* **black eye**.

preparation The process which occurs prior to the reception of an expected stimulus to which a subject has to respond quickly. The subject prepares for the stimulus arrival by a reorganization of *attention and initiates in advance the relevant information processing so that the stimulus can be received and responded to quickly.

preparation period A period of training concerned with preparing an athlete for competition. The preparation period includes conditioning, special training, and specific training. *See also* **periodization**.

preparatory arousal Mental techniques used to get excited, charged-up, psyched-up, and aroused just prior to performance. There is some evidence that preparatory arousal is beneficial for power events, such as weight lifting, but it is not necessarily very good for the execution of complex motor skills. *See also* **zone of optimal functioning**.

prepatellar bursa A superficial bursa at the front of the knee, between the skin and patella.

prepatellar bursitis *See* **housemaid's knee**.

presbyopia A diminished ability to see at close range due to an age-related loss of elasticity in the lens of the eye.

prescribed leader A leader appointed by an external authority. *Compare* **emergent leader**.

prescribed leadership behaviour (required leadership behaviour) A style of *leadership that conforms to the established norms of an organization (e.g., the teaching behaviour expected by a school of its physical education teachers). *See also* **multidimensional model of leadership**.

pressoreceptor A nerve ending in the wall of the *carotid sinus and *aortic arch sensitive to vessel stretching. *See also* **baroreceptor**.

pressure The force acting on a given area (pressure = force/area). Common units of pressure are Newtons per square centimetre and Pascals. The ability to spread forces over a wide area and thereby reduce pressure has important applications to safety in sport. High jumpers, for example, spread their body forces by landing flat on their backs. In other sports, the use of equipment such as helmets also tends to spread forces and reduce pressure. Failure to minimize the pressure on any one part of the body can lead to serious injury.

pressure bandage Bandage used to compress tissues and reduce swelling.

pressure drag *See* form drag.

pressure point The point at which an artery is adjacent to a bone on which it can be compressed to stop blood flow.

pressure receptor *See* baroreceptor.

pressure training A training system, much used in team sports, which consists of deliberately creating intensive conditions for skill practice, much more difficult than those required by the game itself. In soccer, for example, a player may be put under pressure by being made to deal in a particular way with a much more rapid sequence of footballs than would occur in the game itself. Pressure-training can improve the speed of executing skilled movements, and it can help performers retain skills under the duress of competition. If pressure-training continues after the skill breaks down, learners may have their confidence destroyed and the training may be counterproductive.

prevertebral muscles Muscles which have their proximal attachment on the anterior aspect of the *occipital bone and *cervical vertebrae, and their distal attachments on the anterior surface of the cervical and three *thoracic vertebrae. Prevertebral muscles include the rectus capitis anterior, the rectus capitis lateralis, the longus capitis, and the longus colli. Their primary actions are flexion, lateral flexion, and rotation of the cervical region of the spine.

priapism A persistent, painful erection. Priapism has been reported among racing cyclists. The pressure of a badly fitting saddle pushes up against the perineum and compresses the pudendal nerve supplying the penis. Treatment may include sedation to reduce the erection, and the acquisition of a better saddle.

PRICES A mnemonic for the initial management of acute musculoskeletal injuries. P represents protection against further injury (e.g. by using a sling); R represents rest, from absolute rest to relative rest, depending on the severity of the injury; I represents ice (*see* **ice treatment**); C represents compression, for example, with a bandage; E represents elevation of the injured part above the heart to enhance venous return; and S represents support, for example, by taping.

prickly heat (miliaria) A condition characterized by intense itching and a rash of red bumps caused by blockage of sweat glands and an inability to sweat freely. Not surprisingly, it is most common in hot humid environments. People travelling from cool, temperate climates to hot humid ones are particularly vulnerable. Treatment includes avoidance of heat and conditions which encourage sweating, application of calamine lotion, and a daily dose of vitamin C (1 g). Rubbing the juice of a lemon over the body after taking a shower or bath is reputed to reduce the chances of having prickly heat.

primary behavioural involvement The direct participation in sport as a competitor or performer. *Compare* **affective sport involvement**: **cognitive sport involvement**; **secondary behavioural involvement**.

primary consequential injury An injury sustained as a direct result of taking part in a physical activity.

primary deviance The initial act of deviance. *Compare* **secondary deviance**.

primary factors *See* first order traits.

primary group A small group, such as a sports team, family, or professional colleagues, which has its own norms and in which there is much face-to-face interpersonal interaction.

primary mechanical purpose A statement of the main objective of an activity, movement, or skill which can be expressed in mechanical terms. For example, the primary mechanical purpose in the long jump is to project the body for the maximum horizontal displacement. Skills that have the same primary mechanical purpose share some of the mechanical principles which determine their effectiveness.

primary motivation In sport, a source of *motivation derived directly from the activity itself. Hitting a golf ball hard and accurately at a target area provides primary motivation. *See also* **inborn motivation**. *Compare* **secondary motivation**.

primary motor cortex Part of the brain concerned with conscious control of skeletal movements. The primary motor cortex is located in the precentral *gyrus of the cerebral cortex and contains *pyramidal tracts of axons connecting the brain and spinal cord. Specific areas of cortical tissue control particular muscles.

primary ossification centre An area of *hyaline cartilage in the centre of the shaft of a long bone where *ossification typically begins.

primary reinforcement Reinforcement provided by the satisfaction of physiological needs, such as that supplied by food or sleep.

primary sport involvement *See* **primary behavioural involvement**.

prime mover *See* **agonist**.

principal axes (cardinal axes) Three perpendicular axes which pass through the centre of gravity of a human body. They are used to describe rotation of the body. For a person standing upright, the principal axes approximately follow lines drawn through the *centre of gravity and passing from the top of the head to the feet (longitudinal axis), from left to right across the body (transverse axis), and from back to front (frontal or anteroposterior axis).

principal plane *See* **cardinal reference plane**.

principle moment of inertia The *moment of inertia of the whole body with respect to one of the principal axes.

principle of contiguity A principle which posits that classical conditioning is effective only when the conditioned stimulus and unconditioned stimulus are contiguous (i.e. follow one another closely in time). *See also* **classical conditioning**.

principle of developmental direction A principle of development which states that neuromotor organization proceeds from head to foot along the longitudinal axis, and from central to peripheral body segments. Thus, there is a progressive advance of motor control from larger, fundamental muscles to smaller muscles which execute more refined movements.

principle of disuse A basic training principle which states that training effects are gradually lost when training stops. This principle has been summarized by the phrase 'Use it or lose it'. *See also* **detraining**.

principle of functional asymmetry A principle of development based on studies of infant behaviour which recognizes that the infant is equipped and capable of facing the world on a *frontal plane of symmetry and could become perfectly ambidextrous. It suggests that a person comes to prefer the use of one hand, foot, or eye mainly because of the preference for the right hand in our culture, and not because the individual is incapable of learning with the left. Neurologically speaking there is equal facility for developing either side of the body, e.g. right or left handedness. This is demonstrated where an injury forces a person who is normally right handed to use the left hand, and also by people who are right handed for one skill and left handed for another.

principle of individual maturation A principle which suggests that children achieve their individuality by becoming progressively differentiated from their fellows with every new maturational change and accompanying environmental experiences.

principle of individuality A basic *training principle which states that any training programme must take into account the specific needs and abilities of the individuals for whom it is designed. It is based on the fact that heredity plays a major part in determining how a person responds to a training program, therefore no two individuals (except possibly identical twins) will respond in the same way to a given training programme.

principle of levers (principle of moments) A principle which applies to a system of balanced forces about a fulcrum or pivot, in which the total anticlockwise moment is equal to the total clockwise moment. Therefore, a lever will balance or turn uniformly about the point of support when the product of the *force and *force arm equals the product of the *resistance and *resistance arm.

principle of moments See **principle of levers**.

principle of orderly recruitment The principle that *motor units are usually activated in a fixed order of recruitment. The motor units within a given muscle appear to be ranked. The same motor units are recruited for a given force production. Units with higher rankings are recruited as the force needed to perform an action increases. Thus, more units are recruited as the force of a muscle action increases.

principle of overload See **principle of progressive overload**.

principle of progressive overload According to this basic *training principle, training must include overload and progression to be successful. The body must be overloaded so that it has to work harder than normal. As the body adapts to a particular workload, the person should progress to a higher work level. For example, to gain strength, the muscles must be loaded beyond the point at which they are normally loaded. As the muscles become stronger, the load has to be increased to stimulate further strength increases. The load should be increased gradually over a long period of training. If the load is too high, there is a risk of overtraining and overuse injuries.

principle of reciprocal interweaving A principle of development, based on studies of infant behaviour, which refers to the intimate relationship that exists between the growth of an individual's body structures and the behaviour of an individual. Interweaving applies to the development of neural pathways between antagonistic pairs of muscles so that *reciprocal innervation occurs. The development of the neural network results in a progressive spiral of more advanced forms of behaviour.

principle of specificity A basic *training principle which states that in order to improve a particular component of physical fitness, a person must emphasize that component in training. A training programme must stress the physiological systems used to perform a particular activity in order to achieve specific training adaptations. Consequently, a weight lifter who trains only for strength and power will probably be stronger than an untrained person but have no better aerobic endurance. See also **principle of progressive overload**.

principle of variance The training principle that maximum benefits are obtained when a training programme includes a variety of training methods.

principle of work and energy A principle of mechanics which states that the work of a force is equal to the change in energy that it produces in the object on which it acts.

proactive assertion Forceful behaviour which is permitted by the rules of a sport (e.g., tackling and blocking in American football). It is sometimes difficult to distinguish between proactive assertion and *aggression; a player may tackle an opponent legitimately, but with the intent of injuring the opponent.

proactive inhibition The negative effect one learned task has on the retention of a newer task; a type of interference or negative transfer observed in memory experiments and other learning situations. Compare **retroactive inhibition**.

proactive transfer A form of *transfer of training in which the learning and/or performance of one skill influences another skill yet to be learned.

probability The likelihood that a given event will occur. Probability is expressed as values between 0 (complete certainty that an event will not occur) to 1 (complete certainty that an event will occur), or percentage values between 0% and 100%.

probability of success The perceived *probability of succeeding at a task. *See also* **risk-taking behaviour**.

probablistic explanation An explanation in which a specifiable probability (a chance of less than 100 per cent and more than 0 per cent, or, in probability theory, less than 1 and more than 0) is taken as explaining the occurrence of an event.

probe A thin pliable instrument with a blunt, swollen end. It is used to investigate, or introduce things, into body-spaces.

probenecid A drug used to treat gout by reducing levels of uric acid in the blood. Probenecid inhibits the transport of organic acids and antibodies across some tissue barriers, such as the barrier between the blood and the kidney tubule. It has two very important effects on other drugs: first, it can increase the concentration of another drug or antibody within the blood; secondly, it can reduce the amount of drug (e.g., anabolic steroid) released into the urine, making a banned drug much more difficult to detect. Because probenecid may be used to alter the integrity of a urine sample and avoid detection in dope tests, it is categorized as a *banned substance by the International Olympic Committee. Probenecid is relatively easy to detect in a urine sample.

probe technique (reaction time probe) A technique used to study the role of the attention demands of movements of subjects performing a primary task while presented with an occasional stimulus (usually auditory) to which the subjects must respond. The *reaction time to the stimulus is used as a measure of the attention demands of the primary task: low reaction times are assumed to indicate that the amount of *attention required for the primary task is relatively small. The probe technique assumes that there is a fixed capacity for attention.

problem solving The ability to adjust to a situation by acquiring new modes of response. Problem solving applies especially to learning in which a certain amount of insight or reasoning occurs.

procedural skill A skill involving a series of discrete responses each of which must be performed at the appropriate time in the appropriate sequence.

process In sport psychology, the behavioural interactions within a *group which enable the group to use its resources to achieve group objectives. A group with process faults (e.g., lack of coordination between team members, or conflicting motivations) is likely to fall short of achieving its full potential.

processing capacity The amount of space a person has available in the central nervous system for processing information. The use of the term implies individuals have a limited capacity for such processing. It has been used to explain a person's limited ability to do several things at the same time.

process orientation An approach to the study of movement which emphasizes the study of the mental processes underlying movement and motor skills. Researchers using a process orientation approach are usually interested in finding out about the underlying mechanisms that contribute to the performance of a motor skill rather than the outcome of the performance. *Compare* **task-orientation**.

product orientation A *leadership style which is best explained in terms of *initiating structure where the emphasis is on task fulfillment.

professional 1 A person, such as a medical doctor, having an occupation which requires special training. **2** An expert player who gives instruction in a game; for example, golf professional. **3** Applied to any person, such as a professional cricketer, who engages in an activity as his or her means of livelihood, which is generally followed as a pastime.

profile drag *See* **form drag**.

Profile Of Mood States (POMS) A psychological test designed to measure a person's affective states. These include tension, depression, anger, vigour, fatigue, and confusion. Unlike *personality traits, mood states are thought to be transitory and specific to a given situation, although moods can also be measured for recent prolonged periods such as the past several months. POMS is a popular research tool among sport psychologists.

prognosis Forecast of the course and outcome of a disease or injury.

progression *See* principle of progressive overload.

progressive muscle relaxation (progressive relaxation; PMR) A highly effective technique for managing *stress, tension, anxiety, and worry. Muscle groups from head to toe are tensed for a few seconds and then relaxed in sequence. Tensing the muscles really hard seems to enable the muscle to relax fully. With practice it is possible to perform the technique in seconds. PMR is used by many athletes to maintain *arousal at optimal levels before a competition.

progressive part method A method of learning a multi-part task, in which the parts are learned and combined sequentially. After the first two parts are mastered, they are combined and practised together until learned. Then the third part is taught by itself. After it has been acquired the three parts are combined and practised together until learnt. This procedure is followed for each part until all of them can be practised as a whole. The technique is most appropriate when the parts form a natural and meaningful sequence of actions which need to be practised together. For example, a gymnast's floor sequence. *See also* learning method.

progressive relaxation *See* progressive muscle relaxation.

progressive resistance exercise (progression) Exercise in which a load is increased in predetermined steps. Ideally, the increments should be large enough to ensure overloading (*see* principle of progressive overload), but not large enough to cause damage. Progressive resistance exercises in weight-training are generally based on the *repetition maximum (RM). In one session, several sets of exercises are performed, each at a higher intensity than the preceding one. The following example consists of three sets of repetitions with a short rest of 1 to 2 minutes between each: set 1 at 50 per cent 10-RM; set 2 at 75 per cent 10-RM; and set 3 at 100 per cent 10-RM. Between sessions, the 10-Rm is re-evaluated to ensure that the training conforms to the overload principle. *See also* principle of progressive overload.

progressive resistance system A system of training based on *progressive resistance exercises.

projected fatigue An element of psychological or subjective fatigue characterized by sensations such as leg weakness, shaking or aching muscles, palpitations, shortness of breath, and a dry mouth. Projected fatigue shares many of the somatic manifestations of an *anxiety state.

projectile Any airborne object, such as a human body during a jump, a football kicked in the air, and a javelin in flight, that is subject only to the forces of gravity and air resistance. A projectile's motion is determined by three main mechanical factors: angle of projection, the projectile's initial speed (*see* speed of release), and relative height of projection.

projection A mechanism of *ego defense in which an individual transfers personally unacceptable wishes or actions to another person or external object. For example, an athlete who dislikes himself or herself may transfer those feelings to the coach who is then perceived as disliking or even hating the athlete.

projective procedure (projective test) Psychological test that uses relatively unstructured and open-ended tasks. The assumption is that such a test, in which there are no clear right or wrong responses, encourages open and honest responses.

prolactin (lactogenic hormone; LTH; luteotrophic hormone; luteotropin) A hormone secreted by the anterior lobe of the *pituitary gland. Prolactin stimulates the secretion of milk after pregnancy. Prolactin secretion increases during exercise. This may be useful both in conserving water through its antidiuretic effect and in mobilizing fat for energy.

prolapse The displacement of an organ or organ part such as an intervertebral disc.

prolapsed intervertebral disc (herniated disc; slipped disc) Displacement of part of the gelatinous interior of an *intervertebral disc so that it protrudes through the fibrous coat pressing on adjacent nerves. It is usually caused by a combination of disc degeneration over a long period of time and a physical trauma sustained during a single event. The lumbar region is the most commonly affected part of the backbone because it is subjected so frequently to enormous loads. Symptoms include pain in the buttocks and legs, with the pain worsening when coughing and straining. Initial treatment may include icing the back (during the first 48–72 hours; *see* **ice treatment**), rest in bed with the knees bent, and application of a heat pad to reduce muscle spasms. A doctor may prescribe long-term rest (8 to 12 weeks), anti-inflammatories, cortisone injections, and, for persistent problems or in an emergency situation, surgical correction. Once the pain has dissipated and the disc is healed, rehabilitation includes exercises that strengthen the abdominal and back muscles in order to reduce a recurrence of the prolapse. *See also* **sciatica**.

promotively independent goal A situation in which all members of a team can achieve their goals; the achievement of a goal by one individual does not preclude others from achieving their goals. *Compare* **contritely interdependent goal**.

pronation 1 An inward rotation of the forearm so that the palm is facing posteriorly or inferiorly (i.e. backward or downward). During pronation, the distal end of the radius moves across the ulna towards the midline. Pronation is the natural position (but not the anatomical position) of the

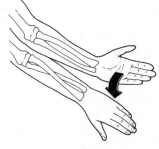

pronation 1

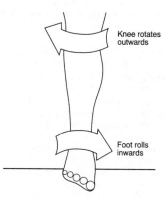

Knee rotates outwards

Foot rolls inwards

pronation 2

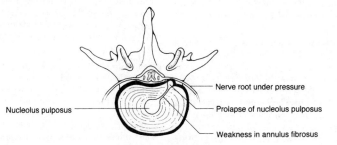

Nerve root under pressure

Nucleolus pulposus

Prolapse of nucleolus pulposus

Weakness in annulus fibrosus

prolapsed intervertebral disc

forearm when a person is standing in a relaxed position. *Compare* **supination**. **2** During the midstance of the weight-bearing phase of running and walking, a tendency for *eversion and abduction to occur as the foot moves into dorsiflexion. Pronation serves as a shock-absorbing and an energy-return mechanism.

pronator 1 A muscle that effects pronation. **2** A person who tends to exhibit excessive pronation during running and walking.

pronator quadratus The deepest muscle of the anterior fascial compartment of the forearm. It has its origin on the lower quarter of the anterior ulna and its insertion on the radius. Its primary action is elbow pronation.

pronator teres A two-headed muscle. The upper head has its origin on the medial epicondyle of the humerus; its lower head has its origin on the coracoid process of the ulna. The heads converge and the common tendon of insertion is on the lateral midpoint of the radius. The primary action of the pronator teres is elbow pronation. It also acts as a weak elbow flexor.

pronator teres syndrome A syndrome consisting of pain and tenderness in the middle anterior part of the elbow, numbness in the second, third, and radial half of the fourth finger, pain during pronation, and weakness during plantar flexion. It is caused by entrapment of the median nerve by overactivity of the *pronator teres, for example, as a result of repetitive throwing.

prone 1 Applied to the body position when lying horizontally, face down. **2** Applied to the forearm when the palm is facing down.

propeller propulsion Motive force produced by the rotation of blades (usually two or three) inclined back from their leading to trailing edges. Although the blades rotate in circular paths, the leading edge of each blade can displace a fluid backwards and thereby drive an object forwards. It has been suggested that swimmers doing the front crawl use their hands like rotating propeller blades within a single armstroke,

with the hands forming a new blade each time they change direction. *See also* **propeller propulsion**.

prophylaxis Any preventative treatment of a disease.

propinquity The nearness, for example, of an athlete to his or her team mates. Propinquity is used in particular to denote the location of an athlete in terms of his or her visibility and observability by team mates.

proportionality In anthropometry, the relationship of body-parts one to another or to the whole body.

proprioception The awareness of body position in space. *See also* **kinaesthetic perception**.

proprioceptive neuromuscular facilitation (PNF) An effective stretching technique for increasing the range of motion of joints. All PNF procedures require a partner and involve some pattern of alternating contraction and relaxation of the muscles being stretched so that the *Golgi tendon organs are stimulated.

proprioceptor A sensory receptor located in muscles, tendons, and joints which conveys information about the physical state and position of skeletal muscles and joints. Proprioceptors provide essential information for smooth coordinated movements and the maintenance of body posture. *See also* **Golgi tendon organs**; **kinaesthesis**; and **muscle spindle organs**.

propulsion (motive force; propulsive force) The force that causes motion. In swimming the front crawl, for example, the propulsive force is provided by the combined actions of the feet and hands pushing water backwards so that the swimmer moves forwards. *See also* **propeller propulsion**.

propulsive drag A drag force acting in the same direction as a body's motion through a fluid. A tailwind, for example, which has a velocity greater than the velocity of a moving body contributes to the forward propulsion of the body. Propulsive drag contributes to movements of swimmers, especially those doing the front crawl.

Backward movements of the hands and arms through the water produce forwardly directed reaction forces which help to propel the swimmer forwards.

propulsive force *See* propulsion.

prosocial behaviour Behaviour in which one individual helps another. *See also* **sporting behaviour**.

prostaglandin A member of a group of organic chemicals derived from the fatty acid, *arachidonic acid. Prostaglandins are found in cell membranes. They have many effects including regulating blood pressure. They are involved in the *inflammation response. They dilate blood vessels and make them more permeable to fluid and proteins, causing oedema (swelling) and a temperature rise. They also sensitize nerve endings, thus promoting pain.

protective muscle spasm A sustained involuntary muscle contraction which occurs after injury to the muscle as a protective mechanism to prevent further movement. Such spasms commonly result in muscle stiffness.

protective protein theory Theory that regular exercise increases the level of fat-carrying high density lipoproteins in the blood thereby reducing the risk of heart disease.

protein A member of a group of organic polymers containing chains of amino acids linked together by peptide bonds. Proteins play a vital part in the structure and function of all cells, comprising 10–30 per cent of cell mass. Structurally, they are divided into two main groups: fibrous proteins and globular proteins. Functionally, they have many varied roles. They act as enzymes, hormones, respiratory pigments, and antibodies. Excess protein cannot be stored in the body and is excreted, mainly as urea in the urine. Each gram of protein contains about 4 kilocalories of energy. Protein can supply up to 10 per cent of the energy needed to sustain an endurance activity. A diet containing 10–15 per cent of calories from protein should be adequate for most athletes. The World Health Organization recommend a daily protein intake of 1g/kg body weight; studies by sports nutritionists indicate that athletes involved in prolonged heavy training require more protein, about 1.2–1.7 g/kg body weight. There is little scientific evidence to support the use of very high-protein diets by athletes. On the contrary, these diets could damage the kidneys, and can cause dehydration and constipation. Protein-rich foods include meat, grains, and legumes.

proteinuria An abnormal presence of serum proteins in the urine. Proteinuria is a feature of renal impairment. Its occurrence after exercise was at one time thought to indicate a serious disturbance of renal function, but it is now recognized that moderate proteinuria is common in healthy young adults after heavy exercise. This condition, unlike pathological conditions, is quickly reversed when the athlete rests in a recumbent posture. *See also* **athletic pseudonephritis**; **orthostatic proteinuria**.

proteoglycan Member of a class of compounds consisting of polysaccharide (95 per cent) and protein (5 per cent). Proteoglycans and water form the ground substance of connective tissue such as cartilage and tendons and are important in determining the mechanical properties of these tissues. Within tendons, for example, the ground substance provides friction that helps collagen fibres to adhere to one another, and also provide the spacing and lubrication that allows the fibres to slide past one another. Different types of proteoglycans are found in areas subjected to compressive rather than tensile forces.

proteolytic enzyme An enzyme which catalyses the breakdown of proteins. Hyaluronidase is a proteolytic enzyme used to treat soft tissue injuries.

protocol The formal technique and procedure for conducting an investigation, such as fitness testing or drugs testing.

protraction Nonangular forward (anterior) movements of a body-part in a transverse plane, such as the forward projection of a mandible when the jaw is jutted out. *Compare* **retraction**.

proxemics The study of how people communicate nonverbally by the way they use the space between themselves and other people.

proximal Closer to the trunk (e.g., the elbow is proximal to the wrist) or the origin of a structure. *See also* **directional terms**.

pruritis ani Intense irritation and discomfort in the anal region often exacerbated by scratching and secondary infections. Pruritis ani is often due to wearing tight clothes and is associated with heavy sweating, therefore it is relatively common among athletes. Treatment consists of scrupulous toilet hygiene, careful washing and drying, followed (in some cases) by the application of hydrocortisone cream.

pseudoanaemia *See* **athletic pseudo-anaemia**.

pseudoarthrosis A false joint formed around a displaced bone after *dislocation.

pseudocoxalgia *See* **Perthe's disease**.

psoas major A long, thick thigh muscle, just medial to the *iliacus. Its origins are on the transverse processes of the twelfth thoracic vertebra and lumbar vertebrae and lumbar intervertebral discs. It shares a tendon of insertion with the iliacus with which it works in combination. Its

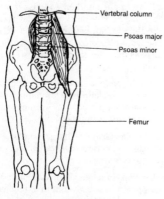

- Vertebral column
- Psoas major
- Psoas minor
- Femur

psoas muscles

primary action is flexion of the femur. It flexes the spine and is an important postural muscle.

psoas minor A small thigh muscle, often absent, that shares the same actions as the *psoas major.

psoas position Position of a person lying on back with knees bent. The psoas position is adopted to relieve back pain, for example, after a prolapsed intervertebral disc.

PST *See* **Psychological Skills Training**.

psyche An ancient Greek word meaning soul or mind, it often refers to the mental as opposed to the physical aspects of an individual.

psyched-out A colloquial term indicating a disruption of flow and a disturbance of mental balance.

psyched-up A colloquial term describing an increased state of *arousal and confidence of an athlete prior to competition.

psychiatrist A medical doctor who specialises in the treatment of mental of behavioural disorders. *Compare* **psychologist**.

psychiatry A branch of medicine concerned with the study, prevention, and treatment of mental illness.

psychic energy A term sometimes used synonymously with *arousal. It refers to the vigour, vitality, and intensity with which the mind functions. It can be either positive or negative. When performers go from low to high levels of psychic energy they are said to become psyched-up; while those who go from high to low levels are psyched-out. As in arousal, there is an optimum level of psychic energy. *See also* **inverted-U hypothesis**.

psyching-up Colloquial term used by athletes and coaches which refers to motivational strategies aimed at enhancing performance by raising arousal and increasing the activation level. Psyching-up often consists of a coach exhorting athletes to make greater efforts (*see* **pep-talk**). Sometimes the process results in heightened levels of *anxiety and poorer performance (*see* **inverted-U hypothesis**).

psychoanalysis A method of treating mental disorders pioneered by Sigmund Freud (1856–1939) which employs the techniques of free association, interpretation, and dream analysis to reveal and release repressed fears so that they can be effectively dealt with.

psychoanalytically based theory Theory of psychosocial behaviour based on the assumption that the current behaviour of a person has developed as a result of past experiences, especially those of early childhood concerned with sex. *See* **psychoanalysis**.

psychobiological model A model of behaviour which incorporates biological and psychological factors. A psychobiological model of *exercise adherence, for example, may include body composition (biological factor) and self-motivation (psychological factor).

psychodynamic theory A major theoretical approach to the study of *personality based mainly on in-depth examination of the whole person and his or her unconscious motives. The most influential proponent was Sigmund Freud (1856–1939) who believed that *personality resulted from a dynamic interaction between its three components: the id, the ego, and the superego.

psychogenic Originating from the psyche rather than the body. For example, an illness which has a psychological basis rather than an organic basis. *See also* **psychosomatic**.

psychogenic dependence A condition in which a drug-taker experiences an irresistible craving or compulsion to take a drug for pleasure or for relief from discomfort.

psychological core The central, internal, and consistent part of an individual's personality. It includes an individual's *self-concept, basic values, attitudes, and motives; a person's true self.

psychological fatigue (false fatigue; subjective fatigue) A feeling of fatigue caused by things such as lack of exercise, boredom, or mental stress that results in lack of energy and depression.

psychological fitness The mental fitness, for example, of an athlete to cope with the stresses of competition.

psychological measuring instrument A technique, usually with proven reliability and validity, for measuring a psychological phenomenon. For example, the *competitive state anxiety inventory for measuring competitive stress.

psychological orientation The mental attitude which a person has towards the value of his or her work and workmates. The psychological orientation includes *interaction orientation, *self-orientation, *task orientation.

psychological preparation Mental preparation in which competitors learn how to deal with psychological *stress and achieve optimum levels of *arousal so that they will be able to perform to the best of their ability.

psychological presence The degree to which a performer feels the presence of an *audience. *See also* **evaluation apprehension**.

psychological profile A distinct pattern of behavioural responses an individual or group displays. The profile is usually based on the results of several inventories which are displayed on a graph or in a table. *See also* **iceberg profile**.

psychological refractoriness *See* **psychological refractory period**.

psychological refractory period (PRP; psychological refractoriness) The delay in the response to the second of two closely spaced stimuli. Ball players often attempt to increase the PRP in their opponents by disguising a shot or 'selling a dummy' (i.e. feinting to go one way and then going another).

psychological reversal *See* **reversal theory**.

psychological skills hypothesis A hypothesis which suggests that *imagery works through the development and refining of psychological skills (for example, by improving concentration, reducing anxiety, and enhancing confidence).

Psychological Skills Training (PST) Training designed to improve mental skills of an athlete, such as self-confidence, motivation, the ability to relax under great pressure, and the ability to concentrate. PST takes many forms but each usually has three phases: the education phase, during which athletes learn about the importance of psychological skills and how they affect performance; the acquisition phase, during which athletes learn about the strategies and techniques to improve the specific psychological skills that they require; and the practice phase, during which athletes develop their psychological skills through repeated practice, simulations, and actual competition.

psychological well-being (mental well-being) A mental condition characterized by pleasant feelings of good health, exhilaration, high *self-esteem, and confidence, often associated with regular physical activity.

psychologist An individual who has completed a programme of study in psychology and is engaged in research, clinical treatment, teaching, or other applications of psychology.

psychology A branch of science which studies the mind, mental activities, and behaviour.

psychometrics 1 Measurement of mental factors **2** Investigation of the time factor in mental processes.

psychomotor (psychomotoric) Pertaining to both mental activity and muscular movement. *See also* **motor**.

psychomotor test Psychological questionnaires and tests which assess psychomotor reaction time and other psychomotor functions.

psychoneuromuscular theory A theory postulated to explain the positive effects of motor *imagery. It suggests that vivid, imagined events produce neuromuscular responses similar to those of an actual experience. That is, the images produced

in the brain transmit impulses to the muscles for the execution of the imagined skill, although these impulses may be so minor that they do not actually produce movement, or the movement may be undetectable. Support for this theory comes from a number of sources. For example, *electromyograph patterns of the muscle activity of skiers who imagine they are performing a downhill run, are similar to the electrical patterns of the skiers' muscles when they have actually been skiing. *See also* **imagery, symbolic learning theory**.

psychophysiological orientation An approach to the study of sport psychology which focuses on the relationship between mental activities and physiological processes (e.g. heart rate and muscle action potentials), and their effects on physical activity. *See also* **behavioural orientation**; and **cognitive-behavioural orientation**.

psychophysiology The study of the relationships between psychological states and physiological measurements (e.g., the relationship between anxiety and heart rate).

psychosocial behaviour Behaviour and mental activities of individuals and groups which influence and determine their relationships, their ability to work together, and their attitudes towards each other.

psychotonic A stimulant, such as *amphetamine, which has its primary effect on the brain and central nervous system. A psychotonic increases psychological tone and delays the subjective feeling of fatigue without actually improving the physical capacity of muscles.

psychotropic drug A drug which affects emotional state. Psychotropics include antidepressants, sedatives, stimulants, and tranquillizers.

psychrometer An instrument that measures relative *humidity.

pternion An anatomical landmark at the most posterior point of the heel of the foot when the subject is standing erect.

PTH *See* **parathyroid gland**.

puberty (pubescence) A period in the *life course between the appearance of pubic hair and, in females, the first menarche, or, in males, the first development of sperm. Puberty varies but in females it usually occurs between 9 and 15 years, while in males it usually occurs between 11 and 14 years.

pubes Pubic hair or the region of the body on which it grows.

pubescence See puberty.

pubic bone See pubis.

pubic symphysis A fibrocartilaginous disc joining the two pubic bones of the pelvic girdle. The pubic symphysis is an *amphiarthrotic joint capable of slight movement. In females, it becomes more mobile during pregnancy.

pubis The two bones making up the anterioventral part of the *pelvis. In adults, the bones fuse at the *pubic symphysis. See also coxal bones.

pudendal nerve Nerve supplying the external genitalia.

pugilist's nose A deformity caused by frequent blows to the nose. It is characterized by septal deviation with old or recent bony or cartilaginous fracture. It is common among boxers and repair is usually delayed until after retirement. However, if the deformity causes breathing problems, repair is made immediately.

pulled elbow A *subluxation of the head of the radius in children, accompanied by paralytic pain and disability of the forearm and the hand. See also elbow dislocation.

pulled muscle See muscle strain.

pulley A wheel-like device for changing the direction of the application of a force. A pulley usually has a groove through which a cord can run in order to change the direction of the force applied to the cord. A pulley-like action is represented in the human body by tendons which wrap around parts of bones and thereby change the line of pull of a muscle, resulting in a line of movement which might otherwise

not have occurred. The *quadriceps tendon, for example, by passing over the patella, inserts on the tibia at a greater angle than would otherwise have occurred. This change in angle increases the rotary component of the force of the *quadriceps muscle and decreases the stabilizing component, thereby achieving a more effective force during movement.

pulmonary Pertaining to the lungs.

pulmonary artery A blood vessel carrying deoxygenated blood from the right ventricle to the lungs.

pulmonary blood pressure The blood pressure within the blood vessels supplying the lungs.

pulmonary capillary blood volume The volume of blood in contact with the gas in the *alveoli of the lungs at any instant.

pulmonary circuit See pulmonary circulation.

pulmonary circulation (pulmonary circuit) Flow of blood from the right ventricle of the heart through the blood vessels of the lungs and back to the left ventricle of the heart.

pulmonary diffusion The exchange of gases between the alveoli and the capillaries in the lungs. Oxygen diffuses from the alveoli into the capillaries and carbon dioxide diffuses in the opposite direction.

pulmonary diffusion capacity The volume of gas that diffuses across the membranes between the alveoli and lung capillaries per minute per torr mean pressure difference. The pulmonary diffusion capacity represents the rate of diffusion of gas between the alveoli and the blood of the lung capillaries. It varies with many factors, but the surface area of contact between the alveoli and the blood in the pulmonary capillary is especially important. The pulmonary diffusion capacity for oxygen increases in an approximately linear manner with increasing workloads. It levels off at near maximum loads when it is up to three times more than at resting levels. Compared with nonathletes, trained athletes tend to have larger diffusion capacities at rest and during exercise.

pulmonary edema *See* **pulmonary oedema**.

pulmonary function The role of the lungs in meeting the demands of muscular activity to deliver oxygen and to eliminate carbon dioxide from the pulmonary circulation. Pulmonary function is accomplished by the flow of blood through lung capillaries, by ventilation, and by the diffusion of oxygen from the lungs into the blood and of carbon dioxide from the blood to the air into the lungs.

pulmonary function test A test of the ability of the lungs to carry out their function of ventilation and gaseous exchange. *See also* **forced expiratory volume**; and **minute ventilation**.

pulmonary hypertension High blood pressure within blood vessels supplying the lungs. Pulmonary hypertension may complicate heart diseases and chronic lung diseases. Regular aerobic exercise can reduce blood pressure.

pulmonary oedema (pulmonary edema) An accumulation of fluid in the alveoli and lung tissues. *See also* **high altitude pulmonary oedema**.

pulmonary perfusion The volume of blood flowing through the lungs.

pulmonary valve A semi-lunar valve which prevents backflow of blood from the pulmonary artery to the right ventricle.

pulmonary vein A vein carrying oxygenated blood from the lungs to the left atrium of the heart.

pulmonary ventilation Breathing; the movement of air in and out of the lungs during inspiration and expiration. *See also* **minute ventilation**.

pulse The rhythmic expansion and recoil of the arteries resulting from a wave of pressure produced by contraction of the left ventricle of the heart. The pulse can be felt in any artery sufficiently close to the body surface which passes over a bone. *See also* **pulse rate**.

pulse pressure The difference between *systolic blood pressure and *diastolic blood pressure.

pulse rate The frequency per minute of pressure waves propagated along superficial, peripheral arteries, such as the carotid and radial arteries (*see* **pulse**). In normal, healthy individuals, the pulse rate and heart rate are identical, but this is not so in patients suffering from some cardiovascular diseases such as arrhythmias.

pump Plimsolls; a type of sports shoe with a rubber sole used in games such as tennis and badminton.

pump bump A rounded swelling on the heel that coincides with rough, close-fitting heel counters of 'pumps' (training shoes). The swelling is due to frictional irritation of a subcutaneous bursa against the heel counter. The bursa overlies the *Achilles tendon which may also become tender and inflamed at its point of insertion onto the heel bone. Pump bump is often complicated by overtraining which causes inflammation of the deep bursa between the lower end of the Achilles tendon and the heel bone. A pump bump due solely to irritation with footwear, can be alleviated by smoothing the heel counter or protecting the heel with padding around the tender area. Anti-inflammatories are usually prescribed, but surgical treatment may be necessary if the condition becomes chronic, particularly if it is accompanied by bossing of the heel bone. *See also* **Achilles tendinitis**; and **bursitis**.

pumping-up A body-builder's term for increasing the apparent size of muscle by lifting comparatively light weights many times in quick succession. The contraction of muscles compresses veins so that less blood leaves the capillaries than enters them through the arteries. The pressure within the capillaries is raised, forcing some of the fluid out into the tissue spaces and thus increasing the size of muscles. Shortly after exercise, the pressure is reduced as the excess fluid in the tissue spaces returns to the blood and the size of the muscle returns to normal.

punch drunk *See* **encephalopathy, traumatic**.

punishment An unpleasant stimulus presented immediately following a particular behaviour. Punishment is applied to weaken the response to which it is associated. *Compare* **negative reinforcement**; and **reward**.

pupillary constriction Reduction in size of the pupil in the eye (the central opening of the iris through which light enters the eye). Pupillary constriction functions with *accommodation and *convergence to enable a batsman, for example, to retain focus on a fast approaching projectile, such as a cricket ball.

Purkinje fibres Modified cardiac muscle fibres consisting of conduction myofibrils which act as a fast conduction system (known as the Purkinje system) from the right and left branches of an *atrioventricular bundle to all parts of the ventricles of the heart.

purpose An intention, expressed as a conscious thought in the present, to realize a future goal or aim.

purposive explanation An explanation of behaviour in terms of the purposes or the conscious intentions of the actors.

purposive sampling A form of sampling in which the selection of the sample is based on the judgement of the researcher as to which subjects best fit the criteria of the study. *Compare* **random sampling**.

purposivism An approach in psychology which claims that, in addition to stimuli, purposes are effective determinants of behaviour.

purulent Resembling, consisting of, or containing pus.

pus A thick yellow product of inflammation consisting of dead leucocytes, bacteria, cell debris, and tissue fluid.

Putti–Platt procedure A surgical procedure for stabilizing the glenohumeral joint after recurrent anterior shoulder dislocations. The subscapularis tendon is detached near its insertion on the humerus, the joint opened, and the stump of the tendon on the lesser tuberosity is sutured to the glenoid labrum. Sometimes the procedure is combined with reattachment of the glenoid labrum. The Putti–Platt procedure tends not to be performed on throwers because it can reduce the range of movement in the shoulder.

P wave Component of an *electrocardiograph which appears as a small positive deflection prior to the QRS complex. At rest, it normally lasts less than 0.12 s and has an amplitude of 0.25 mV or less. It represents atrial depolarization.

PWC$_{170}$ test *See* **physical work capacity**.

pyknomorph A *somatotype in the Conrad system that is equivalent to endomorph in the Heath–Carter system.

pyramid 1 A conical mass of cells in the kidney medulla. **2** A pyramid-shaped area in the medulla oblongata of the brain.

pyramidal cells Pyramid-shaped cells in the *motor cortex of the brain which send nerve impulses to voluntary muscle.

pyramidal system A collection of nerve tracts (*see* **pyramidal tract**) within the pyramid of the medulla oblongata.

pyramidal tract (corticospinal tract) A tract of nerve fibres which transmits nerve impulses from pyramidal cells in the motor cortex through the medulla oblongata to the anterior motor neurones of the spinal cord. *See also* **primary motor cortex**.

pyramid system A type of strength-training in which loads are increased successively in each set while the number of repetitions in a set is reduced. Assuming a 2-RM (*see* **repetition maximum**) of 45 kg, a typical session might consist of seven repetitions at 20 kg; six repetitions at 25 kg; five repetitions at 35 kg; three repetitions at 40 kg; and two repetitions at 45 kg.

pyramid training A formal method of varying the duration and intensity of work and recovery intervals in running, swimming, and canoeing (*see* **locomotives**).

pyrexia *See* **fever**.

pyridoxine *See* **vitamin B$_6$**.

pyrosis See **heart burn**.

pyrrole A five-membered ring structure which contains nitrogen. See also **porphyrin**.

pyruvate A salt or ester of *pyruvic acid.

pyruvic acid An important three-carbon molecule formed as an end-product of *glycolysis. In anaerobic metabolism (oxygen-independent glycolysis), pyruvic acid is converted into lactic acid, but if oxygen is available it is converted to acetyl coenzyme A which enters the *Krebs cycle.

Pythagorean theorem A theorem which states that for any right-angled triangle, the square of the hypotenuse is equal to the sum of the squares of the opposite two sides. Pythagorean theorem is used in biomechanics to solve problems dealing with vector quantities.

Q

Q to quotient

Q See **cardiac output**.

Q-angle (quadriceps angle) The angle formed between the longitudinal axis of the femur, representing the pull of the *quadriceps muscle, and a line that represents the pull of the patellar tendon. A clinical measure of the angle is obtained by connecting the central point of the patella with a line through the anterior iliac spine above and with a line through the tibial tuberosity below. The Q-angle is normally less than 15° in men and 20° in women when the qaudriceps are relaxed. The angle becomes smaller when the quadriceps are contracted. A Q-angle greater than 20° increases the likelihood of the quadriceps pulling the kneecap laterally, increasing the risk of knee disorders such as *patellofemoral pain syndrome.

QO$_2$ See **oxidative capacity**.

QRS complex The largest component of an *electrocardiograph. It corresponds to ventricular depolarization and, at rest, normally lasts less than 0.1 s.

Q–T interval The time interval from the start of the QRS complex to the end of the T wave. It reflects the electrical *systole of the *cardiac cycle.

Q$_{10}$ (temperature coefficient) A measure of the effect of a 10 °C rise in temperature on the velocity of a chemical reaction. The Q$_{10}$ is expressed as the ratio of the velocity of a chemical reaction at a given temperature to that of the same reaction at a temperature 10 °C lower.

quackery The activities or methods of an unqualified person who claims to have medical knowledge.

quadratus In anatomy, a four-sided muscle.

quadratus femoris A short, thick four-sided muscle which has its origin on the ischial tuberosity and extends laterally from the

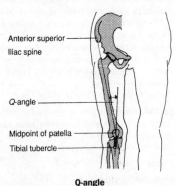

Anterior superior
Iliac spine

Q-angle

Midpoint of patella

Tibial tubercle

Q-angle

pelvis to have its insertion on the greater trochanter of the femur. Its primary action is lateral (outward) rotation of the femur.

quadratus lumborum One of a pair of fleshy muscles forming part of the posterior abdominal wall. It has its distal attachments on the iliolumbar ligament, next to the *iliac crest, and it has its proximal attachment on the last rib and the transverse processes of the first four lumbar vertebrae. Its primary action is lateral flexion of the spine. It also plays a role in maintaining an upright posture.

quadriceps *See* **quadriceps femoris**.

quadriceps angle *See* **Q-angle**.

quadriceps femoris (quadriceps; quads) A muscle at the front of the thigh which has four distinct portions: the rectus femoris, vastus intermedius, vastus lateralis, and vastus medialis. The four muscle heads join in a single tendon which crosses the patella to insert onto the tibial tuberosity. The quadriceps is the main extensor of the lower leg.

quadriceps haematoma *See* **charley horse**.

quadriceps insertion strain An *overuse injury characterized by pain in the tendon of the quadriceps muscle, just above and on top of the kneecap. Quadriceps insertion strain is commonly associated with excessive hill-running or squats.

quadriceps muscle-pull *See* **quadriceps strain**.

quadriceps strain (quadriceps muscle-pull) A relatively common injury involving one of the four *quadriceps muscles (usually the rectus femoris because it crosses two joints, the hip and knee). It is usually caused by overextension (e.g. when kicking) or overuse. Those most at risk are poorly conditioned athletes taking part in sports, such as badminton, squash, soccer, and basketball, which require explosive stop–start actions. Typically, the leg hurts when touched and feels sore when the quadriceps contracts during activities such as walking upstairs, running uphill, or doing squats. The cornerstone of treatment is rest, ice, compression, and elevation (*see* **RICE**). *See also* **muscle strain**.

quads *See* **quadriceps**.

qualitative Pertaining to subjective assessments or descriptions, such as 'bigger' and 'blue'. *Compare* **quantitative**.

qualitative analysis Identification of the components of a system and the description of those components in nonnumerical terms.

quality 1 A fundamental aspect or attribute of sensory experience, which is distinguishable in nonquantitative terms from others in the same sensory field. **2** The value, grade, or standard of excellence a performance. *Compare* **quantity**.

quality training *See* **model training**.

quantification The process of expressing observations in numerical terms to aid analysis and comparison.

quantitative Pertaining to objective, numerical measurements.

quantitative analysis Description of the components of a phenomenon, such as the movement of a mechanical system, in numerical terms. *Compare* **qualitative analysis**.

quantity The degree, amount, or size of a particular thing. *Compare* **quality**.

Quebec ninety-second test A *long-term anaerobic test consisting of a ninety-second maximal effort performed on a bicycle ergometer during which the total work performed is computed by a microprocessor.

Quebec ten-second test A *short-term anaerobic test consisting of a ten-second maximal effort on a bicycle ergometer with a microprocessor to record the total work performed each second.

questionnaire A form containing questions to which a subject or subjects respond. The information gained from the questionnaire is often subjected to statistical analysis. Questionnaires can be used to examine the general characteristics of a population, to compare attitudes of different groups, and to test theories. Questionnaires appear

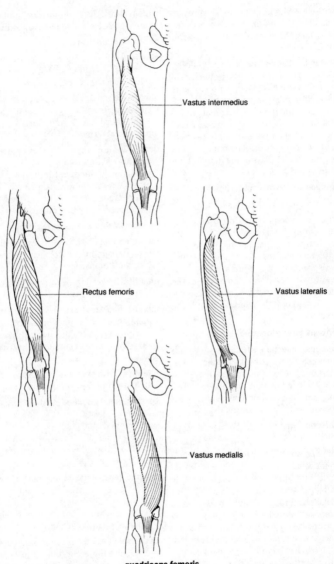

Vastus intermedius

Rectus femoris

Vastus lateralis

Vastus medialis

quadriceps femoris

simple, but they are very difficult to compile in a manner which establishes *reliability and *validity. A question worded in one way, for example, may elicit a differ-ent response from the same question worded slightly differently.

Quetlet index *See* body-mass index.

quiet breathing Relatively noiseless breathing typically performed by a person at rest who is not making forced ventilatory movements.

quinones A group of benzene derivatives. Quinones act as electron-carriers in *mitochondria. *See also* **vitamin K**.

quota sample A sample selected from a population as a proportion of each defined part of the parent population. The parent population is divided into a number of parts on the basis of some relevant factor, such as size, age, sex, or ethnic origin. The sample size for each part reflects the parent population structure. During sampling, the selection of individuals within a category continues until the quota has been filled. Quota sampling does not conform to the requirements of *random sampling.

quota system Restriction of the number of a particular group in a team. For example, in English cricket, each county team is allowed to have only a limited number of overseas players. The quota system is alleged to occur in the USA where the number of black players on some teams is limited.

quotient The result of dividing one number by another. *See also* **intelligence quotient**; and **respiratory quotient**.

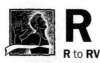

R
R to **RV**

R *See* **respiratory exchange ratio**.

race (racial group) A group of people who share a common ancestry. The use of the term in everyday language often implies that the group are biologically distinct and share qualities which are unalterable; this view of race has been biologically discredited and many sociologists prefer to use the term *ethnic group.

racial discrimination (racism) A prejudicial or unequal treatment of an individual or a group on the basis of their supposed membership of a racial or *ethnic group.

racial stratification Process by which the supposed membership of an individual or a group to a race becomes the basis for *social stratification.

racism *See* **racial discrimination**.

racquet player's pisiform An injury to the wrist involving roughening of the articular cartilage (a chondromalacia) between the *pisiform and triquetral bones (the piso-triquetral joint). It is thought to be due to repeated torsional stresses on the piso-triquetral joint by sharp and powerful supination–pronation movements performed by racquet players. The condition appears to be more common among squash and badminton players who use a lot of wrist action, than among tennis players who tend to make strokes using the shoulder. Golfers may also sustain a similar condition.

rad *See* **radian**.

radial 1 Pertaining to the *radius of the forearm. **2** Pertaining to the radius of a circle or ray.

radial acceleration The component of *angular acceleration which directs a body in angular motion towards the centre of curvature. Radial acceleration can be measured using the following formula: $a_r = v^2/r$, where a_r is the radial acceleration, v is the tangential linear velocity of a moving object, and r is the length of the radius of rotation.

radial artery A branch of the *brachial artery which passes down the forearm from the elbow, across the wrist, and into the palm of the hand.

radial component The component of a given *vector (for example, a force) acting at right angles to the curved path followed by a body. *Compare* **tangential component**.

radial deviation (wrist abduction) Movement of the hand toward the radial side of the arm brought about by the cooperative action of the flexor carpi radialis and extensor carpi radialis.

radiale An anatomical landmark at the upper and lateral border of the head of the *radius.

radial fossa A depression on the *humerus which receives the head of the radius when the elbow is flexed.

radial groove A groove which runs obliquely down the posterior aspect of the *humerus shaft and is the course of the radial nerve.

radial head fracture A fracture of the mushroom-shaped knob at the top of the radius in the elbow joint. Radial head fractures occur most commonly in contact and collision sports when a player falls onto an outstretched hand or arm. A fracture is characterized by excruciating pain on the outside of the elbow which worsens as bleeding swells the joint. Primary treatment involves sending for expert medical assistance, securing the arm to the body in a comfortable position (usually with the elbow at a 90 degree angle) and gentle application of ice for twenty minutes. Further treatment requires the expertise of an orthopaedic surgeon because a fracture in which the bone is displaced may require fixation. A bone fractured with no displacement may require only splinting the arm at a 90 degree angle for a few weeks, but rehabilitation to full mobility may take several months.

radial height A body height measured from *radiale to *base.

radial nerve An important mixed nerve (i.e., it carries both sensory and motor neur-

ones) which is a branch of the brachial plexus in the arm. It is one of three nerves which supply the forearm and hand.

radial pulse The *pulse taken by *palpation at the wrist where the radial artery runs alongside the radius.

radial reflex A *reflex action induced by tapping the lower end of the radius causing the forearm, and sometimes the fingers, to flex.

radian (rad) A unit of angular measure. The radian is the angle subtended at the centre of a circle by an arc equal in length to the radius of the circle. 1 rad = 57.3 degrees. Radians are often quantified in multiples of pi. One complete circle (equal to 360 degrees) is an arc of 2 pi radians.

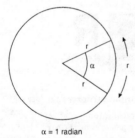

α = 1 radian

radian

radiation The emission or transfer of radiant energy (e.g., heat) as rays, electromagnetic waves, or particles. At rest, radiation is the main method of dissipating body heat. The nude body loses about 60 per cent of its excess heat by radiation.

Radin's rule A rule stating that structures will tear at their weakest point. For example, muscle tears occur most commonly at the musculotendinous junction.

radiocarpal joint The synovial condyloid joint between the *radius and the three proximal *carpal bones. It permits abduction, adduction, circumduction, extension, and flexion of the wrist.

radiography *See* X-ray.

radiohumeral joint *See* elbow joint.

radioimmunoassay A sensitive technique widely used to measure a range of biological substances, and to detect drugs such as peptide hormones and anabolic steroids during dope testing. The technique is based on the ability of an unlabelled form of the substance to inhibit competitively the binding of a radioactively labelled substance by specific antibodies. The concentration of the unknown sample is determined by comparing the degree of inhibition with that produced by a series of standards containing known amounts of the substance. The reliability of the test depends on the precise specification of the conditions under which the tests are made.

radiotelemetry Use of radio-transmitted signals to monitor heart rate, body temperature, and blood pressure during exercise.

radioulnar joint A synovial pivot joint between the radius and the ulna. The head of the radius rotates around a ring-like ligament secured to the ulna permitting pronation and supination of the forearm.

radius 1 A bone of the forearm. The radius is shorter than the *ulna and, in the anatomical position, lies laterally on the thumb side. **2** A line extending from the centre to the circumference of a circle.

radius of gyration In a rotating system, a length representing the distance between the point about which rotation of a body occurs (the axis of rotation) and the point at which the body's mass is distributed and has the maximum effect. It is the horizontal distance between the axis of rotation and a point which represents the sum of all the separate moments of inertia of the parts of the body. It is given by $k = \frac{1}{2}(I/m)$, where k = the radius of gyration, I = moment of inertia, and m = mass of the body.

radius of rotation For a rotating body, the linear distance from its *axis of rotation to a point of interest on the body.

ramus 1 A thin bar projecting from a bone that usually helps to form a joint. **2** A branch, especially or a nerve, artery, or vein.

Randle cycle (glucose–fatty acid cycle) A metabolic pathway linking fat and carbohydrate metabolism. Endurance-trained athletes may have a larger than normal concentration of fat oxidation enzymes and other enzymes involved in the Randle cycle. This would give them the ability to delay fatigue by deriving a major portion of their energy from fat metabolism, with a lower rate of lactate formation and sparing *muscle glycogen.

random Lacking any prearranged order, as if due to pure chance.

random practice Practice in which all components of a multi-task skill are practised in random order within each practice period.

random sample A sample from a population selected in a manner which ensures that each member of the population has an equal chance of being selected.

random sampling A procedure for selecting subjects or items for research on the basis of chance. The subjects or items are chosen from the population in such a way that all of them have the same chance of being selected.

range The spread of values of a set of data. The range is the difference between the maximum and minimum values and is a measure of the dispersion of a set of values. *See also* **descriptive statistics**.

range of motion (range of movement; ROM) The angle through which a joint moves from the anatomical position to the extreme limit of its motion in a particular direction. It is measured in degrees. For example, the ROM for flexion at the elbow is the difference between the angle at the elbow in the anatomical position (fully extended) and the angle at the elbow when it is in maximum flexion. If a knee joint can be extended from 30° at full flexion to 165° at full extension, its ROM is 165 − 30 = 135°. The complete range of motion of a joint is divided into three equal parts (the inner range, middle range, and outer range). *See also* **maximum active range**; **maximum passive range**; and **normal active range**.

range of movement *See* **range of motion**.

range of projectile The horizontal displacement of a projectile from its point of take-off and point of landing.

ranked list (ranked response) A technique, often used in questionnaires, in which the respondent places items in order of importance.

ranked response *See* **ranked list**.

ranking structure A system used to assign a player to a hierarchical position of excellence based on ability in a particular sport.

raphe A line, ridge, or furrow in a tissue or organ.

raptures of the deep *See* **nitrogen narcosis**.

ratchet mechanism The mechanism by which a muscle fibre can shorten. It consists of the attachment, detachment, and reattachment of cross bridges from *myosin onto *actin. *See also* **sliding-filament theory**.

rate control The ability to adjust the speed of movement of the body or body segments. Rate control is important for tasks such as shooting at a moving target, or kicking a ball to a moving team mate. *See also* **timing**.

rate of force development A measure of the rate at which a force is developed. Rate of force development (RFD) is measured in newtons per second or newton-metres per second. The average RFD is sometimes calculated as the *peak force divided by the time taken to reach peak force.

rate of relaxation A measure of the rate at which a force or torque is reduced when a muscle relaxes. It is important in sports which require a rapid cessation of muscle actions.

Rating of Perceived Exertion (RPE) A numerical scale, rating an individual's own subjective assessment of how hard he or she has worked during a physical activity. The Borg scale, devised by the Swedish physiologist Gunnar Borg, originally consisted of 15 grades from very, very light to very, very hard exertion. This has been modified in the New Borg Scale to take into account the fact that exercisers become more sensitive to changes of exertion at higher work rates. The Ratings of Perceived Exertion follow changes in heart rate quite closely and are therefore regarded as reasonably accurate estimates of actual exertion.

rating scale A technique used to measure, among other things, *personality. Typically, an independent judge or judges use a checklist or scale to assess behaviour of the subject in two types of situations: an interview or during the observation of a performance. The checklist contains specific traits and behaviours which are rated in terms of clarity and strength.

ratio 1 The numerical comparison of one class of objects with another, for example the ratio of men to women. **2** In mathematics, the numerical relationship between two quantities of the same type (e.g., the ratio of 30 g and 10 g, and 60 g and 20 g, are both 2:1.

rational choice theory An approach to sociological theorizing which assumes that social life can be explained in terms of the rational choices of individual *actors. That is, social life is the result of individuals choosing options which they believe likely to have the best overall outcome.

rationality The process of using reason or logic to solve a problem.

rationalization 1 The conscious or unconscious explanation of events or *behaviour which avoids giving the true reasons because they would be disadvantageous to the subject or they would be socially unacceptable. **2** The process whereby social organizations increasingly emphasize efficient means and planning in order to achieve their goals. *See also* **ludic institutionalization**.

raw score Score obtained directly from the measuring instrument, and which has not yet been tested by statistical methods.

Raynaud's phenomenon A condition of unknown cause in which the arteries of the fingers become hyperreactive to the cold and go into a spasm. It is more common in women than men, and may affect up to 10 per cent of otherwise healthy female athletes causing them great difficulties in cold environments. Warm gloves and calcium-channel blocking agents (e.g., nifedipine) may relieve the condition.

RBC An abbreviation sometimes used for red blood cell.

reaction board A device for estimating the *centre of gravity of a person. It consists of a board supported horizontally on two very thin edges, one of which rests on a block of wood while the other rests on a platform made of a set of scales. The subject's weight is measured in different body positions on the board and the figures used to estimate the centre of gravity.

reaction board method *See* **board and scales method**.

reaction force A counterforce; an equal and opposite force exerted by a second body on a first in response to a force applied by the first body on the second. *See also* **ground reaction force**.

reaction formation The repression of an unacceptable feeling or condition by reversing it to a directly opposite emotion or condition. For example, an athlete may deny his or her real feelings about a coach and instead reverse the personally less acceptable dislike, or, hate, into liking or even love. Reaction formation is regarded by some as a mechanism of *ego defence where the energies of the id are redirected in the opposite direction.

reaction, law of Newton's third law of motion which states that for every action there is an equal and opposite reaction. Therefore, when one object exerts a force on another, there will be an equal force exerted in the opposite direction by the second object on the first.

reaction potential In an athlete, the level of potential excitement associated with a particular response. Reaction potential is a construct of *drive theory. In any condition of competing responses, for example, one correct and the other incorrect, the selected response is the one associated with the highest reaction potential. This is

called the dominant response and may or may not be the correct response.

reaction time 1 The interval from presentation of a stimulus to the initiation of the response. Reaction time is a simple measure to make. It is used extensively in the *chronometric approach to information-processing to study the different stages of the processing. Reaction time is the sum of all the event-durations that occur between the presentation of a stimulus and the evocation of a response. It depends on the length of the neural path between the receptor organ (e.g. eye or ear) and the responding muscles (e.g. in the leg of runner) together with delays incurred when the information is processed centrally. Reaction times of 14–16 hundredths of a second for acoustic stimuli and 16–18 hundredths of a second for optical stimuli are generally regarded as good. **2** A skill-oriented ability underlying tasks for which there is one stimulus and one response, and for which the subject must react as quickly as possible to a stimulus in a single reaction time situation; for example, a sprint start in swimming. *See also* **choice reaction time**; **response time**; and **simple reaction time**.

reaction time probe technique *See* **probe technique**.

reactive aggression A form of *hostile aggression in which there is a conscious attempt to injure another person, as in a retaliation.

reactive behaviour In studies of coaching behaviour, the responses or reactions of the coach to player or team behaviour. An example of reactive behaviour is a coach verbally correcting an athlete after the athlete has made a mistake. *Compare* **spontaneous behaviour**.

reactive inhibition A term used in *drive theory to describe a depressant variable that is built up during nonreinforced trials and that reduces the quality of a performance. Reactive inhibition has been used to explain why a basketball player, attempting a hundred foul shots, performs better in the middle of the session than at the end, and generally performs better at the beginning of a new day than at the end of a previous session.

readiness The time, resulting largely from maturational factors, when somebody is first capable of responding correctly to a task.

readying mechanism A mechanism that predisposes a person to display *hostile aggression, but which is not the cause of the aggression. For example, hostile aggression is more likely to occur in the presence of a readying mechanism such as high levels of physiological *arousal.

rearfoot valgus A condition in which the rear of the foot tends to curve outwards at the ankle joint (it involves eversion at the subtalar joint). Those with rearfoot valgus usually need to strengthen the foot invertors, and may need instep supports or orthoses if participating in running sports.

rearfoot varus A condition in which the rear of the foot tends to curve inwards at the ankle due to inversion at the subtalar joint. Those with rearfoot varus tend to be more susceptible to ankle sprains when landing after a jump. They usually need to strengthen evertors to help pull the foot back to its neutral position.

reason A faculty of the human mind which enables logical inferences to be made and rational arguments to be undertaken to understand the world and solve problems.

reasoning Solving a problem implicitly, using symbols to represent objects or situations. Reasoning involves thinking through a problem rather than engaging in overt trial and error.

rebound The springing back of an object when it meets a resistance greater than its own. *See also* **angle of rebound**.

rebound hypoglycaemia *See* **insulin rebound**.

rebound rib A relatively uncommon fracture of the first rib, thought to be due to a violent contraction of the anterior scalenus muscle. It is characterized by poorly local-ized shoulder pain. Diagnosis depends on radiography. Treatment is usually conservative (e.g., ice-treatment; immobilization in a sling; and analgesics).

recall Retrieval of past experience; remembering a past event with minimal cues. In free recall, a series of events is recalled in any order; in serial recall, a specific order is required as well.

reception time The period of time between the beginning of a stimulus and the first change in electrical activity in the cerebral cortex of the brain. It is a part of *reaction time.

reception time The period of time between the beginning of a stimulus and the first change in electrical activity in the cerebral cortex of the brain. It is a component of *reaction time.

receptor A cell or group of cells that respond to particular types of stimuli. Receptors enable the body to detect changes in the internal or external environment. All sensory nerve-endings function as receptors. *See also* **exteroceptor**; **interoceptor**; and **proprioceptor**.

receptor anticipation A situation in which an individual anticipates the arrival of an event by watching or listening to relevant parts of the environment; the individual learns to associate critical events with the appropriate environmental stimuli. Receptor anticipation is very common and provides the basis for many motor tasks, enabling individuals to respond to signals at appropriate times. In cricket, for example, a fielder anticipates the arrival time of the ball and makes preparatory movements to catch it by listening to how the ball was struck and watching its progress.

receptor potential A *graded potential in a receptor cell.

receptor site A molecular site on the surface of, or within a cell that recognizes and binds with specific molecules, and which results in a specific change in the cell.

reciprocal determinism A phenomenon in which *self-efficacy is affected by and affects other variables. In sport, the experience of a previous performance (e.g. success or failure) influences the present level of self-efficacy and this in turn influences the next performance and so on.

reciprocal inhibition A process that inhibits the *stretch reflex in antagonistic pairs of muscles. When one muscle contracts it sends inhibitory nerve impulses to its opposing muscle causing it to relax.

reciprocal innervation Nerve interconnections between antagonistic pairs of muscles which enable *reciprocal inhibition to take place. A monosynaptic reflex arc links stretch receptors in each muscle to its opposing partner.

reciprocity An interaction between two parties, for example a coach and an athlete, when there is give and take on both sides and the two parties are working to mutual advantage.

recognition Perceiving something as having been experienced before, as being familiar; a method of measuring memory.

reconstruction surgery Surgery to reconstruct damaged tissue in deep structures, such as the cruciate ligament of the knee.

recovery The physiological processes taking place in the period following an acute bout of exercise when the body is restored to its pre-exercise condition. Recovery processes include replenishment of *muscle glycogen and *phosphagen stores, removal of lactic acid and other metabolites, reoxygenation of myoglobin, and protein replacement.

recovery period Period following exercise, when the body is restored to its pre-exercise condition.

recovery position A position in which an unconscious but breathing patient is placed in order to ensure that the airways are kept open.

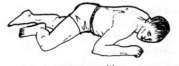

recovery position

recovery principle A major training principle which posits that adaptation takes place during the recovery period after training is completed.

recovery training Training performed the day after a competition or a hard training session. It consists of performing light physical activities, such as jogging, in which the mean heart rate is about 130 beats per minute.

recovery unit A period of time specified in a training schedule for rest and recovery within a microcycle (*see* **periodization**). Recovery is often accelerated if an athlete exercises lightly rather than rests completely.

recreation A term sometimes used synonymously with *leisure. However, recreation is usually used to describe active leisure. Sometimes its use implies that the activities have positive value in terms of mental and physical therapy. *See also* **physical recreation**.

recreational therapy The provision of treatment and recreational services to improve the health and well-being of people with illnesses or disabling conditions. Recreational therapy is designed to help patients regain their independence, and reduce or eliminate the effects of illness or disability.

recruitment The enlistment of different numbers and types of *muscle fibre during the contraction of a whole muscle. Recruitment follows a set pattern: slow-twitch fibres are brought into action first, then *fast-twitch a fibres (fast oxidative glycolytic FOG), and finally *fast-twitch b fibres (fast glycolytic or FG fibres). The level of recruitment is generally determined by the force demanded of a muscle. However, even during maximal efforts, the nervous system does not usually recruit all the available fibres. Normally, only a fraction of muscle fibres are stimulated at any specific time. This prevents damage to muscles and tendons which would probably be torn if all the fibres in a muscle were active at the same instant.

rectal Pertaining to the rectum.

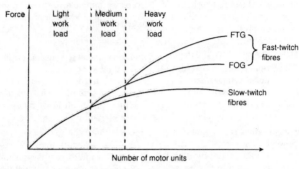

recruitment

rectangular motion *See* **linear motion.**

rectangular reference plane *See* **cardinal plane.**

rectangular test A test of *aerobic fitness in which the athlete exercises at one intensity level only, and maintains that exercise intensity as long as possible.

rectilinear motion Motion along a straight line in which all parts of the system (e.g. human body) move at the same speed and same direction. *Compare* **curvilinear motion.**

rectum Terminal part of the alimentary canal which stores the faeces.

rectus abdominis One of a pair of medial, superficial, abdominal muscles which extend from their proximal attachment of the costal cartilage of ribs 5–7 to their distal attachment on the *pubis. The rectus abdomini flex and rotate the lumbar region of the spine, fix and depress the ribs, stabilize the pelvis during walking, and increase intra-abdominal pressure.

rectus capitis anterior *See* **prevertebral muscles.**

rectus capitis lateralis *See* **prevertebral muscles.**

rectus capitis posterior major *See* **suboccipitals.**

rectus capitis posterior minor *See* **suboccipitals.**

rectus femoris A superficial muscle at the front (anterior) of the thigh. It is part of the *quadriceps femoris. Its origin is on the anterior inferior iliac spine and its insertion at the base of the patella and tibia via the patellar ligament. Its primary action is flexion of the femur about the hip joint and flexion of the tibiofemoral joint about the knee.

recurrent 1 Applied to an injury or illness that tends to occur again. **2** In anatomy, applied to a structure such as a blood vessel or nerve which turns back on itself to form a loop.

recurrent dislocation Repeated dislocations. Recurrent dislocations most commonly involve the shoulder or knee and often result from too energetic early mobilization following an acute dislocation. Once a recurrent dislocation pattern has established, surgical fixation may be necessary, but an alternative for noncontact athletes, such as jockeys and motor cyclists, might be harnessing.

red blood cell (red blood corpuscle; erythrocyte) A cell, normally confined to blood vessels, which is specialized to transport oxygen. When mature, red blood cells are biconcave discs which lack a nucleus and contain *haemoglobin.

red blood corpuscle *See* **red blood cell.**

red bone marrow The blood-forming tissue found within the internal cavities of bone. *See also* **yellow bone marrow.**

red fibre *See* **slow-twitch muscle fibre.**

red muscle *See* **slow-twitch muscle fibre.**

redox A chemical reaction in which there is a simultaneous *oxidation and *reduction.

reduced focus An *attentional style in which the individual has a chronic tendency to concentrate on a few stimuli and ignore other stimuli, even when this is not appropriate. *Compare* **narrow focus**.

reducible hernia An uncomplicated hernia which returns, either spontaneously or after manipulation, to its original site.

reduction 1 Addition of hydrogen or an electron, or removal of oxygen from an atom or molecule. **2** The restoration of a displaced part, such as a dislocated bone, to its original position (*see* **reducible hernia**).

reductionism The analysis of complex things into their simpler parts. It is sometimes used disparagingly of the notion that all complex things can be completely understood in terms of their component parts.

reference group A group used as a basis of self-appraisal or comparison. The use of the term implies that the action and behaviour of people within various social contexts are to some degree influenced by the group with which the individual primarily identifies. *Compare* membership group. *See also* **role theory**.

reference human *See* phantom.

reference man and woman A hypothetical man and woman, based upon the average physical dimensions from detailed measurements of thousands of subjects in anthropometric studies. Reference man has the following characteristics: age 20–24; height 68.5 in; weight 154 pounds; total fat 23.1 lb (15 per cent) of which storage fat is 18.5 lb (12 per cent) and essential fat is 4.6 lb (3 per cent); muscle 69 lb (44.8 per cent); bone 23 lb (14.9 per cent); remainder 38.9 lb (25.3 per cent). Reference woman has the following characteristics: age 20–24; height 64.5 in; weight 125 pounds; total fat 33.8 lb (27 per cent) of which storage fat is 18.5 lb (15 per cent) and essential fat is 15 lb (12 per cent); muscle 45 lb (36 per cent); bone 15 lb (12 per cent); remainder 31.2 lb (25 per cent).

reference point *See* **norm**.

referred pain (synalgia) Pain felt in an undamaged part of the body away from the actual point of injury or disease. It may be a visceral (abdominal organ) pain which is perceived as originating in the body wall due to the nerve impulses from visceral pain receptors travelling along the same pathway as somatic pain impulses, or the pain may arise in body wall structures and be referred distally. Degenerative changes in cervical vertebrae, for example, can cause tendinitis-like pain in the elbow, and degeneration of lumbar facets can cause calf pain.

reflection thesis The proposition that sport mirrors the beliefs, values, and norms that exist elsewhere in the wider society. Sport is therefore viewed, as in the *reinforcement thesis, as maintaining the status quo. *Compare* **resistance thesis**.

reflex *See* **motor reflex**.

reflex arc The essential neural pathway involved in a motor reflex which links the stimulus, the activated sensory receptor, and the response. A motor reflex arc usually consists of five elements: receptor, sensory neurone, an integration centre (e.g., an association neurone in the central nervous system; this may be absent in some reflex arcs), a motor neurone, and a muscle which acts as the effector.

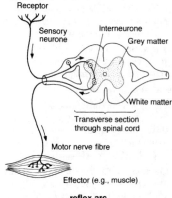

Receptor

Sensory neurone

Interneurone

Grey matter

White matter

Transverse section through spinal cord

Motor nerve fibre

Effector (e.g., muscle)

reflex arc

reflex-reversal phenomenon The phenomenon, observed in the study of locomotion, by which a given stimulus can produce two different reflex actions depending on the location of the limb in a movement. Usually, a reflex action is thought of as a single stereotyped response to a stimulus.

reflex sympathetic dystrophy A disorder of an organ or tissue characterized by pain much more severe than expected for the inciting trauma. It is thought to be due to abnormal activity of the sympathetic nervous system and/or hypersensitization of peripheral mechanoreceptors and/or nociceptors. Reflex sympathetic dystrophy has been recorded in the knee. It is usually presented as a swollen, painful, and immobile knee which is hypersensitive to the touch. There may also be bone and soft tissue changes. The condition may result from a direct blow to or a fall on the knee, or chronic overloading of the knee (e.g. by using weights to build-up the quadriceps). Treatment involves pain relief followed by physical therapy to restore mobility and reverse the bone and tissue changes.

refocusing The return of *attention to relevant stimuli after being distracted.

refractory Applied to a medical condition that does not respond to treatment.

refractory period If absolute, a period of total inexcitability of a nerve or muscle cell immediately following stimulation. After this absolute refractory period, there is a relative refractory period during which only a stronger than normal stimulus can excite the nerve or muscle.

regeneration Replacement of destroyed tissue by proliferation of the same kind of cells. Compare **fibrosis**.

regression See **regression analysis**.

regression analysis A statistical technique for analysing the relationship between two or more variables and which may be used to predict the value of one variable from the other or others.

regression line The 'line of best fit' between two variables, whose slope and intercept are determined by *regression analysis.

rehabilitation Restoration of an injured person to the level of physical fitness he or she had before the injury. In the past, rehabilitation often followed the treatment of the injury, but now it usually begins at the same time as the treatment. The aim of rehabilitation in sport is to facilitate the safe return of the athlete to training and competition at as high a standard and as quickly as the specific priorities of the athlete determines. See also **aggressive rehabilitation**.

rehearsal The repeated mental or physical practice of a motor skill used by an athlete in competition.

rehydration See **water replacement**.

reification The interpretation of an abstract idea or concept, such as the state, as real or concrete.

reinforcement (reinforcer) Anything following an action which tends to increase the probability of that action occurring again. Some workers include only rewards involving the satisfying of basic physiological needs. Others include social approval and similar psychosocial constructs. See also **external reinforcement, internal reinforcer; negative reinforcement;** and **positive reinforcement**.

reinforcement theory See social reinforcement theory.

reinforcement thesis The proposition that sport strengthens social inequalities experienced in the wider society and thereby maintains the status quo. For example, it is argued that sport involvement is perceived by the socially disadvantaged as a means of social mobility, thus reducing their frustration and imposing an element of social control. Compare **resistance thesis**.

reinforcer See **reinforcement**.

Reiter's syndrome A triad of arthritis, urethritis, and conjunctivitis, commonly associated with infection of the urinary tract. Reiter's syndrome can restrict movements; typically, it affects the ankle, knee, or elbow joints. Treatment includes long-term antibiotic therapy. Mechanical stress on the affected joints should be avoided but active exercise, under the direction of the treating doctor, is important to maintain joint mobility.

relapse Recurrence of an illness.

relationship 1 The tendency for variations in one variable to be associated with variations in some other variable. **2** The mutual dealings between two or more people. *See also* **interpersonal relationship**; and **intrapersonal relationship**.

relationship motivation A *leadership style which emphasizes concern with interpersonal relationships. It is regarded as equivalent to consideration. A coach adopting this style gives the needs of the athlete a high priority.

relative angle The angle at a joint formed between the longitudinal axes of the body segments adjacent to the joint. Relative angles are always measured on the same side of a particular joint. A straight, fully extended joint is regarded as having a relative angle of 0 degrees. *Compare* **absolute angle**.

relative body fat The ratio of fat mass to total body mass, expressed as a percentage. Relative body fat is often a better indicator of athletic potential than total body weight. In general, the greater the relative body fat, the poorer the athletic performance (with possible exceptions including swimming and sumo wrestling).

relative body mass The body mass of an individual calculated as a percentage of mean values for a normal population. Élite athletes in power sports tend to have a much higher relative body mass than those in endurance sports.

relative density The ratio of the density of a solid or liquid at a specified temperature (usually 20 °C), to the density of water at the temperature of its maximum density (4 °C). Relative density is generally used in preference to specific gravity.

relative force A hypothesized feature of a *motor program that defines the relationships between the forces produced in the various actions of a movement.

relative frequency of knowledge of results During the acquisition of a skill, the percentage of trials when knowledge of results are given; it is the absolute frequency divided by the number of trials.

relative humidity *See* **humidity**.

relative load In strength tests, a load which is a proportion of the weight of the lifter. *Compare* **absolute load**.

relative motion The motion of one body relative to another. For a body moving in a fluid, it is the difference between the speed of the body and the speed of the fluid. When considering the influence of a fluid on the motion of a body, the relative motion is more important than the absolute speed of either the fluid or the body. Most studies find it convenient to consider the body to be at rest and the fluid to be moving past it.

relative projection height The difference between the height from which an object is initially projected into the air and the height at which it lands or stops. The greater the relative projection height, the longer the flight time and the greater the horizontal displacement of a projectile (assuming a constant projection velocity).

relative refractory period A period following stimulation of a muscle fibre or nerve cell during which only a stronger than normal stimulus can evoke an action potential. *Compare* **absolute refractory period**.

relative strength The maximum force exerted in relation to body weight or muscle size. *Compare* **absolute strength**. *See also* **strength**.

relative velocity The rate at which one system is changing its position with respect to another system. When a body is moving in a fluid, in a direction opposite to the flow of the fluid, the magnitude of the body's relative velocity is the algebraic sum of the magnitude of its own velocity and that of the fluid. The relative velocity of the body will affect the magnitude of the forces (e.g., drag and lift) exerted by the fluid on the body.

relative weight The percentage by which a person is overweight or underweight, as determined by standard weight tables.

relaxation A controlled and relatively stable level of *arousal which is lower than the normal waking state. Relaxation is incompatible with feelings of *tension, worry, and *anxiety. Techniques such as *progressive muscle relaxation can be used to induce relaxation and obtain levels of optimal arousal before *competition (*see* **zone of optimal functioning**). *See also* **behaviour therapy; biofeedback training; desensitization;** and **progressive relaxation**.

relaxation procedure Any technique employed to reduce tension and *anxiety in sport. For example, an *intervention strategy or the use of a *drug.

relaxation response A set of changes in bodily functions such as slowing of the heart rate and breathing rate, and an increase in the brain waves associated with relaxation, that take place as a result of meditating or practising other relaxation techniques.

relaxation therapy Use of muscle relaxation to treat high levels of anxiety. *See also* **progressive muscle relaxation**.

relaxation time The time it takes for an active muscle to revert to its resting, relaxed state.

relaxed-arm girth The circumference of the arm at the midpoint between the *acromiale and the *radiale, when the subject is standing erect and the relaxed arm is hanging by the side. *See also* **body girth**.

relaxin A hormone secreted by the placenta in the terminal stages of pregnancy. It brings about a softening of connective tissues (cartilage and tendons), so that the bones at the front of the pelvis can separate, making it easier for the baby to be born. This can cause the sacroiliac joint to rotate abnormally and lead to pain in the low back and buttocks. Relaxin also affects tissues of other joints, loosening them and making them more susceptible to injury. These effects of relaxin may persist for several weeks after the birth of the baby. Therefore, most physicians advise expectant mothers to avoid vigorous weight-bearing exercises during the later stages of pregnancy and for a few weeks after the birth.

relearning Regaining a *skill that has been partially or wholly lost. The savings involved in relearning compared with original *learning gives an index of the degree of *retention.

release point (point of release) The point at which a projectile, such as a javelin, is released from the hand as the hand moves through an arc. The projectile moves in a line which is tangential to the arc at the point of release.

releaser A stimulus which serves to elicit instinctive behaviour.

releasing factors A chemical factor secreted by the *hypothalamus and transported to the anterior pituitary gland where it stimulates the secretion of a particular pituitary hormone. For example, growth-hormone-releasing-factor from the hypothalamus stimulates the secretion of *human growth hormone.

reliability (reproducibility) A characteristic of a measurement or experimental procedure which produces consistent results on two or more separate occasions. A typical way of testing reliability is to compare the results of two independent recorders. This is termed interrater reliability. High correlations between results (for example 0.80 or better) indicate reliability. Several statistics, such as *standard deviation of repeated tests, can give a measure of reliability. Reliability of tests on human activities is rarely perfect because of biological variance due to factors such as mood, time of day, previous experience affecting the activities. Reliability can be maximized, however, by standardizing as many of these factors as possible (e.g. test at the same time of day). *See also* **objectivity; validity; sensitivity**.

relief interval In *interval training, the time between work intervals as well as between sets.

reminiscence An improvement in later performance due to rest or non-practice. The period of rest is called the retention interval. Thus far, studies yield inconsistent results as to the optimal retention interval for reminiscence. *See also* **inhibition**.

REM sleep A phase of sleep during which dreaming takes place. REM is an abbreviation for 'rapid eye movement'. During this phase the sleeper's eyes move quickly, heartbeat and metabolism speed up, and toes and fingers twitch. Disturbance of REM sleep may result in fatigue and irritability, leaving an athlete less able to cope with physical exertion. *See also* **sleep**.

renal Pertaining to the kidney.

renal buffering A homeostatic mechanism which uses the kidneys to help maintain the acid–base balance by excreting either an acidic or alkaline urine in response to changes in the hydrogen ion concentration of body fluids. Renal buffering involves a complex series of reactions within kidney tubules.

renin An enzyme released by the kidneys in response to exercise, stress, low blood pressure, and reduced blood flow. Renin indirectly increases sodium retention and helps to maintain the plasma volume. When blood pressure is decreased, renin reacts with a substance in the liver (angiotensinogen) to produce two different forms of angiotensin which constricts arterioles (increasing blood pressure) and triggers the release of aldosterone (which increases the reabsorption of sodium from the kidney tubule into the blood). This control of blood pressure by the kidney is called the renin–angiotensin mechanism. Overproduction of renin can cause hypertension.

renin–angiotensin mechanism *See* renin.

rennin An enzyme produced in the stomach to coagulate milk protein and delay the passage of milk into the small intestine. The delay enables other enzymes to break the protein down into absorbable amino acids. Relatively large amounts of rennin are present in the gastric juice of infants.

Renshaw cells Interneurones which make connections with motor neurones in the medial region of the ventral horn of the spinal cord. Renshaw cells act as a link between motor neurones and sensory neurones from muscles and the skin.

repetition 1 In interval training, the number of work intervals in one set. For example, an interval training prescription of 6 × 200 m would constitute one set of six repetitions. **2** In strength training, the number of times an exercise is performed without stopping. *See also* **repetition maximum**.

repetition maximum (RM) The maximum load that a muscle group can overcome for a given number of repetitions before *fatigue prevents further muscle action. The 10RM, for example, is the maximum load that can be overcome for 10 repetitions.

repetition running Running a given distance at a predetermined speed a specific number of times with complete rest and recovery (usually walking) after each run. It is usually performed at, or near, race pace to develop *anaerobic metabolism.

repetition training Training which follows the same pattern as *repetition running, but which may be adapted for swimming, cycling, and other sports.

repetitive method A method of *learning a skill in which the subject learns a part, then combines it with a new part and practises them together until learned. These two are then combined with a third part and practised together until mastered. The procedure is followed for each remaining part until all are practised as a whole. It is a variant of the *progressive part method.

repetitive strain injury An injury to soft tissues, especially tendons, due to repeated use of a muscle or muscle group. In an industrial setting, tenosynovitis of the forearm (colloquially called 'teno') is often regarded as a repetitive strain injury to those tendons that pass through the forearm and cross the wrist to be inserted into the hand. Any activity involving frequent and repeated grasping (e.g., weight-lifting and rowing) may provoke a repetitive strain injury. *See also* **de Quervain's disease**; and **overuse injury**.

replacement drink A drink specifically designed to replace water, energy, and electrolytes and to assist recovery after exertion. *See also* **electrolyte drink**; **energy drink**; and **water replacement**.

replication The folding back of a tissue on itself.

repolarization The process by which a neurone or muscle fibre regains its resting potential after it has discharged an action potential.

representative sample In research, a small group which reflects accurately the characteristics of the total population.

repression An *ego defence mechanism where an unacceptable wish or idea is excluded from the conscious mind.

reproducibility *See* **reliability**.

reproduction *See* **social reproduction**.

required leader behaviour *See* **prescribed leader behaviour**.

RER *See* **respiratory exchange ratio**.

research method The techniques of investigation used by a particular academic discipline.

research question A question posed by a scientist about a previously unknown area of a subject which requires a systematic, scientific investigation to answer.

residual volume The volume of air remaining in the lungs at the end of maximal expiration; a typical value is 1200 ml. The residual volume (RV) equals the difference between the total lung capacity (TLC) and vital capacity (VC) ($RV = TLC - VC$).

resilience A measure of a body's resistance to deformation. Resilience is usually defined as the work required to deform an elastic body to its elastic limit divided by the volume of the body.

resistance The amount of force opposing a movement.

resistance arm The perpendicular distance from the axis of a lever to the point of resistance in the lever.

resistance runs A special form of resistance training consisting of repeated runs against an added resistance, such as a hill, weights on the body, a drag which has to be pulled, or a soft, uneven surface (often sand). *See also* **functional overload**.

resistance thesis The proposition that sport provides an arena for opposing the interests, values, and norms of the wider society. *Compare* **reflection thesis**; and **reinforcement thesis**.

resistance training Training aimed at developing power and strength. Resistance training can use static (isometric) actions, dynamic (ballistic) actions, or both. Dynamic actions include weight-training (with free weights or on a machine, such as a variable resistance device or an isokinetic machine), *plyometrics, and all other forms of training which involves working against loads greater than normally experienced. Resistance training using weights is usually based on an individual's *repetition maximum. Typically, beginners use a weight one half of their 1-RM which they should be able to lift about ten times. Most athletes include resistance training as an important component of their overall training programmes. It is also recognized as important for nonathletes who wish to gain the health-related benefits of exercise. Resistance training can improve the strength and muscle mass of elderly people, reducing the risk of falls, a major source of injury for the elderly. The benefits of resistance training in sport are very specific. When athletes train they should try to use movement patterns and speeds that closely mimic those needed for their particular sport (*see* **principle of specificity**).

resistance vessel A vessel which regulates blood pressure.

resisted active exercise An exercise in which the action of muscles is resisted by an external force, for example weights or a spring.

resisted movement A particular movement attempted by using the appropriate muscle actions but which is resisted by someone or something blocking it. Thus a resisted movement involves a static muscle action and no movement of a joint. Resisted movements are used in the diagnosis of sports injuries to test for muscle or tendon damage.

resocialization A process of socialization in which individuals take up new social identities and make a sharp break with a prior *socialization. It applies to the socialization of an individual who adjusts to retirement from professional sport by taking up another sport (or the same sport at a lower level), and placing sport at a lower priority than work, family, or education.

resolution of forces The mathematical process of dividing forces into components that act in specified directions.

resonance The condition of a body when it is subjected to a periodic series of disturbances having a frequency equal to one of the natural frequencies of vibration of the body. The body is set into vibrations which have a maximum amplitude. A trampolinist who moves in phase with the trampoline will be projected higher than one who is not.

respiration Any or all of the processes used to generate metabolic energy, mainly in the form of adenosine triphosphate, from the breakdown of food. *See also* **cellular respiration**.

respiratory acidosis An increase in hydrogen ion concentration of the blood (*see* **acidosis**) caused by failure to expire carbon dioxide from the lungs as quickly as it is formed in the tissues. Carbon dioxide accumulates in the blood where it forms carbonic acid which dissociates to increase the hydrogen ion concentration. *Compare* **metabolic acidosis**.

respiratory alkalosis A decrease in hydrogen ion concentration (an increase in pH) caused by hyperventilation and a reduction of carbon dioxide in the body fluids. It may occur where partial pressures of oxygen are low (e.g., at high altitude). *Compare* **metabolic alkalosis**.

respiratory centre An area of the *medulla oblongata and pons (part of the brainstem) which controls the rate and depth of breathing in order to maintain respiratory rhythm.

respiratory chain A chain of organic molecules on the inner surface of mitochondria capable of accepting hydrogen atoms

respiratory chain

and electrons derived from the *Krebs cycle during *aerobic metabolism. The hydrogen atoms, and then the electrons, are transferred in an ordered sequence along the chain by a series of redox reactions; the final reaction involves the reduction of oxygen to form water. The redox reactions liberate free energy which is used to manufacture ATP; this metabolic process is known as oxidative phosphorylation.

respiratory dead space See anatomical dead space.

respiratory exchange ratio (gas exchange ratio; R; RER) The ratio of the volume of carbon dioxide eliminated from the lungs per minute to the volume of oxygen taken into the lungs during the same time. RER = VCO_2/VO_2. During rest, the respiratory exchange ratio usually equals the respiratory quotient (RQ), but during exercise an unstable state arises due to expired air containing carbon dioxide and oxygen derived from stores within the body, and the R value is not the same as the RQ value.

respiratory frequency The number of breaths an individual takes per minute. Values vary, but an average figure for a healthy, resting, recumbent young male, breathing air at sea level is 12 breaths per minute. The value may change with position, age, size, sex, altitude, and activity.

respiratory insufficiency A condition in which the respiratory system is unable to meet fully the demands of the body for the supply of extra oxygen and the removal of carbon dioxide during exercise.

respiratory membrane The membrane separating air within the alveoli from the blood within pulmonary capillaries. It consists of the alveolar wall, the capillary wall, and their basement membranes. The respiratory membrane is very thin (less than 0.5 micrometres).

respiratory minute volume See minute ventilation.

respiratory muscles Muscles involved in breathing. The main respiratory muscles are the intercostals and diaphragm, but during exercise other muscles may contribute to ventilation. During inhalation, contractions of the scaleni and sternocleidomastoids assist the actions of the external intercostals and diaphragm to increase the thoracic cavity and draw air into the lungs. During exhalation, contractions of the abdominal muscles combine with contractions of the internal intercostals to reduce the thoracic cavity and force air out of the lungs.

respiratory pump A mechanism which helps to pump blood back to the heart during inspiration. Intrathoracic pressure decreases during inspiration, causing the pressure in the atria of the heart to drop to around 2.1 kPa, aspirating blood towards the right atrium from the thoracic vein.

respiratory quotient (RQ) The ratio of the amount of carbon dioxide produced to the amount of oxygen consumed in tissues of the body (compare respiratory exchange ratio). The RQ can be used to determine which food is being metabolized during cellular respiration. The RQ for fat metabolism is 0.7; for protein metabolism, 0.9; and for carbohydrate metabolism 1.0. An RQ greater than 1.0 indicates anaerobic metabolism.

respiratory rhythm The rhythm of alternating inspiratory and expiratory movements which take place during breathing. Four respiratory centres are thought to control the respiratory rhythm: the inspiratory centre and expiratory centre in the medulla, and an apneustic centre and pneumotaxic centre in the pons.

respiratory surface In humans, the surface of the *alveolus, specialized for gaseous exchange between air in the lungs and gases in the blood.

respiratory system The organs and tissues involved in breathing and gaseous exchange. The system includes the nose, nasal passages, nasopharynx, larynx, trachea, bronchi, and lungs.

respiratory threshold See minute ventilation method.

respiratory tree (bronchial tree) The principal airway from the nose or mouth, through the pharynx, larynx, and trachea into the bronchi which branches and terminates in the alveoli.

respiratory work The work done by the respiratory muscles during inspiration and expiration. Respiratory work consists mainly of overcoming the elastic resistance and flow-resistive forces of the thorax and lungs. At rest, the respiratory muscles require about 0.5–1.0 ml of oxygen per litre of ventilation. With increasing ventilation, the oxygen cost per unit of ventilation becomes progressively greater. It has been estimated that respiratory work uses as much as 10 per cent or more of the total oxygen uptake during heavy exercise. However, under normal conditions, respiratory work is not a limiting factor of exercise unless the oxygen delivered to the circulation by the additional ventilation is less than the corresponding increment in oxygen consumption by respiratory muscles. Under most circumstances, ventilation is well adapted to ensure maximum uptake.

respondent A person who completes a questionnaire.

responders Individuals who benefit significantly from completing a particular training programme when compared with nonresponder. Responsiveness to training seems to be determined mainly by genetic factors.

response The way a person, an organ, or a cell, reacts to a stimulus. In the *social reinforcement theory, the response is not separated from the stimulus and is an alteration of behaviour occurring as the result of the presence of a stimulus.

response-chaining hypothesis An early explanation of movement control which suggested that each action is triggered by *feedback from the immediately previous action. A movement is initiated by an external stimulus which causes a muscle or muscle group to contract. The muscle contraction generates sensory information called response-produced feedback. This feedback serves as a trigger for the next contraction and so on until the movement

sequence is completed. Research has shown that feedback is not essential for all motor actions, therefore the response-chaining hypothesis cannot be universally applicable.

response delay The period of time between a stimulus and the reaction or response of an individual. The response delay is a function of the amount of information which needs to be processed.

response integration An ability underlying tasks for which the utilization and application of sensory cues from several sources must be integrated into a single response.

response orientation An ability to choose rapidly between alternative movement patterns. Response orientation is apparently related to the ability to select a correct movement under *choice reaction time situations.

response-programming stage A stage of information processing in which a previously chosen response is transformed into overt muscular action. The duration of this stage is affected by the response complexity.

response rate The percentage of the total number of subjects sampled who respond to a survey or *questionnaire.

response selection stage A stage of *information processing concerned with translating the decision mechanism which leads to the choice of response associated with the presented stimulus. The duration of this stage is affected by variables such as the number of stimulus–response alternatives and stimulus–response compatibility.

response time The time interval from the presentation of a stimulus to the completion of a movement; it is the sum of reaction time and movement time.

rest 1 In biomechanics, the state of a body with a speed of zero which does not change position; a state of no motion. **2** A state of physical inactivity. Rest is an essential component of the primary management of most sports injuries. The rest required varies from absolute or complete rest to partial or relative rest, depending on the severity of the injury. The need for rest may apply only to an affected limb, not to the whole body.

resting heart rate The heart rate at rest. The average resting heart rate is between 60–80 beats per minute. Regular endurance training can reduce the resting heart rate to less than 40 beats per minute. During initial training, the resting heart rate of previously sedentary subjects decreases by about 1 beat per minute per week. An increase in resting heart rate may indicate stress from overtraining.

resting membrane potential (resting potential) The potential difference between the electrical charges inside a cell and outside the cell when the cell is in a resting state (e.g., when a neurone is not conducting a nerve impulse, or when a muscle fibre is not producing tension). The resting membrane potential is established by an unequal distribution of charged ions on either side of the cell surface membrane. In a *motor neurone, the inside of the cell is negatively charged relative to the positively charged outside, and the resting membrane potential is about –60 mv.

resting metabolic rate The *metabolic rate of a person at rest. When the resting metabolic rate is measured early in the morning in a laboratory under optimal conditions of quiet and relaxation, following an overnight fast and 8 hr sleep, it is regarded as an approximation of basal metabolic rate.

resting potential *See* **resting membrane potential**.

restitution *See* **elasticity**.

restoring force A *force tending to maintain the dimensions of a body and restore the original dimensions of a body once a distorting force is removed. *See also* **elasticity**.

rest recovery A form of recovery used in interval training in which an athlete rests between work periods. *Compare* **exercise recovery**.

rest relief In interval training, a type of relief interval involving moderate moving about,

such as walking and flexing of an arm or leg.

resultant (resultant vector; vector sum) A single *vector, such as a force or velocity, that produces the same effect as that of two or more vectors of the same type acting together.

resultant displacement The position from a starting point, expressed in terms of distance, when there have been two or more specified changes of direction.

resultant moment The sum of moments about the point at which a body, acted on by a number of forces, is tending to rotate.

resultant vector *See* **resultant**.

resuscitation The process of restoring to consciousness someone who appears to be dead. *See also* **artificial resuscitation**.

retaliation hypothesis The supposition that an athlete will not participate in acts of *aggression if he or she fears counter-aggression from a potential victim.

retardation 1 Negative acceleration, or deceleration; the rate of decrease of velocity. **2** The slowing up, or delayed development of a process. For example, mental retardation refers to a delay in intellectual development.

retention The maintenance of learning so that it can be utilized later, as in recall, recognition, or relearning.

reticular Resembling a network.

reticular activating system One of two parts of the reticular formation in the brainstem which maintains the alert state of the cerebral cortex and is concerned with *arousal. The reticular activating system filters out repetitive stimuli, preventing sensory overload.

reticular fibres A network of *connective tissue fibres. Reticular fibres support many structures including muscles, nerves, and blood vessels.

reticular formation A functional brain system that spans the central core of the medulla oblongata, pons, and midbrain. The reticular formation includes the two reticular activating systems which help regulate the sensory input to the cerebral cortex and cortical arousal. It also contains motor nuclei which help to regulate skeletal muscle activity.

reticular tissue Tissue consisting of a network of *reticular fibres, typically in a loose matrix. Reticular tissue forms a soft internal skeleton supporting other cells, for example, in bone marrow.

reticulin Collagen-like protein fibres found in *reticular tissue.

retina Lining of the interior of the eye containing photoreceptor cells (rods and cones) that are connected to the optic nerve. The retina lies below the vascular choroid which nourishes it. *See also* **detached retina**.

retinaculum A band of thick tissue which supports and maintains the position of other tissue. In the wrist, for example, the *fascia are thickened into retinacula that form protective passageways through which tendons, nerves, and blood vessels pass.

retinol *See* vitamin A.

retraction Nonangular backward movement in a transverse plane that returns a protracted bone or body-part to its original position. An example of retraction is squaring the shoulders in a military-like stance. *Compare* **protraction**.

retraining The recommencement of training after a period of no or little training. There is no unequivocal, clear scientific evidence that prior training increases the rate or magnitude of training adaptations.

retrieval The mental process of recalling information from the *long-term memory.

retroactive inhibition The partial or complete obliteration of memory by a more recent event, particularly new learning. *Compare* **proactive inhibition**.

retroactive transfer A form of *transfer of training in which the learning and/or performance of a skill influences the performance of another skill which has already been learned.

retrocalcaneal bursa Bursa between the *calcaneus and the *Achilles tendon. The anterior aspect of the retrocalcaneal bursa consists of a thin layer of cartilage covering a part of the tuberosity onto which the Achilles tendon inserts.

retrocalcaneal bursitis *See* Achilles bursitis.

retrograde amnesia A form of *amnesia in which there is a loss of memory of events occurring before a trauma.

retrospection A systematic recall of what has been experienced in the past.

rev *See* revolution.

reversal theory A theory of *arousal and *personality which combines aspects of *drive theory and the *inverted U-theory. It suggests that although athletes are disposed to be either paratelic (excitement seeking) or telic (anxiety avoiding), they can switch back and forth between these two orientations or states of mind. It is thought that the athletes' state of mind at any particular time will depend on three factors: contingent events, the athletes' degree of frustration, and the athletes' level of satiation.

reverse action muscle A muscle which can move its point of origin towards its point of insertion. Muscles usually move their insertion towards their origin. For example, the *gluteus maximus works in the normal manner when it extends the hip joint: when the leg is pulled backwards, the insertion on the femur moves towards the origin on the pelvis, which remains stationary. However, it exhibits a reverse action when the trunk is bent forwards: the gluteus maximus pulls the trunk upright by moving its origin on the pelvis towards its insertion on the femur, which remains stationary.

reversibility principle A basic principle of training which refers to the gradual loss of beneficial training effects when the intensity, duration, or frequency of training is reduced. Training effects produced over a short term are usually lost more quickly than those produced over a longer term, and strength losses tend to be faster than mobility losses.

revolution (rev) Unit used in the measurement of angular distance. In some sports, such as diving, the unit is not stated but implied; for example, a twist is one revolution about the longitudinal axis of the body, and a somersault is one revolution about the horizontal axis parallel to the end of the diving board. One complete revolution produces an angular displacement of 360 degrees. The term is always used in relation to a particular axis of the body.

revolve Behaviour of a body which has a circular motion around an axis which is outside the body.

reward A positive reinforcement in which the consequences of a particular action have an incentive value to the actor (e.g., an athlete) so that the action is more likely to be repeated.

rewarding behaviour Coaching behaviour which reinforces an athlete by recognizing and rewarding good performance. *See also* **positive feedback**.

Reynold's number A dimensionless quantity named after Osborne Reynolds (1842–1912), applied to a fluid flowing through a tube with a circular cross section. The Reynold's number is expressed by the equation $Re = vpl/n$, where v = velocity of flow, p = density of the liquid, l = diameter of the tube, and n = the coefficient of viscosity of the liquid. When the Reynold's number exceeds a critical value, the flow of the fluid changes from streamline or laminar flow of the fluid to turbulent.

rhabdomyolitis A destructive muscle condition associated with heat exhaustion. It can lead to renal failure, indicated by a dark-coloured urine, and fluid congestion of the heart and lungs. It has been recorded in a weight-lifter who took a sauna 15 minutes after a strenuous weight-lifting session. Exercisers are advised not to take very hot baths immediately after strenuous activity.

rhe SI unit of fluidity; it is the reciprocal of *poise.

rheography A cardiovascular functional test which gives a graphical record of the flow of blood through blood vessels.

rheumatism Any disorder in which aches and pains affect joints and muscles. Rheumatism is marked by inflammation, stiffness, and pain in and around the joints.

rheumatoid arthritis A chronic inflammatory disorder which primarily affects the joints, but may also affect tendons, tendon sheaths, muscles, and bursae. The main symptoms are stiffness, pain, and swelling of the affected joints. Although sufferers may find competitive sport difficult, physical exercise, particularly active mobility exercises, can be beneficial. Because symptoms are similar, rheumatoid arthritis sometimes masquerades as sport-related musculo-skeletal injuries, with a true diagnosis being made only after rheumatological screening.

rhinencephalon Part of the *cerebrum concerned with the reception and integration of olfactory impulses.

rhinitis Inflammation of the nose. Acute rhinitis is a symptom of a common cold and hay fever. Rhinitis usually results in blockage of the nose, but this rarely limits aerobic performance because breathing switches from the nose to mouth when the *minute ventilation volume rises above 25 l. Rhinitis has assumed far greater importance in sports medicine than it really deserves, because many of the drugs used to treat the condition contain banned substances (e.g. codeine). Several élite athletes have been disqualified from competitions because they have used these substances.

rhizopathy An intense, sharp pain with clearly defined limits following the distribution of an affected nerve.

rhomboideus muscles *See* **rhomboids**.

rhomboid major *See* **rhomboids**.

rhomboid minor *See* **rhomboids**.

rhomboids Two rectangular muscles, the rhomboid major and rhomboid minor, in the upper back between the backbone and the shoulder blade. The rhomboids have their origins on the sixth and seventh cervical vertebrae, and their insertions on the inner border of the shoulder blade. They act together and with the trapezius to 'square' the shoulders; they rotate the scapula so that the *glenoid cavity rotates downwards, as when the arm is lowered against a resistance (for example when paddling a canoe); and they also stabilize the *scapula.

rhythm Any sequence of regularly recurring functions or events, such as certain physiological processes (e.g., *see* **circadian rhythm**). Locomotory movements may also have a rhythm as in the regular repetition of a stride sequence in running or the stroke action in swimming. A sense of rhythm and an ability to maintain a regular sequence during locomotory functions is an important skill in sport. *See also* **timing**.

rib One of twelve pairs of long, flat, curved bones forming part of the thoracic cage, attached at one end to a thoracic vertebra. *See also* **false ribs**; **floating ribs**; and **true ribs**.

riboflavin *See* **vitamin B₂**.

RICE An acronym for a simple and effective primary treatment for many sports-related musculo-skeletal injuries: R, rest the injured part (this may require either absolute or relative rest, depending on the severity of the injury); I, apply ice (*see* **ice treatment**); C, apply compression (*see* **bandage**); and E, elevate the injured extremity above the level of the heart to facilitate *venous return. RICE is the cornerstone for treating many sports injuries. For soft-tissue injuries, such as sprains and strains, RICE should begin as soon as the injury occurs, or as soon as symptoms are felt. RICE helps reduce swelling, restricts bruising, and accelerates the healing process.

rickets Deficiency disease of children in which bones do not harden and are deformed due to lack of vitamin D.

rider's bone (rider's thigh) A condition resulting from calcification in the thigh bone (femur) following overuse and inflammation of the thigh adductors (*see* **myositis ossificans**).

rider's strain (adductor strain) A *strain of the *adductor muscle, a thick band of muscle on the inner side of the thigh. It is relatively common among fast bowlers, and footballers who make lunge tackles.

rider's thigh *See* rider's bone.

ridge A long, narrow protuberance on a bone which runs along the shaft as a crest.

right-hand thumb rule A procedure for identifying the direction of a *vector for angular motion. The angular motion vector is represented by an arrow drawn so that if the curled fingers of a person's right hand points in the direction of rotation, the direction of the arrow coincides with the direction indicated by the extended thumb. The magnitude of the vector is indicated by the length of the arrow. Any angular motion vector can be represented in this way and can be either added to a corresponding vector to obtain a resultant or can be resolved into components using a *parallelogram of vectors.

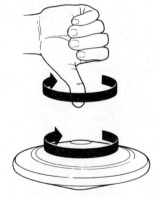

right-hand thumb rule

right spin *See* side spin.

righting reflex A reflex resulting in the body or a body segment tending to regain its former body position when it is displaced. Righting reflexes are strong in performers of physical activities, such as gymnastics, in which the position of the head is altered quickly. Gymnasts need to learn to modify and overcome these responses to perform certain routines.

rigid body A solid object which tends not to change shape when forces are applied to it.

rigidity In the context of *learning, an inability to change behaviour patterns, attitudes, or body postures.

rigor complex A chemical complex formed between *myosin and *actin during a muscle action. In the rigor complex, the myosin head is bent to the 45 degree position and is bound to actin. Unbinding of the head requires ATP and removal of calcium bound to *troponin, so that *tropomyosin can prevent the myosin head from binding to the actin. Muscle cramps may be due to the development of a rigor complex, either because of lack of ATP or an inability to remove calcium. *See also* **sliding-filament theory**.

Ringelmann effect The decrease in average individual performance with increases in group size. It was named after a German psychologist, Ringelmann, who studied groups pulling on a rope. He found that the average *force for 2 persons was 93% of average individual force; the average force for 3 persons 85% of average individual force, and the average force for 8 persons was only 49% of the average individual force. It was once thought that the Ringelmann effect was due to coordination difficulties as group size increases, now it is thought to be primarily the result of motivational losses. *See also* **social loafing**.

Ringman's shoulder Tendinitis at the insertion of the *pectoralis major muscle in the shoulder. It is commonly associated with repeated maintenance of the iron-cross position in gymnastics.

ringworm An infection of the skin, hair, or nails by a microscopic fungus (including *Tinea* and *Epidermophyton*). The infection usually develops as a dry, scaly, circular area on the skin. *See also* **Athlete's foot; and dhobie itch**.

risk factor Any factor, environmental or organic, which has a strong association with the onset and progress of a disease or injury. Risk factors for hypokinetic diseases include poor diet, heavy smoking, an inactive lifestyle, and stress. *See also* **cardiac risk factor**.

risk-taking behaviour Behaviour of a person who tends to choose challenging tasks with relatively low probabilities of success. It has been hypothesized that athletes with high achievement orientation tend to seek out relatively challenging situations, such as those with a 50% chance of failure, while those with low achievement orientation tend to choose very easy or very difficult tasks. Highly motivated athletes tend to perform much better in challenging situations than in situations where there is a high probability of success.

rite of passage A ceremony or ritual which may take place when a person changes *social status and social identity. For example, the presentation of a County cap for a cricketer who has become a regular first-team player.

rivalry Behaviour where defeating opponents has a high priority. *Compare* **competition**.

robust statistic A statistic which gives the same results in spite of some of the assumptions for its use being violated.

rocket jump A test of jumping ability which reflects the dynamic concentric work produced mainly by the ankle, knee, and hip extensors. The jump is initiated from a static position with no counter movement. The subject assumes a crouched position with the trunk vertical and, hands on hips, jumps vertically upwards using only the legs for propulsion.

role The behaviour expected of a particular person by society. Examples are roles of teacher, coach, team captain, and referee.

role conflict (role strain; role stress) Situation which arises as the result of performing two or more inconsistent roles. For example, a coach may have to perform the conflicting roles of teacher, friend, and team selector. *See also* **cognitive dissonance**.

role differentiation The degree to which different members of a group have specialized functions. *See also* **division of labour**.

role model A person whose behaviour and attitude conforms with that which society or other social groups expects of a person in his or her position, and who has become an example for others to copy.

role modelling hypothesis The hypothesis that youths of particular minority or ethnic groups take up specific roles and positions in sports teams because they wish to copy highly successful players from the same group. For example, it is argued that many black youths in North America tend to compete in noncentral positions in sports teams because they are trying to emulate black élite athletes who they previously saw performing successfully in those positions.

role-related behaviour An individual's behaviour which is determined by the *role of the person and the person's perception of how he or she should behave in particular environmental situations. It is rarely a valid indicator of the *psychological core of an individual's personality. For example, an athlete may play the role of a braggart but in truth be rather insecure.

role strain *See* role conflict.

role stress *See* role conflict.

role theory A theory suggesting that a person's behaviour results from him or her conforming or failing to conform to various *roles defined by the social context in which the person finds himself or herself. *See also* action theory.

rolling friction Friction that opposes the motion of a ball (or other object) when it rolls across a surface. Rolling friction occurs because the ball and the surface upon which it rolls are deformed slightly during contact. The magnitude of the rolling friction between dry surfaces is influenced by the *coefficient of friction between the surfaces in contact, the *normal reaction force, the radius of curvature of the ball, and the deformability of the rolling object. The amount of rolling friction is changed dramatically if a liquid occurs between the surfaces. Synovial fluid decreases the rolling friction in a ball-and-socket joint. Presence of a liquid can change the nature of a surface on which a ball rolls. For example, rain makes grass both wet and soft, increasing rolling friction and slowing down a ball.

ROM *See* range of motion.

rope skipping A popular form of exercise and conditioning activity, especially among boxers. Although relatively easy to perform, rope skipping is probably too strenuous for most novice exercisers: the exercise intensity at 60 to 80 skips per minute is approximately 9 metabolic equivalents (METs). This value exceeds the capacity of most sedentary individuals. Also, the exercise intensity of rope skipping is not easily graded: doubling the rate of skipping increases the energy requirement by only two to three METs.

Rorschach test A psychological test in which a subject describes an ink blot. The subject's responses are analysed by the tester in order to measure *personality. Although the test has had much clinical use, recent research suggests that it is not a reliable, objective, and valid measure of an athlete's personality.

rotary force The angular equivalent of a linear or direct force (*see* torque).

rotary component The component of muscle force acting perpendicular to the long axis of the attached bone of joint. It is the only component which actually causes rotation.

rotary motion *See* angular motion.

rotation 1 Angular or circular motion of a system around an axis that is located within the rotating system. *See also* revolution. **2** An angular movement around the longitudinal axis. Rotation of the arm or leg as a unit in the transverse plane is called medial rotation when it is towards the midline, and lateral rotation when it is away from the midline. Rotations in the transverse plane of the head, neck, and trunk are called right rotations or left rotations.

rotational energy Energy stored in a spinning system. Rotational energy depends on both the moment of inertia and angular

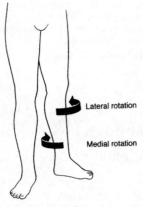

Lateral rotation

Medial rotation

rotation

velocity, and is given by: rotational energy $= \frac{1}{2}Iw^2$ where I = the moment of inertia of the object about an axis through the centre of gravity of the system, and w = the angular velocity of the system about an axis through the centre of gravity of the system.

rotational equilibrium The state of a body in which the sum of all the external torques acting on the body is equal to zero.

rotational inertia A body's resistance to a change in its state of *angular motion. It is also called the *moment of inertia.

rotational movement *See* rotation.

rotator A muscle which effects rotation of a body-part.

rotator cuff Four small muscles (the infraspinatus, subscapularis, supraspinatus, and teres minor) which bind the head of the humerus into the socket of the glenohumeral joint capsule. The rotator cuff provides stability to shoulder movements by synergistically steadying the head of the humerus in the glenoid cavity, thus preventing slippage and skidding. They also contribute to rotation of the humerus.

rotator cuff impingement syndrome *See* shoulder-impingement syndrome.

rotatores *See* deep spinal muscles.

rotatory motion *See* angular motion.

roughage *See* fibre.

round shoulders A postural defect in which the shoulders are protracted (drawn forward), the head is extended, and the chin pokes forward. It may be corrected by strengthening the middle fibres of the *trapezius muscle and the rhomboids, and improving the flexibility of the pectorals and neck extensors.

rowing ergometer *See* ergometer.

RQ *See* respiratory quotient.

rubrospinal system A tract of motor nerve fibres in the ventrolateral column of the spinal cord that carries nerve impulses originating from the cerebral cortex and cerebellum. It plays an important part in the performance of skilled movements.

Ruffini's corpuscle A flattened capsule containing nerve-endings which are thought to be heat receptors sensitive to temperature increases from 25 to 45 °C. Ruffini's corpuscles are deeper than cold receptors (*see* **Krause's end-bulbs**) and occur in joints, suggesting that they might function as mechanoreceptors.

rule A regulation governing conduct or procedure.

ruler drop test A simple test of *response time in which the subject attempts to stop a falling ruler. The distance the ruler drops is converted into response time using the formula: $d = ut + \frac{1}{2}.at^2$; where d is the distance the ruler falls in centimetres, u is the initial velocity of the ruler (if static at the start time, this will be zero), t is the response time in seconds, and a is the acceleration of ruler due to gravity constant (i.e. 981 cm/sec).

rundown A condition characterized by a decrease in physical performance. It may comprise four distinct causal and modal entities: physical fitness and form affected by factors outside the sport, such as lack of sleep; *overtraining; *overstraining which may result in overuse injuries; and *indisposition. *See also* **overtraining syndrome; and stress.**

runner's diarrhoea A gastrointestinal disorder that affects runners, especially just before a competition. It is characterized by a mild but inconvenient diarrhoea (commonly called 'runner's trots') and nausea. Exercise-induced diarrhoea is not confined to runners: activity of any kind is usually associated with increased secretion of sympathetic hormones (e.g. adrenaline) which increases gut motility. However, mild diarrhoea during or after competition appears to be more frequent in runners than other athletes, indicating that there are predisposing factors specific to that activity. Perhaps the bouncing movements performed during running increases mechanical mixing in the gut, increasing motility. Other predisposing factors to diarrhoea include a mild intolerance to milk products or a sensitivity to some other factor (e.g. fructose). Eating a low-fibre diet for 24 to 48 hours before competition will reduce the risk of diarrhoea. If diarrhoea occurs, it is important to ensure that fluids are replaced to prevent dehydration (*see* **water replacement**).

runner's haematuria A condition in which blood is passed in the urine after running a long distance (*see* **march haemoglobinuria**).

runner's haemolysis *See* **march haemoglobinuria**.

runner's high A feeling, usually unexpected, of exhilaration and well-being directly associated with vigorous physical activity. Runner's high is thought to be related to the secretion of *endorphins. *See also* **flow**.

runner's knee A term first used by Dr George Sheehan in the 1970s to describe a rather enigmatic running injury characterized by pain around the kneecap which occurs during running but which is not linked to any specific external trauma. The pain worsens with the distance of the run and makes walking up and down stairs difficult. It is not usually resolved by conventional treatments, such as cortisone injections. It was first thought to be a form of *chondromalacia patellae which would suggest that running may cause degeneration of articular cartilage. However, the pain associated with runner's knee is usually on the inner or outer border of the kneecap. The condition is now thought to be a form of *patellofemoral pain syndrome. The term runner's knee has also been applied to the pain on the outside of the knee associated with *iliotibial band syndrome. Running on cambered roads and excessive pronation increase the risk of suffering from painful knees.

runner's toe *See* **black nail**.

runner's trots *See* **runner's diarrhoea**.

rupture 1 Tearing or bursting apart of an organ or tissue; a tear. **2** A term commonly applied to an *inguinal hernia.

ruptured disc *See* **prolapsed intervertebral disc**.

RV *See* **residual volume**.

 S

S to systolic blood pressure

s *See* **second**.

sac A pouch or sac-like structure.

sacral Pertaining to the sacrum or the region around the sacrum (i.e. lower portion of the back just above the buttocks).

sacral curvature *See* **spinal curvature**.

sacral nerves Five pairs of nerves emerging from the sacrum which supply motor neurones and sensory neurones to the anal and genital regions, and to the leg.

sacral promontory Bulge of the anterio-superior margin of the first vertebra of the sacrum. The *centre of gravity usually lies about 1 cm behind this landmark.

sacroiliac crest A ridge on the bony junction between the *sacrum and *ilium. It is an attachment point for muscles (e.g., the *gluteus maximus).

sacroiliac joint The *synovial joint, consisting of fibrocartilage, between the sacrum of the vertebral column and the ilium of the pelvic girdle. The sacroiliac joint is usually capable of only very slight gliding movements, except during pregnancy when the joint is more mobile (*see* **relaxin**).

sacroiliac mobility test A test performed by asking the subject to stand on one leg and flex the opposite hip. A normal response is a downward (inferior) movement of the posterior iliac spine on the side of the flexed hip. Sacroiliac joint dysfunction is indicated if the posterior iliac spine does not descend, and internal rotation of the hip is often uncomfortable and slightly limited.

sacroiliac stress A pain and dysfunction in the *sacroiliac joint caused by repetitive stress involved in sports such as the steeplechase and hurdles. Typically, the pain is felt over the sacroiliac joint and radiates down into the buttocks and groin. Unlike sacroiliitis, sacroiliac stress is exacerbated by exercise. It may be linked to muscle imbalances (e.g. the rectus femoris may be disproportionately stronger than the gluteals imposing abnormal rotatory stresses on the joint) which must be corrected if the condition is to be resolved. Treatment also includes reducing the stress on the sacroiliac joint for several months. Steroid injections into the joint may also be helpful.

sacroiliitis Inflammation of the sacroiliac joint. It is characterized by low back pain and morning stiffness. Unlike sacroiliac stress, it is unaffected by exercise. It may appear as a component of ankylosing spondylitis. Treatment consists mainly of spinal flexibility exercises.

sacrum Five fused vertebrae forming a triangle-shaped structure at the back of the pelvis. The sacrum articulates superiorly with a *lumbar vertebra, inferiorly with the *coccyx, and anteriorly with the *ilium of the pelvis. The sacrum strengthens and stabilizes the pelvis.

saddle-joint A *synovial joint in which the articulating surfaces are both shaped like a riding saddle (i.e. they have concave and convex areas). The articular surfaces then fit together, convex surface to concave surface, allowing movement in two planes. The carpometacarpal joint in the thumb is a saddle joint.

sagittal axis (anteroposterior axis) An imaginary line (one of the anatomical reference axes) perpendicular to the frontal plane, around which rotations in the frontal plane occur.

sagittal plane (anteroposterior plane) One of the three *cardinal planes, the sagittal plane runs longitudinally down the body, dividing it into right and left halves. It is the plane along which forward and backward movements of the body and body segments occur.

SAI *See* **state anxiety inventory**.

SAID principle (Specific Adaptations to Imposed Demands principle) A principle which proposes that if a human body is placed under stress of varying intensities and duration, it attempts to overcome the stress by adapting specifically to the imposed demands.

salbutamol A drug belonging to the $beta_2$-stimulants. Salbutamol is an effective bronchodilator used to treat exercise-induced asthma and some other forms of respiratory distress. Although stimulants are on the International Olympic committee list of *banned substances, the use of salbutamol is permitted (subject to written notification) by the International Olympic Committee Medical Commission for the treatment of asthma and other respiratory conditions, but they may only be taken by inhalation.

salicylates Drugs which are salts of salicylic acid. Many have anti-inflammatory antipyretic and analgesic effects similar to aspirin (*see* **acetylsalicylic acid**), and are used in the treatment of painful muscle and joint conditions.

salicylic acid A drug which has bactericidal and fungicidal properties. Salicylic acid causes the skin to peel and is used in a concentrated form to remove warts and corns. A number of analgesic, anti-inflammatory drugs, such as acetylsalicylic acid, are prepared from it.

salicylism Poisoning caused by high doses of salicylates such as aspirin (*see* **acetylsalicylic acid**). Salicylism is characterized by dizziness, impaired hearing, drowsiness, sweating and, in very high doses, delirium and collapse.

saline A 0.9 per cent sodium chloride solution, isotonic with blood (*see* **isotonic solution**).

saliva A viscous, transparent, alkaline liquid containing water, salts, mucin (a glycoprotein), immunoglobulins (*see* **salivary Immunoglobulin A**), and enzymes (e.g. salivary amylase). Saliva prevents the buccal cavity from drying out, acts as a lubricant for the passage of food into the oesophagus, and starts the digestion of starch.

salivary Immunoglobulin A An *immunoglobulin present in saliva. Salivary Immunoglobulin A may help protect the upper respiratory tract from infection. Very intense exercise is associated with a drop in salivary Immunoglobulin A concentration, but the level usually returns to normal a few hours after the exercise has stopped. However, *overtraining can prolong the effect, resulting in a chronic state of immunosuppression that makes the overtrained athlete particularly vulnerable to viral infections.

salt A chemical compound formed when the hydrogen of an acid has been replaced by a metal. A salt is produced, together with water, when acid reacts with a base. Salts such as sodium chloride, calcium carbonate, and potassium chloride are common in the body and play vital roles in body functions such as conduction of

nerve impulses and the production of muscle actions.

saltatory conduction The means by which a nerve impulse is rapidly conducted through myelinated fibres. The wave of *depolarization appears to leap from one *node of Ranvier to the next.

salt depletion Loss of salt from the body, either by sweating, persistent vomiting, or diarrhoea. Salt depletion is common after heavy physical exertion and in hot environments, and can lead to muscle weakness and cramps. *See also* **salt replacement**.

salt replacement The replenishment of salts (especially sodium salts) lost from the body. If they are not replaced there is a risk of suffering from a number of disorders, including cramps. Salt replacement is mainly achieved from the diet. Sports men and sports women rarely need to take salt tablets. Sports drinks sometimes contain salts, but their main value is to accelerate the uptake of water from the small intestine. *See also* **water replacement**.

salt substitute A flavour enhancer used in the same way as table salt but which does not contain sodium or has a reduced sodium content. People who are sodium-sensitive and have high blood pressure can take substitutes in which potassium and/or ammonium replaces the sodium. This can make the food taste bitter, but potassium may reduce blood pressures.

salt tablet A tablet containing sodium chloride used to replace the salts lost during sweating. If the tablets are taken without adequate water, there is a danger of a salt imbalance occurring.

saluretic A drug belonging to the *diuretic drugs which are on the International Olympic Committee list of *banned substances. Saluretics act on the kidney to increase the excretion of both salts and water.

sample A portion of a given population of people, objects, or events which accurately reflects all the significant features of that population.

sampling error Differences which occur between the true value of a characteristic of a population and the value estimated from a sample. To reduce the error as far as possible, *random sampling is used.

sampling frame The full list of members of the population to be studied from which a sample can be drawn.

sanction A means by which a moral or social standard is enforced. Sanctions can be either positive (through rewards) or negative (through punishments). They may also be either formal, such as the imposition of a sporting boycott on a country whose policies are disapproved of by other governments; or informal, such as the refusal by one athlete to compete with another who has been found to have taken banned substances.

SA node *See* sinoatrial node.

sarco- Prefix pertaining to muscle.

sarcolemma The cell membrane surrounding a *muscle fibre.

sarcomere The smallest functional unit of a muscle. It is composed mainly of the contractile proteins, *actin and *myosin. A single sarcomere extends from one *z-line to the next.

sarcoplasm The *cytoplasm of a muscle fibre; the gelatin-like substance that fills the spaces between *myofibrils. It differs from the cytoplasm of most cells because it contains *myoglobin and stores of *glycogen.

sarcoplasmic reticulum System of membranous tubules surrounding each *muscle fibre. The sarcoplasmic reticulum transmits the contractile impulse to all parts of a muscle fibre. It does this by releasing and then sequestering calcium ions which are essential for muscle contraction. *See also* **sliding-filament theory**.

sargent jump test A test of muscular power in which the difference between the subject's maximum static reach and maximum reach after jumping is measured. Typically, the subject swings his or her arms downwards and backwards, assumes a crouch position, pauses momentarily to maintain balance, and then leaps upward as high as possible, swinging the arm forcefully forwards and upwards.

sartorius (tailor's muscle) A strap-like superficial muscle running obliquely across the anterior surface of the thigh to the knee. It is the longest muscle in the body crossing both the hip and knee joints. Its origin is on the iliac spine and its insertion is on the medial aspect of the proximal (upper) tibia. It assists with flexion, abduction, and lateral rotation of the femur.

satellite cell A nonfunctioning reserve muscle cell that occurs outside the *sarcolemma (muscle cell surface membrane) but inside the basal lamina. Satellite cells remain quiescent until stimulated to undergo rapid proliferation, for example by injury. They add nuclei to muscle fibres as the muscle fibres increase in size with

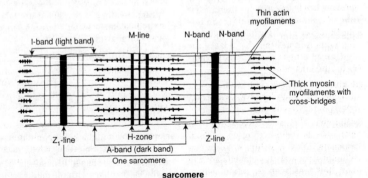

sarcomere

maturity, and they are involved in regeneration of injured muscle fibres. Proliferation of satellite cells may occur in response to heavy resistance training. This could contribute to an increase in muscle bulk by *hyperplasia, but in humans satellite cell proliferation appears to be involved in replacing cells damaged by training, so that there is no significant increase in the net number of muscle fibres.

satiation The fulfillment beyond capacity of a desire. Satiation may occur as the result of an excessive use of a reinforcer which leads to a loss in the effectiveness of the reinforcer (*see* **reinforcement**).

satisfaction The sense of achievement and the fulfillment of a need. It is generally accepted that sport can render possible the expression of satisfaction of many desires: for example, the desire for recreation, social contact, aggression, play, and self-assuredness.

saturated fatty acid A fatty acid that possesses no double bonds, so that it has the maximum amount of hydrogen atoms attached to the carbon atoms. Saturated fats are usually solid at room temperature. They are metabolized along different pathways from polyunsaturated fats. Along with cholesterol, saturated fatty acids are implicated in the deposition of fatty substances on artery walls which may lead to *atherosclerosis. Saturated fats come chiefly from animal sources (such as beef, butter, whole-milk products, the dark meat of poultry, and poultry skin) as well as some tropical vegetable oils (e.g., coconut and palm kernel oils).

Saturday-night arm A condition in which the arm and hand lose sensitivity due to being kept in a cramped position for prolonged periods. It was named Saturday-night arm because it commonly occurs in athletes who make long weekend trips to sports venues, confined in a coach seat.

scabies A skin infection caused by a mite, *Sarcoptes scabei*. The female mite burrows under the skin, particularly around the fingers and genitalia, and lays eggs. Scabies is transmitted by close body contact, especially in crowded and unhygienic places, but the mite is no respecter of social class. Infection does not interfere with physical activity, although it can be transmitted in close contact sports such as wrestling. Treatment is application of a cream which gets rid of the mites. Athletes can return to contact sports the day after the mites have been removed.

scalar A physical quantity that can be described completely in terms of its magnitude (e.g., length, mass, speed, time, and volume). *Compare* **vector**.

scaled response *See* scaling.

scalenus One of four muscles (scalenus anterior, scalenus medius, scalenus minimus, and scalenus posterior) located anterolaterally on each side of the neck, deep to the sternocleidomastoid muscle. They have their origins on the transverse processes of the cervical vertebrae and their insertions posteriolaterally on the first two ribs. They flex and rotate the neck, and elevate the first two ribs during inspiration.

scaling (scaled response) A means of measuring *personality traits and *attitude on a continuum from one extreme to another, for example, from very *introvert through to very extrovert.

scalogram Scale for measuring *attitude which assumes that if a subject agrees with one statement, then the subject will also agree with all statements of a lower intensity.

scan 1 An examination of a human body or body part using a moving detector or a sweeping beam of radiation as in computerized tomography, nuclear magnetic resonance, scintigraphy, or ultrasonography. The term also applies to an image formed from such an examination. **2** *See* **scanning**.

scanning Form of visual *perception in which a person attends to many aspects of the stimulus field. Scanning tends to increase under great *stress. *See also* **focusing, narrowing, selective attention**.

scaphoid A boat-shaped bone of the *wrist which articulates with the radius behind, the trapezium and trapezoid bones in front, and with the capitate and lunate medially.

scaphoid fracture A very common wrist fracture which results mainly from a fall on an outstretched arm. *See also* **carponavicular fracture**.

scapula (shoulder-blade) A flat, triangular bone on the upper posterior part of the thorax. With the clavicle, it forms the pectoral girdle. Many large muscles that move the arm are attached to it.

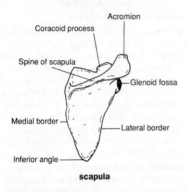

Acromion
Coracoid process
Spine of scapula
Glenoid fossa
Medial border
Lateral border
Inferior angle

scapula

scapulohumeral rhythm The general pattern of coordination between movements of the scapula and humerus during some shoulder movements: rotations of the scapula accompany and facilitate abduction of the humerus.

scapulothoracic joint The joint in the shoulder formed between the anterior surface of a scapula and the tissues between it and the ribs.

scar A mark formed by connective tissue replacing damaged tissue which have failed to heal themselves completely.

SCAT *See* **sport competition anxiety test**.

scattergram A graph on which a subject's score in two tests can be jointly represented as a single datum point.

sceptical argument The proposal that athletic performance cannot be predicted from *personality traits. *Compare* **credulous argument**.

SCG *See* **sodium cromoglycate**.

schema 1 A mental framework or outline which functions as a kind of vague standard that arises out of past experience, growing and differentiating throughout childhood, and places new experiences in their appropriate context and relation. **2** In the schema theory of motor control, a set of operational rules or algorithms that have been acquired from practice or experience, which determine the motor responses in a given situation. It is proposed that there is a separate schema for each class of movement and that skill proficiency is determined by the efficiency of the schema. The use of schema implies there are generalized *motor programs for a given class of movement. It is proposed that the schema would not take up much storage space (storage is a problem with theories positing a one-to-one relationship between stored programs and generated movements) and would help explain the ability to perform relatively novel tasks.

schema theory *See* **schema**.

Scheurmann's disease An *osteochondrosis affecting the distal thoracic and proximal lumbar spine. It causes irregularities in the *epiphyses of vertebra with subsequent propulsion of the *nucleus pulposus into adjacent vertebra bodies (*see* **prolapsed intervertebral disc**) and anterior wedging. It may be painless, but is often associated with back pain during and after physical activity. Scheurmann's disease mostly affects young men between 15 and 20 years old. Although not proven, this disorder may be due to repeated trauma. Treatment includes active back exercises. The condition does not usually preclude participation in sport, though it often results in reduction in the level of strenuous activity during the painful phase.

Schwann cell *See* **myelin sheath**.

sciatica Irritation or inflammation of the *sciatic nerve characterized by a severe pain radiating down the nerve, from the lower back into the leg (true sciatica causes symptoms below the knee and into the foot). The onset of sciatica may be sudden and brought on by a strain to the lower back or a slipped disc (*see* **prolapsed intervertebral disc**), though sometimes no cause can be identified.

sciatic nerve The largest and longest nerve in the body. The sciatic nerve leaves the pelvis via the greater sciatic notch, descends deep to the *gluteus maximus muscle, and continues down the posterior aspect of the thigh. There it supplies the hamstring muscles and part of the adductor magnus. The sciatic nerve divides immediately above the knee to give rise to the peroneal nerve and tibial nerve.

sciatic notch A notch above the triangular spine of the ischium which is converted into a foramen (a hole) for the passage of nerves, blood vessels, and tendons into the thigh region.

science A systematic study, using observation, experiment, and measurement, of physical and social phenomena, or any specific area involving such a study.

scientific approach (scientific method) Set of systematic procedures which enable a problem to be approached or a question answered in a methodical and logical way. Typically, the stages of a scientific approach to the solution of a problem include posing a research question and making a plan, gathering information, interpreting the findings and results, formulating a hypothesis, and testing the hypothesis by experiment.

scientific management Theory of management which focuses on the efficiency of the management process: improved efficiency is assumed to increase production. It is a formal style of *leadership behaviour which is closely related to the *initiating structure.

scientific method *See* **scientific approach**.

scientific realism Assumption that a physical world exists independently of the human senses.

scientific stretching for sport The 3S system; an effective technique for improving flexibility in which a muscle is passively stretched by a partner and then exposed to an isometric muscle action.

scientism Term, often used pejoratively, to describe a doctrine which oversimplifies scientific concepts or has an unrealistic expectation of science.

scintigraphy A technique used to diagnose sports injuries. A radioactive tracer is used in conjunction with a scintillation counter to produce pictures. A diagram, called a scintigram, shows the internal distribution of a radioactive tracer in internal parts of the body. In sports medicine, scintigraphy is particularly useful in the detection of *stress fractures in bones. *See also* **bone scan**.

sclerosis Hardening of organs or tissues, usually due to excessive production of connective tissue after inflammation. *See also* **arteriosclerosis**.

scoliosis An abnormal lateral curvature of the spine which occurs most often in the thoracic region. It may be congenital or acquired, for example, from poor posture or an unequal muscle pull on the spine. Mild cases of scoliosis may have no adverse symptoms but severe scoliosis can be painful and deforming, and usually requires bracing and/or surgery. *See also* **tennis shoulder**.

screener An individual with a good ability to filter out various irrelevant stimuli from their environment. Screeners are selective in the stimuli to which they respond and tend not to be easily distracted or upset. *Compare* **nonscreener**. *See also* **selective attention**.

screening *See* **medical screening**.

scrumpox (herpes gladiatorum) A highly contagious skin disease, usually caused by the herpes simplex virus. Scrumpox is commonly associated with rugby football where the combination of skin lesions and the abrasive effects of facial stubble during scrumming facilitates transmission of the infection. Transmission may also occur through shared towels and equipment. Creams or tablets containing acyclovir, a specific antiviral agent, are used to treat the condition. Scrumpox may also be caused by bacteria (*Streptococcus pyogenes* or *Staphylococcus aureus*) or fungi, in which case antibacterial or antifungal creams or tablets are used in the treatment.

SCUBA An acronym for Self-Contained Underwater Breathing Apparatus, the main means of remaining underwater for diving sports.

scurvy A deficiency disease due to lack of vitamin C. Initial signs include bleeding gums. This may be followed by anaemia, cutaneous haemorrhage, degeneration of muscle and cartilage, and weight loss. The effects are reversed by treatment with vitamin C.

SDH *See* **succinic dehydrogenase**.

second (s) **1** Base unit of time for the SI system; symbol s. It was formerly defined as 1/86 400 of the mean solar day, but it is now defined in terms of periods of radiation from a caesium-133 atom. **2** A unit of angle equal to 1/60 of a minute of an arc.

secondary analysis An inquiry based on data, such as census returns, which have already been collected and analysed.

secondary behavioural involvement (secondary sport involvement) Indirect participation in a sport as a sport producer or sport consumer. *Compare* **primary behavioural involvement**.

secondary deviance The process by which an individual, having once broken a rule, comes to change his or her attitudes and affiliations and begins to associate himself or herself with being outside the normal or socially acceptable. That is, his or her *self-image is changed to one of deviance.

secondary drive An acquired *drive not directly related to satisfying physiological requirements; e.g. the drive to win a medal at the Olympic Games.

secondary immune response Second and subsequent responses of the immune system to an antigen which has been previously encountered. The secondary immune response is more rapid and more effective than the primary immune response.

secondary infection A new infection superimposed on a pre-existing infection.

secondary motivation In sport, a source of *motivation not derived directly from the activity itself. A coach and an audience are sources of secondary motivation. *See also* **inborn motivation**. *Compare* **primary motivation**.

secondary ossification centre An area of bone growth which appears at the junction between the shaft and one or both epiphyses of a long bone; an area from which ossification of the epiphyses occurs. *See also* **epiphyseal plate**.

secondary plane A plane passing through the *centre of gravity of a body segment, through the centre of a joint, or through some other point of reference.

secondary sexual characteristic Any of the several features of a male or female produced when sexually mature but which are not concerned directly with gamete production.

secondary sport involvement *See* **secondary behavioural involvement**.

secondary task method An experimental method in which the subject performs a secondary task simultaneously with a primary task. The method is used to study the attentional demands of the main task during skill learning. *See also* **probe technique**.

second-class lever A lever which has its point of resistance (load) between its fulcrum (point of support or axis of rotation) and point of effort (force application). In the human body, a second class is used when a person stands on tip-toe.

second-degree strain *See* **muscle strain**.

second impact syndrome The rapid development of diffuse brain swelling when the head suffers a second impact before brain injury from the first impact has cleared. A seemingly minor second impact on an already damaged brain can lead to a massive swelling and rapid deterioration of the casualty. Usually within seconds to minutes of the second impact, the initially conscious athlete loses consciousness,

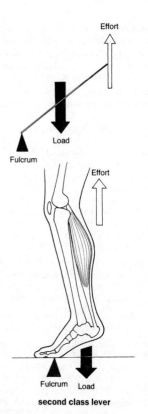

second class lever

clustered traits. In Catell's 16 PF personality inventory, for example, six of the sixteen first-order traits cluster to form the second order trait of *anxiety.

second wind A phenomenon characterized by a sudden transition from an ill-defined feeling of distress and difficulty in breathing during the early stages of prolonged exercise, to a more comfortable, less stressful feeling later in the exercise. There is some debate about the physiological reality of second wind, some scientists believing it to be more psychological than physiological. However, second wind may be due to an initial increase in lactate levels at the beginning of exercise, followed by recovery as a steady state is established; or it may be related to an improvement in the contractility of inspiratory muscles and an improved blood supply to the diaphragm.

secretin An intestinal hormone secreted by the duodenum in response to acid chyme (partly-digested food) from the stomach. Secretin passes into the blood stream and promotes the flow of bile and pancreatic juices into the intestine, and inhibits gastric gland secretions.

sedative A drug, such as *alcohol, which can calm an individual without inducing sleep. Sedatives have been used by marksmen to improve their precision. *See also* **anxiolytic**.

sedentary Applied to a person who is relatively inactive and has a lifestyle characterized by a lot of sitting.

segmental method A procedure for estimating the *centre of gravity of a whole human body from the centres of gravity and weights of individual body segments in the head, trunk, and limbs. The estimate involves quite complex computations and many measurements, but it hinges on the fact that the sum of the moments of the weight-forces of the separate segments is equal to the moment of their resultant.

Segond's fracture An *avulsion fracture involving the meniscotibial portion of the lateral capsular ligament in the knee. The fracture, in which a fleck of bone is chipped

collapses, and shows evidence of respiratory failure. This postconcussion condition is often fatal and emphasizes that conservative guidelines should be followed before athletes are allowed to return to participation in a contact or collision sport after a head injury. *See also* **concussion**.

second messenger A substance that acts as a chemical messenger inside a cell after a nonsteroidal hormone or neurotransmitter binds onto cell surface receptors. The most widely studied second messenger is *cyclic AMP.

second order conditioning In classical conditioning, the use of a conditioned stimulus as the basis of further conditioning.

second order trait A personality trait used to describe a large number of similar, off the tibia, indicates a severe lateral capsular injury that often affects the anterior cruciate and medial ligaments.

selective attention (selectivity) The ability of a person to attend to specific stimuli and exclude other competing stimuli. Selective attention is one of the most important cognitive abilities of a successful athlete. However, this usually useful ability can also have unfortunate consequences. A footballer, for example, may perceive the ball as the only important aspect of the game and ignore all other sources of information. The ball-watching may allow an opponent to move undetected and unmarked into a scoring position.

selective filter A filter, found in most models of *selective attention, that either eliminates or attenuates information of minor importance.

selenium A trace element (*see* **mineral**) found in meat, seafood, and cereals. Selenium acts, often in association with vitamin E, as an *antioxidant. It is also a component of many enzymes. The Reference Nutrient Intake for adults is 75 micrograms per day. Supplements are not recommended because high levels of selenium are toxic.

self A person as perceived by himself or herself in the context of society and his or her relationships with others. Self is an important determinant of motivation and interaction with others.

self-activation The process, performed by an athlete on himself or herself, of increasing the level of activation. Mental strategies, such as positive self-talk, and psyching-up procedures (e.g. thigh slapping) are often used as self-activation methods to enhance strength and muscular endurance, especially when an athlete is feeling lethargic.

self-actualization (self-realization) The realization of a person's full potential whatever it may be and regardless of the rewards involved; doing what one is best suited to do. Self-actualization is only attainable when all other needs have been met (*see* **motivational hierarchy**).

self-assertiveness *See* **assertive behaviour**.

self-attention An athlete's concern about the execution of his or her own skills. With some highly skilled performers, self-attention is higher at home matches than away ones. *See also* **home court advantage**.

self-concept All the elements which make up a person's *self. Self-concept represents how a person sees himself or herself and is thought to have three components: ideal self (the person one would like to be); public self (the image one believes others have of oneself); and real self (the sum of those subjective thoughts, feelings, and needs that the person sees as being authentically theirs). Sometimes there is a conflict between the different components of self, resulting in anxiety. To maintain good mental health, the public and ideal self should be compatible with the real self.

self-confidence A person's belief that he or she has the ability to succeed. Athletes who are self-confident and expect to succeed often *do* succeed. *See also* **self-efficacy**.

self-control The ability to exercise control over one's own feelings and behaviour.

self-directed relaxation An abbreviated form of progressive muscle relaxation used in stress management. The subject achieves full body relaxation by relaxing muscle groups while breathing slowly and evenly and visualizing tension flowing out of the body.

self-disclosure Sharing one's feelings and thoughts with others. Self-disclosure is an important aspect of a coach's behaviour. Some coaches prefer being reserved, and wish to stay detached and objective; others prefer to be open and share with their athletes the way they feel about events, believing that self-disclosure generates trust.

self-efficacy A situation-specific form of *self-confidence. In sport, self-efficacy refers to a performer's belief that he or she can execute a behaviour required to produce a certain outcome successfully. Assuming an athlete has the potential to perform successfully and that there are sufficient incentives to do so, self-efficacy theory asserts that the quality of an actual performance will depend on the athlete's belief in his or her own competence. *See also* **Bandura's self-efficacy theory**.

self-esteem A person's inner conviction of his or her own competency and worth as a human being. Positive self-esteem is viewing oneself as a competent and worthy person, however that is defined, and feeling good about that aspect of oneself.

self-focusing The process of *selective-attention towards information that concerns oneself.

self-fulfilling prophecy A prediction which is confirmed solely because it was suggested. For example, potential spectators may not go to view a match because they have heard it will not be well supported.

self-image *See* **self concept**.

self-orientation A psychological orientation in which an individual wishes to have direct personal rewards regardless of the effects on others working with that individual. A self-orientated person is often dominating, introspective, and socially insensitive. Highly successful athletes tend to be self-oriented while good coaches tend to be lower in self-orientation. *Compare* **task orientation**.

self-paced task A task or skill, the initiation of which is determined by the performer. Self-paced tasks include a golf-drive and a tennis serve. Typically, they occur in stable, predictable environments in which the performer has plenty of time to respond. *Compare* **externally paced task**.

self-perception The way a person sees himself or herself; perceptions of oneself in any domain, such as physical or academic. *See also* **self-concept**.

self-realization *See* **self-actualization**.

self-regulation The regulation of one's own goal-directed behaviour without immediate external control. In sport, self-regulation involves an athlete taking control of and responsibility for his or her own training, performance, and participation in sport.

self-report inventory Questionnaire in which respondents answer questions about themselves. Such inventories are commonly used to measure, among other things, *anxiety.

self-serving attributional bias The tendency to ascribe positive outcomes of performance to internal factors such as ability and effort, and negative outcomes to external factors, such as luck and the weather, in order to maintain *self-esteem. *See also* **functional model of attribution**.

self-serving hypothesis A hypothesis based on the observation that people sometimes make illogical attributions to enhance or protect their egos.

self-talk A mental preparation strategy in which individuals talk to themselves in an attempt to enhance their self-confidence and convince themselves that they can succeed.

self-theory An approach to the study of *personality which emphasizes the role of the individual in shaping his or her own destiny. Particularly important is the individual's self-concept (the person's consistent, organized perception of himself or herself). Supporters of this theory stress the subjective side of human existence, and regard an individual's self-concept as more important than environmental conditions.

self-worth A feeling of positive self-esteem so that a person views himself or herself as competent and worthy.

semicircular canal One of three fluid-filled canals in the inner ear containing cells, sensitive to movement of the head, which serve as an organ of balance.

semilunar cartilage One of two crescent-shaped cartilages in the knee joint between the femur and tibia. *See also* **meniscus**.

semilunar valve (pocket valve) A crescent-shaped valve, present in the *aorta and the pulmonary artery, which prevents blood returning to the ventricles after *ventricular systole.

semimembranosus One of three hamstring muscles. It has its origin in the ischial tuberosity and its insertion on the medial condyle of the tibia. Its primary actions are extension of the femur and flexion and

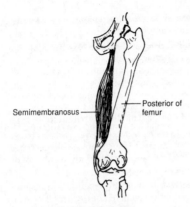

semimembranosus

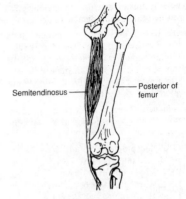

semitendinosus

medial rotation around the tibiofemoral joint of the knee.

semiology (semiotics) **1** The study of signs and symbols, especially the relationship between written and spoken signs. Semiology draws attention to the layers of meaning which may be embodied in a simple set of representations, such as the five interlocking rings of the Olympic flag. It is concerned with the meaning invested in the sign and the signifier (the physical representation of the sign). **2** The scientific study of the signs and symptoms of disease.

semiotics *See* **semiology**.

semispinalis One of a pair of composite muscles (the semispinalis capitis, cervicis, and thoracis) on either side of the vertebral column forming part of the deep layer of back muscles which extends from the thoracic region to the head. The proximal attachments are on the occipital bone and the spinous processes of thoracic vertebrae 2–4; the distal attachments are on the seventh cervical vertebrae and the transverse processes of the thoracic vertebrae. The primary actions of the semispinalis group of muscles are extension, lateral flexion, and rotation (to the opposite side) of the spine.

semitendinosus One of the three hamstring muscles. It has its origin on the medial ischial tuberosity of the pelvis and its

insertion on the medial aspect of the tibial shaft. Its primary actions are extension of the femur about the hip, and flexion and medial rotation of the tibia about the knee.

semivegetarian A person who has a diet mainly of plants supplemented with some animal products. *See also* **vegetarian**.

sensation An irreducible sensory experience such as might occur when a sensory receptor is stimulated. Theoretically, a sensation is devoid of conscious meaning until the process of perception has taken place.

sense One of several faculties, including sight, touch, hearing, taste, and smell by which qualities of the internal and external environment can be appreciated.

sense organ An organ in the body containing cells which respond to particular external and internal stimuli. Messages from a sense organ are conveyed by sensory neurones to the central nervous system where they are processed and where perception takes place.

sensibility The capacity to be affected by, and to respond to, stimuli.

sensible temperature The critical temperature range beyond which a person feels too hot or too cold. The sensible temperature is affected by relative humidity and wind chill. *Compare* **comfort zone**.

sensitivity 1 The aspect of a measurement dealing with the possibility of detecting changes in a dependent measure in relation to varying experimental conditions. *See also* **objectivity**; **reliability**; and **validity**. **2** The ability to respond to stimuli. The term is used especially for the ability to be affected by and to respond to stimuli of low intensity.

sensitization 1 A form of behavioural therapy in which anxiety-provoking stimuli are presented to the subject whenever he or she exhibits unwanted behaviour so that the unwanted behaviour can be suppressed. **2** The process which increases the excitability of receptors to sensory stimuli.

sensorimotor *See* **motor**.

sensorimotor process Any overt motor act initiated by a sensory process.

sensory adaptation Adaptation of some sensory functions, as in dark adaptation when objects not seen at first in dim light gradually become visible. *See also* **adaptation**.

sensory area One of the several areas of the cerebral cortex which process incoming messages conveyed by sensory neurones from sense organs.

sensory information store *See* **short-term sensory store**.

sensory memory *See* **short-term sensory store**.

sensory-motor integration The process by which the sensory and motor systems communicate and coordinate with each other. It involves stimulus reception and transmission to the central nervous system (CNS) where the stimulus is interpreted. The CNS then determines which response to make and transmits its instructions as *nerve impulses along a motor neurone to the appropriate effector (e.g. a group of muscle fibres) which carries out the response.

sensory nerve A *nerve containing processes of sensory neurones and carrying afferent nerve impulses to the central nervous system.

sensory neurone (afferent neurone) A nerve cell conveying impulses from receptor to the central nervous system.

sensory reaction A component of *reaction time during which the subject's attention is directed to the stimulus rather than the response.

sensory receptor Any cell or part of cell specially adapted to respond to a *stimulus.

sensory register *See* **short-term sensory store**.

sensory transduction Transformation of energy from a stimulus into a nerve impulse.

separation *See* **dislocation**.

sepsis The breakdown of tissue by putrefying bacteria or toxins.

septic Pertaining to *sepsis.

septicaemia Blood-poisoning; a condition in which the blood contains many pathogenic bacteria and their toxins. Septicaemia may result from any wound, even a small abrasion, that has become infected.

septic arthritis A bacterial infection of a joint marked by fever, swelling, and pain in the affected joint. It is associated with other infections and requires urgent medical attention. During the acute stage, the joint should be relieved of any load, and the pathogenic organism identified and then eliminated with antibiotics. After the acute stage, isometric exercises may be introduced to offset muscle atrophy. Physical exertion should be resumed only with medical guidance.

septic bursitis *See* **bursitis**.

sequencing A method of learning a multipart motor skill in which the subject repeats the component movements in the proper order.

sequential acceleration *See* **force summation**.

sequentially dependent task A delegated task in which group members must perform their skills in a prescribed order. *Compare* **sequentially independent task**.

sequentially independent task A delegated task in which group members can perform their skills in any order or at any time in relation to each other.

sequential stabilization In the human body, an increase in the stability of some body parts to stabilize the movement of other parts. During a golf swing, for example, the leading leg is stabilized to enable an effective force to be produced by the trunk and arms. *See also* **force summation**.

serial processing A pattern of *information processing in which the stages of processing are arranged sequentially in time, as in spinal reflexes. *Compare* **parallel processing**.

serial skill *See* **serial task**.

serial task (serial skill) A task consisting of a series of several discrete elements strung together to produce an integrated movement. The order in which the elements are performed is important. In the high jump and triple jump, for example, the run-up and take-off phases occur in a particular order. *See also* **continuous task**; and **discrete skill**.

series elastic component A noncontractile component of muscle which lies in series with the muscle fibres. Series elastic components store energy when stretched and make a major contribution to the elasticity of the human skeleton. Tendons are the major representatives of the series elastic component, but the cross bridges between *actin and *myosin may also contribute. *Compare* **parallel elastic component**.

serosa *See* **serous membrane**.

serotonin (entramine; 5-hydroxytryptamine; 5-HT) A *metabotropic neurotransmitter belonging to the biogenic amines. Serotonin is made from the amino acid tryptophan, one of the brain's principal neurotransmitters. Serotonin is secreted in some neurones in the brainstem and *hypothalamus, limbic system, pineal gland, and the spinal cord where its effects are generally inhibitory. It acts as a vasoconstrictor and is thought to play an important role in the inflammation response. When a person eats a meal, the level of serotonin is raised or lowered, depending on the type of food eaten. Serotonin levels may affect mood and motivation. The activity of serotonin is blocked by lysergic acid diethylamide (LSD).

serous Pertaining to serum or another watery fluid.

serous fluid A clear, watery fluid secreted by cells of a serous membrane.

serous membrane (serosa) A double-layered membrane forming a sac which lines large body cavities. The outer, parietal membrane lines the walls of the cavity and the inner, visceral membrane lines the organ. The inner surface of the sac is moistened by fluid which reduces friction of the organs within their cavities.

serratus anterior (anterior serrated muscle) Muscle of the anterior thorax which lies deep to the scapula and inferior pectoral muscles on the lateral ribcage. The serratus anterior forms the medial wall of the axilla (armpit). The muscle has its origins (which resemble the teeth of a saw) on the first eight or nine ribs, and its insertions on the inner border of the scapula. The serratus anterior is the main muscle responsible for pushing and punching movements; consequently, it is sometimes referred to as the boxer's muscle.

serum The clear watery body fluid exuded by a serous membrane. Blood serum is the amber-coloured, noncellular, fluid part of blood, excluding fibrinogen and platelets.

serum creatine A biochemical parameter used to measure the effects of exercise. Normal levels are between 0.7 and 1.5 mg per cent; levels increase slightly after hard efforts.

serum urea The amount of urea present in the serum. The serum urea level is a biochemical indicator of protein metabolism. The level is often increased by hard training and long-duration exercise. Its determination the day after intensive training can be used to estimate residual metabolic fatigue and metabolic recovery.

servo An abbreviation for servomechanism (*see* **closed-loop system**).

servomechanism *See* **closed-loop system**.

sesamoid bone A special type of short irregular bone, such as the patella, embedded within a tendon or joint capsule. Sesamoid bones vary in size and number in different individuals. Some alter the direction of pull of a tendon (*see* **pulley**); the function of others is unknown.

sesamoiditis Inflammation around the sesamoid bone in the great toe, probably due to chondromalacia, which causes pain under the metatarso-phalangeal joint. It is usually relieved by the application of a doughnut pad, and resolved by a steroid injection, but it is sometimes necessary to remove the bone surgically.

set In *interval training a group of work and relief intervals.

set point *See* **norm**.

set point theory A theory which postulates that body weight is regulated around a given set point using a homeostatic mechanism similar to that which regulates temperature. Preliminary studies indicate that people who lose weight through semi-starvation or gain weight by overfeeding return to their normal body weight quickly when they revert to normal eating patterns. It has been suggested that the body has the ability to balance caloric intake and expenditure to within plus or minus 10 to 15 kcal per day. It appears that the body attempts to maintain its normal weight when overfeeding or underfed by changing the three components of expenditure (*see* **resting metabolic rate, thermic effect of food, and thermic effect of activity**). If the set point theory is correct, it explains why some athletes have great difficulty losing or gaining body weight for weight-classification sports, such as wrestling and horseriding.

Sever–Haglund disease (apophysitis calcanei; os calcis apophysitis; Sever's disease) An *apophysitis affecting the heel, resulting in inflammation and breakdown in the attachment point of the Achilles tendon to the calcaneus. The condition is characterized by pain, swelling, and tenderness in the calcaneus when running and walking. The condition is probably caused by overloading and overuse. It tends to occur in active individuals between 8 and 15 years and usually resolves spontaneously when the afflicted athlete reaches 16 to 18 years, when ossification of the skeleton is complete. Until resolved, it is important to reduce mechanical stress on the heel. This can be done by moderating activity and using a shock-absorbing heel cushion.

Sever's disease *See* Sever–Haglund disease.

severe strain A third degree strain involving a total muscle tear (*see* **muscle strain**).

sex The biological differences between males and females, especially differences in genitals and reproductive capabilities. *Compare* **gender**. *See also* **sex determination**; and **sex-specific differences**.

sex discrimination The practice whereby an individual is disadvantaged or advantaged on the basis of sex. *See also* **sexism**.

sexism Values, beliefs, and norms that support the process of defining one gender as less worthy and capable than the other, and discriminatory practices which support these beliefs. *See also* **sex discrimination**.

sex-specific differences In sport, differences of performances between males and females determined by physiological and anatomical differences. Although there is an overlap between body build and physiological functions, women tend to have a higher proportion of adipose tissue, lower maximal oxygen consumption, lower bone density, and lower absolute muscle mass than men. These and other differences tend to make them less powerful than men and is one explanation why women are outperformed by men in most sports and physical activities. However, cultural and psychological differences are also contributory factors to the differences in performance.

sex stratification A ranking system in which sex is the basis for making the evaluations, so that *gender becomes the basis for social stratification. *See also* **sex discrimination**.

sex typed An individual whose sex and gender role orientation are the same. For example, a sexual female with female gender role orientation.

sex typing The process of ascribing certain activities as being appropriate for only one sex.

sexuality 1 The innate attributes of an individual, including sexual desires, roles, and identities, which find expression in sexual relationships and sexual activities with others. **2** An individual's preferences for specific forms of sexual expression; an individual's sexual orientation.

sexual orientation *See* sexuality.

shadowing A procedure, used to study *selective attention, in which a subject is exposed to two different spoken messages at the same time through earphones. The subject is instructed to repeat the messages coming through the right earphone and is later asked to recall the information received in the left ear.

shaft *See* diaphysis.

shaping (method of successive approximations) A procedure used to acquire complex skills. Shaping is used to develop athletic skills by starting with what the athlete is capable of doing and gradually requiring a more skillful level of performance before positive reinforcement is given. The complex skill is acquired gradually in small achievable steps so that the athlete can master them.

shapism An emphasis on body shape in the projection of a desirable body image by those with a vested interest in acceptance of this image. In western societies, the emphasis for women is on slimness; and for men the emphasis is on muscularity. Shapism is closely associated with *mesomorphism.

Sharpey's fibres Strong fibres which attach a tendon or ligament to the *periosteum, and secure the periosteum to the underlying bone. Sharpey's fibres consist of dense tufts of collagen fibres that extend from the fibrous layer into the bone matrix.

shaving down Removal of body hair by shaving, commonly performed by swimmers and runners to improve performance. In addition to making the athlete feel more energetic, scientific studies have shown that shaving reduces passive *drag forces, resulting in lower energy costs.

shear An angular deformation of an object without a change in its volume.

shear force 1 A force directed parallel or at a tangent to a surface. A shear force tends to cause one portion of an object to slide, displace, or shear with respect to another portion of the object. **2** A force identified on the basis of the formula: force = mass × acceleration, in which the mass component, or resistance to be overcome, is more important than acceleration. Shear force is particularly important in weightlifting.

shear strain *See* strain.

shear stress A system of shear forces in equilibrium producing or tending to produce shear. Shear stress occurs across a section of bone loaded transversely and also across sections of the shaft of the bone subject to torque. The magnitude of stress across the section depends on the shape of the section.

sheath Layer of connective tissue surrounding structures such as blood vessels, muscles, nerves, and tendons.

Sheldon's constitutional theory *See* constitutional theory.

Sheldon somatotype classification The classification of body types into three basic types: endomorphy (roundness), mesomorphy (muscularity), and ectomorphy (linearity). Sheldon based his classification on thousands of photographs of naked individuals taken from three different perspectives. From these photographs, measurements were taken and each individual ascribed a three-number classification. Each number has a value from one to seven designating the amount each component contributes to the individual's physique: one represents the least contribution and seven the most. The first number represents the amount of endomorphy, the second number the amount of mesomorphy, and the third number the amount of ectomorphy. Thus 7-1-1, represents extreme endomorphy; 1-7-1, extreme mesomorphy; and 1-1-7, extreme ectomorphy.

shin bone *See* tibia.

shin splints A term applied to a number of *overuse injuries characterized by a dull aching pain felt on the inner or outer surface of the shin bone (tibia) and brought on by exercise. It is often associated with overtraining (particularly at the start of a season's training), running on hard surfaces, or poor running technique. Although the term 'shinsplints' is still used by athletes, it is no longer used by most doctors because it is too vague. The conditions embraced within the term include *stress fractures of the tibia or fibula, inflammation on the outer side of the ankle (peroneal tendinitis), increased pressure within the muscle compartments (*see* compartment syndrome), and inflammation of the membrane covering the tibia (*medial tibial stress syndrome). In all of these conditions, the irritation and pain spreads and continues throughout activity. The symptoms stop when activity ceases and the leg usually remains tender to the touch. Treatment depends on the precise cause, but usually includes a long period of rest, ice treatment, anti-inflammatory medication, and stretching exercises.

shivering Involuntary muscular contractions which generate body heat.

shock General term for a life-threatening state of weakness brought about by a circulatory disturbance when arterial blood pressure is insufficient to maintain an adequate supply of blood to the tissues. A person in shock has cold moist skin, a weak rapid pulse, irregular breathing, dilated pupils, and is distressed, thirsty, and restless. Shock may be induced by many causes including dehydration, heart attack, bacterial infection, allergic reactions, drug overdose, severe injury, or haemorrhaging.

shock-box *See* Buss aggression machine.

shock exercises Exercises that involve jumping from an object several feet above the ground. Immediately on landing, the jumper rebounds upwards. Shock exercises are designed to stimulate the *stretch-shortening cycle in muscles and improve the power output from the legs. *See also* **plyometrics**.

shoe-motif pain A pain caused by wearing training shoes with relatively inflexible motifs. A sore area of skin develops, usually on the inside of the shoe where the motif exerts pressure on the foot near the motif's attachment to the sole of the shoe.

short bone A small roughly cuboidal bone. Short bones include the *sesamoid bones, tarsals of the ankle, and carpals of the wrist.

short leg *See* anatomical short leg; and functional short leg.

short saphenous vein A principal vein at the back of the calf.

short-term anaerobic performance Maximal exercise lasting about 10 s, which is supported by the *ATP–PCr system.

short-term anaerobic performance capacity The total work output during maximal exercise lasting about 10 s.

short-term anaerobic tests A test, generally lasting 10 s or less, designed to evaluate the capacity of the *ATP–PCr system in the muscles used to accomplish the test, for example, the *Margaria staircase test and the Quebec ten-second test.

short-term endurance The ability to sustain a strenuous activity which has a duration of 35 seconds to 2 minutes. Short-term endurance is associated with high levels of activity of the brain and high recruitment of fast twitch muscle fibres. The energy for the activities is supplied mainly by the anaerobic system with the ATP–PCr system being important for the initial 10 seconds of the activity.

short-term memory (STM) According to the black-box model of memory, short-term memory is a component of the information-processing system in which new information must remain for a minimum of 20–30 s or the information will be lost. The STM acts as a link between the short-term sensory store (STS) and the long-term memory (LTM). The short-term memory is thought to be analogous to consciousness and has been described as the 'work space' where information from the STS and LTM can be brought together for processing.

short-term motor memory A short-term store for motor information or motor tasks which is analogous to verbal short-term memory. Its functions include storage for a short-time of sensory information acquired from feedback of movements.

short-term sensory store (STS) According to the black box model, the first of three memory compartments involved in *information processing. It is regarded as a functionally limitless short-term store of massive amounts of sensory information without much recoding; that is, the information is recorded in the same way as it came into the system in terms of spatial location and form. Information is held in the STS for perhaps as little as one second. Selected information may be passed onto the short-term memory for further processing.

short-term store *See* short-term sensory store.

short-wave diathermy *See* diathermy.

shoulder Part of the body where the arm joins onto the trunk. The shoulder is a very complex structure because it has five joints (*see* **acromioclavicular joint, coracoclavicular joint, glenohumeral joint, scapulothoracic joint, and sternoclavicular joint**).

shoulder blade *See* scapula.

shoulder blade spine (spina scapula) A bony projection on the scapula which is an attachment point for muscles. The shoulder blade spine forms the origin of the deltoids and the supraspinatus muscles, and an insertion for the trapezius.

shoulder-girdle Two gliding joints: the *sternoclavicular joint and the *acromioclavicular joint. *See* **pectoral girdle**.

shoulder-girdle abduction A movement of the shoulder girdle, primarily involving the scapula and clavicle, forward and upward away from the spinal column.

shoulder-girdle abductor A muscle which effects *shoulder girdle abduction (e.g., the serratus anterior and pectoralis muscles).

shoulder-girdle adduction Movement of the shoulder-girdle (mainly scapula and clavicle) back towards the spinal column.

shoulder-girdle adductors Muscles which effect *shoulder girdle adduction (e.g., the trapezius and rhomboideus).

shoulder-girdle anterior tilt Movement of the inferior angle of the scapula towards the chest.

shoulder-girdle depression Movement of the shoulder girdle from an elevated position (e.g. when shrugging shoulders) back to the anatomical position.

shoulder-girdle depressor A muscle which effects *shoulder-girdle depression (e.g. lower trapezius, pectoralis minor, and serratus anterior).

shoulder-girdle downward rotation Movement of the shoulder girdle which usually accompanies shoulder-girdle depression, bringing the inferior angle of the scapula towards the spinal column and the glenoid cavity to its anatomical position.

shoulder-girdle elevation Movement of the shoulder girdle, mainly of the scapula and clavicle, which results in upward shrugging of the shoulders.

shoulder-girdle elevator A muscle which effects shoulder-girdle elevation (e.g., the upper trapezius and levator scapulae).

shoulder-girdle posterior tilt Movement of the inferior angle of the scapula away from the thoracic surface.

shoulder-girdle rotator A muscle which effects rotation of the shoulder girdle. Upward rotation is effected mainly by the upper fibres of the trapezius and lower fibres of the serratus anterior. Downward rotation is effected mainly by the rhomboids.

shoulder-girdle upward rotation Rotation of the shoulder girdle (mainly scapula and clavicle) which results in moving the inferior angle of the scapula away from the spinal column and increasing the angle of the glenoid cavity with respect to its *anatomical position.

shoulder impingement syndrome (rotator cuff impingement syndrome; swimmer's shoulder) A common overuse injury of those who engage in forceful overhead arm movements (e.g. front crawl swimming). The *rotator cuff muscles and adjacent soft tissues catch repeatedly on the coracoacromial arch (the arch formed between the coracoid process, the acromion process and the coracoacromial ligament). Repeated pinching causes *bursitis and *tendinitis and the rotator cuff muscles become scarred and degenerate. A bone spur may also develop underneath the *acromion process. Symptoms include gradual onset of pain and tenderness exacerbated by rotatory movements of the humerus. Diagnosis includes the 'impingement sign'; intense pain when the physician holds the patient's arm straight out in front and pushes it upwards. Treatment includes application of ice at the first signs of the condition, specific conditioning exercises to strengthen and stretch the rotator cuff muscles, anti-inflammatories, and, in extreme cases surgical repair of the muscles and tendons.

shoulder joint *See* glenohumeral joint.

shoulder movements The shoulder is a highly complex, very mobile region of the body containing several anatomically distinct joints. However, the joints are functionally inseparable: movements of the shoulder-girdle extend the range of motions of the glenohumeral joint allowing, for example, circumduction. All the shoulder muscles help to steady the shoulder when the humerus (arm) is moved and to adjust the angle of the glenoid cavity, allowing a great range of motion. The main shoulder muscles are the *levator scapulae, *pectoralis minor, *rhomboids, *serratus anterior, *subclavius, and *trapezius. In addition, the *rotator cuff

muscles are essential for keeping the head of the humerus within the glenoid cavity.

shunting The diversion of blood from one region of the body to another. During exercise, special vessels, called *shunt vessels, enable blood to be diverted from the intestines to skeletal muscle.

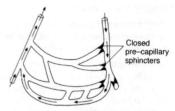

Capillary network in resting muscle

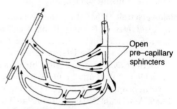

Capillary network in active muscle

shunting

shunt muscle A skeletal muscle with its proximal attachments near the joint or joints at which it acts, and its distal attachments at some distance from the joints, so that the greater part of its force is directed along the bones, tending to pull joint surfaces together. This makes shunt muscles good stabilizers. *Compare* **spurt muscles**.

shunt vessel A blood vessel which enables *shunting to take place. The shunt vessels forms a by-pass channel in the blood circulation, connecting two anatomical channels and diverting blood from one region to the other. *See also* **anastomosis**.

shuttle run test (leger test; multistage fitness test; shuttle test) A test of *aerobic endurance performed by running back and forth between two lines 20 metres apart on a flat, even, and slip-resistant surface. The subject runs at a set pace, which is increased at one minute intervals, and continues until he or she can no longer maintain the set pace. Scores based on the highest pace achieved and maintained are used to estimate maximal oxygen uptake (VO_2 max).

shuttle test *See* **shuttle run test**.

sibling Brother or sister.

sibling influence The affect of a brother or sister on an individual's *socialization into sport. *See also* **significant other**.

sickle cell anaemia An hereditary blood disease characterized by abnormal red blood cells which are sickle-shaped. The red blood cells are inefficient at carrying oxygen and are rapidly removed from the circulation, causing *anaemia.

sickle cell trait An hereditary disease which is a mild version of sickle cell anaemia. The disease is endemic in Africa where the trait confers some resistance to malaria. Consequently, there is a high incidence of sickle cell trait among black people of African origin: for example, 8 per cent of Black Americans have the trait, but less than 0.01 per cent of whites. The red blood cells of people with sickle cell trait appear normal, and only about 40 per cent of the *haemoglobin is abnormal. This produces only mild anaemia and those with the trait can usually lead an active life and can participate in sport, even at the highest level. However, extreme conditions (such as maximal exercise in hot weather, or exercising at high altitude before complete acclimatization) can precipitate a life-threatening syndrome called fulminant exertional rhabdomyolysis. Blood cells in limbs become sickle shaped, and may lead to kidney failure, collapse, and even death. To avoid this syndrome, athletes with sickle cell trait should train wisely, ensure that they do not become dehydrated, and rest at the first signs of environmental stress.

side spin Spin imparted to a ball by an oblique impact which makes the ball kick or break to one side or the other. The spin may be to the left, with the angular rotation in a counter-clockwise direction

around the horizontal axis, or to the right, with the angular rotation in a clockwise direction around the horizontal axis. A ball with a right side spin, on hitting a surface, will rebound to the left, while a ball with a left side spin will rebound to the right.

sign 1 An objective indication (that is, one found by examining a patient) of a disease, physiological malfunction, or injury. *Compare* **symptom**. **2** A gesture or body movement which communicates an idea or intention.

signal 1 A variable parameter, such as frequency of nerve impulses or hormone levels, which conveys information through a system. **2** A specific *stimulus. **3** A sign or gesture to communicate information.

signal detection The ability to detect a particular *stimulus.

signal detection theory A theory explaining how a person is able to respond to one or more specific stimuli, usually against a background of noise. The theory suggests that individuals are actively involved in the response so that it depends not only on the subject's ability to discriminate between the signal and noise, but also on the subject's response bias or response criterion. For example, in experiments where subjects are asked to respond 'yes' when they receive a signal and 'no' when they hear no signal or when there is only noise, some have a rigid response criterion and respond 'yes' only when they are absolutely sure they have heard the signal, while others are less rigid and respond even when they are not certain.

signal substance In the nervous system, a *neurotransmitter.

signal-to-noise ratio The ratio of one parameter of a wanted *signal to the same parameter of noise in a system. The signal-to-noise ratio has an important effect on the ability to detect a signal (*see* **signal detection theory**).

significance In statistics, a description of an observed result that shows sufficient deviation from the expected or hypothesized result to be considered different from the expected result and not attributable to chance.

significant other A person, such as a family member, close friend, teacher, or coach, who is likely to influence an individual's values, beliefs, and behaviour, and to act as a role model.

simple carbohydrate A refined, highly processed carbohydrate which consists mainly of disaccharides or monosaccharides. Foods rich in simple carbohydrate usually lack minerals, vitamins, and roughage.

simple fracture Fracture in which the bone breaks cleanly but does not penetrate the skin; sometimes called a closed fracture.

simulator A training device which provides specific, controlled conditions so that skills can be practised under circumstances closely resembling those experienced in actual performance.

simultaneous conditioning A method of classical conditioning in which the conditioned stimulus is always presented at the same time as the unconditioned stimulus.

simultaneous force summation In humans, the production and combination of forces from different parts of the body to work together at the same time.

Sinding–Larsen–Johansson syndrome A juvenile form of jumper's knee; a *patellar tendinitis. It is an *overuse injury most common among élite basketball players who are tall and have high-riding patellae and elongate tendons. Their jumping and cutting movements subject the tendons to a whip-like action. Often small fragments of bone just below the lower part of the patella are visible on X-rays. Treatment includes reduction or temporary cessation of exercise for some months.

single-blind procedure In research, any method used to prevent a subject from knowing what treatment, such as a drug, he or she has received.

single-channel hypothesis A hypothesis of attention which posits that the information-processing system is structured as a single channel which, at any one time, can only deal with a single stimulus leading to a response. The hypothesis does not seem to account for the possibility of processing in two stages simultaneously or for parallel processing of two signals in one stage.

sinoatrial node (SA node; sinus node) The main pacemaker region of the heart. The sinoatrial node is a specialized area of cardiac tissue, located in the right atrium of the heart, which initiates the electrical impulses that determines the *heart rate.

sinus 1 A cavity within a bone filled with air and lined with mucus. **2** A dilated channel allowing the passage of blood, pus, or lymph from deeper tissues to the exterior.

sinus node *See* sinoatrial node.

sinusitis Inflammation of the paranasal sinuses due to bacterial infection. In order to avoid prolonging the illness, athletes with sinusitis should not take part in hard physical activity until the illness is resolved. Swimmers susceptible to sinusitis may be advised to wear nose-clips during training and competition in water.

Siri equation *See* densitometry.

SIQ *See* Sport Imagery Questionnaire.

SI system Le Système Internationale d'Unites (the International System of Units), an internationally agreed coherent system of units derived from the metric system. The basic units are the metre (m), kilogram (kg), ampere (A), Kelvin (K), mole (mol), and candela (cd). Derived units that are important in sports science include the newton (N), joule (J), watt (W), and pascal (P).

sit-and-reach test *See* sitting toe-touch test.

sit-down-and roll principle Principle of maximizing the area of the body in contact with a landing surface such as a floor or gym mat, to spread the force of landing over as wide an area as possible. It reduces the pressure applied to any particular part of the body and so reduces the risk of injury on landing.

sitting-toe-touch test (sit-and-reach test) An indirect test of flexibility in which the subject sits on the floor with back upright and legs straight, and bends forwards as far as possible. The distance of the fingertips beyond a zero mark on the floor is used as a measure of flexibility.

situation The objective set of conditions towards which a person acts or reacts.

situational approach A theoretical viewpoint which emphasizes the importance of the environmental situation, rather than his or her innate personality disposition, in determining a person's behaviour.

situational behaviour A form of *leadership which is effective in one set of conditions but not another.

situational factor Any factor, such as an environmental factor or the equipment a person is using, which contributes to the set of conditions to which a person acts or reacts. *See also* **display**.

situational leadership theory A theory which proposes that coaches ought to vary their leadership style according to the changing needs of their athletes. Immature and inexperienced athletes, for example, require more emotional support and direction than mature and experienced athletes. Also, the coach should not emphasize skills training until an athlete has gained the maturity and confidence to be successful. Once the athlete has gained sufficient maturity to become self-sufficient, the coach should become less directive.

situational trait A *leadership trait that is effective in one situation but not another.

sit-up An exercise to improve strength and endurance of *abdominal muscles. There are many variations, some do more harm than good. Harmful versions include those in which the legs are kept straight and too much strain is imposed on the neck and lower back. Typically, the subject lies on his or her back, usually with hands on top of the head, knees bent, and soles of the feet flat on the floor about hip-width apart. The subject than curls up, either just lifting the shoulders off the floor or up to a sitting position, touching the elbows to the knees.

sixty-second vertical jump *See* Bosco jump test.

size principle A principle of neurobiology which states that, during the reflex activation, motor neurones with the smallest cells bodies have the lowest threshold, and motor neurones with the largest cell bodies have the highest threshold. Thus, motor units are recruited according to their size as a voluntary contraction increases from zero force to a maximal voluntary force level (100 per cent maximum contraction).

skeletal Pertaining to the bony frame of the body.

skeletal age A measurement of maturity using X-rays of bones, usually of the left hand or wrist; age approximations are based on the extent to which ossification of the epiphyses has occurred.

skeletal connective tissue *See* bone; and cartilage.

skeletal muscle Voluntary muscle attached to bone or occasionally skin. When stimulated, skeletal muscle moves a part of the skeleton, such as an arm or leg. *See also* **striated muscle**.

skeletal system System in the body consisting of *bone and *cartilage which provides the basic framework through which muscles act.

skeletomuscular system Body system composed of muscles, bones, and their attachments.

skeleton Structures that make up the rigid framework of the body, support and protect the soft tissues, and provide a system of levers for locomotion. Some parts of the skeleton also manufacture red blood cells and store materials, such as fat, calcium, and phosphate. The skeleton includes cartilage and over 200 bones which make up the appendicular and axial skeleton, accounting for about 20 per cent of body mass.

skew A measure of dispersion which estimates how far a set of values varies from the symmetry of a *normal distribution curve. A deviation to the right of the curve indicates a negative skew value, deviation to the left indicates a positive value.

skewed distribution Distribution of a set of values which deviates from a normal distribution curve. *See also* **skew**.

skier's thumb (gamekeeper's thumb; goalkeeper's thumb) A sprain of the ulnar collateral ligament of the thumb adjacent to the web between the thumb and forefinger. It can result from any falling accident, but it occurs most commonly when a skier falls on an outstretched arm with the ski-pole forcing the thumb upwards and outwards. It accounts for about 10 per cent of all skiing injuries seen by a doctor. Primary treatment immediately after sustaining the injury includes gentle application of ice for 20 to 30 minutes (*see* **ice treatment**) and analgesics to relieve the pain. Further treatment depends on the degree of the sprain: mild sprains are immobilized in a splint for about three weeks, after which physical therapy is applied; complete ruptures are usually treated surgically.

skill A movement dependent on practice and experience for its execution, as opposed to being genetically defined. It is a learned movement, and is an essential component of sport. Skill enables athletes to produce predetermined results with maximum certainty, often with the minimum expenditure of energy. Three important components of skill are effectiveness, consistency (the ability to reproduce the skill), and efficiency. *See also* **cognitive skill**; **motor skill**; and **perceptual skill**.

skill acquisition The learning process by which a skill is gained.

skill effectiveness A characteristic used to define a *skill; it refers to the accuracy of response and the economy of effort used in performing a skill. *Compare* **skill flexibility**.

skill flexibility A defining characteristic of *skill; it is the ability to perform the skill successfully in different circumstances.

skin cancer Uncontrolled proliferation of skin cells. Skin cancer can be caused by excessive, unprotected exposure to the sun. All outdoor athletes are at risk, especially if they compete for long periods in the summer during the middle part of the day. Professional golfers, for example, have a higher than normal incidence of basal cell skin cancers. Most types of skin cancer are curable if treated early. Outdoor athletes are advised to protect their sun-exposed skin with sunscreens and clothing. *See also* **cyclist's melanoma**.

skin conductance The ability of the skin to conduct electricity, measured as the ratio of the current flowing through the skin to the potential difference across it. Skin conductance varies with the moisture on the skin and has been used to evaluate *arousal levels.

skinfold measurement A widely applied technique for estimating body density, fat-free mass, and relative body fat. Special calipers are used to measure the thickness of a double layer of skin and its underlying *adipose tissue (but not muscle) held by the left thumb and index finger at specific points on the body (e.g., on the back of the arm and below the scapula). Skinfold thicknesses increase with increasing amounts of fat and multiple skinfold measurements are used in equations to give good estimates of body composition (correlations range from about 0.90 to 0.96).

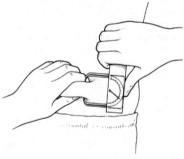

skinfold

skin friction *See* **surface drag**.

skin temperature Temperature on the body surface. Skin temperature varies considerably according to environmental conditions and exercise intensity. *Compare* **core temperature**.

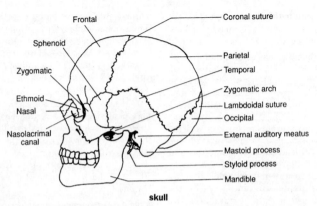

Frontal — Coronal suture

Sphenoid

Parietal

Zygomatic — Temporal

Zygomatic arch

Ethmoid — Lambdoidal suture

Nasal — Occipital

Nasolacrimal canal — External auditory meatus

Mastoid process

Styloid process

Mandible

skull

skull Bones of the head and face. The skull is composed of the cranium enclosing and protecting the brain, and the facial bones.

sledge apparatus Equipment used to investigate the mechanical efficiency of isolated concentric and eccentric exercises, and exercises involving *stretch-shortening cycles. The apparatus consists of a sledge with a mass of 33 kg to which the subject is fixed in a sitting position; a slow-friction aluminium track down which the sledge slides; a force plate paced perpendicular to the track; and apparatus for recording oxygen consumption and muscle activity.

sleep A physiological condition of relative immobility and natural unconsciousness when there is an increased reluctance to respond to stimulation and when many bodily functions are maintained at a minimum level of activity. There is much controversy concerning the significance of sleep. Traditional views emphasize its restorative value; another view emphasizes the advantages of the associated immobility (for example, in conserving energy expenditure). *See also* **REM sleep**; and **sleep deprivation**.

sleep apnoea A potentially dangerous condition in which breathing stops temporarily during sleep. It is often associated with deep snoring when breathing resumes.

sleep deprivation A disruption and reduction in the number of hours of sleep normally needed by a person. There is no standard or minimum number of hours per night regarded as necessary for everyone. Athletes appear to be able to adapt to sleep losses of up to 2 hours per night without impairing their exercise performance. Greater losses of sleep, however, are associated with reduced reaction time, poorer coordination, and lower vigilance, all of which adversely affect some athletic performances. Complete sleep deprivation for 1 to 3 nights can produce distinct alterations in *personality with subjects exhibiting psychotic-like symptoms and bizarre behaviour. Exercise often restores normal sleep patterns in people who suffer sleep disorders.

sliding-filament theory A theory which explains how muscles contract. Each *sarcomere (the functional unit of the muscle) contains overlapping thin (*see* **actin**) and thick (*see* **myosin**) filaments which can be interconnected by cross bridges. According to the theory, a shortening of sarcomere length is brought about by the two types of filaments sliding past each other by means of a rachet-like mechanism of the cross bridges. Strong intermolecular forces occurring between the myosin head and cross bridge, cause the head to tilt. By means of this so-called power stroke, the thin filaments are pulled into the space between the thick filaments in each sarcomere. Contraction is triggered by a stimulatory *nerve impulse which causes an *action potential to spread across the

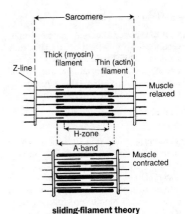

sliding-filament theory

sarcomere. The action potential causes calcium ions to be released around the filaments, enabling the cross bridges from myosin to attach onto the actin (in the absence of calcium, the attachment sites are blocked by *tropomyosin). *Adenosine triphosphate provides the energy used by the rachet mechanism. *See also* **rigor complex**.

sliding friction Friction that occurs during the time two surfaces are in contact and sliding relative to one another.

slipped disc A misnomer; discs do not slip they herniate or rupture (*see* **prolapsed intervertebral disc**).

slipped epiphysis An *overuse injury in young athletes in which there is a disruption of the *epiphyseal plate. *See also* **epiphysiolysis**.

Sloan–Weir formula A formula which uses a combination of anthropometric measures, including *skinfold measurements, for predicting *body density and total body fat.

slope *See* **gradient**.

slow oxidative fibre *See* **slow-twitch fibre**.

slow-twitch fibre (slow oxidative fibre; ST fibre; SO fibre; Type I fibre) A type of *muscle fibre characterized by a relatively slow contraction time, low glycolytic or *anaerobic capacity, and high oxidative or aerobic capacity, making the fibre suitable for low power, long duration activities. ST fibres have a high density of mitochondria, high myoglobin content, and a rich blood supply. *Compare* **fast-twitch fibre**.

Smith's fracture Wrist fracture in which the distal end of the radius is displaced forwards. It is usually caused by a violent forward flexion (palmar flexion) of the wrist. It is often unstable and frequently requires surgical fixation. *See also* **Colles' fracture**.

smelling salts *See* **ammonia salts**.

smoking The act of inhaling the products of combustion from tobacco which contains carbon monoxide and *nicotine. Smoking is harmful to health and athletic performance. It can cause lung cancer. Smoking is the main risk factor for heart disease and peripheral vascular disease.

smooth muscle (involuntary muscle) Muscle consisting of spindle-shaped cells with no obvious striations. Smooth muscle lines the walls of hollow organs such as the stomach, intestines, and blood vessels. It is particularly well adapted to producing long, slow contractions which are not under voluntary control. *Compare* **striated muscle**.

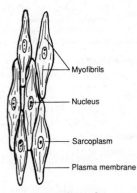

smooth muscle

snapping hip syndrome A symptom of a variety of disorders, usually caused by snapping of the *iliotibial band over the outside of the hip bone. It may lead to *trochanteric bursitis. It is common in gymnasts, hurdlers, and long-distance runners.

sensory store *See* **short-term sensory store**.

snow blindness Inflammation of the cornea and conjunctiva. Snow blindness develops in localities where sunlight is reflected strongly from snow. Ultraviolet radiation is absorbed by DNA in the superficial corneal epithelium, and, 4–6 hours after exposure, the epithelium sloughs off leaving the cornea inflamed and painful. Other symptoms include photophobia and profuse secretion of tears. The photophobia may be so great that the patient is rendered temporarily blind. Similar conditions may occur whenever there is chronic exposure to strong light.

SO fibres *See* **slow twitch fibres**.

soccer toe *See* **black nail**.

sociability Any form of social interaction in which people become involved solely for its own sake. For example, having a drink with a friend in the sports club bar. Although pursued for the sake of the pleasure it gives to the individual, sociability may have a serious underlying purpose, for example, in reinforcing social bonds.

social 1 Pertaining to the interaction humans have with one another, either as individuals or in groups. **2** Pertaining to mutual support and welfare.

social action theory The suggestion that individuals have the capacity to make their own interpretations of a situation and are not dictated to by circumstances, although they are aware of the circumstances. *See also* **role theory**.

social actor *See* **actor**.

social adjustment The ability to integrate successfully with others. *See also* **socialization**.

social approval theory Behaviour directed at gaining approval from significant others (e.g. coaches and parents). Social approval behaviour is particularly apparent in young children and is characterized by the way children often work hard for approval from significant others.

social bonding *See* **bonding**.

social categories theory A theory of mass communication which argues that individuals within broad subgroups (such as age classes, sex, social, or educational class) react similarly to the mass media. *Compare* **individual difference theory**.

social change Any major alteration in the pattern of social interactions in society.

social class A division of society which shares a similar social and economic status, and, in some societies, ancestry. Social class is used as an indicator of an individual's position, status, or power in society. Social mobility of individuals is generally easy within a given social class, but more difficult between different social classes.

social cohesion The degree to which the members of a team like each other and enjoy each other's company. It is a major dimension of team cohesion. *See also* **cohesion**.

social competence The ability to form social relationships easily and to mix with other people. It is often regarded as an objective of physical education.

social conflict A struggle between two or more contesting groups over values or scarce resources.

social contagion The transmission of a corrupting influence from one person to another. Social contagion tends to occur when people are together in large crowds. When aggression is carried out in a sports arena, there observers may be urged to join in and to complete the hostility that has built up. *See also* **audience effect**.

social control The use of negative and positive sanctions (punishment and reward) by control agents to enforce conformity with the norms and expectations of the society. In sport, social control would include the means by which the rules are enforced.

social control agency An organized agency, such as the police, of *social control. In sport, officials such as referees and umpires act as social control agencies.

social Darwinism Term, often used disparagingly, for any theory which attempts to apply Darwin's principles of natural selection to society.

social death A concept applied to the social and psychological changes involved in retirement from sport.

social demarcation The social separation of individuals on the basis of social class. For example, in cricket, there used to be a clear social demarcation between players, who played professionally, and gentlemen who were amateurs.

social development Any change in society which leads to new or more complex relations between individuals or groups within that society. For example, the removal of apartheid in South Africa which is resulting in greater social mixing (including participation in sport) of the population of individuals from different ethnic and social backgrounds.

social distance The degree of separation of one group from another in terms of cultural development and social relationships, which may result in one group not joining in activities with another group. The term applies particularly to social classes and is taken to its extreme in systems such as apartheid.

social distribution In sport sociology, the extent to which a sport has permeated into a particular society, and spread through different societies. Studies of social distribution usually include determining the origin of the sport, in terms of time and place, and tracing the pattern of cultural diffusion.

social evaluation The evaluation of an individual's performance by others. Social evaluation has a powerful influence in sport, especially for top-class sportspeople whose performances are scrutinized by the mass media (*see* **competitive stress**). Sports which focus directly on individual performances tend to be more evaluative than team-sports in which responsibility for performance and outcome is shared.

social exchange theory *See* **exchange theory**.

social facilitation The beneficial or detrimental effects on performance of the presence of an audience which does not interact verbally or emotionally with the performers. Social facilitation occurs whenever an athlete performs differently in front of a noninteractive audience than when working alone. *See also* **audience effect**; **coaction**; and **Zajonc's model**.

social identity (social self) The sense of *self derived from membership and interaction in a social group.

social imitation theory A theory which proposes that the process of *socialization is more or less passive. The individual learns how to behave in specific social situations by observing and modelling the behaviour, perceived values, beliefs and norms exhibited by *significant others. *Compare* **symbolic interaction perspective**.

social indicators Statistics which relate to society and are regularly collected (such as crime rate or birth rate figures) that can be used as general indicators of changes in society.

social interactive force An influence on the learning and performance of a task derived from a person doing the task in a group rather than in isolation. *See also* **audience effect**; **coaction**; and **social facilitation**.

socialization (enculturation) A complex process by which individuals learn skills, attitudes, values, and patterns of behaviour that enable them to function within a particular culture. These patterns are learned from agencies such as school and home. Socialization enables members of a society to interact with one another and so pass on skills, values, beliefs, knowledge, and modes of behaviour pertaining to that society. Sport is generally regarded as playing a significant role in socialization.

socialization into sport 1 The learning process by which individuals acquire behaviour appropriate for a specific sport. It includes the acquisition of attitudes, values, and beliefs, such as sporting behaviour. **2** The process by which a person becomes involved and assumes a particular role in sport as coach, athlete, or spectator.

socialization through sport The process of acquiring, by participating in sport, beliefs, values, norms, and dispositions, such as sportsmanship, that are applicable in other social situations.

socializing agent Any agent that brings about the process of *socialization.

socializing situation The setting or environment in which *social learning occurs. *See also* **situation**.

social-learning theory The theory that, within the constraints of the social environment, individuals behave according to how they have learned to behave by observing others. Other people serve as models and the learner is prompted to imitate them, especially when the models' behaviour has favourable consequences. The social learning theory supports the notion that an athlete's immediate and past experiences influence his or her behaviour more than innate physiological drives; for example, it is proposed that acts of *aggression which are rewarded or go unpunished lead to more aggression, and that aggression in sport does not act as a catharsis against more aggression. *Compare* **frustration–aggression theory**; and **instinct theory**.

social loafing The reduction in individual effort and motivation as group size increases. Social loafing may help to explain performance losses in the Ringelmann's effect, and may be due to a diffusion of responsibility and loss of individual motivation.

social mobility The process by which people move between different social layers such as social classes or economic groups. High social mobility requires that there is a relatively open access to valued positions. Low social mobility exists where the valued positions are transmitted mainly through a system of inheritance.

social movement A collective action to promote or resist change. Social movements (such as feminist movements, civil rights movements, and fitness and health movements), are usually characterized by having an organization with leaders and followers who share similar values and understandings, and who have a sense of membership. Sport has often been used by social movements to publicize their activities and policies.

social pathology A condition or phenomenon in society, such as a widespread and deep civil unrest, generally regarded as unhealthy.

social problem Any aspect of society that might cause concern and a general desire for the society to intervene. Social problems in sport include inequality, oppression, discrimination, scandal, deviant behaviour, and violence. They are usually a reflection of (and therefore a part of) the problems of society in general.

social psychology Study of how a person's thoughts and behaviour are affected by others. Social psychology contains elements of both sociology and psychology.

social psychology of sport An area of sport psychology which brings together a number of important topics which cannot be classified as either entirely sociological or psychological. Social psychology of sport deals with areas of sport which affect both individuals and groups.

social reinforcement A form of reinforcement that consists of intangible, positive or negative evaluation, comments, and actions from others. Social reinforcement can take the form of verbal praise or criticism, or nonverbal communication such as smiles, frowns, and gestures.

social reinforcement theory The theory that social behaviour results from situations and encounters which are either rewarded or punished as an individual matures from childhood to adulthood. The theory includes the idea that rewarded behaviours are likely to be repeated. *See also* **classical conditioning**; **hedonism theory**; and **instrumental conditioning**.

social relationship An interaction between individuals which affects every participant. Social relationships include the interactions which bind people together into sports teams and groups.

social relationships theory A theory of mass communication which suggests that informal social relationships, particularly with significant others, have an important effect on an individual's response to the mass media.

social reproduction The processes by which societies reproduce their social structures and social institutions. *Socialization plays an important part in social reproduction.

social science A discipline which involves the systematic study of society and individuals, or social phenomena. There is some disagreement on how far some disciplines, such as the history of sport, can be regarded as a social science or can be studied in a scientific manner.

social scientist A person who studies a social science or who approaches a discipline concerned with some aspect of society in a scientific manner.

social self *See* **social identity**.

social setting A location, defined in terms of both space and time, which provides the contexts in which social interactions can occur.

social status A position to which an individual has been assigned in a social group determined by the attitudes towards him or her of other members of the group. The attitudes may be influenced by a number of factors, including the individual's income, occupation, and family.

social stratification The process by which people are assigned different social ranks in society. Social stratification forms the basis of inequalities within a society: higher social ranks tend to have more power, prestige, and privilege than the lower ranks. Social stratification is based on social or biological characteristics, such as social class, age, gender, ethnic group, rather than natural ability. It is possible for a person to be assigned a high social rank with respect to one factor, such as economic status, and a lower rank with regards another factor, such as gender.

social stratum A distinguishable layer within a hierarchical social system. *See also* **social stratification**.

social structure The more or less enduring structural elements and cultural components of a sport or other social activity.

social support behaviour A coaching behaviour characterized by concern for the welfare of individual athletes, a positive group atmosphere, and warm interpersonal relationships with members of the group or team.

social theory Any theory which attempts to systematically account for the development and organization of the structure of a society.

social thought The thoughts and views of different segments of society concerning the social value and significance of a social activity such as sport.

society A group of people connected to one another by shared customs, institutions, culture, and, to a lesser extent, territory.

sociocultural aspects of sport Aspects of sport which focus on the interactions between sport, society, and culture.

sociobiology The study of social organization and behaviour in humans and other animals which uses biological explanations based on the premise that all behaviour is adaptive.

socioeconomic status Categorization of an individual's position in society by means of his or her level of education, income, and occupation. *See also* **social status**.

sociogram Diagrammatic representation of data gathered to show how individuals, such as team members, relate to each other. *See also* **sociomatrix**; **sociometry**.

sociologist A person who studies *sociology.

sociology The study of every aspect and type of society in a scientific way. It encompasses elements of the other social sciences, but views society in a holistic way.

That is, sociology does not separate a study of society into areas such as history, economics, or politics but sees how all these aspects relate to one another.

sociomatrix A tabular representation in matrix form of data collected using a sociometric method to measure interpersonal relationships. The information in the matrix is often transformed to a sociogram.

sociometric cohesion The contribution to the *cohesion of a group made by interpersonal attraction between members of the group. *See also* **sociometry**.

sociometric measurement *See* sociometry.

sociometric method *See* sociometry.

sociometry (sociometric measurement; sociometric method) An observational field study method used mainly to measure what people in a group think and feel about each other. It uses a given criterion to gain a subjective measure of how members of a group view one another. For example, a question about who was the best player could be asked of each member of a team. The data gathered can be shown diagrammatically on a sociogram and it can be used to reveal who is generally highly thought of, which individuals form mutually supportive and attracted groups, and those who are isolated.

SOD *See* superoxide dismutase.

soda loading *See* bicarbonate loading.

sodium A metallic element that plays a major role in the regulation of the volume of water in the body. Deficiency is rare but it can occur if losses from heavy sweating are not replaced. Deficiency leads to nausea, dizziness, and muscle cramps. An excessive intake of sodium (e.g. by eating too much table salt) has been linked with high blood pressure and heart disease.

sodium bicarbonate A salt of sodium that neutralizes acids. Sodium bicarbonate is used in tablet-form as an ergogenic aid in the hope that it will augment the body's alkaline reserves against lactic acid and thereby delay fatigue (*see* **bicarbonate loading**). Sodium bicarbonate is also

taken to treat stomach disorders, acidosis, and sodium deficiencies.

sodium chloride (common salt) A salt of sodium. It is an important constituent of the human body.

sodium cromoglycate (SCG) A beta$_2$ agonist used to treat asthma and hay fever. It also helps prevent exercise-induced asthma. SCG has no reported effect on the cardiovascular system and no ergogenic value. Its use by inhalation is permitted by the International Olympic Committee. However, a mixture of cromoglycate and isoprenaline is banned.

sodium pump An active mechanism by which sodium is transferred against a concentration gradient from the inside to the outside of cells. The sodium pump plays an important role in maintaining the *resting potential of muscle fibres and nerve cells. Its operation depends on energy from ATP.

SO fibres *See* slow-twitch fibres.

soft tissue A tissue which has not been hardened (e.g., by ossification). The soft tissues surrounding a joint are muscle, tendons, fasciae, ligaments, and skin.

solar plexus The network of sympathetic nerves, situated behind the stomach, that supply the organs in the abdomen.

solar radiation Electromagnetic radiation, including the light-waves within the visible spectrum, from the sun.

sole 1 The underside of the foot. **2** The underside of a shoe.

soleus A flat muscle that extends along the back of the calf behind the gastrocnemius with which it forms the triceps surae. The soleus has extensive, cone-shaped origins on the superior tibia, fibula, and interosseus membrane. Its insertion is on the calcaneus via the *Achilles tendon. It has a high proportion of slow-twitch fibres which make it relatively fatigue-resistant. Its primary action is *plantar flexion. It is also an important postural muscle during locomotion.

soluble fibre Dietary *fibre found especially in oat bran. Soluble fibre may chemically prevent or reduce the absorption of *cholesterol and some other substances into the bloodstream. It may also help regulate blood glucose levels.

solute A substance dissolved in a solvent to form a solution.

solution A homogeneous mixture of two or more dissimilar substances. Most solutions are liquid and consist of a liquid solvent and a solid solute.

solvent A substance that has the ability to dissolve a solute. A solvent is the component of a solution which has the same physical properties as the solution itself.

somatic Pertaining to the body.

somatic anxiety Anxiety demonstrated by actual physiological responses such as increased heart rate and sweating. *Compare* cognitive anxiety. *See also* somatic state anxiety.

somatic nervous system Portion of the peripheral nervous system which carries efferent motor nerves to skeletal muscles.

somatic pain Pain arising from the skin, muscles, or joints, as distinct from pain arising from the viscera.

somatic sense Sense that enables people to feel pain, temperature change, touch, pressure, and the body's position in space.

somatic-state anxiety The somatic or body-related dimension of state anxiety. Somatic state anxiety is increased when a person feels threatened and becomes increasingly aware of his or her heart rate, ventilation rate, and sweating. *Compare* cognitive-state anxiety.

somatic stress management A procedure involving the relaxation of body musculature, used to cope with *stress. *See also* progressive muscle relaxation; *compare* cognitive stress management.

somatochart A diagram that can be used to display the somatotype of an individual or group.

somatocrinin A *hormone which promotes the secretion of *human growth hormone from cells in the anterior pituitary gland.

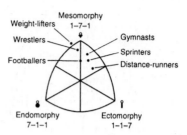

somatochart

Somatocrinin is produced by the *hypothalamus.

somatogram A triangular pattern for recording individual physique using the three-figure classification of somatotyping. All possible somatotypes can be recorded on a somatogram.

somatomedin *See* insulin-like growth factor.

somatostatin A peptide secreted in the retina, the *hypothalamus, and some other areas of the brain where it may function as a *neurotransmitter. Somatostatin is also secreted by the pancreas. It inhibits the release of *human growth hormone.

somatotonic trait A *personality type which, according to Sheldon's constitutional theory, has a strong correspondence with the mesomorph somatotype. Somatotonics are regarded as bold, competitive, risk-taking, and adventure seeking extroverts.

somatotype (body-type) The characteristic shape and physical appearance of an individual, disregarding size. There are several methods of somatotyping. The most commonly used is based on Sheldon's somatotype classification in which there are three types: endomorph, mesomorph, and ectomorph. Typically, individuals are rated on a scale of 1 to 7 for each type, according to the degree of dominance. The descriptive sequence of numbers refers to components in the following order: endomorph, mesomorph, and ectomorph. Thus, 1–7–1 indicates extreme mesomorphy. Successful athletes of particular sports tend to share the same somatotype: for example, discus-throwers, shot-putters,

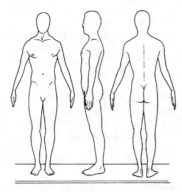

somatotype

and hammer-throwers tend to have a somatotype of about 3–6–3, while middle- and long-distance runners tend to have a somatotype of about 2.5–4–4. However, somatotypes of individual élite athletes sometimes deviate from the average somatotype of their group, indicating that although a certain somatotype may contribute to success in specific activities, it is by no means essential. Skill attainment depends on many factors and a disadvantageous somatotype may be overcome by emphasis on other factors.

somatotyping Rating a person's physique along three dimensions: endomorphy (roundness), mesomorphy (muscularity), and ectomorphy (linearity). *See also* **somatotype**.

sore Any open wound of the skin or mucous membranes.

source trait *See* **first-order trait**.

spaced practice *See* **distributed practice**.

spasm (muscle spasm) A sudden, involuntary muscle twitch ranging in severity from merely irritating to very painful. A spasm may be due to chemical imbalance. Massaging the area may help to end the spasm.

spasmolytic A drug which inhibits spasms.

spasticity Resistance to the passive movement of a limb which is maximal at the beginning of the movement and which

becomes less as more pressure is applied. Spasticity is a symptom of spinal injuries. It is usually accompanied by weakness in the affected limb (spastic paralysis).

spatial perception The ability to perceive or otherwise react to the size, distance, or depth aspects of the environment.

spatial planes and axes Planes and axes identified according to their relationship with the ground. Axes are designated as the x-axis, y-axis, and z-axis. The axes may be used to describe the direction of movement of a body.

spatial summation A phenomenon occurring at the *synapses between different neurones and at neuromuscular junctions in which the responsiveness of the postsynaptic neurone or muscle fibre depends on the additive effect of numerous stimuli coming from different afferent neurones or dendrites. *See also* **summation**.

Spearman rank correlation coefficient A test which uses a ranking system to assess the degree of correlation existing between two sets of data. The two sets of data are placed in rank order next to each other so that they can be compared statistically.

special training (sport-related training) Training (e.g., hill running for sprinters) aimed at perfecting individual components of sports techniques and sport specific fitness.

specific adaptations to imposed demands principle *See* SAID.

specific dynamic action Former name for the *thermic effect of food.

specific gravity The former name for *relative density.

specific heat capacity The quantity of heat required to raise the temperature of unit mass of substance by one degree. It is measured in $Jkg^{-1}K^{-1}$.

specificity *See* **principle of specificity**.

specificity of fitness principle The principle that athletes need to develop the right kind of fitness for their particular activity because different sports vary in their physical demands.

specific muscle training Training which involves exercising muscles in isolated movements. This form of training is specific for the muscle groups that are being trained, and adaptation is limited to the kind of movement performed. Specific muscle training can be divided into muscle strength training, muscle speed endurance training, and flexibility training.

specific strength The strength of a particular type of muscle action. A person who has a high level of strength for one type of muscle action does not necessarily have a high level of strength for other types. *See also* **principle of specificity**.

specific training (competition-specific training) Training in which techniques and skills are rehearsed in situations similar to those expected in competition.

spectator A group of individuals actually observing a sport. *See also* **audience**.

speed 1 Distance travelled per unit time, measured in m s^{-1}. It is a *scalar quantity. In running and walking speed is a product of stride length and stride rate. **2** The ability to perform a movement quickly. Speed of movement of either the total body (e.g., in sprinting) or of a particular body part is an important component of performance related fitness (*see also* **reaction time**). **3** *See* **amphetamines**

speed-accuracy trade off The general principle that the accuracy of a movement tends to decrease when its speed is increased. *See also* **Fitt's law**.

speed endurance training A form of *anaerobic training which has two main components: production training which improves the ability to perform maximally for short periods of time, and maintenance training which increases the ability to sustain exercise at a high intensity.

speed of arm movement A skill-oriented ability underlying tasks, such as a boxer's jab, for which a limb must be moved from one place to another very quickly.

speed of release The speed of a projectile at the instant of release. In throwing events (such as discus, shot, and javelin), the speed of release is proportional to the average force exerted through the projectile's *centre of gravity. Generally for a given angle and relative projection height, the displacement of a projectile increases with the speed of release. As the angle of release is lowered, the speed of release needs to be increased to achieve the same displacement. Speed of release depends on the speed of the last part of the body involved in the action at the time of release.

speed play *See* **fartlek training**.

speed–time curve A curve or line which best fits the points on a graph on which speed is plotted on the y-axis and time on the x-axis. A speed–time curve may be used to identify different levels of *acceleration; for example, during different phases of a 100 m race.

speed training A form of anaerobic training which involves sprinting. In team games such as soccer, speed training not only improves a player's sprinting ability, but also improves a player's ability to perceive, evaluate, and act quickly in competitive situations. *See also* **speed endurance training**.

SPF (sun protection factor) An indication on sunscreen products of the relative degree of protection it provides against sunburn as compared with using no sunscreen. A product with an SPF of 15, for example, is claimed to enable a person to be exposed to the sun fifteen times longer on average than if no sunscreen were applied. *See also* **skin cancer**.

sphincter A circular muscle the contraction of which can close an opening. Sphincter muscles in blood vessels play an important role in *shunting blood from one part of the body to another.

sphygmomanometer (blood pressure cuff) An instrument for measuring *blood pressure in the arteries. It usually consists of an inflatable cuff which incorporates a pressure gauge. The cuff is wrapped around the arm and pumped up sufficiently to stop the pulse as felt at the wrist or heard with a stethoscope placed on the artery at the bend of the elbow. As the applied pressure is reduced, blood starts to flow again in the artery and the pressure reading on the gauge at this point represents systolic pressure. The pressure at which there is a full flow of blood, indicated by a marked change in the sound heard through the stethoscope, represents the diastolic pressure.

sphyrion An anatomical landmark on the distal tip, but not the outermost point, of the *malleolus.

spin Rotation of a ball or other projectile around its central axis. Friction tends to impart some spin on a ball. If a ball is spinning when it makes contact with another surface, the rate and direction of the spin will affect the magnitude of friction. Consequently, the speed and direction of the ball after impact will also be modified. *See also* **back spin**; **side spin**; and **top spin**.

spinal canal Canal formed by vertebrae through which the spinal cord passes.

spinal column *See* **vertebral column**.

spinal cord Part of the central nervous system which extends down the back as a relatively uniform tube. The spinal cord is enclosed and protected by the vertebrae. Pairs of spinal nerves leave the cord in each segment of the body. The cord is continuous with the brain.

spinal curvature The normal S-shaped curvature in the vertebral column which increases its strength, resilience, and flexibility. Viewed from the side, there are three principal curvatures that give the back its normal S-shape. The cervical and lumbar curvatures are concave posteriorly; the thoracic curvature and the sacrum are convex posteriorly. *See also* **kyphosis**; **lordosis**; and **scoliosis**.

spinale height A body height measurement made from the *iliospinale on the hip to base.

spinal extension Return of the spine to its anatomical position after spinal flexion.

spinal extensor A muscle that effects spinal extension. Spinal extensors include the *splenius, *erector spinae, and *semi-spinalis muscles.

spinal flexion Anterior (forward) movement of the spinal column.

spinal flexor A muscle that effects spinal flexion. Major spinal flexors include the *external oblique, *internal oblique, and *rectus abdominis muscles.

spinal generator A mechanism in the spinal cord consisting of a complex network of neurones capable of producing oscillatory behaviour (a rhythmical output of activity) thought to be involved in the control of certain basic movements in locomotion.

spinal hyperextension Extension of the spine backwards, beyond the *anatomical position. Hyperextension is greatest in the cervical and lumbar regions. Extreme lumbar hyperextension is important in many sports such as the high jump, pole vault, and gymnastics (during the back handspring, for example, the curvature of the lumbar region may increase twenty-fold).

spinalis The most medial muscle in the *erector spinae group. The spinalis has its origins on the neural spines of the lumbar and lower thoracic vertebrae. Its insertions are on the upper thoracic and cervical vertebrae. The spinalis is involved in trunk extension.

spinal lateral flexion Sideways movement of the spine in the frontal plane, left or right away from the anatomical position. The greatest range of lateral movement occurs in the cervical region. Spinal lateral flexion is effected by the *quadratus lumborum, *laevator scapulae, and many other back muscles when they contract on one side of the body only.

spinal movements Although the spinal column can move in all three planes, movement between adjacent vertebra is very limited and the range of movement varies throughout the length of the column. Spinal movements are usually accompanied by pelvic and hip movements to move the trunk as a whole.

spinal nerve A nerve originating from the spinal cord. There are 31 pairs of spinal nerves. Each contains thousands of afferent (sensory) and efferent (motor) fibres.

spinal process A projection rising from a bone; for example, the neural spine on a *vertebra.

spinal reflex A somatic *reflex action mediated by the spinal cord. It is the simplest type of reflex, requiring a minimum of two neurones, and may not involve the higher brain centres. An afferent neurone carries a sensory impulse via the dorsal root of the spinal cord, and the impulse is transmitted along a motor neurone to the effector organs. Usually, a third neurone, the association neurone in the spinal cord, occurs between the sensory neurone and motor neurone.

spinal rotation Rotation of the spine about its longitudinal axis. The greatest range of spinal rotation is in the cervical region and it decreases progressively down the spine until the lumbrosacral region where it increases slightly. For structural reasons, spinal rotation is always accompanied by lateral rotation although this may be so slight that it is not observable with the naked eye. Rotation is a complex movement often brought about by a combination of muscle contractions, some of which function as *neutralizers. Some muscles (e.g., the internal obliques and the splenii)) contract unilaterally to rotate the body to the same side, but other muscles (e.g., the external obliques and erector spinae) unilaterally contract to rotate the trunk to the opposite side.

spinal traction A method of separating vertebrae in the neck and back, and stretching spinal muscles, ligaments, and joint capsules. Spinal traction is used to treat whiplash and certain other spinal conditions, such as degenerative joint disease and joint hypomobility. It may be performed by manipulation or mechanically. The long-term resolution of spinal problems usually requires special exercises, and posture modification.

spine See **vertebral column**.

spinner's finger An injury commonly caused by spin bowling in cricket, baseball, and other ball sports. Although the skin in the hand becomes hardened with use, the forces used to impose spin on the ball can crack the skin, leaving open wounds susceptible to infection. If this happens, the skin must be allowed time to harden and heal.

spiral fracture An angulated break which occurs when excessive twisting forces are applied to a bone. Spiral fractures of the long bones are common in sport.

spirometer A device for measuring the volume of gases inspired into and expired from the lungs during ventilation.

splanchnic shunt Diversion of some blood from internal organs such as the intestines, liver, and kidneys, to active muscle during exercise. These internal organs normally can survive on a reduced blood supply for at least a few hours of exercise. See also **shunting**.

spleen A large, highly vascularized organ situated beneath the stomach. It is part of the reticuloendothelial system producing white blood cells, and removing worn out red blood cells and some foreign bodies. It is the most commonly injured organ in the abdomen. Its position just below the ninth and eleventh ribs makes it very susceptible to puncture by a fractured rib or a direct blow to the trunk. It can even be ruptured during a noncontact sport as a result of very strenuous activity, especially if it has become enlarged during a viral infection. About 40 per cent of sport-related splenic ruptures are associated with *infectious mononucleosis, emphasizing the need to avoid strenuous activity during the febrile stage of an illness. A splenic rupture often results in massive internal bleeding, which can lead to a potentially fatal lowering of blood pressure. Usually, surgical removal of the spleen is the only viable course of action. Splenic ruptures can easily go unnoticed. Expert medical assistance should be sought whenever an athlete is suffering from persistent abdominal discomfort after a blow or extreme physical exertion.

splenic rupture See **spleen**.

splenius A broad superficial muscle divided into two parts, the capitis and cervicis, extending from the upper thoracic vertebrae to the skull. The capitis portion is known as the 'bandage muscle' because it covers and holds down deeper neck muscles. Its origin is on the ligamentum nuchae (the ligament which runs down the side of the neck) and the neural spines from the seventh lumbar and sixth thoracic vertebrae. The insertions of the capitis are on a nipple-shaped extension (called the mastoid process) of the temporal bone and the occipital bone; the insertions of the cervicis are on the transverse processes of the second to fourth cervical vertebrae. The splenius muscles act simultaneously as a unified group on both sides of the neck to extend or hyperextend the head; when the muscles on one side are activated, the head is rotated and bends laterally towards the same side.

splint A rigid device used to support or immobilize an injured body-part. Splints may be used to hold broken bones or ruptured ligaments in place, and to ensure conformity between the broken ends during the healing process.

spondylitis Inflammation of the *synovial joints of the vertebrae. *See also* **ankylosing spondylitis**.

spondylolisthesis A fracture of the pars interarticularis (the weakest part of the neural arch of a vertebra) resulting in complete separation of the anterior region of the vertebra from the region below it. The most common site for this injury is the lumbosacral joint. Spondylolisthesis reduces flexibility and results in tightening of the hamstrings.

spondylolysis A stress fracture in the pars interarticularis (the weakest part of the neural arch) of a vertebra. It is sometimes congenital, but may also be caused by mechanical stress. The condition is characterized by acute pain on one side of the lower back, worsened by twisting and hyperextension. Spondylolysis is unusually common among participants in sports involving repeated hyperextension of the lumbar spine (e.g., fast bowlers, weightlifters, female gymnasts). Treatment may include bed-rest and a special exercise programme incorporating hamstring stretching.

spondylosis A degenerative condition of intervertebral discs. Symptoms include pain and restriction of movement. Sometimes stress at vertebral margins above and below the disc produces an X-ray image characteristic of spondylosis (including narrowing of the space occupied by the disc, and *osteophytes), without any association with pain or a painful syndromes. This entity is known as 'radiological spondylosis'.

sponging Application of a wet sponge to the body surface to aid cooling or to treat minor injuries. During exercise, the skin temperature rises causing peripheral blood vessels to dilate and blood to pool in the extremities. Sponging is an effective way of cooling the body surface so that the vessels constrict and blood is returned to the general circulation. However, although sponging may have circulatory benefits and help an athlete to feel cooler, it does not seem to aid heat loss. Sponging is a traditional primary treatment of minor injuries in sports such as rugby and soccer. Application of cold water may have an analgesic effect, but sponging should not use water from a communal bucket because of the risk of transmission of bloodborne diseases. Athletes suffering from oozing or bleeding wounds should be removed from the field of play and the appropriate treatment given under hygienic conditions.

spongy bone (cancellous bone; trabecular bone) Type of bone found at the ends of long bones and in the vertebrae. It has a honeycomb structure consisting of small needle-like or flat pieces of mineralized bars called trabeculae, in between which are spaces filled with marrow and fat. *Compare* **compact bone**.

sponsored mobility A process whereby a higher social status is acquired through the efforts and help of others. *Compare* **contest mobility**.

spontaneous behaviour Coaching behaviour initiated by the coach and which is not a response to player behaviour. *Compare* **reactive behaviour**.

spontaneous pneumothorax *See* pneumo- thorax.

sport Any highly structured, goal directed physical activity governed by rules, which has a high level of commitment, takes the form of a struggle with oneself or involves competition with others, but which also has some of the characteristics of play. Sport involves either vigorous physical exertion or the use of relatively complex physical skills by individuals whose participation is motivated by a combination of the intrinsic satisfaction associated with the activity itself and the external rewards earned through participation. *See also* **play**; and **recreation**.

sport cohesion instrument Multidimensional questionnaire which measures four dimensions of *team cohesion: attraction to the group, sense of purpose, quality of teamwork, and valued roles. It was originally designed for basketball but its versatility has allowed it to be used for other team sports. *See also* **sport cohesiveness questionnaire**.

sport cohesiveness questionnaire A popular sport-related test of *team cohesion composed of seven questions. Two questions ask team members to assess other members of the team relative to feelings of friendship and team influence; three questions ask the athlete to assess his or her relationship to the team in terms of a sense of belonging, value of membership, and enjoyment; and the remaining two questions ask the athlete to evaluate the team as a whole in terms of teamwork and closeness. The findings of some studies indicate a strong association between cohesion and sport performance, and between cohesion and satisfaction.

sport competition anxiety test (SCAT) A test measuring the propensity of an athlete to experience *anxiety when competing in a sport. It is used to measure *competitive trait anxiety. Test scoring is based on ten questions that ask individuals how they feel when competing in sports and games.

Each item is answered on a three-point scale (often, sometimes, hardly ever) and a summary score ranging from 10 (low competitive trait anxiety) to 30 (high competitive trait anxiety) is computed for each respondent.

sport confidence The belief or degree of certainty individuals have about their ability to be successful in sport. *See also* **Vealey's sport-specific model of confidence**.

sport consumer An individual who consumes sport either directly as a spectator attending a sporting event, or indirectly via the mass media. The direct consumer tends to have an audience effect. There is a strong relationship between sport producers and sport consumers of a particular sport. A survey of adults in the United States concluded that people tend to watch what they play and play what they watch.

sport for all Slogan used in Britain which encourages physical performance opportunities for all members of the community, where emphasis is on participation more than performance standards.

sport-general dropout A person who discontinues involvement in all of sport. *Compare* **sport-specific dropout**.

Sport Imagery Questionnaire (SIQ) A questionnaire that measures athletes' abilities to experience different senses, emotions, and perspectives during imagery. The SIQ refers to four experiences common in sport: practising alone, practising with others, watching a team mate, and playing in a contest. After spending a minute imaging scenes including each of these experiences separately, ratings are made on a five-point Likert scale from 'no image present' to 'extremely clear and vivid image' for three sense modalities (hearing, vision, and kinaesthesis). Some variations of the SIQ include ratings on a five-point Likert scale for controllability of the image (e.g., from 'no control at all of image', to 'complete control of image'). SIQ is used widely in applied sport psychology, but its validity and reliability have not been established.

sporting behaviour (sportsmanship; sports-personship; sportswomanship) Behaviour exhibited by someone who respects and abides by the rules of a sport and responds fairly, generously, and with good humour when winning or losing. It is demonstrated by the competitor who chooses an ethically correct strategy in preference to the success strategy which can be summed up as 'win at all costs'.

sport intelligence A concept recently introduced to describe the particular types of mental ability needed to complete the demands of a sport task successfully. Sporting intelligence includes knowledge of the sport, knowledge of where and when important cues are likely to occur, the ability to search for and detect task-relevant cues, identification of cue patterns, short term memory recall, and decision-making ability.

sport mastery (sport orientation) The ability to perfect a skill and perform it well. Sport mastery may form an intrinsically motivated *achievement goal in which an athlete evaluates success or failure on how well he or she has performed, regardless of winning or losing.

sport orientation *See* sport mastery.

Sport Orientation Questionnaire A questionnaire developed as a multidimensional measure of *achievement motivation. It is composed of 25 items measuring three different orientations: competitiveness (the desire to enter and strive for success in sport-specific situations); win orientation (the desire to win interpersonal competitive sporting events); and goal orientation (the desire to achieve personal goals in sport).

sport personology The study of the *personality of individuals involved in sport. The study often includes three dimensions of personality: personality structure, personality dynamics, and personality development.

sport physiology The application of *exercise physiology to the special demands of sport. Concepts derived from exercise physiology are used to optimize the training of athletes and enhance their performance.

sport population The number of people within a country, community, or some other grouping who physically participate in sporting activities. Different criteria are used by different nations to calculate their sport population. For example, in the old Soviet Union, it was calculated on the basis of those engaged in organized physical culture activities more than twice a week, with each session being at least 1 hour long. In the United States of America and Europe its calculation is usually based on activities which are performed at least three times a week for more than 30 minutes each time.

sport producer Anyone actively involved in the production of a sporting event. Sport producers include coaches, managers, officials, team doctors, promoters, and sponsors. They include direct producers who perform tasks that have direct consequences for the outcome of the sport (for example, games officials, referees, coaches, and medical personnel), and indirect producers who have no immediate impact on the outcome of the sporting event (e.g., sponsors, and ticket-sellers). *Compare* **sport consumer**.

sport psychologist A professionally trained person who observes, describes, and explains the various psychological factors that influence diverse aspects of sport and physical activity. Sport psychologists support sportspersons with behavioural problems, but much of their time is devoted to helping psychologically well-balanced athletes acquire extraordinary psychological skills in order to cope with the unusual demands of competition.

sport psychology The scientific study of behaviour in sport and the application of the principles of psychology to sport situations and people involved in sport. These principles may be applied to enhance performance and improve the quality of sport experience.

sports adrenal medulla An adaptation of the *adrenal medulla to regular, prolonged endurance training. It is characterized by an increased capacity to secrete *adrenaline in response to various stimuli (e.g., hypoxia, hypoglycaemia, and hypercapnia) and, possibly, an increase in the size of the adrenal medulla. Since adrenaline increases mental alertness and muscle contractility, sports adrenal medulla is probably advantageous in competitive sports.

sports anaemia *See* **athletic pseudo-anaemia**.

sports group A group within sport which has a sense of unity or collective identity, a sense of shared purpose or objectives, structured patterns of interaction, structured modes of communication, personal and/or task interdependence, and interpersonal attraction.

sports haematuria *See* **runner's haematuria**.

sports injuries Damage to the body due to physical trauma associated with sport. Many sports injuries differ little from injuries arising from domestic or industrial situations. There are, however, subtle differences in the nature of the damage, the form of treatment, and the rehabilitation required, due to the level of fitness an athlete has before injury, and the need to regain that high level of fitness after injury. There are also a number of *overuse injuries (including *shin splints, *spinner's finger, and *thrower's elbow) peculiar to certain sports and rarely met elsewhere.

sportsmanship *See* **sporting behaviour**.

sports medical examination A medical examination of an athlete specifically to monitor the athlete's fitness to participate in sport. A sports medical examination typically includes full personal details of competition and training performances as well as a clinical examination. The physician needs to know of such problems as epilepsy, asthma, and major allergies, not only because of periods of disablement and inactivity, but also because of any drug therapy.

sports medicine A branch of medicine which is concerned with the welfare of athletes and deals with the science and

medical treatment of those involved in sports and physical activities. The objectives of sports medicine include the prevention, protection, and correction of injuries, and the preparation of an individual for physical activity in its full range of intensity. Sports medicine includes the study of the effects of different levels of exercise, training, and sport on healthy and ill people in order to produce information useful in prevention, therapy, and rehabilitation of injuries and illness in athletes. The information is used to optimize performance in sports. Sports medicine originally dealt with medical aspects of sport, and its foremost objective was the welfare of the athlete. Recently, there has been an emphasis by some practitioners on the possible contribution of medical science to improving athletic performances, sometimes at the expense of morality and ethics.

sports nutrition A subdiscipline of sport physiology that deals with how foods and drink affect performance in sports. It includes the study of how to use commonly available foods to support sportspersons during their preparation for participation in and recovery from sport and exercise.

sport socialization The process by which a person becomes involved in physical activity and sport. *See also* **socialization**.

sport sociology A young, dynamic subdiscipline of sociology which has not yet been clearly delineated. Sport sociology includes the study of sport in society as it affects human development, forms of expression, and value systems. It also includes the study of social systems and social relationships within sport settings.

sport-specific dropout A person who withdraws from participation in a particular sport, but who takes part in another sport. *Compare* **sport-general dropout**.

sport specific ergometry A multidisciplinary science-based evaluation of the energy expenditure of an athlete in conditions that simulate as closely as possible the conditions of competition. Factors considered include the physical and psychological conditions of the competition environment, the body position of the athlete, and the typical work rate, power output, and frequency and duration of activity during competition. Sport-specific ergometers include *treadmills for runners and walkers, *cycle ergometers for cyclists, and *flumes for swimmers.

sports personship *See* sporting behaviour.

sports science The pursuit of objective knowledge gleaned from the observation of sports and those taking part in sport whether as performers, coaches, or spectators. Sports science involves the systematic acquisition and evaluation of information about sport. It includes any discipline which uses the scientific method and relies on observed information and experimentation rather than biased judgement and vague impressions to explain and predict sports phenomena.

sports womanship *See* sporting behaviour.

spot reduction theory The notion that exercising a specific area of the body reduces the fat content in that area. This is incorrect. Exercising one arm, for example, may result in that arm becoming more muscular, but it will have the same fat content as the unexercised arm. Exercise draws fat from stores throughout the body, not from one specific site.

sprain An acute injury to a ligament (a dense band of tissue connecting one bone to another in a joint). Sprains are usually caused by a sudden, forceful movement taking a joint beyond its normal physiological range of movement without dislocation of subluxation. Sprains are classified according to the degree of injury. In a first-degree sprain, few ligamentous fibres are damaged. Symptoms include mild tenderness, slight swelling, but no or very little loss of joint range of motion and no joint instability. In a second-degree sprain, more fibres are damaged, there is swelling, bruising, localized tenderness, moderate pain, and some loss of joint mobility but little to no joint instability. In a third degree sprain, ligamentous fibres are torn or ruptured. This causes swelling and a

variable amount of pain, but disability is severe and there is extreme joint instability. The cornerstone of the primary treatment for sprains is rest, ice, compression, and elevation (*see* **RICE**). *Compare* **strain**.

sprint A run of a short distance which can be covered at top speed in one continuous effort.

sprint training A form of *anaerobic training involving very brief bouts of very fast running.

spurt muscle A skeletal muscle which has its origin some distance from the joint about which it acts and its insertion near the joint. It directs the greater part of its force across the bone rather than along it, and provides the force that acts tangentially to the curve traversed by the bone during movement. Spurt muscles tend to be prime movers. *Compare* **shunt muscles**.

squat Weight-training exercise for conditioning muscles in the legs and buttocks. There are many types of squats. Typically, the subject places a barbell on the shoulders either behind or in front of the neck and grasps the barbell with a palms-upward position of the hands. The subject then squats down to two-thirds of knee bend, keeping the back straight, and then returns to starting position.

squat jump A jump performed from a starting position in which the subject squats down to two-thirds of a knee bend before executing the jump. *See also* **jump height**.

squat thrust (burpee) An exercise to develop lower-body muscles and aerobic fitness. From a standing position, the subject squats down with arms outside the knees and body supported on hands and toes. The legs are thrust backwards into the press-up position with the back kept straight. Then the legs are moved forwards so they come to rest under the arms. The backwards and forwards movements are repeated a variable number of times, but the hands are kept in the same position. The subject finishes the exercise by standing up.

squinting patellae A condition, usually associated with femoral torsion, in which the patellae face inward slightly instead of facing outward.

S–R approach (S–R viewpoint) An approach to behavioural research which focuses upon stimulus–response relationships. The approach, often adopted for the study of motor behaviour, focuses on the responses produced as a function of the stimuli presented, without regard to the intervening mental events or processes.

S–R inventory A list of situations, and the behavioural responses of an individual to each of the situations. Originally, the S–R inventory was designed to study general anxiety but recently it has been used to study dominance, hostility, and interpersonal behaviour. Sometimes physiological responses, such as heart rate, are recorded in addition to the subjects being asked how they feel in different situations. An S–R inventory of anxiousness, for example, contains 11 anxiety-eliciting situations and 14 modes of response varying from 'heart beats faster' to 'feel anxious'. Each mode of response is paired with each of the eleven situations providing 154 inventory items.

S–R viewpoint See S–R approach.

stability 1 Tendency of an object to maintain its resting position or maintain a constant linear velocity or angular velocity. Factors affecting stability include the mass and height of the object, and the position, size, and shape of its supporting base. The stability of an object is inversely related to the height of its centre of gravity above its supporting base. The object tends to be more stable as its line of gravity falls closer to the centre of the base of its support. The further one part of the object moves away from the line of gravity, the less stable the object will be unless another part of the object makes compensatory movements. The stability of an object in motion is directly proportional to its momentum. *See also* **equilibrium**; **2** *See* **joint stability**. **3** In groups, the turnover rate for group-membership, and the length of time members of a group have been together. High stability is associated with high *cohesion. **4** A dimension of *causal attribution

theory which extends from stable to unstable, indicating whether the attributions are liable to change or remain unchanged. Athletes tend to attribute stable factors (such as level of ability) to expected outcomes, and unstable factors (such as luck) to unexpected outcomes.

stabilization (stabilizing the subject) A procedure used in strength-measuring studies to ensure that only the muscle or muscles primarily responsible for a particular motion contribute to the effort being measured. Other muscles which can contribute to the effort are rendered ineffective, for example by strapping down the relevant segments on which they act.

stabilizer See **fixator**.

stabilizing component At certain joint angles, the component of muscle force directed towards the joint centre, bringing the ends of articulating bones closer together. *Compare* **dislocating component**.

stabilizing the subject See **stabilization**.

stable equilibrium Condition of a stationary body which tends to return to its original position of equilibrium when slightly displaced. A body in stable equilibrium has a position of minimum potential energy. *Compare* **unstable equilibrium**.

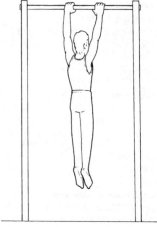

stable equilibrium

stable factor In *causal attribution theory, a factor tending to remain relatively unchanged from competition to competition (e.g., innate athletic ability).

stacking (positional segregation) The assignment of athletes to positions on a sports team on the basis of ascribed characteristics, such as ethnic group, rather than on the basis of merit. In North America, for example, central positions tend to be assigned to whites and noncentral positions to black players.

stage-training A variation of *circuit-training. Athletes perform exercises in sets with the same exercise repeated a number of times before moving on to the next exercise. Stage training tends to make more demands on *anaerobic metabolism than circuit-training.

STAI See **state trait anxiety inventory**.

staleness Mental fatigue and loss of enthusiasm, often associated with *overtraining or unimaginative, repetitive training sessions.

stall angle (angle of stall) A critical, maximum *angle of attack beyond which a projectile tends to fall toward the ground because drag forces are increased and lift forces are decreased.

stamina See **endurance**.

standard bicarbonate See **alkali reserve**.

standard deviation A statistical index of the variability of data within a distribution. It is the square root of the average of the squared deviation from the mean; that is, it equals the square root of the variance. See also **descriptive statistics**.

standard error A statistical measure of the dispersion of a set of values. The standard error provides an estimation of the extent to which the mean of a given set of scores drawn from a sample differs from the true mean score of the whole population. It should be applied only to interval-level measures.

standard error of difference A statistical index of the probability that a difference between two sample means is greater than zero.

standard error of the mean A statistical index of the probability that a sample mean is representative of the mean of the population from which the sample was drawn.

standardization A criterion for effective testing or assessment of two or more test situations. Standardization demands that the test conditions need to be vigorously controlled and must be the same for each test situation. Thus, if the performance of one athlete is to be compared with another, or a comparison be made of performances of the same athlete at different times, all the test conditions should be the same.

standing broad jump Test of muscular *power in which the subject toes a line and jumps forward with both feet simultaneously. The jump is measured from the take-off line to the nearest point touched by any part of the body at the end of the jump. Compare **sargent jump**.

standing toe-touch An indirect test of *flexibility in which the subject stands with hands by the side and knees straight, then leans slowly forward to touch the floor with the fingertips. In one test of minimal flexibility, men should be able to touch the fingertips to the floor and women should be able to touch the palms to the floor.

starch A carbohydrate which acts as a storage product of plants. It is a *polysaccharide made of alpha glucose units, forming amylose and amylopectin. Starch is very difficult to digest, but heating breaks down the starch molecules to smaller compounds called dextrins which are more digestible.

Starling's law (Frank–Starling law) A law which states that the *stroke volume of the heart increases in response to an increase in the volume of blood filling the heart (the end diastolic volume). The increased volume of blood stretches the ventricular wall, causing cardiac muscle to contract more forcefully (the so-called Frank–Starling mechanism). The stroke-volume may also increase as a result of greater contractility of the cardiac muscle during exercise, independent of the end-diastolic volume. The Frank–Starling mechanism appears to make its greatest contribution to increasing stroke volume at lower work rates, and contractility has its greatest influence at higher work rates.

starting strength The strength recorded 30 ms after the start of a muscle action.

state A transitory emotional condition.

state aggression A transitory, conscious feeling of *aggression, often expressed in overtly aggressive acts against a human target.

state anxiety A temporary emotional condition characterized by apprehension, tension, and fear about a particular situation or activity. State anxiety is usually accompanied by physiological arousal and observable behavioural indicators, such as nervous fidgeting, licking the lips, and rubbing the palms of the hands on a shirt or trousers. However, the correlation between physiological and psychological measures of state anxiety are quite low and can produce conflicting results.

state anxiety inventory (SAI) A test of *state anxiety which consists of twenty questions related to how the subject feels.

state trait anxiety inventory (STAI) A standardized pencil and paper questionnaire which enables researchers to measure both A-trait and A-state levels of anxiety.

state bound learning A law of psychology which states that the use and benefits of learning are greater if the external situation and/or the state of mind during recall are similar to that of the learning situation. Therefore, athletes will perform better during competition if they learn skills in a training environment which is similar to the competition environment.

static action (isometric action) A muscle action in which tension increases but the joint angle remains unchanged and no external mechanical work is done. The force generated by a static action equals the force of the resistance. *Compare* **concentric action**, and **eccentric action**.

static action exercise (isometric exercise) An exercise in which the action of a

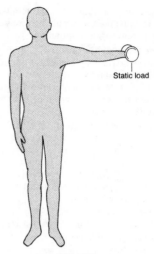

Static load

static action

muscle group produces no movement of the joint to which the muscles are attached. Such exercises include pressing the hands together at the chest and pushing against an immovable object. Isometric exercises produce good strength gains, but only at the specific angle of muscle action. For best results, static action exercises should involve maximal or near maximal static actions against a resistance for at least 5 s. These exercises can be performed almost anywhere and require no specialized equipment. However, they have little beneficial effect on *cardiovascular fitness. In fact, such exercises are contraindicated for individuals with cardiovascular disease because the exercises can increase intra-abdominal pressure and blood pressure and put a strain on the heart.

static endurance The ability of a muscle to remain in tension for a long period of time. This may be measured by the length of time an individual can hold a body position. *Compare* **dynamic endurance**.

static equilibrium The state of an object at rest when the resultant forces acting on it are zero (i.e. the sum of the vertical forces is zero; the sum of the horizontal forces is zero, and the sum of all the torques is zero). A gymnast performing a hand-stand maintains a static equilibrium.

static flexibility The *range of motion of a joint when a body segment is passively moved (e.g. by an exercise partner) and held in position. It is measured using a flexometer or goniometer. See also **flexibility**.

static friction Friction that acts at the interface between two motionless surfaces. Static friction acts in the direction opposite to the external force tending to produce motion, and increases with the external force until motion is initiated. See also **limiting friction**.

statics A division of mechanics dealing with systems in a constant state of motion, that is either at rest or moving with a constant velocity.

static strength (isometric strength) The *force or torque of reaction achieved when a maximum effort is exerted by a voluntary static action of a muscle for 2–6 s. Static strength is important in many activities including a rugby scrum, tug-of-war, and weight-lifting.

static stretching A form of stretching in which a stretched position is held for a given duration (6–60 s). Static stretching avoids forced movements which can provoke a stretch reflex. During static stretching, the *golgi tendon organs are stimulated resulting in relaxation of the muscles being stretched (see **inverse stretch reflex**). Therefore, there is less danger of damaging the tissues. Compare **ballistic stretching**.

statistic A single piece of information capable of exact numerical representation, such as the arithmetic *mean of a sample.

statistical significance A measure of the *probability that an observed numerical result in a test occurred by chance. When a difference between two means is said to be statistically significant to the 0.05 level, this statement means that the probability of obtaining a difference this large or larger would occur by chance less than 5 times in a 100 trials.

statistics A branch of mathematics concerned with the collection, classification, and interpretation of numerical data. It usually involves the application of *probability theory in the analysis of information.

stature (height; skeletal height) Height of a person usually measured as the distance from the bottom of both feet with heels together, to the highest point on the head. However, there are several techniques for measuring stature. The subject may be standing freely, stretching up, or even recumbent. Each technique gives slightly different measurements.

status A social position or rank held by a person in a *group or *society, and the respect, reputation, and power associated with the position. See also **achieved status**; **ascribed status**; **horizontal status**; **vertical status**.

status reward Any form of non-tangible *positive reinforcement which enhances a person's reputation and *status. Status rewards include acquiring a desirable nickname, such as 'Magic', and receiving verbal praise from *significant others.

status symbol Any article or service whose intrinsic value is supplemented by the prestige it bestows on the person who acquires it, either in their own perception, or those of others.

staying power See **endurance**.

steadiness The ability to maintain the body or limb in a fixed position, or to execute smooth movements without any deviation from the desired direction. Steadiness is affected by muscle tremors and muscle tension. Generally, as the force of a muscle action increases, steadiness decreases. Steadiness is an important ability in target sports such as pistol marksmanship. See also **beta blockers**.

steady state The condition of a system or physiological function which remains at a relatively constant (steady) value. After a few minutes of submaximal exercise, for example, a person reaches a steady state in which heart rate and rate of oxygen consumption tend to remain constant at a constant rate of work (*compare* **cardiovas-cular drift**). Generally, endurance-trained athletes have lower steady state heart rates at a given level of work than those who are untrained.

steady state heart rate *See* **steady state**.

Steiner's model A model of the relation between individual abilities or resources on a team and how the team members interact. It is summarized by the equation: actual productivity = potential productivity–faulty group processes. Potential productivity refers to the team's best possible performance if all members perform to their full potential. Group processes refer to the complex interactions that are required to transform a group of individuals into a collective unit. The model implies that teams rarely perform to their full potential because of the negative effects of faulty group processes (e.g., poor communication). Team sports which require high levels of cooperation (e.g., basketball and football) are more affected by faulty group processes than sports requiring less cooperation. *See also* **Ringelmann effect**; and **social loafing**.

stenosis The abnormal constriction or narrowing of an opening such as a blood vessel or heart valve.

stepping-stone test A test of dynamic balance in which the subject leaps onto successive marked spots on the floor, maintains balance on the landing foot for a few seconds, then leaps again, and so on over an irregular pattern. Scoring for the test considers both time taken and the error rate.

step test (bench test) A test of cardiorespiratory fitness which evaluates changes in pulse rate in response to standard workloads. The step test is based on the ability of the subject to recover from the workload as determined by the time required for the pulse rate to return to a predetermined percentage of the resting pulse rate. There are several different step tests, each with its own protocol, but one of the first to be used on a wide scale was the *Harvard step test.

stereotype Preconceived, simplistic description of all members of a given group which leads to having certain expectations, often inaccurate and prejudicial, about members of that group without regard to individual differences.

stereotyping The process of ascribing a stereotype to an individual.

sternal Pertaining to the sternum (breastbone).

sternal body Mid-part of the sternum, the sides of which are notched where it articulates with the cartilage of the third to seventh ribs.

sternal notch A v-shaped structure on the sternum.

sternoclavicular joint A modified *ball-and-socket joint between the manubrium of the sternum and the proximal end of the clavicle. With the acromioclavicular joint it forms the pectoral shoulder girdle. Most of the motion of the girdle takes place at the sternoclavicular joint.

sternocleidomastoid (sternomastoid) A two-headed muscle deep on the anterolateral surface of the neck. The muscle has one of its origins on the manubrium of the sternum and the other on the medial aspect of the clavicle; its insertion is on the mastoid process (a nipple-like extension) of the temporal bone. The primary actions of the sternocleidomastoid are flexion of the neck, extension of the head, and lateral flexion about the spine. It also acts as an accessory inspiratory muscle, elevating the sternum.

sternocostal joint Cartilaginous, amphiarthrotic joint between the sternum and ribs 2 to 7. The joint permits slight movements only.

sternomastoid *See* **sternocleidomastoid**.

sternum (breastbone; breastplate) A flat bone in the anterior midline of the thorax. The sternum consists of three parts: the manubrium at the top, the main sternal body, and the xiphoid process at the bottom.

steroids Lipid-soluble hormones that can pass through cell membranes. Once inside the cell, a steroid hormone binds to specific receptors which can enter the nucleus and activate certain genes. Steroids include testosterone and oestrogen. They may occur naturally or be synthesized.

sterol A group of chemicals derived from *steroids. They include cholesterol and the several compounds which make up vitamin D.

sticking point *See* cheating.

stick-lengthwise test *See* balance tests.

stiffness 1 A characteristic of muscles and springs defined as the change in tension divided by the change in length. A very stiff spring requires a great deal of tension to increase its length. Muscles behave in some ways like a spring. For example, they provide a compliant (springy) interface between a runner and the ground. **2** The subjective experience of restricted mobility caused, for example, by muscle overuse.

stigma 1 A mark or spot which acts as a sign of a particular disease. **2** Any mark or lesion in the skin.

stimulants A pharmacological class of agents banned by the International Olympic Committee (*see* **doping classes**). Stimulants have been used as appetite-suppressants and weight-reducing drugs, and to obtain a feeling of well-being. They have been misused in sport, particularly in endurance events, to increase mental alertness, to conceal feelings of exhaustion, and to increase aggressiveness. Athletes using stimulants may force the body beyond safe limits. Several deaths have been associated with the use of stimulants such as *amphetamines. In addition, use of stimulants may result in loss of judgement and increase the risk of injury to both the user and others taking part in sport. Stimulants include psychotonics and analeptics. *See also* **sympathomimetic amines**.

stimulus (pl. stimuli) **1** Any factor inside or outside an organism, but external to a sensory receptor, which initiates activity of some kind. **2** An internal or external event that tends to alter the behaviour of an organism.

stimulus generalization *See* generalization.

stimulus identification (detection) The process of picking out a particular stimulus among many other stimuli which may be present. *See also* **cocktail party phenomenon**.

stimulus-identification stage A stage of information-processing in which the stimulus is identified, and features or patterns are abstracted.

stimulus–response compatibility The degree to which the set of stimuli and associated responses are naturally related to each other. For example, stimulus–response compatibility occurs if, when coloured lights and coloured balls are presented to a subject, the response required is to hit the ball of the same colour as the flashing light rather than one of a different colour.

stimulus threshold *See* threshold.

stinger *See* brachial plexus neurapraxia.

stitch A sharp pain commonly in the side of the abdomen or ribcage. Stitch often occurs early during exercise and subsides as exercise is continued, but the pain may be so severe that the exerciser is forced to stop. The exact cause of a stitch is unknown, but it may be due to lack of oxygen in respiratory muscles, particularly the diaphragm and intercostals, due to insufficient blood flow. Stitches are also associated with jolting the body, and are made worse by eating a meal before exercising. There is no simple remedy but a stitch can sometimes be relieved by supporting the abdominal wall (e.g. by pressing a hand against the abdomen), or by lying down with the hips raised. Although stitches have no serious medical significance, they are a great inconvenience to athletes. *See also* **cramp**; and **caecal slap syndrome**.

Stockholm swimming flume A sophisticated *ergometer in which a swimmer has to swim to maintain a static position against a water current produced by the thrust of propellers.

storage fat Fat contained within *adipose tissue of the skin. It acts as an energy store, thermal insulation, and also offers the internal organs some protection against mechanical damage.

storage problem A problem with early notions of *motor programs, because the number of necessary programs required by early theories was so large that the storage of such programs in the central nervous system seemed impossible.

stork stand test *See* blind stork test.

storming *See* team.

strain 1 The condition of a material being distorted by forces acting on it. Strain is measured as the ratio of deformation of the material to the dimension of the material in which the forces are being applied. Therefore, compressive strain is the ratio of contraction of the material to the original length of the material; tensile strain is the ratio of elongation of the material to its original length; and shear strain is the ratio of the deflection of the material in the direction of the shear force to the distance between shear forces. **2** *See* muscle strain.

strain energy (elastic energy) The ability of a body to do work because of its deformation and its tendency to return to its original shape. A fully extended bow, for example, has strain energy by virtue of the change in its shape. Strain energy is measured in joules and is given by the equation: $SE = 1/2kd^2$, where SE is strain energy, k is a spring constant representing a material's ability to store energy on deformation, and d is the distance over which the material has been deformed.

strapping *See* taping.

strategic interaction Interaction, such as in a competition, when one participant must lose if another is to win.

strategy The art of planning a campaign. The term is usually used in a military context, but it has been adopted in sport to describe the overall game plan of coaches and managers. *Compare* tactics.

stratified random sample *See* stratified sample.

stratified sample (stratified random sample) A sample drawn from a population which is divided into tiers or strata specifically relating to the study being undertaken. For example, in a study of peoples' exercising habits, age, sex, and social class might be relevant. A random sample will then be taken from each stratum to ensure greater precision in the results.

streamline A contour on the body that offers the minimum of resistance to a fluid flowing around it. It is technically described as a line in a fluid such that the tangent to it at every point follows the direction of the velocity of the fluid particle at that point at a given instant.

streamline flow *See* laminar flow.

streamlining Making the overall shape of a body moving through a fluid streamlined so that it offers the minimum resistance to the fluid flowing around it. Streamlining, for example by cyclists, skaters, and skiers who assume a more crouched body position, reduces the amount of turbulence created, especially at the rear, and also reduces the area of the body oriented perpendicular to the fluid flow.

strength The ability of a muscle to exert force and overcome resistance. Strength is essential for physical activity. There are a number of different types of strength (*see* absolute strength; dynamic strength; elastic strength; explosive strength; one-repetition maximum; relative strength; specific strength; starting strength; strength deficit; strength endurance; and static strength). The value obtained for the strength of a muscle or muscles depends on the type of action, the velocity of the action, and the length of the muscle or muscles. Although early gains in absolute strength are influenced by neural factors, long-term gains depend mainly on increases in muscle size (*see* hypertrophy).

strength curve A plot of the resultant moment exerted about an axis through a joint (or the external force exerted on a joint) against an appropriate measure of joint configuration (usually the *included joint angle or the *anatomical joint angle). The resultant joint moment (Nm) forms the y-axis, and the joint configuration (in degrees) forms the x-axis. Strength curves are used clinically to determine the status of patients before giving them an exercise prescription, and to monitor rehabilitation. They have also been used by sports scientists to determine the effects of different training regimes.

strength deficit A strength parameter defined as the difference between maximum strength (when measured as a maximum voluntary eccentric muscle action) and maximum *static strength.

strength endurance The ability of a muscle to withstand fatigue while performing repeated *muscle actions. See also **muscular endurance**.

strength maximum See **absolute strength**.

strength training Exercises performed specifically to develop strength. Strength training often involves weight training using progressive resistance exercises incorporating a *repetition maximum which ensures overload (see also **pyramid system**; **multi-set system**; **super-set system**; and **multi-poundage system**). Other strength training exercises include body resistance exercise, exercises with a *medicine ball, *circuit-training, and *plyometrics. Strength training has both *myogenic and *neurogenic effects which are generally slow to develop. The time taken to improve strength varies according to genetic factors, age, sex, and the muscle groups being exercised. But it may take several weeks to make even moderate strength gains. The effects of strength training include muscle hypertrophy; increased muscle capillarization; toughening of connective tissue, joints, and bones; and reduction of body fat. To be effective, strength training needs to take place at least two to three times a week for 45 minutes each time.

stress 1 The magnitude of a distorting *force, expressed as force per unit area of the surface on which it is applied. If the stress on an object, such as bone, exceeds the tolerance load, a fracture may occur

(see also **stress fracture**). A compressive stress results from squeezing or pressing objects together; tensile stress results from pulling forces (see **tension**); and shear stress results from sliding forces (see **shear force**). **2** Any factor, physical or psychological, that tends to disturb *homeostasis and has a detrimental effect on body functions. **3** A psychological condition occurring when individuals perceive a substantial imbalance between demands being made on them and their ability to meet those demands, where failure to do so has important consequences. See also **distress**; **eustress**; **general adaptation syndrome**; and **state anxiety**.

stress fracture (fatigue fracture; insufficiency fracture) A microscopic break in a bone caused by repeated loading and unloading. Stress fractures are usually slow to develop and are not usually linked to any single injury. They occur when forces applied repeatedly to a bone exceed its structural strength. According to the fatigue theory, bones are more likely to have stress fractures if they are not supported adequately by surrounding muscles; lack of support results in impact forces being transmitted directly to the bones. Consequently, stress fractures tend to be more common in poorly conditioned athletes. Those with brittle bones, such as older people and females with menstrual irregularities (see **amenorrhoea**) are also more susceptible to stress fractures. Stress fractures are characterized by local pain exacerbated by activity and relieved by rest. Most bones can become stress fractured, but most stress fractures affect the tibia. Stress fractures may be difficult to diagnose, except by bone scan, because they may not appear on an X-ray until well established. Those with a stress fracture should avoid high-impact activities (e.g. running) which impose a lot of mechanical stress on the bone, and replace them with low impact activities (e.g. pool running) to maintain fitness. Ice massage, nonsteroidal anti-inflammatories, stretching and strengthening exercises may also be prescribed.

stress injury *See* **overuse injury**.

stress inoculation training (SIT) A form of cognitive stress management which athletes have used to overcome competitive stress. The athlete produces a hierarchy of stressors and identifies the type of negative thoughts associated with each stressor. The athlete then develops positive self-statements as substitutes for the negative thoughts. Finally, the athlete imagines each stressor, starting with the least stressful, and attempts to feel the stress while practising physical relaxation techniques as well as replacing the negative thoughts with positive ones.

stress management Procedures designed to control or reduce stress. *See also* **autogenic training**; **intervention strategy**; **progressive muscle relaxation**.

stress modelling The inclusion in a training programme of stressors which an athlete is likely to encounter just before or during competition, so that the athlete can cope more easily with the stressors. *See also* **isolation stress**.

stressor An internal or external factor which makes demands on an individual and which tends to disrupt *homeostasis. Stressors include physical trauma, disease, social events and situations, and the demands of exercise and competition.

stress process The process by which the objective demands of a situation result in an increase in the *state anxiety of an individual if the situation is perceived as threatening. The stress process is dependent to a large extent on how the individual perceives the demands. This perception will be a product of a variety of factors including the individual's emotional disposition, previous experiences, abilities, the need for success, and the perceived importance of the situation.

stress reaction A reaction in bones to a constant repetitive stressing resulting in the development of microscopic fractures called pre-stress fractures. These fractures generally heal if the athlete decreases the intensity of activities. However, if the force on the bone is continued, an actual *stress fracture may result.

stress test *See* **electrocardiogram**; and **exercise stress test**.

stretching A linear deformation of tissue that increases its length. Exercises involving muscle stretching are performed to maintain or improve flexibility. *See also* **ballistic stretching**; **proprioceptive neuromuscular facilitation**; **static stretching**.

stretch receptor A receptor which detects stretching in a muscle. There are two main types: *Golgi tendon organs at the junction between a muscle and its tendon; and *muscle spindle organs in the belly of a muscle. Stretch receptors are essential for coordinated muscle activity, passing information about the state of muscles to the central nervous system (*see* **kinaesthesis**).

stretch reflex (myotatic reflex) The reflex contraction of a muscle in response to a sudden longitudinal stretching of the same muscle. The stretch reflex is mediated by *proprioceptors and is an important mechanism for maintaining muscle tone. Clinical tests of neuromuscular functioning sometimes include observing a stretch reflex provoked by a quick forceful tap with a rubber hammer on a tendon (e.g., patellar tendon).

stretch-shortening cycle A common movement pattern which increases the power generated by a muscle group. The stretch-shortening cycle consists of a combination of the three types of muscle action: an eccentric action followed by a static (isometric) action, and then a concentric action of the same muscle group. The combined actions exert greater force or power output than movements produced by concentric actions alone. The enhanced force generation is probably due to the elastic behaviour of muscle components during and immediately after the eccentric action. The stretch-shortening cycle is taken advantage of in many sport activities, for example when a counter movement or bob-down movement is performed before a jump, and when a wind-up movement is performed before a throw.

stretch-shortening cycle test Measurements of strength and power movements which incorporate the *stretch-shortening cycle. Such movements include jumping, and the test may involve a subject jumping from a platform that can measure the force, work, and power produced during the jump.

striated muscle (skeletal muscle; striped muscle; voluntary muscle) Contractile tissue consisting of fibrils with marked striations at right angles to the longitudinal axis. Each multinucleated muscle fibre consists of *sarcomeres. The muscle fibre may be a fast-twitch fibre or a slow-twitch fibre. Striated muscle is involved in voluntary movements of skeletal parts.

stride length The length between each step in running or walking. Stride length is an important component of speed (speed = stride length × *cadence). Stride length depends on strong leg muscles and a good range of motion in joints, especially those of the hip and knee.

striped muscle *See* **striated muscle**.

stroke (apoplexy; cerebrovascular accident) An interruption in the blood supply to the brain. Causes include a blood clot, a head injury, or an aneurysm, but the primary cause is usually disease of the heart or blood vessels, with the effects on the head being secondary. A stroke results in a part of the brain being deprived of oxygen. Small strokes may occur without symptoms and go unnoticed by the victim, but the most common manifestation is some degree of paralysis; large strokes may be fatal. Regular aerobic exercise produces a number of benefits (e.g., reduction of blood pressure in those with moderate hypertension) that can reduce the risk of a stroke.

stroke cycle 1 The complete cycle of a swimming stroke, including the propulsive and recovery phases. **2** Any one of the repeated movements used by a swimmer.

stroke rate In swimming, the number of stroke cycles per minute.

stroke velocity The *velocity of a swimmer in water.

stroke volume The volume of blood pumped out of the left ventricle of the heart per beat. It is the difference between the end diastolic volume and the end systolic volume. Typically, the stroke volume is 75 ml for an untrained man at rest, and 105 ml for a trained athlete at rest. The resting stroke volume varies according to whether the person is supine, sitting, or standing. Stroke volume increases as the intensity of exercise increases (*see* **Starling's law**). It may reach 200 ml in highly trained endurance athletes during maximal exercise.

structural assimilation The incorporation into society of an ethnic group so that it has equal access to the major associations and institutions. *See* **cultural assimilation**.

structural functionalism A theoretical approach to the study of social systems in societies in which social structures are described in terms of how they contribute to the maintenance of these systems. For example, sport may be described in terms of its contribution to social integration.

structural interference Interference which occurs among tasks and is caused by the simultaneous use of receptors, processing systems, and effectors. A decrease in the quality of performance occurs when different tasks, which use the same structures, are performed simultaneously.

structuralism A theoretical approach in sociology which views social structures as being of greater importance than human actions. It often involves searching for the social reality which lies below outward, superficial structures.

structural rating scale A structured method of measuring *causal attribution in which the subject is asked to rate several attributions, such as ability, effort, difficulty, and luck, in terms of how each applies to a particular outcome. It is felt by some researchers that this method is too constrained. *Compare* **open-ended attributions**.

structure **1** Any institutionalized social arrangement. The governing bodies of various sports can be regarded as structures. **2** The rules which underlie and create the outward features of a society; the social relations which underpin these superficial features.

structured interview Type of interview in which each interviewee is asked the same questions, in the same way. Consistent responses are obtained by posing questions in such a way that the response to each question is limited to choices which can be recorded numerically through the use of scaled response systems or checklists.

strychnine An alkaloid drug belonging to the *stimulants which are on the International Olympic Committee list of *banned substances. Strychnine is obtained from seeds of *Trychnos nuxvomica* and was formerly used in small amounts in 'tonics'. The drug blocks the action of *glycine. High doses cause muscular spasms similar to those resulting from *tetanus; death can occur due to spasms of the respiratory muscles.

studded footwear *See also* **cleated footwear**.

Student's t-test A statistical significance test for comparing one set of data with another, by comparing two *means to see if they are significantly different.

style An individual adaptation of a technique.

stylion An anatomical landmark located at the most distal point of the *styloid process of the radius. It is located in the *anatomical snuff box.

styloid process A pointed pen-like projection; for example, the process at the wrist end of the ulna.

subacromial bursitis Inflammation of the *bursa that lies between the rotator cuff tendons and the shoulder blade. The *bursitis is due to excessive, repeated shoulder movements. It is characterized by pain in the front and upper part of the shoulder, especially when the arm is raised. The condition is common among swimmers and javelin throwers. It often occurs in conjunction with an *impingement syndrome or rotator cuff tendinitis. Usually conservative treatment (rest, ice, and anti-inflammatories, and, sometimes, a steroid injection) are sufficient to resolve the condition. In severe cases, immobilization in a sling or surgery may be necessary.

subacute Applied to a disease or injury which develops more quickly than a chronic injury but does not become acute.

subclavius Small, cylindrical muscle extending from its origin on the first rib to its insertion on the clavicle. The subclavius helps to stabilize and depress the pectoral girdle.

subconscious In psychology, that part of the mind containing memories and motives of which the subject is not personally aware except with much effort.

subcultural resistance Opposition to a dominant culture which can occur when subcultures are created. For example, subcultural resistance can occur when new or adapted forms of sport are created. People within the new sport subcultures may dislike or oppose the existing sporting opportunities.

subculture An identifiable subgroup of society with a distinctive set of behaviour, beliefs, values, and norms. Though a subculture is subordinate to the dominant culture of a society, it sometimes allows individuals greater group identification. Those who take part in particular sports, for example, racing cyclists, professional footballers, are sometimes referred to as a subculture. *See also* **idioculture**.

subcutaneous Pertaining to areas beneath the skin.

subjective competitive situation An athlete's thoughts and feelings about a particular *objective competitive situation. It refers particularly to whether or not the athlete perceives the situation as threatening. This will depend to a certain extent on the athlete's *competitive A-trait and will affect precompetitive *anxiety.

subjective danger An avoidable and manageable danger that is potentially under the control of an athlete (e.g., by the correct use and choice of equipment). *Compare* **objective danger**.

subjective fatigue (mental fatigue; perceived fatigue) A mental condition characterized by a need for rest, and a feeling of exhaustion. It is caused by psychological factors, such as boredom or mental stress, not physical or physiological ones. It usually results from repetition of the same behaviour. An athlete who is subjectively fatigued (i.e. feels tired) can often continue to use a particular muscle group if the type of activity is changed or if the athlete is psychologically encouraged. *See also* **projected fatigue**; **task aversion**; and **poor motivation**.

subjective reinforcement A form of *reinforcement in closed-loop theories of motor learning, which enables an individual to be able to report to himself or herself the errors made in the execution of a skill. It is suggested that the subject acquires a reference of correctness (called the perceptual trace). When a movement is completed, the subject can compare the feedback received against the perceptual trace; the deviation represents the error that the subject could report to themselves or an experimenter as subjective reinforcement.

subjectivity The perception an individual has about a situation or phenomenon. *Compare* **objectivity**.

sublimation A mechanism of *ego defence by which energy of the id is directed from a primary but unacceptable object to one that is socially acceptable. The term was originally conceived by Sigmund Freud (1856–1939) to describe behavioural mechanisms that channel sexual energies into more socially beneficial forms. In sport, sublimation may consist of directing energies to training hard and achieving excellence or seeking perfection in competition.

subliminal Applied to a stimulus below the level of awareness and below the absolute threshold of stimulation, as when an auditory or visual presentation is too weak to have an effect, or at least any effect of which the subject is aware.

subluxation Movement of a joint beyond its maximum passive range so that the alignment between the joint surfaces is distorted. Unlike a complete dislocation, partial contact is maintained between the articulating bones. It is often a transient condition with the joint going back to its normal position without any special treatment, but sometimes a deformity persists. A subluxation of the collar bone at the acromoclavicular joint, as a result of a badly timed tackle in a contact sport, for example, commonly leaves a deformity if not treated properly. Subluxations often recur because they are usually linked with an inherent weakness of the surrounding structures or an anatomical abnormality.

submaximal test A test which evaluates the adaptation of *oxygen transport system to exercise below maximal intensity, so that main energy system used is aerobic. *See also* **increasing intensity test**; **periodic load test**; **rectangular test**; **time test**; **trapeziform test**; and **triangular test**.

submuscular bursa A *bursa found between muscles.

suboccipitals A group of neck muscles which have their proximal attachment on the occipital bone and transverse process of the first cervical vertebra, and their distal attachments on the posterior surfaces of the first and second cervical region. They are the obliquus capitis superior, obliquus capitis inferior, rectus capitis posterior major, and rectus capitis posterior minor. Their primary actions are extension, lateral flexion, and rotation, of the cervical region of the spine.

subroutine A component of a *motor program which consists of a group of commands for the execution of a simple, discrete element or movement that is thought to be combined with other subroutines to form the basis of larger, more complicated movements.

subscapularis A *rotator cuff muscle in the shoulder. It has its origins on the entire anterior surface of the scapula, and its insertion on the lesser tubercle of the humerus. The primary action of the subscapularis is medial rotation about the shoulder.

subscapular neuropathy A shoulder injury involving denervation of the *infraspinatus which leads to loss of strength during external rotation of the humerus. It sometimes occurs among competitive volleyball players because of repeated stretching of the nerve during the serving motion.

substance P A peptide found in the central nervous system and gut tissue, thought to be a *neurotransmitter and involved in transmission of impulses from pain receptors.

subtalar joint A joint in the ankle formed between the lower anterior and posterior facets of the talus and the superior calcaneus. The joint is essentially uniaxial and is bound together by four talocalcaneal ligaments.

subungual exostosis A bony outgrowth under the nail usually caused by repeated impact to a toe, commonly the big toe. It may be painful and the nail or the bony outgrowth (exostosis) may need to be removed to relieve pressure.

subungual haematoma *See* black toe.

success The achievement of a goal. In sport, the concept of success can be very personal (*see* **perceived success**) and is not always dependent on winning a competition or obtaining a very high standard of performance .

success cycle A cycle showing the relationships between how an athlete feels about himself or herself and how he or she is likely to perform in competition. A positive self-image is likely to promote a positive attitude which in turn leads to high expectations. An athlete with high expectations is likely to improve behaviour (e.g., eat a well-balanced diet and abstain from excessive alcohol consumption) so that performance in competition is enhanced. Successful performances improve self-image, and so on. A negative self-image

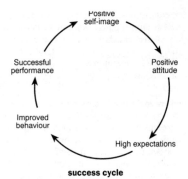

success cycle

leads to opposite effects, reducing the chances of success in competition.

successive force summation In the human body, the combination of forces resulting from the sequential acceleration of different body parts. *See also* **force summation**.

succinic dehydrogenase (SDH) A mitochondrial enzyme involved in *Krebs cycle. There is a direct relationship between SDH activity and the oxygen capacity of muscle fibres. SDH occurs in higher concentrations in slow-twitch muscle fibres than in fast-twitch fibres. The muscles of endurance athletes have SDH activities up to four times those of untrained individuals.

sucrose A *disaccharide formed from fructose and glucose. It is a valuable energy source but it can encourage the growth of oral bacteria which cause tooth decay. Refined sucrose made from sugar cane and sugar beet, forms white table sugar.

sudden death An unexpected death, not caused by physical trauma, that occurs instantaneously or within minutes of an event which changes the clinical status of an individual. Exertional sudden death occurs during a medically unsupervised activity or within 1 hour after completion of the activity. Cardiac abnormalities (especially *hypertrophic cardiomyopathy, an abnormal enlargement of the ventricular septum of the heart) are the most common causes of exertional sudden death in people under 35 years of age; *coronary artery disease is the most common cause for those over 35 years of age. The overall incidence of death during athletic activity has been estimated as a rate of 0.003 to 0.006 per year. Although sudden death is more likely during exercise than at rest, those who do not exercise regularly have the greatest risk of death during exercise and at rest.

sudden immersion injury An injury caused by the sudden entry into very cold water. Freezing water can incapacitate muscle actions and disturb the heart rate and breathing, making it impossible to swim. Sudden immersion can result in loss of consciousness which may lead to death from drowning, a stroke, or heart attack. Participants of water sports, such as canoeing, are at obvious risk, and should always wear wet- or dry-suits to retain body heat. Safety procedures should ensure quick removal of someone who has fallen into cold water, a change into dry clothing, and warm drinks. Alcohol should never be given because it encourages heat loss.

sudden strenuous exercise Vigorous exercise performed suddenly without any warm-up. Sudden strenuous exercise increases the risk of musculoskeletal injury and cardiovascular problems. Exercise intensity should be increased gradually. See also **warm-up**.

sudomotor Pertaining to the activation of the sweat glands.

sudor See **sweat**.

sudoriferous gland An epidermal gland that produces sweat. See also **sweat gland**.

sugar A group of simple carbohydrates which share the characteristics of being sweet, crystalline, and soluble in water.

sulcus 1 A groove in the tissue on the surface of the cerebral hemispheres in the brain **2** An infolding of soft tissue in the mouth.

sulphur A nonmetallic element which, as a constituent of the amino acids methionine and cystine, is an essential component of a healthy diet. These sulphur-containing amino acids are readily available from meat, eggs, and legumes. They are particularly abundant in mucopolysaccharides, cartilage, tendons, and bone. Sulphur also forms part of the vitamins thiamin and biotin.

sulphur dioxide A common air pollutant which irritates the upper airway. Levels above 1.0 ppm cause discomfort and are detrimental to athletic performance.

summation The summing of all the individual changes elicited by different stimuli on the membrane potential of a neurone or muscle fibre. Summation may involve two or more excitatory stimuli, inhibitory stimuli, or a combination of excitatory and inhibitory stimuli.

sunburn (actinic dermatitis) Damage to the skin due to overexposure to the sun's rays. Sunburn may vary from a mild redness to wide-spread blistering. See also **skin cancer**; and **SPF**.

sun-protection factor See **SPF**.

sunstroke Overheating effect of the direct rays of the sun on the head or back of the neck. Symptoms include red skin, swollen face, buzzing in the ears, dizziness, nausea, elevated pulse rate, and rapid breathing. If overheating persists, there is a risk of *heatstroke. Athletes with sunstroke should stop any activity and should rest in the shade, and preferably be fanned with cool air. They should have their clothes loosened or removed, and cold water applied to the forehead and back of the neck.

superability A general ability thought to have a position above all specific abilities in a particular domain. In the motor domain, for example, it has been hypothesized that general motor ability is a superability which lies above all specific motor abilities and has relevance to any motor task.

super-adherer An exerciser (typically, a runner, swimmer, cyclist, or triathlete) who expends significant long-term effort and commitment, constantly training so that he or she can participate in endurance events.

supercompensation A physiological response to a special exercise-diet procedure in which the amount and rate of *glycogen resynthesis in skeletal muscles during recovery from exercise is increased to values much higher than normal. *See also* **carbohydrate loading**.

superego Part of the mind which acts as a moral conscience and controls the ego by placing moral restrictions on it. The superego is thought to develop as an infant becomes aware of restrictions, controls, and reprisals emanating from parents and others close to the infant. Consequently, the child adopts for itself the moral standards of parents and society. The superego is one of the three chief psychic forces of Freud; the others are the *ego and the *id.

superficial Toward the surface of the body or body structure. *See also* **directional terms**.

superficial muscle Muscle, lying close to the skin, which can be palpated.

superior (cranial) Toward the head or upper end of the body or body part; above (e.g. the forehead is superior to the nose). *See also* **directional terms**.

superoxide dismutase (SOD) An enzyme widely distributed in the body, which destroys superoxide (O_2^-) radicals released during aerobic metabolism. These free radicals have been linked with cancer and degenerative diseases. Some athletes believe that they have insufficient SOD to deal with the large amounts of free radicals produced during vigorous aerobic activities. Consequently, they take supplements of SOD to protect the body against the adverse effects of the radicals. However, when taken orally, this enzyme is digested and made useless.

super-set system A strength training schedule in which two exercises are performed in the same session to develop opposing muscle groups of the same limb (e.g. one exercise involves flexion at a joint, and the other extension).

supination 1 An outward rotation of the forearm so that the palm faces anteriorly or superiorly (i.e. forwards or upwards). The forearm is supinated when in the *anatomical position. **2** A combination of plantar flexion, inversion, and adduction of the foot during walking and running. The rear part of the foot inverts to some ex-

tent when the heel strikes the ground, and plantar flexion and adduction occurs as the foot rolls forward and the forefoot makes contact with the ground.

supinator 1 A deep muscle in the posterior fascial compartment of the forearm. It has its origin on the lateral epicondyle of the humerus and its insertion on the lateral upper third of the radius. Its primary action is elbow supination. **2** A runner who tends to rotate the foot outwards during running. The inside edge of the heel strikes the ground and the foot rolls forward towards the outside edge of the toes to push off. *Compare* **pronator**.

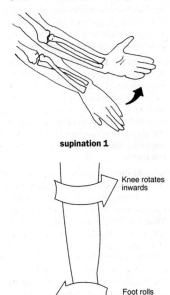

supination 1

Knee rotates inwards

Foot rolls outwards

supination 2

supine The position of a person lying horizontally on his or her back, with face upward. *Compare* **prone**.

suppleness An ability to bend easily without causing damage, and to move easily and gracefully. *See also* **flexibility**.

supra- A prefix used in anatomy to denote above or over.

supramaximal exercise Exercise that requires energy production exceeding that which can be sustained by purely oxidative metabolism, that is, it requires an oxygen consumption greater than the maximal aerobic capacity. Sprinting is a supramaximal exercise. A 100 m sprint run at 36 km/hr would require an oxygen consumption of approximately 140 ml/kg/min, far greater than the highest recorded VO_2max. Supramaximal exercise requires energy from anaerobic metabolism.

suprascapularis A muscle in the front of the shoulder which rotates the arm inwards. It has its origin on the inner surface of the shoulder blade and its insertion on the lesser tuberosity of the humerus.

supraspinatus tendinitis Inflammation of the tendon of the supraspinatus muscle. Supraspinatus tendinitis is a frequent cause of shoulder pain in throwers, wrestlers, racket players, and others who repeatedly use the shoulder muscles with the arm at or above shoulder level. *See also* **shoulder impingement syndrome**; and **tendinitis**.

supraspinatus A *rotator cuff muscle of the shoulder which has its origin on the supraspinous fossa of the scapula and its insertion on the greater tuberosity of the humerus. The primary action of the supraspinatus is abduction about the shoulder. In addition to working with the other rotator cuff muscles to stabilize the shoulder and prevent downward dislocation of the humerus (e.g., when carrying heavy loads), the supraspinatus also assists with lateral rotation.

sural Pertaining to the calf region of the lower leg.

surface drag (skin friction; viscous drag) Resistance derived from friction between the surface of a body and the fluid through which it is moving. The fluid particles adjacent to the body slow down, causing turbulent flow. The magnitude of surface drag depends on a number of factors: it increases with the relative velocity of fluid flow, the surface area over which the flow occurs; the roughness of the body surface; and the viscosity of the fluid. Surface drag is generally more pronounced for bodies moving in air than for those moving in water. Athletes can reduce surface drag by making their body surface smoother, for example, by wearing tight-fitting clothing made of a smooth fabric and streamlined headgear. Swimmers shave off body hair to reduce surface drag and improve their ability to feel the water and coordinate movements.

surface tension A property of a liquid due to the forces of attraction between its molecules. Surface tension exists at the boundary surface of a liquid and leads to the apparent presence of a surface film which has properties similar to those of a stretched elastic film. Surface tension is measured as the tension across a unit length of a liquid surface.

surface traits Personality characteristics which are readily apparent, such as sociability or shyness.

surfer's ear *See* **otitis externa**.

surgery A branch of medicine which specializes in treating injuries and disease by operative measures or manipulation.

surgical Pertaining to surgery.

surgical decompression The reduction of pressure on an organ or body part by using a surgical procedure. For example, an abnormal pressure on a nerve root by a prolapsed intervertebral disc (commonly called a 'slipped disc') may be released by excising the offending disc fragment.

surgical neck A point just below the head of the humerus; so named because it is the most frequently fractured part of the humerus.

surgical spirit A liquid containing mainly alcohol which is used to sterilize the skin before surgery and the administration of injections. Surgical spirit is also applied to the soles of feet to harden the skin and prevent *blisters.

survey A research technique which is primarily descriptive. It is used most commonly to gather information about individuals, for example the beliefs, attitudes, and values of different athletes. Surveys take many forms but often use questionnaires and interviews.

sustained force contraction A gross body movement made when a force is applied against a resistance by contracting *agonists while antagonists are relaxed. The initial leg thrust in a sprint start is achieved by a sustained force contraction.

suture 1 An immovable joint. Most skull bones are interconnected by sutures since any movement of the joints could severely damage the brain. **2** A surgical sewing thread or stitch.

sway back *See* lordosis.

sweat (sudor) A clear watery fluid secreted by the sweat glands. Sweat contains salts (mainly sodium chloride and urea) but it is less concentrated than blood plasma. Sweat plays a minor role in nitrogenous excretion. Its main function is to provide a cooling effect when it evaporates from the skin surface. Urocanic acid in sweat may protect the skin against ultraviolet radiation.

sweat glands Coiled tubular glands in the dermis of the skin which secrete sweat onto the skin surface. There are two main types: apocrine glands and eccrine glands. Apocrine glands secrete fatty acids in addition to salts and water. They are less numerous than eccrine glands, occurring mainly in the axillae (arm pits). Apocrine glands are not important in thermoregulation. Eccrine glands are distributed over most of the body surface, but occur in greatest density on the palms of the hands, soles of the feet, in the axillae (arm pits), and forehead. They are supplied with sympathetic nerve fibres and play a major role in *thermoregulation.

sweating The secretion of sweat onto the skin surface. Sweating plays a major role in dissipating the excess heat produced during exercise. Because of the high latent heat of vaporization of water, sweat provides effective cooling as it evaporates, but it provides little or no cooling if it just

drips off the body. Evaporation of each litre of sweat removes about 58 kcal of heat. Sweat rates may reach 3 litres per hour, with maximal daily sweat rates reaching up to 15 litres. Sweating can cause weight losses as high as 15–30 g per kg of body weight per hour. Soccer players have lost as much as 5 kg during one match on a hot day. If sweating continues without adequate water replacement, overheating and dehydration occur. In addition to increasing with physical activity and body temperature, sweating also increases during periods of mental and emotional arousal. *See also* **water replacement**.

sweet spot The spot on a racket or bat that produces the least initial shock to the hand of the player when a ball is hit; in physics it is called the centre of percussion.

swimmer's back *See* kyphosis.

swimmer's ear *See* otitis externa.

swimmer's shoulder *See* shoulder impingement syndrome.

swimming flume An *ergometer that measures the work output of swimmers under controlled conditions which are similar to those used in free swimming. The flume contains propeller pumps that circulate water past the swimmer who attempts to maintain body position in the flume. The circulation of the water can be increased or decreased to alter the resistance against which a person must swim in order to maintain position.

swimming propulsion *See* propeller propulsion.

symbolic interactionism A study of communication between individuals, and between individuals and society, based on symbols and meanings, as in the use of language. Central to the concept of symbolic interactionism is that the shared meanings are actively constructed through social interactions between people. Symbolic interactionism has made an important contribution to the analysis of roles, *socialization, communication, and actions in sport. *See also* **symbolic interaction perspective**.

symbolic interaction perspective A viewpoint which emphasizes the importance of interpersonal interactions in socialization. The perspective has as its basis the communication of symbols and shared meanings between individuals who tend to acquire more or less similar ways of behaving in specific social situations. Through talking with peers, for example, adolescent athletes often reinterpret expectations of a coach and may publicly or privately question demands which in the past they had automatically accepted.

symbolic learning theory A theory, proposed to account for the effectiveness of *imagery, which suggests that the imagery helps to develop a mental blueprint by creating a *motor program in the central nervous system. *See also* **psychoneuromuscular theory**.

sympathetic nervous system (adrenergic nervous system) Part of the autonomic nervous system that prepares the body for physical activity. Stimulation of the sympathetic nervous system results in a number of responses including constriction of blood vessels supplying the skin, dilation of blood vessels supplying the heart and skeletal muscles (*see* **shunting**), dilation of the bronchioles to facilitate increased ventilation, and release of glucose from the liver. The nerve-endings use *adrenaline and *noradrenaline as a neurotransmitter. *Compare* **parasympathetic nervous system**.

sympathetic tone State of partial *vasoconstriction of blood vessels maintained by impulses from the *sympathetic nervous system.

sympathomimetic amines A group of *stimulants which include ephedrine (adrenaline), phenylpropanolamine, and pseudoephedrine. They stimulate the *sympathetic nervous system, increase mental alertness, and increase blood flow to muscles. Adverse effects of high doses include raised blood pressure, increased heart rate, and increased *anxiety. Use of sympathomimetic amines by athletes is banned by the International Olympic Committee. Low doses are often present in

cold and hay fever preparations, thus no athlete should use any product to relieve a cold, flu, or hay fever without first ensuring that the product does not contain a drug of the banned stimulants class.

sympathy 1 An emotional feeling of regret for a person experiencing troubles. *Compare* **empathy**. **2** In physiology, the relationship between different parts of the body where a change in one part affects the other part or parts.

symphysis 1 A joint in which the bones are united by *fibrocartilage. Symphyses, such as the pubic symphysis and the joints formed by intervertebral discs, allow only slight movement. **2** The line of union between two bones which were separate during early stages of development.

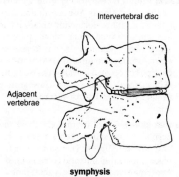

Intervertebral disc

Adjacent vertebrae

symphysis

symphysium A *landmark located on the *superior border of the *symphysis pubis at the mid *sagittal plane.

symptom Any indication of a disease or injury perceived by the patient. *Compare* **sign**.

symptomatic treatment The treatment of the symptoms of an illness.

synalgia *See* **referred pain**.

synality The relationship and similarity of a social group to an individual's psychosocial functioning. Synality traits are analogous to *personality traits and include such things as *aggression towards another group. *See also* **group personality**; and **synergy**.

synapse The connection or junction of one neurone to another. Most synapses consist of a gap, the synaptic cleft, across which a neurotransmitter diffuses to facilitate transmission of a *nerve impulse but some synapses are electrical (*see* **electrical synapse**). *See also* **neuromuscular junction**.

synaptic cleft A fluid-filled gap, approximately 40 nm wide, which separates a presynaptic membrane of one neurone from a postsynaptic membrane of another neurone or a muscle fibre, across which neurotransmitter substances diffuse.

synaptic delay The time (typically 0.3–0.5 ms) required for a neurotransmitter to be released from a presynaptic membrane, diffuse across the synaptic cleft, and bind to a receptor site on the postsynaptic membrane. Synaptic delay is a rate-limiting factor in the transmission of a nerve impulse from one neurone to the next or to an effector cell, and is a component of *reaction time.

synaptic knob The expanded *distal end of small terminal branches of a *neurone.

synarthrosis An immovable joint formed of fibrous tissue connecting two bones. Examples occur between some bones of the cranium, with the synarthroses forming sutures.

synchondrosis A slightly movable *joint in which the bones are united by *hyaline cartilage, such as the joint between the ribs and the sternum.

syncope (fainting) Loss of consciousness due to an insufficient blood supply to the brain. Syncope may occur in otherwise healthy people because of emotional shock, overheating, or because of a sudden reduction in blood pressure on standing up quickly (*see* **orthostatic hypotension**). However, it may also be due to severe injury or loss of blood. Syncope on exercise is a classical warning of severe heart disease and may indicate a low fixed *cardiac output which cannot increase to compensate adequately for the increased demands of oxygen during exercise. Syncope can occur in normal, fit athletes after exertion due to *pooling of blood in the legs.

syndesmology A branch of anatomy which deals with the study of joints and related structures.

syndesmosis An immovable *joint formed by *connective tissue between two bones. For example, the articulation between the *fibula and *tibia at the ankle is formed by strong ligaments.

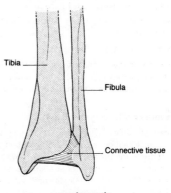

Tibia

Fibula

Connective tissue

syndesmosis

syndrome A combination of symptoms and signs which form a distinctive clinical picture characteristic of a particular disease or injury.

syndrome X A set of signs and symptoms associated with the accumulation of fat in the abdomen. It is commonly associated with middle-aged males with a pot belly or paunch. It is linked to a number of disorders including gout, impaired glucose metabolism, raised blood pressure, and elevated cholesterol levels. Those with syndrome X have a high risk of heart disease.

synergist 1 A *muscle that aids the action of a *prime mover by effecting the same movement or prevents undesirable movements by stabilizing joints across which the prime mover acts. **2** A drug that interacts with another drug so that the combined effects of the two drugs is more than the sum of their separate effects.

synergy 1 The total psychological energy available in a group. It includes the energy needed to hold the group together (maintenance synergy) and the energy exerted to meet outside goals (effective synergy). In a sports team, if internal conflicts require a lot of energy to maintain the group together, there may be little effective energy left to deal with opponents. **2** Coordinated activity, in an antagonistic pair of muscles, of agonist and antagonist resulting in smooth, well-controlled movements.

synostosis A completely ossified *joint; fixed joint.

synovia *See* **synovial fluid**.

synovial bursa A flattened sac found between two tissue surfaces which slide over each other; the synovial bursa reduces friction.

synovial cavity *See* **synovial joint**.

synovial fluid (synovia) A transparent, slightly yellow viscous fluid contained within a membrane enclosing a movable joint, a *bursa, or a tendon sheath. Synovial fluid contains *hyaluronic acid secreted by the synovial membrane, and interstitial fluid derived from blood plasma. Synovial fluid has many functions: it lubricates and nourishes cartilage in the joint; it bears most of the weight at joint surfaces, preventing the articular cartilages from touching each other, thereby minimizing friction and damage; and the fluid contains cells that can devour microbes and the cell debris resulting from wear and tear during joint activity (*see* **phagocytosis**).

synovial joint (diarthrosis) A joint in which the articulating bones are separated by a fluid-containing joint cavity which permits substantial movement. The ends of the bone are covered with articular cartilage. The bones are interconnected by ligaments lined with synovial membrane. Synovial joints can be classified according to the number of *axes of rotation they permit and the type of movement they allow (*see* **ball-and-socket joint**; **condyloid joint**; **gliding joint**; **hinge joint**; **pivot joint**; and **saddle joint**). Synovial joints that allow one, two, and three axes of rotation are called uniaxial, biaxial,

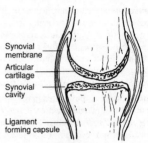

Synovial membrane
Articular cartilage
Synovial cavity
Ligament forming capsule

synovial joint

and triaxial joints, respectively. Synovial joints that permit only limited movement are called nonaxial joints.

synovial membrane Loose *connective tissue lining the inside of a joint capsule and covering all the internal joint surfaces not covered by hyaline cartilage. The synovial membrane secretes *synovial fluid.

synovial sheath An elongated, closed sac forming a sleeve around a *tendon.

synovitis Inflammation of the *synovial membrane of a joint. A healthy joint contains only a small volume of fluid, but when it is inflamed (for example, as a result of a blow or infection), copious amounts may be produced, leading to swelling and limitation of joint movement.

synovium *See* **synovial membrane**.

synthesis Formation of a complex substance from simpler components.

syringe An instrument consisting of a hollow tube with a tight fitting piston. A syringe is used for injecting a fluid, washing out a body cavity, or removing substances from a part of the body.

system 1 Any kind of organized structure within society which contributes to society. (e.g., education system). **2** An organized set of interrelated and interactive parts which has a definite purpose. The human body can be viewed as a system in that it is a set of elements which works together, responding to changes in the *environment (*see also* **homeostasis**). **3** In biomechanics, a mechanical system chosen for study. The system may be the entire human body, a part of the body, a projectile, or some other object.

systematic desensitization *See* **desensitization**.

system goal *See* **norm**.

systemic Pertaining to the whole body.

systemic circulation The flow of arterial blood from the heart to the body tissues (such as muscles, but excluding the lungs) and of venous blood from the tissues back to the heart. *Compare* **pulmonary circulation**.

systems theory An approach to behavioural studies which regards human beings as systems. That is, a human contains wholeness, organization, interactive parts, and the potential to interact with other systems. Systems can be closed or open. A closed system engages in repetitive activity and is rather limited. An open system is versatile and creative. Humans reveal capabilities of both types of system, with the type depending on the demands of the task and the level of the skill.

systole The phase of the *cardiac cycle during which cardiac muscle contracts. Atrial systole concerns simultaneous contraction of the two atria and produces the pressure which pumps blood into the ventricles; during ventricular systole, the ventricles contract and pump blood to the lungs and rest of the body. Typically, systole lasts about 0.3 s in a resting adult man.

systolic blood pressure The maximum pressure in the arteries during *systole. Systolic blood pressure is represented by the top number in the fraction of a *blood pressure reading. A typical value for a young adult man at rest is 120 mmHg.

T

tachycardia to tyrosine

tachycardia A fast resting heart rate (more than 100 beats per minute, or 20 to 30 beats above normal heart rate). Simple sinus tachycardia occurs just before athletic competition or during periods of excitement, but other forms of tachycardia may be associated with a pathological condition.

tachypnoea Excessive frequency of breathing (*see also* **hyperventilation**).

tachypnoeic drift The gradual increase in breathing rate during prolonged, continuous submaximal exercise of constant intensity. The tachypnoeic drift is analogous to and coincidental with the *cardiovascular drift.

tackle shuttle test A fitness test designed specifically for rugby in which the player has to move around a designated circuit and, at specific points, drive tackle bags a predetermined distance (usually 5 metres). Typically the player completes three circuits with no rest. The time is started on a whistle and completed when the player has returned to the start position.

tactics The detailed directions and instructions which control movements or manoeuvres designed to achieve an aim. *Compare* strategy.

tactile Pertaining to the sense of touch.

TAI *See* **Trait Anxiety Inventory**.

tailor's muscle The common name for sartorius muscle, so-named because it helps effect the cross-legged position which was often adopted by tailors (*see* **sartorius**).

tail suction *See* **eddy resistance**.

Taiwan acute respiratory disease An infectious disease caused by the virus-like bacterium, *Chlamydia pneumoniae*. The bacteria can attack the heart making strenuous activity during infection highly dangerous; *myocarditis caused by the bacterium was shown to have caused the sudden death of an élite Swedish orienteerer.

talar Pertaining to the *talus.

talar tilt test A test which, when positive, indicates a sprain of the anterior talofibular and the calcaneofibular ligament in the ankle. With the foot in the anatomical position and the knee in 90 degree flexion, the distal tibia and fibula are stabilized with one hand and an inversion stress applied to the ankle (an adduction force is applied with the hand cupped under the heel) in an attempt to displace the mortice laterally. The test is positive if, when compared with the opposite ankle, the talar tilt is 10 degrees or more. A twenty degree talar tilt indicates a positive test, regardless of comparison with the opposite ankle.

talent An individual's special aptitude or above-average ability for a specific function or range of functions. Physical talents may be functional, expressive, or athletic.

talent identification The identification of new athletic talent.

talus (astragalus) A large bone which forms part of the ankle. The talus articulates with the tibia above, the fibula to the side, and the calcaneus below.

tangent A line that touches a curve at a single point but does not cross the curve. The tangent of a circle at any point is at right angles to the radius of the circle at that point.

tangential acceleration The component of *angular acceleration directed along a tangent to the path of a body travelling in angular motion that indicates change in linear speed: $a_t = v_2 - v_1/t$; where a_t is the tangential acceleration, v_1 is the tangential linear velocity of the moving body at an initial time, v_2 is the tangential linear velocity of the moving body at a second time, and t is the time interval over which the bodies are being assessed.

tangential component A component of a given vector acting at right angles to a given radius of a given circle.

tangible reward A reward which has physical substance, such as money or a trophy. *Compare* **status reward**.

taper period A period of reduced training which enables the body to recover from a long period of intense training. During the taper period damaged tissues can be healed and the body's physical and mental energy reserves replenished.

tapering A reduction in training intensity prior to an important competition. Tapering gives the body and mind an opportunity to benefit from a break from the rigours of intense training. *See also* **Zatopek phenomenon**.

taping Use of tapes, straps, or bandages to support a weakened body part without limiting its function, by preventing movements which stress the weakened area. The tapes generally used are rather inelastic and 38–50 mm in width. Taping may also be used as a preventative measure to improve stability and decrease injuries. There are two main attitudes towards preventative taping. One is that it is always wise to tape joints prior to activity, thus preventing damage and maintaining joint stability by spreading the load onto other joints. The other attitude is that joints should always be left untaped because an immobilized joint cannot take its share of the load and therefore overloads other joints.

tapotement A massage technique in which the fingertips, palms, or sides of the hands create tapping and slapping movements.

tapping a joint *See* joint aspiration.

target cell A cell capable of being affected by a particular hormone.

target game A game, such as darts or archery, where a person tries to hit an object or an area with a projectile.

target heart rate The *heart rate recommended for a fitness work out. The heart rate is a good indicator of intensity of effort and the target heart rate is set at a level above the adaptive threshold ensures overload (*see* **principle of progressive overload**) but is also within limits of safety. There are various methods of determining the target heart rate for different individuals (*see* **Karvonen method**).

target organ Cell tissue or organ upon which a *hormone has an effect.

tarsal 1 Pertaining to the ankle. **2** *See* **tarsal bone**.

tarsal bone One of seven bones in each foot which forms part of the *tarsus. The tarsal bones are the medial cuneiform, intermediate cuneiform, lateral cuneiform, navicular, cuboid, talus, and calcaneus bones.

tarsalgia An aching pain in the ankle.

tarsal tunnel A passage just below the *medial malleolus through which pass the plantaris lateralis nerve and plantaris medialis nerve.

tarsal tunnel syndrome A condition associated with excessive pronation of the foot. Tissues (the retinaculum, abductor hallucis, and flexor hallucis muscles) in the sole become inflamed, swell, and press against the posterior tibial nerve within the tarsal tunnel causing symptoms similar to *plantar fasciitis. The pain follows the course of the nerve and is felt from the area of entrapment and radiates along the inside of the foot along the sole towards the toes. Treatment is similar to that for plantar fasciitis. Surgical decompression of the nerve has had variable results and is generally not recommended.

tarsometatarsal joint A nonaxial synovial gliding joint between the tarsus and metatarsals.

tarsus (ankle bone) The seven *tarsal bones of the ankle and proximal part of the foot. The top of the tarsus articulates with the tibia and fibula, and the front articulates with the metatarsals.

task A specific activity which is to be completed. In sport, tasks usually require the performance of motor skills. The terms task and skill are often used synonymously.

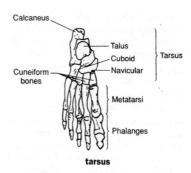

tarsus

task analysis A process of determining the underlying abilities required and the structure of motor skills that need to be performed to complete a task.

task aversion An element of psychological or subjective fatigue characterized by increased sweating, general discomfort, and a desire to do something other than train or compete. Task aversion increases in unpleasant or unfamiliar environments.

task cohesion The degree to which members of a group work together to achieve a specific identifiable goal. Task cohesion is a major dimension of *team cohesion. *See also* **sociometric cohesion**.

task dependence The amount of interaction required between team mates for a task to be completed. In baseball, pitching is an example of a task requiring low interaction while a double play requires high interaction.

task irrelevant cognitive activity (tica) *See* **cognitive state anxiety**.

task motivation A style of *leadership behaviour in which the successful completion of the task is the critical factor. It is consistent with *initiating structure.

task orientation A psychological orientation in which an individual is concerned primarily with completing the job, solving the problem, and working persistently and doing the best job possible. Those with task orientation tend to compare their performances with personal standards. They usually work well within a group, perceiving that contribution to the group effort will contribute to overall success in the task. *Compare* **interaction orientation**; **outcome goal orientation**; **and self-orientation**.

taste The sense of flavour in the mouth by which it is possible to identify food substances. There are four basic taste sensations: sweet, bitter, sour, and salt.

taste culture A subculture which reflects the preference of a group for a particular cultural product. Membership of the group may be determined by many factors including ethnic origin, social class, age, gender, and country or place of residence. In sport, preference for particular activities often depends on the taste culture with which a person identifies. For example, polo and boxing are the preferred sporting activities of particular social classes. *See* **high culture**; and **popular culture**.

taxis Manipulation by the hand to restore a body-part to its normal position, as used to treat a dislocation or a hernia.

Taylor manifest anxiety scale A means of measuring differences in chronic anxiety between different subjects using a standardized paper and pencil questionnaire with items such as 'I am easily embarrassed', and 'I have few headaches', to which the subject responds with the answer either true or false.

T-cell A type of lymphocyte produced in bone marrow that counteracts the presence of foreign antigens by a process of cell-mediated immunity. The antigen is slowly destroyed by the T-cell or by a toxin released from T-cells.

team A social unit which has a relatively rigid structure, organization and communication pattern. The task of each member of a team is usually well defined and the successful functioning of the team depends on the coordinated participation of all or several members of the team. Typically, the development of a team takes place in four stages: forming (members familiarize themselves with each other and start to form interpersonal relationships); storming (characterized by rebellion against the leader and interpersonal conflict); norming (during which hostility is replaced by cooperation with team members striving for economy of effort and task effectiveness); and performing (during which team members clarify roles and channel energies to achieve team success). *Compare* **group**.

team building The art of developing *team cohesion so a team can work together more effectively. Team building depends on the ability to blend the styles and temperaments of different people so that the skills of each can be used to the full. It involves improving communication, reducing conflict, and generating the desire among team members to achieve a common purpose. Although team building often involves individual members subordinating their needs to the interests of the team, good team building should also provide opportunities for individual needs to be satisfied.

team chemistry A colloquial term for *team dynamics.

team cohesion A dynamic process that is reflected in the tendency of a team to stick together and remain united in pursuit of its goals and objectives despite difficulties and set-backs. It is distinguished from *group cohesion by the importance in team cohesion of dynamic processes and the pursuit of team goals. *See also* **social cohesion**; and **task cohesion**.

team cohesion questionnaire A questionnaire incorporating a 9-point *Likert-type scale which measures six dimensions of *team cohesion including satisfaction, value of membership, leadership, task cohesion, desire for recognition, and affiliation cohesion.

team culture The attitudes, beliefs, and norms of a team. Team culture is concerned with how the team operates, including its selection procedures and power structure; how rewards are given; practice procedures; game protocols; acceptable behaviour; and dress code. Team culture often depends on the traditions, or lack of them, of a team. *See also* **idioculture**.

team development *See* team.

team dynamics Often referred to colloquially as 'team chemistry'; the patterns of interaction among team members that determine team spirit, harmony, cohesion, and morale. Some coaches believe that team dynamics are beyond their control, resulting from the unpredictable mixture of the personalities. Others believe that one of the most important tasks of a good coach is to create the best possible team dynamics for success.

team homogeneity Team mate similarity in terms of such things as culture, ethnic, and religious background, and socioeconomic status. *See also* **determinants**.

team psyche The spirit of a team, including sense of loyalty and dedication, which is determined in part by the team culture.

team satisfaction A measurement of how good a team feels, or how good a team member feels being part of a team. *See also* **consequences**.

team stability The degree to which the membership of a team remains the same. Team stability can be defined in terms of length of time that the team members remain together. *See also* **determinant**.

technical competency An individual's knowledge and expertise in the specific group task and its processes, that is, knowledge of the skills, strategies, and tactics of a sport and its rules and regulations. Technical competency is a managerial competency which a coach or other leader requires to be successful.

technical model An exemplar, used in coaching, of a technique in action. Technical models may be visual, verbal, or in writing.

technique A pattern of movement which is technically appropriate for a particular skill and which is an integral part but not the whole part of that skill. The Fosbury flop, for example, is a particular technique used in the skill of high jumping.

teeter-totter An unstable platform used to test *balance.

teleceptor *See* telereceptor.

telemetry The use of radio waves to transmit the readings of measuring instruments to a device which can record the readings. Telemetry is used in exercise physiology to monitor the heart rate and other functions of an athlete in motion.

telencephalon The anterior part of the forebrain which develops into the olfactory lobes, cerebral cortex, and corpus striatum (part of the basal ganglia).

teleological explanation An explanation (for example, of human behaviour) in terms of its outcomes or goals. Such explanations are usually in terms of the purposes, reasons, or motives underlying a particular behaviour.

teleology The concept that phenomena such as human behaviour are directed and determined by a goal or a purpose.

telereceptors (teleceptor) Specialized sense receptors, such as those in the eyes, ears and nose, that respond to distant external stimuli.

telic Applied to an athlete who has a goal-directed, anxiety-avoiding personality orientation. While athletes are in a telic state of mind, they tend to be serious and regard increased arousal as being unpleasant and stressful. *Compare* **paratelic**. *See also* **reversal theory**.

temperament Emotional aspects of *personality, such as joviality, moodiness, tenseness, and excitability.

temperature A measure of hotness; a property which determines the rate at which heat will be transferred between bodies which are in direct contact: heat flows from regions of high temperature to regions of low temperature. In science, temperature is expressed in terms of degrees kelvin or degrees Celsius.

temperature coefficient *See* Q_{10}.

temperomandibular joint A synovial, biaxial joint between the mandible (lower jaw) and the temporal bone at the base of the skull. It is capable of the following joint movements: elevation, depression, protraction, and retraction.

temperomandibular joint syndrome (TMJ) A painful condition of the temperomandibular jaw characterized by grinding, clicking, soreness, and limitation of jaw movement when chewing.

tempolauf A form of training which emphasizes high intensity effort equalling or approaching that required in competition. Tempolauf may take the form of continuous or intermittent work, as in a time trial, or brief repetitions at the competitive distance with adequate intervening rest periods. The aim of such training is to accustom the athlete to the tempo or pace of competition.

temporal 1 Pertaining to the temple. **2** Pertaining to time.

temporal awareness An awareness of the passage of time; an essential ingredient of pace judgement and a sense of rhythm.

temporal summation The summative effect of repeated stimulation of one presynaptic neurone on the response of a postsynaptic membrane. Each stimulus causes a release of *neurotransmitter from the presynaptic membrane which produces a *graded potential in the postsynaptic membrane. The graded potentials evoked by a rapid succession of two or more stimuli are added together until a *threshold level is reached and an *action potential occurs in the postsynaptic membrane.

ten per cent rule A training rule for runners which states that training distances (or training durations) should be increased by no more than 10 per cent per week. Increases of more than 10 per cent increases the risk of *overtraining injuries.

tendinitis Inflammation of a *tendon that usually occurs from *overuse especially in those who perform one sport or movement regularly and intensely. The tendon becomes swollen, red, and tender to the touch; motion may be impaired by pain. Treatment may include rest and modification of tendon function so that the range of movement through which the tendon moves is altered (for example, a heel pad may be used in cases of Achilles tendinitis). Surgical decompression may be necessary.

Treatment by injection of *steroids such as hydrocortisone into the paratenon may be helpful, but injection into the tendons themselves can result in a tendon rupture. *See also* **Achilles tendinitis**.

tendinosus A symptomatic *tendon degeneration due to ageing, accumulated microtrauma, or both; it is subclassified into microscopical failures, central *necrosis, and partial *rupture.

tendon A band of white tissue connecting a muscle to a bone. It consists mainly of numerous bundles of parallel collagen fibres which provide mechanical strength, and a little elastin which provides some elasticity. Tendons resist tensile stresses very well and have a tensile strength of about $50-100$ newtons/mm^2. But they resist shearing forces less effectively and provide little resistance to compressive forces. The tendons contribute to effective muscle action by concentrating the pull of the muscle on a small area of bone.

tendon organs *See* **Golgi tendon organs**.

tendon injury Damage to a *tendon. Tendons have a poor blood supply, therefore injuries are generally slow to heal. Tendon injuries include ruptures which may be partial or complete, *tendinitis and *tenosynovitis. The main aims of treating acute tendon injuries are: (i) to avoid disruption of the repairing tendon early in healing, (ii) prevent atrophy of associated joints and muscles, and (iii) encourage the tendon tissue to heal. Initial treatment (for the first 5 or 6 days after the injury) includes *RICE and anti-inflammatories, followed by a gradual introduction of stress.

tendon rupture Loss of continuity of some or all fibres of a *tendon. Tendon ruptures commonly occur after the sudden application of an unbalanced load. The injury can be very dramatic with the victim feeling as if he or she has received a severe blow. A tendon rupture may be classified as complete (third degree strain, resulting in complete loss of function) and partial ruptures (first degree strain and second degree strain). They heal slowly because of the poor blood supply to the tendon. *See* *also* **tendinitis; tenosynovitis**; and **tenoperiostitis**.

tendon sheath A fibrous sheath lined with synovial membrane and containing *synovial fluid which surrounds the paratenon of some tendons which are close to bones. Tendon sheaths surround many of the long muscle tendons crossing the wrist and fingers.

tennis elbow (enthesitis; lateral epicondylitis) A form of tendinitis affecting the common extensor tendon attached to the lateral *epicondyle of the humerus. It is characterized by a pain which originates in the outer part of elbow but which may pass from the shoulder to the wrist. Tennis elbow is a common *overuse injury of the elbow joint which can occur in any sport where the elbow is constantly bending while the hand is gripping an object; for example, canoeing, racquet sports, baseball, ten pin bowling, fly fishing. It is often caused by a technical fault. *See also* **Mills' manoeuvre**.

tennis leg A condition characterized by a sudden sharp pain in the upper calf which feels like a 'shot in the leg'. It is due to a rupture of the musculotendinous junction of one of the heads of the gastrocnemius muscle. The injury is caused by a sudden extension of the knee while the foot is dorsiflexed, or by a sudden dorsiflexion when the knee is extended. The injury occurs most often in middle-aged athletes after some degeneration of the tendon, who play sports such as tennis, squash, and basketball.

tennis shoulder A condition caused by excessive performance of a one-sided activity, such as tennis, which leads to an increase in the size of bones and muscles, and an increased laxity of the joint capsule and ligaments in the more active side. This can result in a dropping of the shoulder, a relative lengthening of the arm, and, in extreme cases, can cause scoliosis (abnormal lateral curvature of the spine). Players of one-sided sports should make a special effort to strengthen both sides of the body during training.

tennis toe *See* **black nail**.

tenoperiostitis An inflammation at the point where a *tendon inserts into, or originates from, bone. It usually arises from overuse and causes pain at the insertion during active motion. It is not common in adults but in adolescents occurs as Sever–Haglund's disease when there is pain at the insertion of the Achilles tendon into the *calcaneus, and as Osgood–Schlatter's

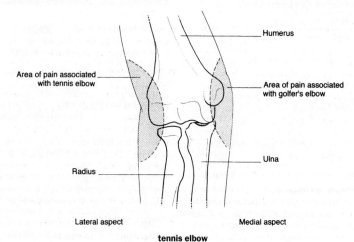

tennis elbow

disease when there is pain at the tendon insertion at the tibial tuberosity.

tenosynovitis (peritendinitis; tenovaginitis) Inflammation of the soft membrane surrounding a tendon (paratenon). Tenosynovitis causes pain and swelling. It can be a very disabling condition, commonly due to overuse. Primary treatment consists of rest, ice, compression, elevation (see **RICE**), and anti-inflammatories. It is important for the injury to heal completely before training is resumed, otherwise an easily resolved acute condition can develop into a recalcitrant, chronic condition. Chronic tenosynovitis may result in scarring which increases the thickness of the paratenon, reduces mobility, and may require surgery to correct.

tenosynovitis cyst A cyst or *ganglion formed as a result of inflammation of a tendon and accumulation of *synovial fluid within a sac. See also **wrist ganglion cyst**.

tenovaginitis See tenosynovitis.

TENS See **Transcutaneous Nerve Stimulation**.

tensile force See tension.

tensile strain See strain.

tensile strength The ability to resist tension (pulling and stretching forces).

tensile stress See tension.

tension 1 The state of an object being pulled or stretched. Tension is created by a pulling or stretching force (the tensile force) directed axially through an object. The distribution of tension within an object is called tensile stress, and it is usually measured as the force per unit area exerted by a stretched material on a support. **2** An overt muscular contraction caused by an emotional state or an increased effort. See also **stress**.

tensor A muscle that stretches a body part.

tensor fasciae latae Muscle of anterior compartment of thigh which has its origins on the anterior aspect of the *iliac crest and anterior superior iliac spine and its insertion on the *iliotibial tract. It acts as a *synergist of the *iliopsoas, *gluteus medius, and *gluteus minimus muscles during flexion and abduction and medial rotation of the thigh, steadying the trunk by making the iliotibial tract taut. It also takes part in knee extension.

teres major A thick rounded muscle at the back of the axilla (arm pit). It has its origin on the posterior surface of the scapula and it shares an insertion tendon with the *latissimus dorsi on the lesser tubercle of the humerus. Its primary actions are extension, adduction, and medial rotation of the upper arm around the shoulder.

teres minor A small, elongated, *rotator cuff muscle of the shoulder joint which lies inferior to the infraspinatus. It has its origin on the lateral border of the dorsal scapular surface and its insertion on the greater tubercle of the humerus, inferior to the infraspinatus. It acts with the infraspinatus holding the humerus in the glenoid cavity and rotating the humerus laterally, that is outwards.

terminal cisternae Sac-like channels of the sarcoplasmic reticulum at the junction between the light and dark bands in a *sarcomere of a muscle. The terminal cisternae contain calcium ions which are released from the sac immediately before a muscle contraction (see **sliding filament theory**).

terminal feedback Feedback given after a movement or performance has been completed. Compare **concurrent feedback**.

terminal velocity A constant velocity reached by an object falling through a resisting medium and being acted upon by a constant force. A body falling through the atmosphere under the force of gravity accelerates until its terminal velocity is reached. It is the velocity at which the upward drag force is equal to the weight of the falling object. The terminal velocity varies with the weight and orientation of a falling body. An ability to vary terminal velocity is very important in sky-diving.

terminal threshold See threshold.

terminal fibril See axon terminal.

terpenoids Compounds, including *steroids, made up of repeating units of isoprene (a 5-carbon organic chemical).

test 1 An examination designed to reveal the relative standing of an individual in a group; for example, with respect to achievement or fitness. **2** A chemical or other form of analysis to determine the composition of a substance.

test-anxiety approach A theory of *achievement motivation which proposes that test-anxiety is a critical factor in determining whether or not an individual approaches or avoids an *achievement situation.

test-anxiety A fear of taking a test or of failing a test.

testicle One of a pair of male sex organs within the scrotum.

testicular feminization *See* testicular feminizing syndrome.

testicular feminizing syndrome A rare condition in which a person has testes, is genetically male (having XY chromosomes), but has female organs. Those with the syndrome lack the protein, coded for by a gene on the Y-chromosome, which prevents the development of female organs. The condition causes difficulties of sex determination. The person is by virtually all definitions female, but by having a Y-chromosome, could be defined as a male.

testis Gamete-producing organ of male which also produces male sex hormones.

Test of Attentional and Interpersonal Style (TAIS) A self-report inventory which is used to assess *attention. It is based on the idea that attention has two independent dimensions: the first is width (narrow–broad), and the second is direction (internal–external). The original TAIS does not predict specific skill levels as well as sport specific versions such as the tennis-TAIS (T-TAIS), and the baseball-TAIS (B-TAIS).

testosterone An androgenic and anabolic hormone which occurs naturally in both males and females (it is secreted by the adrenal cortex and ovaries in small amounts). It is the main male sex hormone secreted by the testes that induces

testosterone

and maintains the changes that take place in males at puberty. The testes continue to produce *testosterone throughout life, though there is some decline with age. Synthetic testosterone preparations have been designed to emphasize anabolic effects while minimizing androgenic properties. Injections of testosterone or related drugs have been banned by the International Olympic Committee (IOC) since 1984. Testosterone is usually excreted in the same amounts as epitestosterone. Consequently, the ratio of testosterone to epitestosterone in the urine is used by the IOC as an indicator of testosterone misuse. The IOC regards a ratio of 6:1 (testosterone: epitestosterone) as constituting an offence unless there is evidence that this ratio is due to a physiological or pathological condition. Detection of testosterone abuse is fraught with difficulties, for example, alcohol can increase the ratio, and athletes trying to avoid detection may take mixtures of epitestosterone and testosterone. *See also* **human chorionic gonadotrophin**.

tetanic contraction *See* tetanus.

tetanus 1 Lockjaw; a particularly dangerous infection by a bacterium (*Clostridium tetani*), that can result from a laceration. Even when not fatal, this is a most unpleasant condition characterized by muscle stiffness and rigidity requiring prolonged and painful treatment. The infective organism can be found anywhere but is most common on ground which has been used by animals. It is possible to use anti-tetanus serum but this carries the risk of allergic reactions and active immunity is better. **2** Sustained contraction of muscle due to fusion of many small contractions (twitches) following one another in rapid succession. Tetanus produces sustained maximal tension and results from high frequency stimulation.

tetany Spasm and twitching of muscle due to lack of calcium which increases the excitability of nerves. Tetany usually affects the hands and feet. It may be caused by *alkalosis.

tethered swimming A method of controlling the resistance against which a person swims while maintaining a constant body position in a pool. The swimmer is attached to a harness connected to a rope and a series of weighted pulleys. As weights are increased the person must swim faster and therefore work harder to maintain position. Tethered swimming is used as an *ergometer for measuring work output of swimmers under controlled conditions, but it suffers from the disadvantage that the swimming technique is not similar to that used in free swimming (*compare* **swimming flume**).

tethering of scar A scar which adheres to deeper structures. Tethering scars commonly occur around the eyes of boxers where the scar tissue adheres to underlying bone.

thalamus A mass of grey matter in the diencephalon of the brain through which most sensory impulses pass before being transmitted to the cortex.

thanatological model A model of sport retirement based on thanatology, the study of death and dying. It adopts the concept of social death as explaining the social and psychological changes involved in retiring from sport. Social death is the condition of being treated as if one were dead although still intellectually and physiologically active.

theatre sign *See* **patellofemoral pain syndrome**.

thelion An anatomical landmark located on the breast nipple.

thematic apperception test A *personality test in which the subject is encouraged to make up an oral or written story about a particular picture presented to him or her.

thenar Pertaining to the palm of the hand.

thenar muscles Four short muscles in the palm of the hand that act exclusively to circumduct and oppose the thumb.

theoretical mechanical advantage *See* **mechanical advantage**.

theoretical sampling *See* **purposive sampling**.

theoretical square law A law which states that the resistance a body creates as it moves through a fluid (*see* **drag**) varies approximately with the square of its *velocity. The law applies to a swimmer doing the front crawl who, by doubling the speed of arm movements, increases by fourfold the resistance to forward motion.

theory A set of hypotheses or propositions, logically or mathematically linked, which is offered as an explanation in general terms for a wide variety of connected phenomena.

theory of games A treatment of competitive games in which probability theory is used in relation to the advantages and disadvantages of decisions that have to be made in situations involving conflicting interests.

therapy Treatment of an illness or injury.

thermic effect of activity The energy expended during an activity in excess of that required for resting metabolism. *See also* **metabolic equivalent**.

thermic effect of food An increase in *metabolic rate (reflected by an increase in oxygen consumption) associated with the digestion, absorption, transport, and assimilation of ingested food. The thermic effect of food accounts for about 10 per cent of our total energy expenditure per day. The thermic effect of a particular food seems to be variable, even within the same individual.

thermodynamic laws Laws which are believed to govern processes that involve heat changes. The two laws which are most relevant to sport science are the law of conservation of energy and the law of entropy. Conservation of energy applies to a system of constant *mass in which energy can be neither created nor destroyed. A consequence of the law of entropy is that heat cannot be transferred by any continuous self-sustaining process from a colder to a hotter body. Which means that the efficiency of energy transformations is imperfect and some free energy will escape from the system, usually as heat.

thermodynamics The science of the transformation of heat and energy.

thermogenesis The production of body heat. Most body heat is a by-product of *metabolism. These reactions increase during exercise, consequently there is a greater risk of overheating. During cold weather, extra internal heat may be generated by increasing metabolism (nonshivering thermogenesis), and by uncontrolled muscular contractions (shivering thermogenesis). Nonshivering thermogenesis involves stimulation of metabolism by the *sympathetic nervous system. *See also* **thermic effect of food**.

thermography Use of infra-red photography to measure thermal emissions from the skin and subcutaneous tissue. The thermograph is the picture produced. It provides a visual means of identifying areas of inflammation associated with some sports injuries and *ischaemia.

thermolysis The removal of body heat (for example by evaporation of body sweat).

thermoreceptor A sensory nerve-ending that responds to changes in temperature. Skin thermoreceptors (hot and cold receptors) detect changes in environmental temperature. Some scientists believe that Ruffini's corpuscles and Krause's end bodies act as skin thermoreceptors. Other scientists are convinced that the receptors are naked nerve-endings and that Ruffini's corpuscles and Krause's end bodies are mechanoreceptors. Thermoreceptors in the *hypothalamus detect changes of body core temperature.

thermoregulation The maintenance of a relatively constant body *core temperature.

Thermoregulation may involve behavioural and physiological processes (*see* **thermotaxis**). Skin thermoreceptors monitor environmental temperatures for behavioural thermoregulation involving voluntary behavioural responses initiated by the cortex of the brain. The *hypothalamus contains thermoreceptors involved in physiological responses.

thermoregulatory centre Part of the *hypothalamus responsible for regulating body core temperature. It relays information through the autonomic system, for example, to sweat glands.

thermotaxis The normal physiological responses, such as changes in the rate of sweating and metabolic rate, which help to keep a balance between heat losses and heat gains in the body.

thermotherapy *See* **heat treatment**.

thiamine (aneurine, vitamin B_1) Water soluble organic compound found in cereals (for example, rice husks) and yeast, whose main function is to act as a coenzyme in sugar breakdown by forming part of the molecule of *nicotinamide adenine dinucleotide.

thick filament The thicker of the two main types of filament in a muscle sarcomere. Each thick filament contains approximately 200 *myosin molecules bundled together so that its central portion is smooth and its ends are studded with cross bridges. *Compare* **thin filament**; *see also* **C-stripes**.

thigh The region between the knee and the hip.

thigh abductor Muscles which effect abduction of the thigh. The most important are the *gluteal muscles.

thigh adductor One of three fleshy adductor muscles (the adductor magnum, adductor longus, and adductor brevis muscles) in the medial part of the thigh. All three adductors are involved in movements which press the thighs together.

thigh extensor A muscle which effects extension of the thigh. The most important are the massive hamstring muscles and, during forceful extensions, the gluteus maximus.

thigh flexor A muscle which effects *flexion of the thigh. Thigh flexors include the *iliopsoas, *tensor fasciae latae, and the *rectus femoris, which are among the most powerful muscles of the body. These are assisted by the *thigh adductors and the strap-like *sartorius.

thigh girth An anthropometric measurement which is the circumference of the thigh (usually the right) 1–2 centimetres below the protuberance of the gluteal muscles on the thigh. The measurement is taken when the subject is standing erect with feet slightly apart and with weight equally distributed on both feet.

thigh lateral rotator A muscle which rotates the thigh outwards, that is laterally away from the mid-line of the body. The thigh lateral rotators include the *piriformis, *obturator externus, *gemellus, *quadratus femoris, and the *obturator interna.

thigh length In anthropometry, either the difference between the *trochanterion height and the *tibiale (laterale) height; or, the difference between the stretched stature and the sum of the sitting height and the tibiale (laterale) height.

thigh medial rotator A muscle, such as the *tensor fasciae latae or the *gluteus medius, which rotates the thigh inwards on the hip, towards the midline of the body.

thigh movement A movement which occurs either at the knee (mainly extension and flexion) or at the hip (which includes abduction, adduction, circumduction, extension, flexion, inwards and outward rotation).

thin filament The thinner of the two main types of filament seen in electron micrographs of a muscle *sarcomere. Thin filaments are composed mainly of helically arranged actin along with *nebulin and the regulatory proteins *tropomyosin and *troponin. *Compare* **thick filament**.

third class lever A lever which has its point of effort (force application) between the

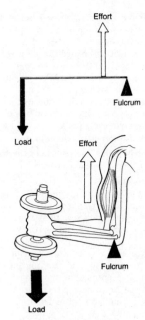

third class lever

fulcrum (point of support or axis of rotation) and the resistance or load. It is the most common type of lever used in the human body. Since the distance between the resistance and the fulcrum is usually greater than the distance between the effort and fulcrum, the effort is greater than the load, but such levers provide a good range of movement at speed.

third degree strain A complete rupture of a muscle or a tendon which often occurs in athletes attempting a power activity. The tendons most commonly affected are the Achilles tendon, the biceps tendon, patellar tendon, quadriceps tendon, and the supraspinatus tendon. *See also* **strain**.

thirst An uncomfortable feeling of dryness in the mouth and throat accompanied by a desire to drink.

thirst mechanism An uncomfortable feeling of dryness in the mouth and throat accompanied by a strong desire to drink. Unfortunately, the thirst mechanism does not come into play until after an athlete loses significant amounts of body fluids. Therefore, to ensure that they do not become dehydrated, athletes should drink plenty of watery fluids during and after exercise, even if they do not feel thirsty. *See also* **dehydration**.

Thomas model A model of *psychological skills training (PST) used by applied sport psychologists to enhance the performance of athletes. It consists of seven phases: an orientation phase, during which the purpose of the PST is clarified, objectives identified, and commitment determined; analysis of the physical, psychological, and biomechanical demands of the sport in relation to the individual or team; an assessment phase, when the psychological strengths and weaknesses of the individual or team are assessed; a conceptualization phase, during which the results so far gathered are discussed with the athlete so that their accuracy can be checked and the athlete can be made more aware of the situation; a psychological skills training phase, during which the athlete learns to develop a variety of skills (e.g. self-awareness and self-confidence) and techniques (e.g. physical relaxation and imagery); an implementation phase, during which the various skills and techniques are used in training and competition; and an evaluation phase, during which the effectiveness of the intervention by the applied sport psychologist is evaluated.

Thompson's test A clinical test used to assess the integrity of the *Achilles tendon. The patient is placed in the prone position with feet dangling off the end of an examination table and the calf is squeezed. Tendon rupture is indicated if *plantar flexion does not occur (the heel does not move).

thoracic Pertaining to the chest.

thoracic cage *See* **bony thorax**.

thoracic cavity The chest cavity. *See* **thorax**.

thoracic curvature *See* **spinal curvature**.

thoracic duct A large duct that receives *lymph drained from the lower body, the left upper extremity, and the left side of the head and thorax, and drains into the left subclavian vein and then into the heart.

thoracic injury Damage to the structures in the thorax. Injuries to the thorax are often serious since they can affect the vital organs of the lungs and heart. A fall from a horse, a crush in a rugby scrum, or any other direct hit on the thorax can result in fractured ribs with the potential risk of a punctured lung. *Stress fractures of the rib occasionally occur, especially in those, such as tennis players, who use mainly one arm.

thoracic vertebra One of twelve vertebrae which articulate with the ribs. Each thoracic vertebra has a roughly heart shaped centrum, a long spinous process, and bears costal facets which receive the ribs.

thorax The chest; the portion of the body trunk above the diaphragm and below the neck which contains the heart and lungs and is enclosed by the thoracic cage.

Thorndikes stimulus–response theory of learning A theory which proposes that all learning consists primarily of the strengthening of the relationship between the stimulus and the response. In developing this theory, Thorndike proposed three laws: the *law of effect, the *law of exercise, and the *law of readiness.

thought stopping A technique used to overcome negative attitudes when performing. The performer is trained to recognize and become aware of negative thoughts and to replace them with constructive ones. A skier at the start of a slalom, for example, who starts to think about the consequences of misjudging turns, stops these thoughts and replaces them with thoughts of how the descent can be successfully completed. *See also* **centring procedure**; and **refocusing**.

threonine An essential amino acid which is found in beans and other legumes, corn, and other grains.

threshold (limen) A term which usually refers to the weakest value of any stimulus or other agency which will produce a specified effect. This is sometimes called the absolute threshold or stimulus threshold. The term may also refer to the smallest difference between two stimuli (the just-noticeable difference), in intensity, magnitude, or pitch which can be discriminated. This is more precisely referred to as the difference threshold or differential threshold. The terminal threshold is the upper limit of sensitivity; the point beyond which further increases in the intensity of stimulation have no typical effect. The typical effect refers to a change in the type of experience being studied. For example, increases of light intensity above the terminal threshold may cause pain, but this is not the usual effect of that stimulation.

threshold of training The minimum amount of exercise that will improve physical fitness. For exercise to be effective, it must be done with sufficient frequency, intensity, and for a long enough duration. As fitness improves the threshold level gets higher. See also **principle of progressive overload**.

thrombin An enzyme that catalyses the formation of *fibrin from *fibrinogen during the clotting of blood.

thrombocytes See **blood platelet**.

thrombosis A condition in which a thrombus forms in a blood vessel.

thrombus A blood clot that remains at its point of formation.

thrower's elbow (pitcher's elbow) A term given to a number of conditions of the elbow associated with round arm throwing. Thrower's elbow includes damage to the ligaments, typically the medial ligaments, and the olecranon process which may suffer a *stress fracture or an *osteochondritis. Thrower's elbow is caused by putting too great a load on the elbow (for example, in forceful straightening of the elbow when serving in tennis or throwing a ball). It often requires correction of faulty technique as well as treatment of the damaged tissue. See also **golfer's elbow**.

thrower's fracture A fracture of the humerus when the muscular force generated by a

hard throw may be enough to snap the bone.

thrust 1 A *force which produces motion. **2** A continuous force applied by one object on another.

thumb See **pollex**.

Thurstone scales Measures of *attitude consisting of about twenty statements, each representing a different degree of favourableness or unfavourableness toward an attitude object, arranged to present a continuum of equally spaced levels of favourableness.

thymus An *endocrine gland in the neck in which lymphocytes active in the immune response become differentiated. Its function reaches a peak during puberty and then declines with age.

thyrocalcitonin See **calcitonin**.

thyroglobulin A protein in the thyroid gland from which the thyroid hormones thyroxine and triiodothyronine are derived.

thyroid gland A large, bilobed endocrine gland located along the midline of the neck, immediately below the larynx (Adam's apple). The thyroid gland secretes the hormones triiodothyronine and thyroxine which regulate metabolic rate, and calcitonin which helps regulate calcium metabolism.

thyroid hormone A hormone secreted from the thyroid gland. There are at least two separate iodine-containing hormones: thyroxine and triiodothyronine. These hormones have similar effects (see **thyroxine**).

thyroid stimulating hormone (thyrotropin; TSH) A hormone secreted by the anterior pituitary gland which stimulates production of thyroid hormone from the thyroid gland.

thyrostatic Applied to a medication that reduces the production of thyroid hormones.

thyrotoxicosis A condition due to excessive secretion of thyroid hormone. It is characterized by an increased metabolic rate and is usually accompanied by an enlargement of the thyroid gland.

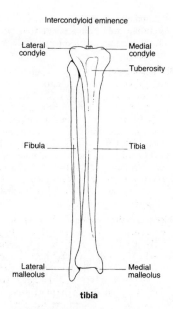

Thyroxine   Triiodothyronine

thyroid hormone

thyrotropin *See* **thyroid stimulating hormone.**

thyroxine An iodine-containing hormone secreted with triiodothyronine from the thyroid gland. These two thyroid hormones share similar functions. They increase the metabolic rate of most cells within the body, and can raise the *basal metabolic rate by as much as 60 per cent. They increase the size and number of mitochondria in most cells. They also enhance *glycolysis, *gluconeogenesis, and *fat mobilization. They are important regulators of tissue growth and development, particularly of nervous and skeletal tissue. Deficiency results in sluggish muscle action, cramps, and *myalgia; excessive secretions produce muscle atrophy and weakness, and, in adults, demineralization of bones. Exercise increases the secretion of these thyroid hormones. Trained athletes have a higher concentration of thyroid hormones at rest, and a higher turnover during exercise, than untrained individuals.

tibia (shin bone) The inner and larger bone in the lower leg extending from the ankle to the knee. It articulates with the talus below and the femur above. It is triangular in cross-section. The sharp anterior crest

tibia

and medial surface of the tibia are unprotected by muscle and can be felt just underneath the skin.

tibiale laterale An anatomical landmark located on the superior extremity and the lateral border of the head of the *tibia.

tibiale mediale An anatomical landmark located on the superior extremity and the medial border of the head of the tibia.

tibial height A body height measurement made from the head of the tibia to the *base.

tibialis anterior A long, superficial muscle in the anterior compartment of the lower leg. It has its origin on the lateral condyle and upper two-thirds of the tibia, and its insertion on the medial surface of the first cuneiform and first metatarsal. Its primary actions are dorsiflexion and inversion.

tibialis anterior syndrome Pain and tenderness felt during ankle dorsiflexion and when pressure is applied to the lateral side of the tibia at the front of the lower leg. It is due to an acute inflammation of the tendon of the *tibialis anterior muscle.

The syndrome commonly arises from overuse of the ankle, for example from prolonged running and jumping on a hard surface.

tibialis posterior A thick, flat, deep muscle in the posterior compartment of the lower leg. The tibialis posterior has extensive origins on the posterior, proximal surface of the tibia, fibula, and interosseus membrane. Its insertion is on the tarsal and metatarsal bones via a tendon which passes behind the medial malleolus and under the arch of the foot. Its primary actions are plantar flexion and inversion. It also helps to stabilize the longitudinal arch, especially during skating.

tibialis posterior syndrome Pain and tenderness associated with movement or loading of the tendon of the tibialis posterior muscle. The tendon runs behind the tibia and the *medial malleolus, through a narrow groove to insert onto the navicular bone. Over-pronation of the foot results in an increase in pressure on the tendon which may cause the tendon, its attachment, or its sheath to become inflamed. The injury is common in skating and skiing.

tibial torsion A rotation of the femur on the tibia so that the midsagittal plane of the femur is directed forward and the midsagittal plane of the tibia is rotated outwards. External tibial torsion is usually associated with internal *femoral torsion. The condition may develop because of an imbalance of the hamstring muscles. Tibial torsion increases stress on the medial structures of the knee-joint and pain in the lateral aspect of the knee; it usually causes the toes to be pointed outwards (laterally) during weight bearing.

tibial tuberosity A large rounded prominence on the tibia.

tibial valgus Curvature of the tibia outwards from its proximal to distal end. The condition is usually combined with a femoral varus and results in a knock-kneed appearance. Tibial valgus results in extra tensile stress being placed on the medial side of the knee and the lateral side of the

ankle. However, this can be at least partly compensated for by strengthening the *quadriceps muscles which stabilize the knee, and strengthening the muscles which support the lateral side of the foot.

tibial varus Curvature of the tibia inwards from its proximal to distal end. Tibial varus is often accompanied by rearfoot valgus. It increases the tensile stress on the lateral aspect of the knee joint and may cause *iliotibial-band friction syndrome.

tibiofemoral joint *See* **knee-joint**.

tibiofibular joint One of two fibrous joints (the inferior and superior tibiofibular joints) between the tibia and fibula. It permits only limited movement, for example, during ankle dorsiflexion.

TICA *See* **cognitive state anxiety**.

tidal volume The volume of air inspired into the lungs or expired out of the lungs during one breath. The typical resting value is 500 ml but it increases dramatically during exercise.

tidal volume inspiratory capacity ratio The ratio of the actual volume of air inhaled and exhaled during a single breath to the total lung capacity.

time A quantity measuring duration. Time is measured in *seconds in *SI units. Time is often an independent variable used in scientific investigations to which other physical magnitudes are related. An example is the change in oxygen consumption with respect to time where the origin in time can be any arbitrarily selected instant; negative values refer to events occurring before and positive values to events occurring after that instant.

time-dependent ageing The loss of function resulting from increasing chronological age. *Compare* **acquired ageing**.

time of flight (flight time) The duration in time a projectile is airborne, which is equal to the sum of the time it takes the projectile to reach its peak and the time the projectile takes to return from the peak to the landing point. When release and landing points are at the same level, the projectile takes the same time to reach its peak as it does to return to its original level.

time test A test of aerobic fitness in which the subject exerts maximum sustained power for a defined period (usually corresponding to the average duration of competition).

time trial Situation in which an athlete (e.g., runner, swimmer, or cyclist) races against the clock to establish how fast he or she can cover a given distance. Time trials may be performed at the competition distance, above that distance, or below it. They may be performed with or without the assistance of other athletes. Time trials form an important part of most training programmes, offering important feedback about the value and effects of training.

timing The ability to perform movements and actions of the body or body-part at a particular moment to produce the best effect. Timing is a quality which characterizes most motor skills. Timing may be facilitated by external stimuli, such as visual or auditory stimuli caused by the movements of team mates, or it may be facilitated by internal rhythmic stimuli. See **rhythm**.

tinea pedis See **athlete's foot**.

tip-to-tail method See **vector chain method**.

tissue A group of cells with a similar structure performing a specific function. The primary types of tissue in the body are epithelial, connective, muscle, and nervous tissue.

tissue–capillary membrane The thin barrier separating the capillaries from respiring tissues. The tissue–capillary membrane is the site at which *gaseous exchange occurs.

tissue fluid A fluid formed by the ultrafiltration of blood plasma which surrounds cells. The tissue fluid acts as the internal environment of cells.

titin A large muscle protein found in sarcomeres (see **elastic filament**).

TLC See **total lung capacity**.

TLV:RV ratio The ratio between total lung volume (TLV) and residual volume (RV).

TMAS (Taylor Manifest Anxiety Scale) A scale used to measure *anxiety. It is based on fifty items to which the subject answers either yes or no. It was most commonly used in the 1950s.

TNS See **transcutaneous nerve stimulation**.

tocopherol See **vitamin E**.

toe extension Straightening of the toes from a flexed position to the *anatomical position.

toe extensor A muscle that effects *toe extension. Toe extensors include the extensor digitorum brevis, extensor digitorum longus, and (for extension of great toe) the extensor hallucis longus.

toe flexion Curling of the toes downwards.

toe flexor A muscle that effects toe flexion. Toe flexors include the flexor digitorum longus, flexor digitorum brevis, quadratus plantae, and lumbricals. The flexor hallucis longus and brevis produce flexion of the hallux (great toe).

toe joint See **interphalangeal joint**.

tolerance 1 The capacity to endure pain or hardship, such as harsh environmental conditions or psychological stress. **2** Condition in which increasing doses of a drug are required to maintain the same response. See also **drug tolerance**. **3** Failure of a body to mount a specific immune response against a particular antigen. Such immunological tolerance usually results from the body having difficulty distinguishing between its own materials which should be tolerated, and foreign materials which should be attacked by antibodies.

tomogram The visual record produced by *tomography.

tomography A process by which an image is produced through different planes of a body part using X-rays or ultrasound. See also **computerized tomography**.

tone See **muscle tone**.

tonic 1 A drug used to give a sense of wellbeing. Tonics may contain stimulants, banned by the International Olympic Committee Medical Commission. **2** Pertaining to *muscle tone.

tonicity 1 The state of normal partial contraction of a muscle. *See also* **tonus**. **2** A measure of the ability of a solution to cause a change in the volume or tone of a cell by promoting osmotic flow of water (*see* **osmosis**).

tonic muscle *See* **anti-gravity muscle**.

tonic stretch The type of muscle stretch described by the amount of muscle extension, rather than its rate of the extension (*compare* **phasic stretch**).

tonus *See* **muscle tone**.

topical application Application of a drug directly to the part of the body being treated, usually the skin surface.

top spin A spin, typically of a ball, during which the top of the spinning body travels forward and the bottom of the spinning body travels backward relative to the centre. The top spin modifies the angular rotation in a clockwise direction around the horizontal or transverse axis. When a ball is hit by a bat or some other implement, a top spin results from the back of the ball (that is, the part in contact with the bat) being lifted upward and forward during the strike. Generally, the spin will make the ball come off another surface with a greater horizontal velocity than it possessed when it hit the surface, and the angle of reflection is also greater than if no spin had been imparted to the ball.

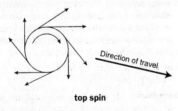

Direction of travel

top spin

torn cartilage *See* **meniscal tear**.

torn meniscus *See* **meniscal tear**.

torque (force moment; moment of force; moment of couple) A *force which produces a twisting or rotary movement in any plane about an axis of motion; it is the rotary effect of an eccentric force. Torque occurs when bones move around each other at joints which serve as the axes of movement. Thus, a muscle force when applied over a range of motion is measured as torque. Torque is a measure of the turning effect of a force on a lever, so that: torque of lever = force × lever arm (or moment arm) distance; also: torque = moment of inertia × angular acceleration. A torque is sometimes called a moment. The SI unit for torque is the newton-metre.

torque arm The force arm, lever arm, or moment arm. *See* **moment arm**.

torr A unit of pressure equal to 1/760 standard atmospheric pressure, approximately 1 mmHg.

torsion A mechanical strain set up in an object when the object is twisted around its longitudinal axis, typically when one end is fixed. The external twisting forces are resisted by the shear stresses induced in the material of the object.

torsional modulus The ratio of *stress to *strain in an elastic material when that material is being twisted. *See also* **elastic modulus**.

torsional rigidity The applied torque needed to produce a unit angle of twist in a circular elastic material; a measure of a body's resistance to torsion.

torticollis (wryneck) A rigid spasm of the *sternomastoid and *trapezius muscles causing the head and neck to be drawn painfully to one side. Torticollis may be congenital but it can occur in young athletes after violent twisting of the neck (e.g. when heading in soccer).

torus fracture An outward buckling of the cortex of the distal end of a bone shaft. The most common torus fracture is of the distal radius. *See also* **fracture**.

total lung capacity Volume of air in the lungs at the end of maximal inspiration. It has a typical value of 5 litres.

total lung volume *See* **total lung capacity**.

touch (tactile sense) The sense by which the size and shape of objects are perceived when they come into contact with the body surface. Touch commonly refers to a number of other senses which are diffused all over the body in addition to the touch sense proper. These are: the pressure sense, by which the heaviness and hardness of objects are perceived; the heat sense, by which increases in cutaneous temperature are perceived; the cold sense, by which reductions in cutaneous temperature are perceived (*see* **thermoreceptors**); and the pain sense, by which pricks, pinches, and other painful effects are perceived.

toxic Applied to poisonous substances.

toxicity The degree to which a substance is poisonous. Almost any substance in food, air, and water can become toxic if taken in a high enough concentration.

toxin A poisonous protein formed by bacteria, plants, and animals. Toxins act as *antigens in the body.

toxoid Toxin which has had its poisonous element removed but which retains its ability to act as an *antigen and stimulate the production of antibodies against the actual toxin.

trabecula (pl. trabeculae) **1** Small needle-like mineralized piece of tissue from which spongy bone is formed. **2** A fibrous band of *connective tissue which supports functional cells and extends from the outer part to the interior of an organ, dividing the organ into separate chambers.

trabecular bone *See* **spongy bone**.

trace conditioning Method of *classical conditioning in which the conditioned stimulus is removed before the appearance of the unconditioned stimulus.

trace element *See* **micromineral**.

trace mineral *See* **micromineral**.

tracer A material, usually a radioactive isotope, which can be used to trace the course of an element or compound through the body.

trachea (windpipe) A tube, reinforced with cartilage and lined with ciliated *epithelium, which extends from the larynx to the bronchi.

tracking *See* **guide movement**.

tract 1 A group of nerve fibres having the same origin, destination, and function in the central nervous system. **2** A system of functionally integrated structures (e.g., the digestive tract).

traction The use of a pulling force, especially a force that counteracts the tension surrounding a broken bone (*see* **fracture**) so that the bone is kept correctly positioned during healing.

tragus The cartilage which projects over the external auditory meatus of the outer ear.

trainability principle A basic principle of training which states that the more fully a person is trained with respect to a given fitness component, the less there remains of that component to be trained in the future. Therefore, benefits are more easily obtained during the early stages of training than later.

training An exercise programme designed to assist the learning of *skills, to improve physical fitness, and thereby to prepare an athlete for a particular competition. Training includes *conditioning, *specific technical training, and psychological preparation (*see* **psychological skills training**). *Compare* **practice**.

training adaptations *See* **aerobic training adaptations**; and **anaerobic training adaptations**.

training cycles *See* **periodization**.

training dose *See* **training impulse**.

training duration 1 The length of time that a training session lasts. The optimum duration of training will depend on the intensity of the session and the level of fitness of the individual, but a minimum period of 15 minutes is recommended for the improvement of health. **2** The length of time for a particular training programme. The minimum period required for improvements to occur varies considerably, but tends to be longer for aerobic activities (at least 12 weeks) than anaerobic activities (at least 8 weeks).

training effects The functional physiological adaptations which have been linked with training and physical exercise. Research has shown that regular training tends to increase the following: *articular cartilage thickness; *adenosine triphosphate (ATP) in muscle; *arterial–venous oxygen difference at maximal workload; *blood lactate at maximal workload; *blood volume; *capillarization of muscle (including cardiac muscle); *creatine phosphate in muscle fibres; *diffusing capacity of the lungs at maximal workload; *diphosphoglycerate in the blood; fibrolytic activity (*see* **fibrinolysis**); *haemoglobin content; heart volume (*see* ***athlete's heart**); heart weight; *high density lipoproteins in the blood; joint mobility; lean body mass; muscle cross-sectional area; *muscle glycogen content; muscle strength; myocardial contractility; *myoglobin in muscle; mitochondrial size and density in muscle cells; *phosphofructokinase activity in muscle mitochondria; *potassium in muscle; *pulmonary ventilation at maximal workload; *respiratory rate at maximal workload; speed of limb movement; strength of bones and ligaments; *stress tolerance; *stroke volume; and *succinic dehydrogenase activity in mitochondria. Regular training tends to decrease arterial *blood pressure; blood *cholesterol; *blood lactate at a given workload; *glycogen utilization; *heart rate at submaximal workloads; *heart rate at rest; *low density lipoproteins in the blood; *myocardial infarction risks; *obesity; oxygen uptake at a given workload; *platelet stickiness; pulmonary ventilation for a given workload; *stress; and triglycerides in the blood. Many of the effects are produced by regular, progressive aerobic training, but it must be emphasized that no one form of training will produce all the effects listed.

training frequency The number of times per week training is undertaken. Some coaches advocate training on seven days a week, but recommended frequencies vary considerably. As a rough guideline, it has been suggested that aerobic training should occur at least four to five times a week, anaerobic training three times per week, and training for health at least three times per week.

training heart rate (THR; training target heart rate) The heart rate which indicates

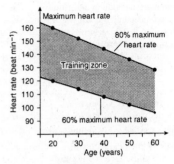

training heart rate

a level of intensity of exercise that produces maximum training effects. There are a number of methods of computing the training heart rate but the method commonly used is to take a range between sixty per cent and eighty per cent of maximum heart rate. The target heart rate will vary for the type of activity and the fitness level of the individual. Anaerobic training requires higher heart rates (up to 95 per cent maximum heart rate) sustained for short periods, while aerobic training requires lower heart rates sustained for long periods. Unfit people should train at the lowest end of the range. Individuals with health problems need to obtain medical advice before taking part in a vigorous physical activity. *See also* **Karvonen method**.

training impulse A measure of an athlete's level of training during a training session assessed from the changes in heart rate during the exercise, the duration of the training session, and the intensity of effort during the session. The training impulse is expressed in arbitrary units.

training intensity *See* **intensity of training**.

training principles Basic principles that can be applied to all forms of physical training to optimize its effects. *See* **principle of individuality; principle of specificity; principle of disuse;** and **principle of progressive overload**.

training programme A plan or schedule for training. *See also* **periodization**.

training session A continuous period of time devoted to training. A single session might include several training units.

training shoe Footwear designed specifically for protection during training. There are many different models and types but most incorporate features to cope with the stress caused by the forces which occur when the foot strikes the ground and the forces exerted by the sideways movements of the foot whilst still in contact with the ground. The parts of the training shoe include the arch support, external heel counter support, heel counter, heel tab, insock, midsock, midsole, and outsole.

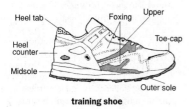

Heel tab, Foxing, Upper, Toe-cap, Heel counter, Midsole, Outer sole

training shoe

training target heart rate See target heart rate.

training time The rate at which exercise is to be accomplished during an exercise or work interval in an *interval training programme. A training time of 30 seconds for 200 metres, for example, would mean that an athlete aims to complete the 200 metres in 30 seconds.

training unit A single period of training aimed at achieving a specified objective. The objective may be to develop *aerobic endurance in which case the unit might be a steady run of 16 km. See also **training session**.

training volume Total amount of training, usually expressed as total distance covered during a given period (e.g. 8 km during an interval training session, or 40 km week^{-1}) or energy expended during a given period (e.g. kcal week^{-1}, or k calday^{-1}). Studies indicate that the optimal aerobic training volume for distance runners is about 80 km of running per week, and for swimmers is about 5000 m day^{-1}.

training zone A range of heart rates indicating an intensity of effort which should be undertaken if training is to be beneficial. See also **aerobic training zone**; **anaerobic training zone**; and **training heart rate**.

trait A relatively stable predisposition to act in a certain way. Traits are usually applied to *personality. Each trait is often represented as a two dimensional construct (e.g. honest–dishonest, assertive–nonassertive) represented by a scale along which an individual can be rated. Traits are viewed as being consistent across a wide variety of different situations (see **trait theory**).

trait aggression A relatively stable *personality predisposition to respond to certain situations with acts of *aggression. Compare **state aggression**.

trait anxiety (general trait anxiety) A general tendency to exhibit *anxiety. Individuals with high trait anxiety are predisposed to perceive a wide range of situations as dangerous or threatening, and to respond to those situations with increased *state anxiety. See also **competitive A-trait**.

Trait Anxiety Inventory (TAI) A measure of *trait anxiety which consists of twenty items to which the subject responds using a Likert-type scale. TAI is often used as a companion test to SAI (see **State Anxiety Inventory**).

trait perspective A view of *personality which suggests that personality traits are relatively enduring qualities which can be used to predict an individual's behaviour in a variety of situations.

trait theory A theory which describes individual differences of personality in terms of traits. See also **trait perspective**.

trait theory of leadership The theory that successful leaders have certain *personality characteristics or leadership traits which make it possible for them to be successful leaders in any situation. This theory is also known as the 'great man' theory of leadership. There seems to be little support for a universal set of personality traits common to all successful leaders. See also **universal behaviours**.

trajectory The flight path of a projectile.

tranquillizer A drug that has a calming effect, reduces anxiety, and relieves tension.

transcendental meditation A relaxation method that features the repetition of a *mantra. It has been used by some athletes to attain a state of calmness before competition.

Transcutaneous Electrical Nerve Stimulation See **Transcutaneous Nerve Stimulation.**

Transcutaneous Nerve Stimulation (TENS; TNS; Transcutaneous Electrical Nerve Stimulation) A technique used to relieve pain. A weak electrical current is discharged through electrodes placed at strategic points on the skin in order to inhibit information about tissue injury from pain receptors reaching the central nervous system. Research shows that transcutaneous nerve stimulation results in the release of encephalins and *endorphins.

transducer A device that transforms energy from one form into another.

transfer design An experimental design for measuring learning effects in which all treatment groups are transferred to a common level of the independent variable; that is, all groups practise the relevant task with the same value for the independent variable.

transfer of learning The effect that learning one skill has on the subsequent learning of another skill. The learning of the new skill may be speeded up, slowed down, or may not be affected at all by previous learning. See also **bilateral transfer; negative transfer; positive transfer;** and **transfer of training.**

transfer of momentum The process whereby *momentum is transferred from one part of a body to another in accordance with the conservation of momentum principle. Airborne movements which include somersaulting and twisting generally involve a transfer of the somersaulting angular momentum, initiated during the takeoff, for the twisting angular momentum performed during the flight.

transfer of training The effect of one form of training on another form of training. See also **transfer of learning;** and **transfer principle.**

transfer principle A principle of training which states that the effects of one form of training on another will depend on the similarity between the two. The transfer principle emphasizes the independent nature of factors such as strength, endurance, and flexibility, and suggests that positive transfer will only occur for those factors that are shared by the two forms of training.

transferrin (siderophilin) A protein which transports iron in the blood.

transfusion The administration of a fluid, such as saline, plasma, or blood, into the circulatory system. The fluid is allowed to drip into the subject's vein under gravity. See also **blood doping.**

transient hypertrophy See **hypertrophy.**

transition period A period of a training programme which allows an athlete to recover both physically and mentally following training or competition. During the transition period, there is a gradual reduction of training intensity but the athlete continues to exercise to maintain a reasonable level of general fitness. Emphasis is usually on physical and emotional relaxation involving leisure pursuits. See also **periodization.**

translation (linear motion; translatory motion) Form of motion in which all parts of a body travel exactly the same distance, in the same direction, in the same time. Compare angular motion. See also **curvilinear translation;** and **rectilinear translation.**

transmitter See **neurotransmitter.**

transverse In anatomy, situated at right angles to the longitudinal axis of the body or an organ.

transverse axis (frontal axis) An imaginary line (one of the anatomical reference axes) that runs perpendicular to the sagittal plane, along which sagittal rotations occur. During running, for example, the major axes of rotation are the transverse axes passing through the shoulders and hips.

transverse chest width The distance across the lateral aspect of the thorax, at the level of the most lateral aspect of the fourth rib. *See also* **body breadths**.

transverse foramina *See* **cervical vertebra**.

transverse plane (horizontal plane) A *cardinal plane running horizontally at right angles to the longitudinal axis of the body, dividing it into superior (top) and inferior (bottom) halves.

transverse process The long projections that extend laterally from each *neural arch of a vertebra.

transverse tubules (T tubules) Extensions of the sarcolemma of a muscle fibre that run between the terminal cisternae of the sarcoplasmic reticulum and penetrate deep into the *muscle fibre. The tubules allow an electrical stimulus and substances carried in the extracellular fluid (e.g. glucose, oxygen, and ions) to reach the deep regions of a muscle fibre.

transversus abdominus (transversus) The deepest of the four pairs of abdominal muscles. The transverse abdominus has its origins on the *inguinal ligament, lumbodorsal fascia, and cartilage of the last six ribs. It has its insertion on the *linea alba and pubic symphysis. The main action of the transversus abdominus is compression of the abdominal contents.

transversus *See* **transversus abdominus**.

trapeziform test A test of aerobic fitness which consists of a step-wise increase in exercise intensity and duration until a desired heart rate is reached after which the intensity is kept constant.

trapezium A wrist bone which articulates with the first metacarpal in front, the trapezoid and second metacarpal on the side, and the scaphoid bone behind.

trapezius The most superficial muscle of the posterior *thorax. The trapezius is flat and triangular in shape with its origins on the occipital bone, the ligamentum nuchae, and the spines of the vertebrae. It has a continuous insertion along the acromion

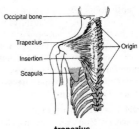

trapezius

and spine of the scapula, and the lateral part of the clavicle. The trapezius adducts and rotates the scapula upwards (via the upper fibres) and downwards (via the lower fibres). It also assists in turning the head and extending the neck backwards.

trapezoid bone A wrist bone which articulates with the second metacarpal in front, the trapezium on one side and the capitate on the other, and the scaphoid in front. *See also* **carpus**.

trauma 1 Physical damage caused by a blow, often the result of an external force. **2** An event causing psychological shock that may have long-lasting effects and lead to a neurosis.

traumatic arthritis Inflammation of a joint due to an injury; it is the most common form of *arthritis in sport.

traumatic injury An acute injury resulting in physical damage. *See also* **trauma**.

traumatology The study of injuries, including recovery from injury. Sport traumatology is especially concerned with enabling an athlete to be sufficiently rehabilitated that he or she can participate in competitions at maximum capacity.

traveller's diarrhoea A notoriously disabling condition which often inflicts a touring sports team when the dietary and hygiene environment is poor. It is usually caused by an unaccustomed strain of the bacterium, *Escherichia coli*. Anxiety and change of diet may also induce diarrhoea.

travel sickness (motion sickness) A condition caused by stimulation of the organ of balance in the ear which gives rise to nausea, vertigo, and vomiting. *Adrenergic and *anticholinergic drugs tend to diminish travel sickness. *Antihistamines, which have an anticholinergic effect, are commonly used to treat travel sickness but they can cause drowsiness which detracts from performance. Travel sickness can be a considerable handicap in sports such as sailing and motor racing.

treadmill A device consisting of a large belt on which a person walks or runs. The belt is moved by the person or by an electric motor. A treadmill is used as an ergometer to measure a person's work output under controlled conditions. Workload is varied by changing the speed and/or the angle of inclination (gradient) of the belt. Most people find treadmills easy to use and they can produce their peak performances on these devices. However, treadmills are not very good for measuring physiological responses to work output in people whose weights have changed, because resistance is directly related to body weight. Also, measuring blood pressure and taking blood samples becomes difficult when a person is jogging on a treadmill (*compare* **cycle ergometer**).

tremor A rhythmical quivering movement that may affect any part of the body. Tremor may be a normal accompaniment of isometric contractions which maintain posture. These physiological tremors tend to increase in states of fatigue or anxiety. Tremor may also be due to disease.

trench foot *See* **non-freezing cold injury**.

Trendelenburg's sign A sign of dislocation of the pelvis. The subject stands on one leg while flexing the knee and hip of the other leg. Dislocation is indicated if the pelvis is lower on the side of the flexed leg, the reverse of the normal situation.

treppe The staircase effect of successive increases in the extent of contractions following rapid, repeated stimulation of a muscle.

triacylglycerol (triglyeride) An ester of three fatty acids and glycerol. Triacylglycerols are the main components of animal and plant *lipids. They are the most concentrated source of energy in the human body and are stored in subcutaneous fat deposits where they contribute to insulation. Fat deposits contain over 70 000 kcal of stored energy, but the triacylglycerol is not immediately accessible for muscle respiration because it must be broken down into its basic components for transport in the blood (*see* **fat mobilization**) and then oxidized before entry into the *Krebs cycle (*see* **beta oxidation**).

triad In medicine, a group of three closely associated structures, or three symptoms

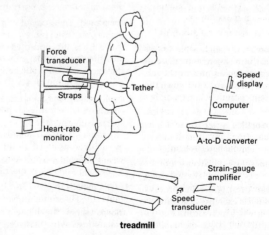

treadmill

which tend to occur together. *See also* **triad response**.

triad of O'Donahue A sports injury that includes anterior ligament tear, medial collateral ligament tear, and medial meniscal tear.

triad response A set of three nonspecific general responses to prolonged stress observed in laboratory animals: enlargement of the adrenal cortex; shrinking of lymphatic tissue; ulceration of the stomach lining and duodenum. These responses have also been observed in some athletes under stress.

triad vesicle (T-vesicle) A sac in a *muscle fibre which contains cellular secretions, such as calcium ions, needed to initiate muscle contraction.

trial A single response in a test.

trial-and-error Learning, common in non-human animals, which is marked by the performance of successive, apparently random responses to a situation until one response achieves a successful outcome. Trial-and-error learning is believed to involve classical conditioning followed by operant conditioning.

trials-delay technique Procedure in which knowledge of results for a particular response are given after one or more other responses. Research has found that this has a detrimental effect on motor performance, but a positive effect on motor learning.

triangle of forces A triangle which can be drawn when the magnitude and direction of three *forces, represented by the sides of the triangle, are in equilibrium and acting at the same point. *See also* **triangle of velocities**.

triangle of velocities A triangle which can be drawn when the magnitude and direction of three component *velocities of a body at rest are represented by the sides of a triangle. *See also* **triangle of forces**.

triangular test A test of aerobic fitness in which the subject exercises at an intensity and duration which increase in a step-wise manner until the point of maximum

tolerable intensity of maximum oxygen consumption is reached. *See also* **shuttle test**.

tribology The science of friction and lubrication.

tricarboxylic acid cycle *See* **Krebs cycle**.

triceps A muscle which has three heads of origin. *See also* **triceps brachii**.

triceps brachii (triceps) A large fleshy muscle in the posterior compartment of the upper arm. It has three heads: the long head originates from the infraglenoid tubercle on the scapula (shoulder blade), the lateral head originates from the upper half of the posterior humerus, and the medial head originates from the lower two-thirds of the posterior humerus. The triceps has a common tendon of insertion on the *olecranon process of the ulna. The long head stabilizes the scapula and assists with extension and adduction of the upper arm about the shoulder. The primary action of the medial and lateral heads is extension of the forearm around the elbow.

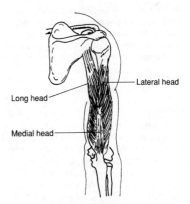

Lateral head
Long head
Medial head

triceps brachii

triceps skinfold A skinfold measurement of a vertical fold of tissue midline between the *acromiale and the *radiale on the posterior surface of the arm.

triceps surae The name given by some anatomists to the *gastrocnemius and the *soleus muscles which shape the posterior calf and insert via a common tendon into the calcaneus of the heel. The gastrocnemius has two heads and the soleus one head.

tricuspid valve A valve with three flaps which occurs between the right atrium and right ventricle of the heart. It ensures that blood flows from the atrium to ventricles by closing and preventing backflow during *ventricular systole.

Triesman model A complex model of *selective attention which contains elements of both the *Broadbent model and the *pertinence model. The model proposes that all sensory information reaches the memory for analysis, but that irrelevant cues are attenuated while relevant information is attended to.

triggered reaction A prestructured response to an environmental stimulus that is thought to be triggered into action by the sensations produced by *stretch receptors. Triggered reaction time is faster than *reaction time.

trigger finger Thickening and hardening of the flexor tendon or its tendon sheath at a metacarpophalangeal joint. The affected finger can flex but it then yields quickly and extension is impaired.

trigger point A localized palpable spot of deep hypersensitivity which, when irritated, results in pain being referred to another area of the body (*see* **referred pain**). A trigger point in the shoulder, for example, might cause a headache. This condition is referred to as myofascial pain syndrome, and is often caused by muscle tension, fatigue, or strain. The trigger point usually coincides with a tight band or 'knot' in a muscle or the *fascia of a muscle.

triglyceride *See* triacylglycerol.

triiodothyronine *See* thyroxine.

triple jumper's heel A *strain of the tissues in the heel, sometimes accompanied by a bone spur in the calcaneus. Triple jumper's heel is commonly caused by

banging the heel in the landing phase of a jump.

triquetral bone (triquetrum) A wrist bone which articulates with the hamate in front, the lunate and pisiform to the side, and the ulna behind. *See also* **carpus**.

triquetrum *See* triquetral bone.

tritium A radioactive isotope of hydrogen which has been used as a *tracer.

trochanter A large blunt, irregularly shaped prominence on the *femur. *See also* **greater trochanter**; and **lesser trochanter**.

trochanteric bursa A *bursa lying above the greater trochanter.

trochanteric bursitis Pain over the bony prominence on either side of the upper thigh due to inflammation of the *bursa which is interposed between the greater trochanter towards the top of the femur and the overlying muscle. Trochanteric bursitis usually results from poor muscular coordination and an abnormal gait during running. *See also* **Ober's test**.

trochanterion An anatomical landmark which is the most superior point on the greater trochanter of the femur.

trochanterion height A body height measured from *trochanterion to base.

trochlea A structure which is shaped like a pulley or functions like a pulley. Examples are the trochleas at the distal ends of the humerus and femur, which are smooth depressions between the condyles.

trochoidal Applied in anatomy to a structure resembling or functioning as a pivot or pulley.

trochoides *See* trochoid joint.

trochoid joint (pivot joint; trochoides) A freely movable joint in which the bone movement is limited to rotation around a central axis (e.g. the joint between the atlas and axis vertebrae).

trophic Pertaining to nutrition or nourishment.

tropic hormone A hormone which has a regulatory effect on another *endocrine gland.

tropomyosin A tube-shaped protein found in thin *actin filaments of muscle fibres. Tropomyosin has a control function: when calcium ion concentration is low within a muscle fibre, the tropomyosin inhibits muscle contraction by blocking the binding site on actin, thereby preventing myosin cross-bridges from attaching. *See also* **troponin**.

troponin A complex of three polypeptides found in muscle fibres. One polypeptide (TnI) binds to actin, another (TnT) binds to tropomyosin, and the third (TnC) binds to calcium ions. When calcium ions bind to troponin, the troponin changes shape, forcing tropomyosin away from the actin filaments. This allows myosin cross-bridges to attach onto the actin and contractions can occur. *See also* **sliding-filament theory**.

true ribs (vertebrospinal ribs) The upper seven rib pairs attached to the sternum by individual costal cartilages. *Compare* **false ribs**.

trunk Body excluding the head, neck, and limbs.

trunk circumduction A sequence of circling movements of the trunk occurring in the sagittal plane, frontal plane, and oblique plane so that the movement as a whole describes a cone.

trunk extension A movement which returns the trunk to the *anatomical position from trunk flexion, or which produces a backward movement of the spine. Muscles involved include the *quadratus lumborum and *erector spinae.

trunk extensor A muscle which effects *trunk extension.

trunk flexion A movement which returns the trunk to the *anatomical position from trunk extension, or which produces a forward movement of the spine. Muscles involved include the obliquus externus abdominis, the obliquus internus abdominis, and the rectus abdominus.

trunk flexor A muscle which effects *trunk flexion.

trunk lateral flexion Movement of the trunk to the left or right, which involves movement of the shoulder towards the hip on either side. The movement is brought about by the action on one side of the body of the external and internal oblique muscles, and the quadratus lumborum.

trunk movements Movements of the trunk involving the lumbar and thoracic regions of the spinal column, with additional motion often resulting from movements of the pelvis and hips. *See also* **spinal movements**.

trunk rotation A rotary movement of the spine in the horizontal plane. Trunk rotation may be to the left or to the right.

trunk strength The strength of muscles, particularly the abdominal muscles, in relation to their ability to move the trunk repeatedly or to support the trunk for a period of time. Trunk strength is an important component of *physical fitness.

truth value The credibility of data acquired through a *naturalistic approach to research. To possess truth value, the interpretation of data must accurately reflect what the subjects have reported.

trypsin An enzyme which acts in the duodenum to continue the digestion of *proteins into amino acids.

trypsinogen An inactive precursor of *trypsin secreted by the pancreas.

tryptophan An *essential amino acid found in some grains (such as corn) and some legumes (such as beans).

TSH *See* **thyroid stimulating hormone**.

T-TAIS A sport-specific *Test of Attentional and Interpersonal Style which has been adapted for use in tennis. The inventory includes a series of questions which are specific to that sport. It is thought to have greater validity and predictive value than the more general TAIS.

t-test *See* **Student's t-test**.

T-tubules *See* **transverse tubules**.

tubercle A nodule or small rounded process on a bone, smaller than a tuberosity.

tuberosity A large rounded projection on a bone, larger than a *tubercle.

tumor A swelling; one of the signs of inflammation. *See also* **tumour**.

tumour An abnormal swelling due to the growth of cells. Tumours may be benign or malignant.

tunica A membrane layer; a covering or tissue coat.

tunica adventitia (tunica externa) The external covering of an artery or vein.

tunica externa *See* **tunica adventitia**.

tunica intima The inner lining of an artery or vein.

tunica media The middle layer of the wall of an artery or a vein. The tunica media contains smooth muscle and elastic fibrous tissue.

tunnel A canal or hollow groove which may form a passageway for nerves or blood vessels through a body structure.

tunnel of Guyon (pisiform-hamate tunnel) The smaller of two anatomical tunnels in the palm of the hand (the bigger tunnel is the carpal tunnel). It is bordered by the pisiform and hamate bones. The ulnar nerve and ulnar artery pass through the tunnel of Guyon.

turbulent flow The flow of a fluid in which the motion of particles at any point varies rapidly in both magnitude and direction. Turbulent flow is characterized by mixing of adjacent fluid layers.

turf toe syndrome Swelling and pain at the base of the big toe caused by the foot sliding forward in a shoe (e.g. when stopping suddenly on artificial turf). The big toe (*see* **hallux**) is bent upward, stretching the ligaments, injuring the articular surface and the joint capsule. Sliding of the foot in the shoe may also result in black nail and even a fracture of the toe.

turgid Distended and congested, usually with blood.

turgor The state of being distended and congested.

turned-in thigh bones *See* **femoral anteversion**.

TV *See* **tidal volume**.

T-vesicles *See* **triad vesicle**.

TWAR *See* **Taiwan acute respiratory disease**.

T-wave A deflection of an *electrocardiogram which follows the QRS complex. The T-wave represents repolarization of the ventricles.

twelve-minute test A test of *aerobic capacity in which the subject runs as far as possible in twelve minutes. *See also* **Cooper test**.

twin method The use of genetically identical twins to study the effects of inheritance and environmental factors on an individual trait. The twin method may involve comparing differences between genetically identical twins who have been brought up in distinctly different environments when differences in traits are hypothesized to be due to the effects of environmental factors. Another procedure involves subjecting one of the identical twins to a test while the other member is held as a control. The difference between the two during and after the test is used as a measure of the effect of the test (assuming other variables are constant). Genetic control of a trait may be studied by comparing a trait in a large sample of identical twins and nonidentical twins in comparable environments. If the similarity between the identical twins is more than that for the nonidentical twins, the trait is assumed to be under genetic control.

twisting In a biomechanical system, a complex movement of rotation around the longitudinal axis which is derived from rotation about the other two cardinal axes. In diving, the body may rotate around its own transverse axis (rotation); the body's own axis of rotation may describe a curve round another axis (precession); and the angle between these axes of the body's own rotation and precession may vary (nutation).

twitch 1 A brief contraction of muscle in response to a stimulus. **2** The response of a motor unit to a single brief threshold

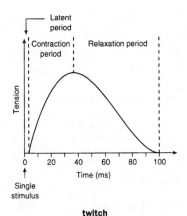

twitch

stimulus. A twitch has three phases: a *latent period; a period of contraction; and a period of relaxation. *See also* **refractory period**.

two-process theory A theory which proposes that both *classical conditioning and *operant conditioning are usually present in any learning situation, and that classical conditioning provides the motivation for operant conditioning.

two-tailed t-test Type of *t-test used when, in a comparison of the *means of two groups, it has not been anticipated which will be the greater or lesser.

two-third strength hypothesis A hypothesis based on the suggestion that changes of muscle strength are proportional to the muscle's diameter and thus to the square of body height $(BH)^2$; and that changes of body mass (BM) are proportional to $(BH)^3$; thus muscular strength is proportional to $(BM)^{2/3}$, i.e. $(BM)^{0.667}$.

tympanic membrane The eardrum, a tight membrane separating the outer ear and middle ear, and connected to the ear bones, which vibrates when sound pressure waves pass along the outer ear towards the middle ear.

type Any class or category with shared characteristics.

Type A behaviour A form of behaviour characterized by a high level of *aggression, competition, drive, time urgency, and vigorous voice stylistics. Type A behaviour has been linked with increased risk of coronary heart disease. However, it may be possible to alter type A behaviour patterns by taking aerobic exercise so that the risk of heart disease is reduced. *Compare* **type B behaviour**.

Type B behaviour A form of behaviour characterized by an easy-going, non-aggressive, and non-competitive attitude. *Compare* **type A behaviour**.

Type I diabetes *See* **diabetes mellitus**.

Type II diabetes *See* **diabetes mellitus**.

type I fibre *See* **slow-twitch fibre**.

type II fibre *See* **fast-twitch fibre**.

type IIa fibre *See* **fast-twitch fibre**.

type IIb fibre *See* **fast-twitch fibre**.

type IIc fibre A *fast-twitch fibre with contractile characteristics intermediate between slow-twitch fibres and fast-twitch fibres.

typical response The manner in which a person usually responds to particular environmental situations. Typical responses, when distinguished from play-acting, may be valid indicators of the *psychological core of an individual's *personality.

typical value In a pulmonary function test, the value obtained from a healthy, resting, recumbent young male (1.7 m² square metres of surface area), breathing air at sea level. The results of pulmonary function tests vary with changes of position, age, size, sex, and altitude.

typology The study of symbolic representations.

tyramine An amine found in cheeses, game, broad bean pods, yeast extracts, wine, and strong beer which has effects similar to those of *adrenaline.

tyrosine A nonessential amino acid which can substitute for phenylalanine.

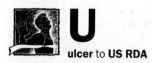

U

ulcer to US RDA

ulcer Lesion or erosion of the skin or mucous membrane (e.g., of the stomach).

ulna A long bone in the forearm. In the anatomical position, the ulna lies medially, away from the thumb side. The ulna articulates proximally at the elbow with the radius and humerus, and distally at the wrist with the radius and carpals.

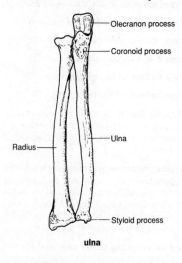

Olecranon process

Coronoid process

Ulna

Radius

Styloid process

ulna

ulnar Pertaining to the *ulna.

ulnar collateral ligament A triangular shaped band of *ligament which helps to stabilize the elbow joint. The ulnar collateral ligament consists of three parts: an anterior portion running from the medial epicondyle to the *coronoid process; a posterior portion which runs from the medial epicondyle to the *olecranon; and a transverse band connecting the olecranon part of the posterior portion to the coronoid part of the anterior portion.

ulnar compression syndrome (cubital tunnel syndrome) A disorder of the elbow caused by direct trauma to the ulnar nerve in the cubital tunnel (a groove behind the elbow), repetitive elbow flexion, hypermobility of the ulnar nerve, and a loose body impingement of the ulnar nerve. The disorder is characterized by aching posteromedial elbow pain, a feeling of 'pins and needles' in the arm, weakness of the thumb-index finger pinch, pain with forced elbow flexion, and, in chronic cases, wasting of the intrinsic musculature of the hand. Treatment includes rest, anti-inflammatories, elbow protection, and (for golfers, weightlifters and racket players who shave the disorder) a change in technique. Severe cases may require surgical decompression and transposition of the ulnar nerve.

ulnar deviation (wrist adduction) Movement of the hand towards the *ulna brought about by the cooperative action of the flexor carpi ulnaris and the extensor carpi ulnaris muscles.

ulnar nerve One of three nerves supplying the lower arm and hands. The ulnar nerve runs along the medial edge of the elbow just behind the *epicondyle to which the flexor muscles of the wrist are attached. The ulnar nerve is susceptible to entrapment in throwing or racket sports when the nerve can be compressed within its groove with subsequent mechanical irritation.

ulnar neuritis Inflammation of the ulnar nerve which may occur when the nerve is subjected to pressure. Vulnerable points are at the level of the elbow and where the nerve crosses the wrist on the inner aspect of the hand. The pressure can be caused by friction of local tissues on the nerve, as happens during cycling. Ulnar neuritis is marked by muscular weakness on attempting to spread the fingers, tingling, and numbness in the little finger. *See also* **ulnar compression syndrome**.

ulnar neuropathy *See* **handlebar palsy**.

ulnar palsy Paralysis or weakness in the hand due to pressure on the ulnar nerve. *See also* **ulnar neuritis**.

ultimate strength *See* **ultimate stress**.

ultimate stress (ultimate strength) The load required to fracture a material expressed as force per original unit area of its cross-section at the point of fracture.

ultracentrifuge Machine capable of spinning at more than 50 000 revolutions per minute. It is used to separate cellular components.

ultrafiltration Process by which small molecules and ions in blood are separated from larger molecules to form glomerular filtrate in a kidney tubule, or tissue fluid.

ultrasonics The study and application of very high frequencies of sound beyond the limits of human hearing (that is, frequencies of about 20 kHz and above). *See also* **ultrasound treatment**.

ultrasonography The use of sound frequencies above 30 kHz to produce images of structures within the human body. A beam of ultrasound is directed into the body and its echoes are electrically analysed to produce the image.

ultrasound Sound frequencies beyond the limits of human hearing (i.e., frequencies above 20 kHz).

ultrasound treatment The use of ultrasonics to treat disorders such as deep, soft tissue injuries. Ultrasound treatment is believed to have a mechanical effect, accelerating the healing process, vibrating and loosening scar tissue, and encouraging the reabsorption of blood and lymph which has escaped into surrounding tissue. The vibrations may reduce sensory stimulation and relieve pain; they also produce heat at a deep level.

ultraviolet light Electromagnetic radiation with short wave-lengths and lying outside the visible spectrum of light. Sunlight contains ultraviolet light which causes sunburn.

uncertainty A major situational source of stress. The greater the degree of uncertainty an individual feels about a situation, the greater the *state anxiety and stress.

unciform bone *See* **hamate bone**.

unconditioned response An original or inborn response such as salivation stimulated by food in the mouth, withdrawal from an injurious stimulus, or contraction of the pupil to light. In *classical conditioning, an unconditioned response is elicited by an unconditioned stimulus.

unconscious Part of the mind dealing with mental processes which are below the level of awareness. According to proponents of Freudian theory, the unconscious plays a major part in mental functioning and contains instincts, memories, and emotions which have been repressed (*see* **repression**). These repressed feelings are the stimuli for actions and behaviour. *Compare* **subconsious**. *See also* **id**.

unconscious motivation Urges (such as fears, hopes, and desires) of which the individual is not aware and which are presumed to be repressed.

unconsciousness Loss of conciousness. It may be due to a head injury caused by a blow (e.g., in boxing). *See also* **concussion**.

underload principle A principle of training which suggests that if regular muscular activity levels are less than normal, muscle strength decreases. *Compare* **principle of progressive overload**.

unfitness A condition in which an individual is unable to meet the demands of that individual's work or way of life. Unfitness may be caused by an organic illness, physical defect, malnutrition, lack of muscular strength, or social, emotional, and psychological maladjustment.

unhappy triad Classic knee injury, first described in American Football, in which there is tearing of the medial collateral ligament, the anterior cruciate ligament, and medial cartilage.

uniarticular muscle A muscle which takes part in the movement of one joint only.

uniaxial movement Movement in one plane only.

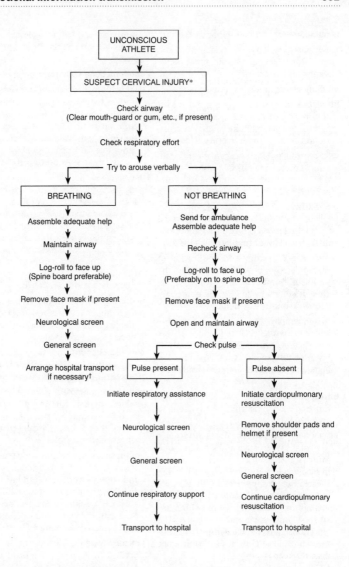

Decision matrix for on-site management of the unconscious athlete.
* Any significant suspicion of cervical injury should prompt all spinal precaution and arrange for transport to medical facility. †Other than very transient loss of consciousness or grade I to II concussions, full assessment at hospital is advisable.

unconsciousness

unidirectional information transmission One-way transmission of informational cues from one or more members of a group to another member or members of the group. *Compare* **omnidirectional information transmission**; and **social facilitation**.

uniform acceleration The condition of a body which maintains the same magnitude and direction of *acceleration.

uniform angular motion The motion of a body which rotates at a constant angle per unit time.

uniform speed Speed of a body which is constant over a certain period of time.

unilateral Pertaining to one side of the body or body-part.

unilateral muscular hypertrophy Development of muscle bulk on one side of the body more than the other, commonly occurring in sportspeople with 'one arm' action; for example, shot putters, tennis players, and oarsmen and women who row on one side of the body. *See also* **tennis shoulder**.

union The healing together of tissue, such as the broken ends of a fractured bone, which has been separated.

unipennate muscle *See* **pennate muscle**.

unipolar neurone A *neurone from which only one main process extends from the cell body.

unisex reference human *See* **phantom**.

unit Quantity adopted as a standard for measurement. *See also* **SI system**.

unitary task Task in which all participants perform in the same or a very similar manner. *Compare* **divisible task**.

universal behaviours A certain set of *leadership behaviours believed to be possessed by all successful leaders. Unlike traits, these behaviours can be learned. *See also* **trait theory of leadership**.

universal donor An individual with blood group O who has no A or B antigens. Consequently, the blood type of a universal donor will not react with the recipient's and the blood can be given to any other ABO type. The term applies only to the ABO blood grouping; other blood groups are important in blood transfusion and the term universal donor is, therefore, rather misleading.

universal functionalism *See* **postulate of functional indispensability**.

universal trait One of a certain set of *personality traits believed to be shared by all successful leaders.

unmyelinated fibre *See* **myelin sheath**.

unobtrusive measure A method commonly used in qualitative sociological research in which data is obtained without the knowledge of the subject and without affecting the data collected (e.g., the recording of player behaviour during a football match using hidden cameras).

unsaturated fatty acid A *fatty acid that contains one (monounsaturated) or more (polyunsaturated) double bonds between carbon atoms. Each double bond takes the place of one hydrogen atom. The double bond imposes a kink in the molecule making unsaturated fatty acids less easy to pack together. Consequently, unsaturated fats are usually liquid (oil) at room temperature.

unstable equilibrium The state of a body which, when slightly displaced, tends to be displaced further. *Compare* **stable equilibrium**.

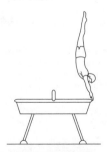

unstable equilibrium

unstable factor In *causal attribution theory, a factor which may be assumed to change over a period of time; for example, weather conditions, the amount of effort an individual applies to a task, or random chance (luck). *Compare* **stable factor**.

unstable joint A joint in which there is abnormal movement and which is unable to support normal loads. A joint may become unstable because ligaments are ruptured or congenitally very lax, or because muscles which normally support the joint are malfunctioning.

unstructured data Data gathered without regard to the way it is to be analysed and interpreted. Much qualitative data, for instance, verbal answers to open-ended questions, are of this nature.

unstructured interview An interview in which the interviewer relinquishes control over the content and pattern of the questions and in which the interviewee is not limited to a set of fixed responses. *See also* **open-ended question**.

upper limb Part of the body which includes the arm, forearm, and hand. The upper limb is relatively light compared with the lower limb, and is adapted for flexibility rather than strength.

uppers *See* **amphetamines**.

up-regulation An increase in the sensitivity of cells to a particular *hormone, probably by increasing the number of specific receptors on the cell surface membrane which bind with that hormone. Up-regulation occurs, for example, in response to regular exercise when cells become more sensitive to insulin. *Compare* **down-regulation**.

upward mobility A form of social mobility which results in a person moving to a higher social class or socioeconomic status. The term is also applied to a sportsperson moving from a lower level of sport to a higher level at which there is an increase in *status among peers.

urea An organic molecule which is the major excretory product of protein metabolism. Urea is formed in the liver from carbon dioxide and ammonia during the *ornithine cycle. Urine is eliminated in urine and, to a much lesser extent, in *sweat.

uric acid An end-product of the metabolism of nucleic acids (e.g., DNA) which is a normal constituent of urine. Excessive amounts of uric acid in the blood are associated with gout.

urinalysis The laboratory examination of a urine sample to test for the presence of bacteria or chemicals such as sugar and alcohol.

urinary system A body system consisting of a pair of kidneys and their associated blood supply and tubes. The urinary system helps to maintain fluid and electrolyte balance, provides long-term regulation of blood pressure, and eliminates nitrogenous waste products (e.g., urea) from the blood while helping to retain useful substances (e.g. glucose).

urine An aqueous solution of inorganic and organic salts, which include urea, representing the nitrogen waste products of metabolism excreted by the kidneys.

uriniferous tubule Kidney tubule which extends from the Bowman's capsule to the collecting duct.

urocamic acid An acid in *sweat which is believed to provide the skin with some protection against ultraviolet radiation.

urokinase An enzyme in urine which causes *fibrinolysis.

urticaria (hives; nettle rash) An acute or chronic condition characterized by the appearance of itchy weals on the skin. The cause may be an allergy to certain foods (such as strawberries), infection, drugs, emotional stress, or local skin irritation resulting from contact with certain plants. Athletes sometimes develop hives while exercising (exercise-induced urticaria). The hives (punctate skin lesions) are small and seem to develop in response to the release of histamines associated with the increase in body temperature produced by exercise.

US RDA A version of the figures for recommended daily allowances used by the United States Food and Drug Administration for the legal regulation of food labelling in the United States. The values, based on RDAs, are expressed in percentages and are used for all persons over four years old.

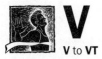

V

V to VT

V A symbol commonly used by pulmonary physiologists to refer to the volume of a gas.

V A symbol commonly used by pulmonary physiologists to refer to the volume of a gas per unit time (usually one minute).

v A symbol commonly used by physiologists to refer to venous blood.

vaccination The administration of a vaccine to confer immunity against a specific disease. Originally, the term was confined to the use of vaccinia (cowpox virus), but it is now used synonymously with inoculation.

vaccine A preparation containing killed or attenuated microorganisms (i.e. microorganisms that have lost their virulence) such as viruses, that is introduced into the human body to stimulate the formation of antibodies and thereby confer immunity against subsequent infections of the microorganism.

vagus nerve One of a pair of nerves which originate in the medulla oblongata and extend down into the thorax and abdomen to innervate the heart, lungs, and parts of the alimentary canal. The vagus nerve carries motor neurones to the muscles which facilitate swallowing, and to both afferent neurones and efferent neurones of the *parasympathetic nervous system.

valgus A condition in which a body segment is curved outwards from its *proximal to its distal end. *Compare* **varus**. *See also* **femoral valgus**; **forefoot varus**; **rearfoot valgus**; and **tibial varus**.

valgus stress A force applied to a joint which causes the distal aspect of a limb to be moved away from the midline of the body.

validation The process of determining the *validity of a test or investigation.

validity The extent to which a test, measurement, or other method of investigation possesses the property of actually doing what it has been designed to do.

valine An *essential amino acid found in grains (e.g., corn) and legumes (e.g., beans).

Valsalva manoeuvre A technique for increasing the intrathoracic and intra-abdominal pressure by trying to breathe out forcibly (using the diaphragm and abdominal muscles) when the glottis (the opening between the vocal cords) is closed. It was named after the Italian anatomist A. M. Valsalva (1666–1723). The manoeuvre is often performed during isometric exercises and weight-lifting. Air is trapped and pressurized in the lungs, causing blood pressure to rise. The great veins may collapse, reducing the flow of blood returning to the heart. Immediately after the manoeuvre, a reflex *bradycardia can occur which may cause dizziness and fainting. Valsalva's manoeuvre is potentially dangerous. It can cause a heart attack in people with high blood pressure or cardiovascular disease.

value-added-theory of collective behaviour The theory that collective behaviour develops only when several elements are present in a social situation. Each element adds to the likelihood of collective behaviour occurring, but all must be present for it to occur. The elements are structural strain (perceived or real social conflicts); structural conduciveness (an acceptance by the collective, such as a crowd, that their grievance cannot be resolved through the normal channels); a shared belief about how to respond to the situation together with precipitating factors which reinforce the shared belief; mobilization of participants to action by leaders and by communication among the crowd; and a lack of adequate social control.

value-alienation The way in which an individual's system of values conflicts or is inconsistent with a system of values the individual is expected to hold. Thus, the individual develops feelings of estrangement from a situation, group, or culture because of the values he or she holds.

value-free approach 1 An approach to research which aims to exclude a researcher's own values when conducting research. Therefore, the aim of a value-free approach is to make the observations and interpretations as unbiased as possible. Some people believe that it is impossible for researchers to adopt a pure value-free approach. In this case, they argue, the researchers should at least make clear what their values are and how they affect their work. **2** An approach to research, particularly sociological research, which aims to establish facts and is not concerned with settling questions of values. *Compare* **normative approach.**

value freedom *See* **value neutrality.**

value judgement An ethical or moral evaluation of what should be done.

value neutrality (value freedom) Applied to a piece of research which has been conducted using a *value-free approach.

values The accepted standards or moral principles of a person or a group. Values are similar to *norms in having a moral and regulatory role, but values have a wider significance than norms in going beyond specific situations. Values are viewed as informing norms in different contexts.

valve A device that ensures that a fluid flows in one direction only. Valves in the blood circulatory system of the human body are flap-like structures that ensure that the blood maintains its unidirectional flow around the body and through the heart. Valves also occur in the *lymphatic system.

vanillylmandelic acid (VMA) A product of *catecholamine metabolism found in urine. Levels of vanillylmandelic acid are used to estimate catecholamine levels; high values after exercise correlate with high physiological and psychological *stress which affects the adrenal glands.

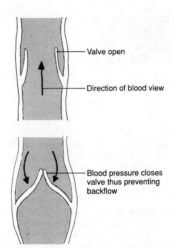

valve open

Direction of blood view

Blood pressure closes valve thus preventing backflow

valve

variability 1 A key training principle which states that athletes can reduce the risk of overtraining and psychological fatigue by ensuring that their long-term training programme incorporates a variety of exercises. **2** The degree of variation in statistical data; measures of variability include range, standard deviation, and variance.

variable 1 A changeable aspect of a situation which can be manipulated or measured, as in the case of a dependent variable and an independent variable in an experiment. **2** A mathematical symbol which is used to represent some undetermined element from a given set.

variable error A measure of the inconsistency of responses produced by a subject who is striving for accuracy at some target (such as a force, a speed, or a location in space) with each response having a measurable dimension (e.g. kilograms, k). The variable error is expressed as a *standard deviation of a set of responses about a subject's own *constant error.

variable resistance exercise An exercise, usually performed on an exercise machine, in which the resistance varies throughout the range of movement of the muscles involved. Since the difficulty of overcoming the load varies with the angle of the joint, variable resistance exercise imposes a relatively constant stress on the muscles.

variance A measure of the extent to which interval values are clustered around a *mean. Variance is calculated by averaging the squared deviations from the mean, and in so doing it takes into account both negative values and the occurrence of unusually high and unusually low values. A low variance indicates high homogeneity and high variance low homogeneity of data.

varices *See* **varicose veins**.

varicose veins (varices) Veins, commonly in the legs, which have become abnormally distended and twisted as a result of incompetence of internal valves. Varicose veins may bleed heavily if ruptured, in which case the application of firm pressure easily controls the bleeding. As long as varicose veins are not associated with other symptoms, a controlled programme of physical exercise may improve circulation and benefit sufferers.

varix A varicose vein.

varus Inward curvature of a body segment from its proximal to its distal end. In varus conditions, extra tensile stress is placed on the lateral side of the segment's proximal articulation and on the medial side of its distal articulation. *Compare* **valgus**. *See also* **femoral varus**; **forefoot varus**; **rearfoot varus**; and **tibial varus**.

varus stress A force applied to a joint which causes the distal aspect of a limb to be moved towards the midline of the body. *Compare* **valgus stress**.

vas A duct or vessel.

vascularization The development of new blood vessels within a tissue or organ.

vascular system A body system containing specialized organs and tissue for transporting substances. *See also* **cardiovascular system**.

vasoactive Applied to factors, such as carbon dioxide, emotions, or pressure, which affect the diameter of blood vessels.

vasoconstriction A decrease in the diameter of blood vessels (usually arterioles) resulting in a reduction of blood flow to the area supplied by the vessel. Factors causing vasoconstriction include pain, loud noises, fear, a fall in temperature, and a fall in blood pressure.

vasoconstrictor An agent, such as *epinephrine, that causes constriction of blood vessels.

vasodilation An increase in the diameter of blood vessels (usually arterioles) resulting in an increase in blood flow to the area supplied by the vessel. Factors causing vasodilation of blood vessels supplying muscles, include exercise, high external temperatures, stress, and a rise in blood pressure.

vasodilator An agent that causes an increase in the diameter of a blood vessel. Drugs such as *calcium channel blockers, glyceryl trinitrate, and hydrazine, are vasodilators commonly prescribed for the treatment of cardiovascular disorders such as hypertension.

vasomotion An increase or decrease in the diameter of a blood vessel.

vasomotor Applied to factors acting on the smooth muscles of blood vessels, thus affecting the diameter of the vessels.

vasomotor centre An area in the *medulla oblongata of the brain which contains neurones concerned with the regulation of the diameter of blood vessels and heart rate so that blood pressure can be controlled.

vasomotor fibres *See* **vasomotor nerve**.

vasomotor nerve A nerve containing sympathetic nerve fibres which regulates the contraction of smooth muscle in the walls of blood vessels, particularly the *arteries, thereby regulating blood vessel diameter and blood flow.

vasopressin *See* **antidiuretic hormone**.

vasospasm A spasm in the smooth muscle of a blood vessel causing the vessel to constrict.

vastus intermedius A component muscle of the *quadriceps at the front of the thigh.

It has its origin on the anterior femur and its insertion on the tibia via the *patellar tendon. Its primary action is knee extension.

vastus lateralis A component muscle of the *quadriceps on the front, lateral aspect of the thigh. It has its origin on the greater trochanter and lateral linea aspera of the femur. Its insertion is on the tibia via the *patellar tendon. Its primary action is knee extension.

vastus medialis A muscle which is part of the *quadriceps at the front of the thigh. It has its origin on the linea aspera and intertrochanteric line of the femur. Its insertion is on the tibia via the *patellar tendon. Its primary action is knee extension.

VC A symbol commonly used by pulmonary physiologists to refer to the vital capacity.

VE A symbol commonly used by pulmonary physiologists to refer to the volume of expired gas during pulmonary ventilation.

Vealey's sport-specific model of confidence A theory of *achievement motivation based on the concept of sport confidence. It suggests that an athlete who is successful in one sport thereby enjoys a general feeling of sport confidence which he or she will be able to transfer to new sport situations. The theory predicts that an athlete will develop self-confidence as he or she experiences task mastery and an expectation of success.

vector 1 A physical quantity that possesses both magnitude and direction. *Velocity and *acceleration are vector quantities. A vector is often represented graphically by an arrow drawn so that its length represents its magnitude, the tail of the arrow represents its origin, and the head represents its direction. *Compare* **scalar**. *See also* **component vector, and resultant vector**. **2** An animal which carries a parasite from one host to another.

vector addition *See* **vector composition**.

vector chain method (tip-to-tail method) Method of obtaining the resultant vector of two or more component vectors that are in the same plane. The vectors are all represented by arrows. The tail of each successive vector is placed on the tip of the previous vector, and the resultant vector is drawn with its tail on the tail of the first vector, and its tip on the tip of the last vector. *See also* **vector, triangle law of**.

vector composition (vector addition; vector sum) Method of determining the resultant vector from two or more component vectors. The sum of the component vectors gives the resultant vector, so that, for example, if two component vectors are oriented in exactly opposite directions, the resultant has the direction of the longer vector and its magnitude is equal to the differences in the magnitudes of the two component vectors. *See also* **vector chain method**.

vector resolution A method of determining component vectors from a resultant vector. A graphical operation replaces a single vector with two perpendicular vectors in such a way that the vector composition of the two perpendicular vectors yields a resultant equal to the original vector. *See also* **vector chain method**.

vectors, parallelogram of *See* **parallelogram of vectors**.

vectors, triangle law of A law which states that if a body is acted upon by two vectors represented by two sides of a triangle taken in order, the resultant vector is represented by the third side of the triangle.

vector sum *See* **vector composition**.

vegan *See* **vegetarian**.

vegetarian A person who consumes mainly or wholly plant or fungal products. Basic types include semi-vegetarians, who omit all animal foods except milk, milk products, and eggs, and vegans who omit all animal products.

vegetarian diet A well-balanced vegetarian diet does not impair endurance capacity or physical fitness. However, vegetarian athletes should be aware that vegetable nonhaem iron is less readily absorbed than animal haem iron, and that a high fibre diet may reduce the absorption of some essential nutrients such as iron and calcium. They should make the appropriate dietary adjustments. Many successful athletes are vegetarians, but strict vegans have to be very careful to ensure that their food provides adequate sources of all the vitamins and amino acids. This applies particularly to vitamin B_{12} which may need to be obtained from supplementation.

vein Vessel carrying blood to the heart. A vein usually has thin walls and a series of one-way valves.

velocity Rate at which a body moves, measured as the length per unit time, in a given direction. Velocity is a vector quantity. *Compare* **speed**.

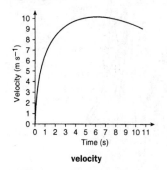

velocity

velocity ratio Ratio of the distance moved by the effort to distance moved by the load in a machine.

velocity–time graph Graphical representation of the motion of a body plotted on the x-axis and velocity on the y-axis. In the velocity–time graph, acceleration of the body is obtained from the gradient of the curve. The area beneath the graph represents the distance travelled.

vena cava One of the two major veins leading into the right atrium of the heart.

venomotor control Regulation of blood flow by changing the diameter of veins. The muscle within the wall of a vein receives neurones from the *sympathetic nervous system and the *parasympathetic nervous system (*see* **venomotor tone**).

venomotor tone The degree of tension in the muscle coat of a vein which determines

the shape of the vein. Changes in venomotor tone can alter the capacity of veins without affecting the vein's resistance to blood flow.

venous return The volume of blood returning to the right atrium of the *heart. The heart can only pump as much blood as it receives, therefore increases in *cardiac output (for example, during exercise when cardiac output may exceed 30 litres per minute) are dependent on venous return increasing to that amount. The *muscle pump, *respiratory pump, and venoconstriction contribute to the increase in venous return during exercise. *See also* **Starling's law**.

ventilation The passage of air into and out of the lungs. *See also* **alveolar ventilation**; and **pulmonary ventilationb**.

ventilation–perfusion ratio A ratio of the volume of air which reaches the *alveoli to the volume of blood supplying the alveoli. Gas exchange in the lungs is most efficient when there is a good match between ventilation and perfusion; an imbalance can cause *anoxia and cyanosis.

ventilation rate The volume of air breathed per minute. Ventilation rate is a product of *tidal volume and *respiratory frequency.

ventilatory breakpoint *See* **minute ventilation method**.

ventilatory buffering A homeostatic mechanism (*see* **homeostasis**) involving changes in *ventilation which help to maintain the *acid–base balance in body fluids. Ventilatory buffering is particularly important during exercise when products of respiration (especially carbon dioxide and lactic acid) decrease the pH (increased acidity) of body fluids. Ventilation of the lungs increases, helping to remove carbon dioxide from the lungs. This reduces the partial pressure of carbon dioxide in the blood and body fluids, resulting in an increase in pH (decrease in acidity).

ventilatory efficiency *See* **ventilatory equivalent for oxygen**.

ventilatory equivalent for carbon dioxide The ratio of the volume of air ventilating

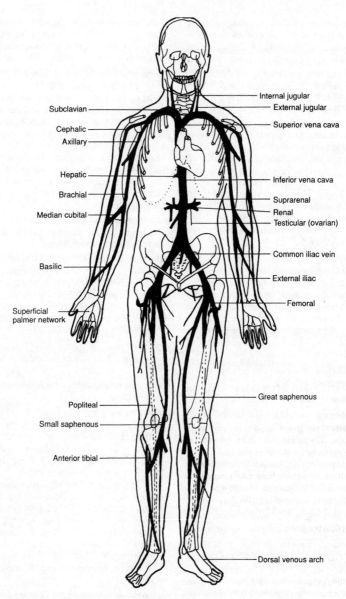

veins

the lungs to the volume of carbon dioxide produced.

ventilatory equivalent for oxygen The ratio of the volume of air ventilating the lungs to the volume of oxygen consumed. It represents the amount of *ventilation required for the consumption of each litre of oxygen and reflects ventilatory efficiency. It is measured as the ratio of the volume of gas expired per minute to the volume of oxygen consumed per minute (i.e., VE/VO_2). At rest the ventilatory equivalent for oxygen ranges from about 23 to 28 litres of air per litre of oxygen consumed. It usually remains relatively constant during submaximal exercises, but the value may increase above 30 litres of air per litre of oxygen consumed during maximal exercise.

ventilatory reserve (breathing reserve) The difference between maximal *ventilation rate (i.e. highest possible ventilation rate) and the maximum ventilation rate during a particular activity. The resting ventilatory reserve indicates the potential for increasing ventilation rate, and therefore the potential for increasing the intensity of activity.

ventilatory threshold *See* **minute ventilation method**.

ventral *See* **anterior**.

ventricle 1 One of a pair of chambers in the *heart. The ventricles lie inferior to the atria. The right ventricle receives deoxygenated blood from the right atrium and pumps this blood to the lungs. The left ventricle receives oxygenated blood from the left atrium and pumps the blood through the dorsal aorta to the rest of the body. **2** A fluid-filled chamber in the brain.

ventricular systole The phase of the *cardiac cycle during which the ventricles contract to pump the blood to the lungs and rest of the body. *See also* **systole**.

venule A small vein which, unlike a *capillary, has some connective tissue in its wall.

verbal feedback *Feedback presented in a form which is spoken or capable of being spoken.

verbal guidance Coaching technique in which athletes are instructed to do exactly what they hear the coach (or cassette, etc.) say they should do. Verbal guidance often involves the use of simple, clear, and meaningful cues.

verbal pretraining The use of simple words, usually given by a coach, to help remind athletes of the sequence of moves they need to make when performing a complex skill. Once mastered, these words (also known as labels) help the athlete to learn skills more easily.

verruca *See* **plantar wart**.

vertebra One of the 33 bones which collectively form the vertebral column. A typical vertebra consists of a bony mass which forms the main weight-bearing component (the body or centrum), a hollow ring known as the neural or vertebral arch, and several bony processes (the transverse processes and, in some vertebrae, the neural spine, a spinous posterior extension of the neural arch). The neural arches and posterior surfaces of the vertebral bodies and intervertebral discs form a passageway for the spinal cord and blood vessels (the spinal or vertebral canal). The bony processes serve as attachment points for muscles, improving the mechanical advantage of the muscles.

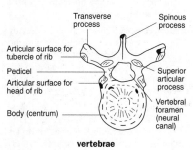

vertebrae

vertebral Pertaining to the spine.

vertebral arch Composite structure in each vertebra consisting of two lamina and two pedicles which help to enclose and protect the spinal cord. Pedicles are short bony cylinders projecting posteriorly from the vertebral body.

vertebral column (backbone; spinal column; spine) A complex and functionally significant segment of the body consisting of a curved stack of 33 vertebrae divided into five regions: the cervical (7 vertebrae), thoracic (12 vertebrae); lumbar (5 vertebrae), sacral (5 fused vertebrae), and coccygeal (4 small fused vertebrae) regions. The vertebral column mechanically links the upper and lower extremities, enabling motion in all three planes.

vertebral rib *See* **floating rib**.

vertex An anatomical landmark located at the most superior point in the midsagittal plane on the skull when the head is held in the *Frankfort plane.

vertical displacement Total height reached by a projectile measured at an angle of 90° to the ground surface.

vertical projection The upward displacement of a projectile at 90° to the ground followed by the downward fall of the object.

vertical status The *status of a person in relation to others at a different hierarchical level. Vertical status on a team, for example, may involve a comparison of ground staff to players, or players to administrators. *Compare* **horizontal status**. *See also* **status**.

vertical velocity The rate at which a body moves upwards at an angle of 90° to the ground. It is the component of a projectile's velocity which is concerned with lifting the projectile. *Compare* **horizontal velocity**.

vertigo (dizziness) A feeling of unsteadiness. There are two main types of vertigo. In the first type the sufferer feels that his or her body or the environment is spinning. It is commonly caused by motion sickness or a viral infection of the organs of balance (*see* **vestibular apparatus**). The second type of vertigo is characterized by weakness and is commonly caused by low blood sugar or low blood pressure. As long as low blood pressure is not the result of shock or blood

loss, a sufferer of the second type of vertigo may benefit from physical activity. Anyone prone to vertigo should take great care when taking part in sports where a fall may be dangerous.

vertobrochondral rib *See* **false rib**.

vertobrocostal joint A synovial, gliding joint between a vertebra and rib.

vertobrospinal rib *See* **true rib**.

very low calorie diet (VLCD) A diet containing less than 800 kcals per day specifically designed for the treatment of severe obesity. Usually, food substitution in the form of a drink made from powder and water is used. Ingredients in the powder are designed to provide nutrients in sufficient quantities to sustain health, and consist mainly of high quality protein such as egg whites, minerals, and vitamins. These diets require medical supervision and are not recommended for people with a *body-mass index (BMI) of less than 30.

very low density lipoprotein (VLDL) A lipoprotein found in blood that is thought to increase the risk of *atherosclerosis by carrying *cholesterol to tissues.

vesicle A small liquid-filled sac or bladder.

vested interest A strong personal concern in producing or maintaining a particular state of affairs. In sport, for example, coaches have a vested interest in maintaining a system of rewards so that they can maintain compliance from, and power over, their players.

vestibular apparatus The equilibrium receptors of the inner ear, consisting of the utricle, saccule, and semicircular canals, that are sensitive to the orientation of the head with respect to gravity, to the rotation of the head, and to balance. Impulses from the vestibular apparatus are conducted along vestibular nerve fibres to the vestibular complex in the brain stem and cerebellum. The complex initiates visual and motor responses which help maintain balance.

vibration A repeated motion that moves back and forth over the same general path.

See also **angular vibration**; **harmonic motion**; and **linear vibration**.

vibratory motion *See* **harmonic motion**.

vicarious experience Experience gained by watching another person perform a skill.

vicarious learning *See* **modelling**.

vicarious punishment Refers to the tendency not to repeat behaviours that we observe others punished for performing. *See also* **modelling**; and **vicarious reinforcement**.

vicarious reinforcement Refers to a tendency to repeat behaviours that we see others rewarded for performing (for example, copying the *aggression of a player who is rewarded for that aggression by winning a match and gaining public acclaim). *See also* **modelling**; and **vicarious punishment**.

vicious cycle A situation in which an action leads to another situation in which all gains brought about by the first action are lost. Typically, the initial problem may be worsened, or a series of actions and situations leads back to the initial problem. For example, an athlete with an overuse injury wants to get back to fitness after a short period of rest so overtrains, leading to further overuse injuries. *See also* **pain cycle**.

victimization In sociology, the institutionalized pressure to participate in a form of violent behaviour which can be dangerous to health and safety. In some contact sports this is regarded as largely normative by those involved, and injuries are regarded as a natural consequence of participation.

victimology The study of victims of crime, including the relationship between the offender and victim. Similar studies have been conducted on players who are victims of foul play.

villus Finger-like projections from the surface of some membranes (e.g. those of the small intestine) that increase the surface area for the absorption of nutrients.

violence Infliction of physical damage on person or property. In sport, the term violence usually refers to serious types of overt aggression.

viral myocarditis Inflammation of the muscle wall of the heart, caused by a viral infection. A cold or influenza virus, for example, may attack, inflame, and irritate the cardiac muscle causing varying degrees of pain and disturbance of the rhythmical beating of the heart. Viral myocarditis can cause circulatory collapse if the sufferer exercises at a high intensity, no matter how fit the person was before infection. *See also* **myocarditis**.

virilization *See* **masculinization**.

virulence The capacity of a microorganism to generate disease.

virus A member of a group of minute infectious agents which have a relatively simple structure and which can reproduce only within living cells. Viruses consist of genetic material (either DNA or RNA) surrounded by a protein coat. They are responsible for many diseases including the common cold, influenza, and AIDS. They are not affected by antibiotics, but many viral diseases can be effectively treated by vaccines.

viscera (singular, viscus) Internal organs of the body cavity.

visceral Pertaining to the internal organs of the body or the inner part of a structure.

visceral fat deposition Adipose tissue found within the body cavity surrounding the liver and intestines. This type of deposition is predominant in *android fat distribution, and has been linked with a higher risk of heart disease and diabetes. The mechanism of risk is unclear but the proximity of fat deposition to the hepatic vascular system is thought to be implicated.

visceral nervous system *See* **autonomic nervous system**.

visceral pain A pain which results from stimulation of pain receptors in the thoracic and abdominal organs. Stimuli include extreme stretching of tissue, ischaemia, irritating chemicals, and muscle spasms. *See also* **referred pain**.

visceral pericardium (serous pericardium) The inner part of the pericardium which lies adjacent to the myocardium. The visceral pericardium contains a small amount of fluid which reduces the friction between the two surfaces as the heart beats.

visceral pleura A thin membrane lining the lungs which secretes *serous fluid. *See also* **pleura**.

visceral reactions Responses of visceral organs, including contractions of the muscular wall of the stomach and secretion of adrenaline from the adrenal glands, which underlie such experiences as nausea and butterflies in the stomach.

visceroceptors *See* **interceptors**.

viscerotonic traits Psychological characteristics which are believed to correlate with *endomorphy. Viscerotonics are typically easy going, sociable people who take pleasure in food and eating. *Compare* **cerebrotonic traits**; and **somatonic traits**. *See* **constitutional theory**.

viscoelastic substance A solid or liquid which can store and dissipate energy during mechanical deformation.

viscometer An instrument for measuring the viscosity of a fluid.

viscosity A measure of the tendency of a fluid to resist relative motion within itself. A liquid with a high viscosity is sluggish and flows in a treacle-like manner. *See also* **coefficient of viscosity**.

viscous drag *See* **surface drag**.

viscous work In human movement, the work done against an internal or external resistance. For example, the viscous work done by a cross-country skier is calculated as the product of distance travelled and the resisting force (the product of gravitational acceleration, the mass of the skier plus skis, and the coefficient of sliding friction for a given wax, temperature, and snow condition).

vision 1 Sight; the ability to perceive with the eye. The eye is the most important sense organ for supplying information about the external world and is classified as an exteroceptor. It has also been shown to be an important proprioceptor (*see* **visual proprioception**). **2** The ability of a coach to set realistic goals and to understand the steps that lead to achieving these goals.

visual accommodation Changes in the lens of the eye so as to focus light from sources at different distances from the eye and thus form sharp images on the retina. *See also* **accommodation**.

visual field The area in front of the eyes within which objects can be seen without moving the eyes. It is usually an advantage to have a wide visual field for sports involving open skills, and a narrow visual field for sports involving *closed skills.

visual guidance A coaching technique in which the coach instructs athletes to copy the actions they see someone else perform. It is a particularly effective form of training for young athletes.

visualization A form of mental practice in which an athlete creates a vivid, controlled visual image of a game situation and imagines how he or she will cope successfully with it. *See also* **external imagery**; and **internal imagery**.

visual proprioception Visual information about a person's own body movements in relation to the environment. Vision can serve as a strong motion detector, particularly in balancing movements.

Visuo-Motor Behaviour Rehearsal (VMBR) A form of *stress management that uses *imagery and relaxation techniques to help athletes reduce anxiety, focus attention, and enhance performance. The procedure involves the use of mental practice in conjunction with progressive muscular relaxation (PMR) then, when a relaxed state is established, the subject imagines himself or herself successfully performing a difficult skill.

vital Pertaining to life.

vital capacity (VC) The maximum volume of air forcefully expired after maximal inspiration. Values vary from 3.5 to 6.0 litres at rest. The value decreases slightly during exercise.

vital centre Collection of nerve cells in the medulla oblongata responsible for ensuring basic functions, such as heart beat and ventilatory movements, are maintained. Injuries to the vital centres are usually fatal because of the nature of the activities for which they are responsible.

vital sign A measurable indicator, such as heart rate or body temperature, of essential body functions.

vitamin A member of a group of potent non-protein organic compounds required in minute amounts for good health and growth. Vitamins (except vitamin D) cannot be synthesized by the body and are therefore essential constituents of the diet. They are classified as fat-soluble vitamins (e.g. vitamins A, D, E, and K) or water soluble vitamins (e.g. vitamins B and C). Many vitamins seem to act as coenzymes or are involved in the production of coenzymes. Each vitamin has a specific function; one vitamin cannot substitute for another. Many metabolic reactions require several vitamins and lack of one may hinder the activity of others. There is much disagreement about the effects of exercise on vitamin requirements. Many coaches believe that the added stress experienced by élite athletes makes greater demands on their vitamin requirements, and that they suffer a greater risk of vitamin deficiency than sedentary people. Currently, there is much research being undertaken to establish the precise vitamin needs of athletes.

vitamin A (retinol) A fat-soluble vitamin which helps with normal functioning of the mucous membranes of the eye and respiratory tract, and the formation of visual pigments in the eye. Vitamin A can be manufactured in the body from *beta-carotene, found in a variety of foods particularly green vegetables and carrots. Vitamin A deficiency increases the risk of infections of the respiratory, digestive, and urinogenital tracts, and causes a number eye disorders, including night blindness. Although it is the most prevalent vitamin deficiency in the world, most people can acquire adequate amounts from a well-balanced diet. There is little evidence to support the use of vitamin A supplements, even for athletes whose demands would be expected to be considerably higher than normal. Excessive intakes of vitamin A can lead to nausea, vomiting, anorexia, headaches, hairlessness, bone and joint pain, and bone fragility. In the UK, the adult Reference Nutrient Intake is 700 micrograms for males and 600 micrograms for females; in the USA, the 1989 Recommended Dietary Allowance is 1000 micrograms for males and 800 micrograms for females.

vitamin B complex A group of vitamins including thiamin (vitamin B$_1$), riboflavin (vitamin B$_2$), niacin (B$_3$), pyrodoxine (vitamin B$_6$), pantothenic acid, folic acid, cyanocobalamin (vitamin B$_{12}$), and biotin. These vitamins play an essential role in the release of energy from food, making them of great interest to exercisers. Prolonged aerobic exercise depends on a sustained production of energy, so deficiencies impair endurance performance. It is not surprising that vitamin B supplements improve the performance of athletes with deficiencies, but there is little scientific evidence to support the use of supplements in those not showing signs of vitamin deficiency.

vitamin B$_1$ (thiamine) A water-soluble vitamin first extracted and isolated from rice polishings. It is also found in lean meat, liver, eggs, wholegrains, and milk. It plays a very important role in releasing energy from foods rich in carbohydrates. Gross deficiency causes the potentially fatal disease known as beri-beri. Mild deficiencies cause fatigue, loss of appetite, muscle weakness, and digestive disturbances. Vitamin B$_1$ is rapidly destroyed by heat and is stored in the body in very small amounts. In the UK, the Reference Nutrient Intake for adults is 1.0 mg each day for males and 0.8 mg for females; in the USA, the 1989 Reference Dietary Allowance is 1.1 mg in females and 1.5 mg in males. Physically active people may require more thiamine than inactive people.

vitamin B$_2$ (riboflavin) A water-soluble vitamin quickly decomposed by heat. When exposed to light it is converted to lumiflavin which destroys vitamin C. Riboflavin is obtained from a wide variety of foods including wholegrains, yeast, liver, eggs, and milk. It is present in the body as co-enzymes which play a central role in releasing energy from food. In the UK, the Reference Nutrient Intake (UK) ranges from 0.4 mg in babies to 1.6 mg in breast-feeding women. In the USA, the Recommended Dietary Allowance for adults is 1.3 mg for females and 1.7 mg for males. Deficiency causes ariboflavinosis, characterized by cracked skin, and eye problems including blurred vision.

vitamin B$_3$ *See* niacin.

vitamin B$_5$ *See* pantothenic acid.

vitamin B$_6$ (pyridoxine) A water-soluble vitamin obtained from meat, poultry, and eggs. It acts as a co-enzyme to over 60 enzymes and plays a vital role in protein metabolism. Vitamin B$_6$ is essential for efficient nerve and muscle function. It is also involved in the initial breakdown of glycogen, and in the formation of antibodies and haemoglobin. Deficiency, although relatively rare, causes nervous irritability, *anaemia, convulsions in infants, and sores around the eyes and mouth in adults. Excessive intake results in depressed tendon reflexes and loss of sensation in the fingers and toes. In the UK, the Reference Nutrient Intake for male and female adults is 1.5 mg; in the USA, the Recommended Dietary Allowance is 1.6 mg for females and 2.0 mg for males.

vitamin B$_{12}$ (cobalamin; cyanocobalamin) A complex water-soluble vitamin containing cobalt. Vitamin B$_{12}$ can be obtained from liver, fish, and some dairy products. It is the only member of the B complex that cannot be obtained from yeast. Vitamin B$_{12}$ acts as a coenzyme. It is involved in DNA synthesis and the formation of red blood cells. Vitamin B$_{12}$ and folic acid work interdependently; deficiency of one can lead to deficiency of the other. In addition, a glycoprotein (known as intrinsic factor) produced by the stomach is needed for absorption of Vitamin B$_{12}$ across the membrane of the intestine into the blood stream. Lack of B$_{12}$, or intrinsic factor, or folic acid, may cause *pernicious anaemia, weight-loss, and degeneration of the nervous system. Vitamin B$_{12}$ is regarded as an ergogenic aid by many coaches who believe it improves energy metabolism in muscle cells. Supplementation to athletes, often by injection into the buttocks, is common even though most research has shown no significant benefits where a B$_{12}$ deficiency does not exist. Toxic effects of vitamin B$_{12}$ are virtually unknown, but allergic reactions occasionally occur from injections. In the UK, the daily Reference Nutrient Intake for adults is 1.5 mg/day; in the USA, the Recommended Dietary Allowance is 2.0 mg.

vitamin B$_{15}$ *See* pangamic acid.

vitamin B$_{17}$ *See* laetrile.

vitamin C (ascorbic acid) A water-soluble vitamin essential for the formation of collagen (a major component of skin, muscles, and bone) and the healthy functioning of tissues containing collagen. It is required for the repair of joint tissues which are often damaged during high levels of physical activity. Vitamin C acts as a stimulant for body defence mechanisms, and protects vitamin A, vitamin E, and dietary fats from oxidation. Vitamin C also plays an important role in the absorption of iron from nonanimal sources. Mild deficiencies can cause fleeting joint pains, poor tooth and bone growth, poor wound healing, and an increased susceptibility to infection. An extreme deficiency of vitamin C causes scurvy. In the UK, the Reference Nutrient Intake (RNI) is 40 mg/day for adults, but this should be increased for those under any stress and those who are physically active. The RNI for pregnant women is 50 mg/day, and for lactating mothers is 70 mg/day. The USA Recommended Dietary Allowance (1989) is higher at about 60 mg. Vegetables (especially green peppers) and citrus fruits are good sources of vitamin C.

vitamin D (anti-rachitic factor) A fat-soluble vitamin containing a number of distinct chemicals that enhance the absorption of calcium and phosphorus from the intestine and, with parathyroid hormone, mobilizes their deposition in bones. Vitamin D is relatively stable when exposed to heat and light. It is stored in the liver and, to a lesser extent, in the fatty tissue in the skin. Vitamin D occurs in two forms: vitamin D_2 and vitamin D_3. Vitamin D_2 (ergocalciferol or calciferol) is obtained in the diet from foods such as oily fish, eggs, and margarine. Vitamin D_3 (cholecalciferol) is the main form of the vitamin and is produced in the skin by the action of ultraviolet light on another compound, 7-dehydrocholesterol. Vitamin D deficiency causes a loss of muscle tone, restlessness, and irritability. It also causes rickets in children, and demineralization and softening of the bones (osteomalacia) in adults. In the UK, there is no daily Reference Nutrient Intake (RNI) for most adults because the main source of vitamin D is from the action of sunlight on skin, but 10 micrograms is the RNI for pregnant, lactating mothers, and adults confined indoors. In the USA, an intake of 10 micrograms throughout life is recommended. As with vitamin A, vitamin D can be toxic if large amounts are consumed over a long period of time. Calcium may be deposited in the organs and soft tissues of the body forming obvious growths. Total intake should not exceed 400 IU (10 micrograms) per day. Vitamin D supplements have been used to treat *osteoporosis and rheumatoid arthritis.

vitamin deficiency disease A disease due to a lack of a vitamin in the body. It may be caused by a dietary deficiency or as a secondary disease associated with anorexia, vomiting, or diarrhoea. Vitamin deficiency disease may also result from the increased metabolic demands for vitamins imposed by fever or stress, including the stress of vigorous, prolonged physical exertion. A substance which interferes with the activity of a vitamin may also cause a deficiency disease. It is now generally recognized that certain groups within the population have a greater risk of deficiency diseases because of their increased vitamin requirements. They include pregnant women, nursing mothers, those following a weight-reducing diet, convalescents, the elderly, athletes in hard training, and those in physically demanding jobs. These groups may benefit from carefully managed vitamin supplementation.

vitamin E (anti-sterility factor; fertility vitamin) A group of related compounds called tocopherols, believed to maintain the integrity of cell membranes. Vitamin E is an *antioxidant and mutually protects vitamins A and C. It also acts as an anti-blood-clotting agent and has been used in the USA to treat some heart diseases. Some coaches claim that it increases muscular development and function; this claim is hotly disputed, but there is considerable support for the suggestion that vitamin E reduces the oxygen requirements of muscles and so enhances performance. Vitamin E is widely available in the diet. The richest sources include wheatgerm oil, sunflower oil, and roasted peanuts. Natural sources of vitamin E are almost twice as effective as synthetic vitamin E. Natural and synthetic forms can be identified by subtle differences in the names of their main components: natural forms are known as 'd-alpha tocopherol' and the synthetic ones as 'dl-alpha tocopherol'. Deficiencies are rare, but when they do occur they may lead to destruction of red blood cells and anaemia. Deficiencies impair the reproductive ability of rats and cause muscle wasting in pigs. There is no strong evidence that vitamin E supplementation can help infertile human females, but large doses have been used to prevent miscarriages. In the UK, because of insufficient information, there is no daily Reference Nutrient Intake. In the USA, the Recommended Dietary Allowance (1989) is 8 mg for females and 10 mg for males.

vitamin F *See* **linoleic acid**.

vitamin H *See* **biotin**.

vitamin K (anti-haemorrhagic vitamin) A fat-soluble vitamin which occurs in two main forms: one of plant origin (phytomenadione), and the other of animal origin (menaquinone). Dietary sources include green leafy vegetables, some vegetable oils, and liver. About half the requirement is derived from the activities of bacteria in the gut. Vitamin K is needed to manufacture prothrombin, a substance essential for the normal clotting of blood. It is also thought to be involved in oxidative phosphorylation, the chemical reactions which release most of the energy from food during aerobic respiration. Deficiency is rare but may result from taking antibiotics which interfere with the activity of gut bacteria. Symptoms include easy bruising and prolonged clotting time, leading to excessive bleeding and haemorrhage. In the UK, there is no Reference Nutrient Intake. In the USA the Recommended Dietary Allowance is 65–80 micrograms

vitamin supplementation Additional vitamins taken to make up a deficit, to avoid a vitamin deficiency disease, or to enhance athletic performance. There is much controversy concerning the value of vitamin supplements as ergogenic aids. There is little evidence to support the notion that extra vitamins improve the physical performance of athletes already eating a balanced diet and not suffering from a vitamin deficiency. However, high doses of vitamins may improve athletic performance by acting as drugs in, as yet, undefined ways. Taking supplements of fat-soluble vitamins can be dangerous because they can be stored in adipose tissue and may be toxic in high concentrations.

VLCD *See* **very low calorie diet**.

VLDL *See* **very low density lipoprotein**.

VMBR *See* **Visuo-Motor Behaviour Rehearsal**.

volition In decision making, the conscious adoption by an individual of a line of action.

Volkmann's contracture Shortening of muscles in the hand and forearm with loss of power caused by an inadequate arterial blood supply resulting from an injury or a constriction (e.g. from a bandage that is too tight). A similar condition can occur in the foot. The condition is named after a German surgeon, R. von Volkmann (1830–1889).

volt The SI unit of potential difference, electromotive force, and electric potential. One volt is the difference in potential between two conducting points carrying a current of one ampere when the power dissipated between these points is one watt.

volume Measure of the amount of space occupied by a body.

volumeter A tank filled with water and used to measure the volume of a body. When the body (which may be a human body) is completely submerged in the water, the volume of the water displaced equals the volume of the body. The volumeter is usually combined with scales so that the weight of the body in and out of the water can be measured. The measurements are used to determine density and specific gravity.

volumetric analysis The measurement of the volume of a body or part of a body to estimate its density. Volumetric analysis is based on *Archimedes principle.

voluntary muscle Muscle under conscious control. *See also* **skeletal muscle**.

voluntary reflex A reflex which originates in the motor cortex of the brain.

vomiting A reflex ejection of the stomach contents through the mouth. It is a common symptom of gastrointestinal infections, abdominal disorders, and a number of diseases. Fluid loss from vomiting can cause *dehydration.

VO₂ max *See* **maximal oxygen uptake**.

VT A symbol commonly used by pulmonary physiologists to refer to the *tidal volume.

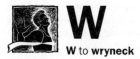

W

W to **wryneck**

W *See* **watt**.

waist girth In anthropometry, the circumference of the waist at the level where the waist noticeably narrows, about midway between the costal border and the iliac crest. *See also* **body girth**.

waist–hip ratio The circumference of the body at the narrowest part of the waist divided by the circumference at the widest part of the hips. The waist–hip ratio is used as a convenient method of assessing body fat distribution. The higher the figure, the greater the tendency towards the higher risk *android fat distribution. The lower the score, the greater the tendency towards *gynoid fat distribution.

waking hypnosis An hypnotic stage during which a subject is instructed to carry out suggestions that are alerting and arousing.

walking Locomotion in which the body is moved in a particular direction while maintaining foot-contact with the ground.

war Violent, open, armed conflict between two or more nations or peoples. Violent outbursts in sport have been linked with the start of war. In June 1969, Honduras played El Salvador in three World Cup soccer games. Riots occurred during the games and, following the games, diplomatic relations were severed between the two countries.

warm-down (cool-down) Gradual, controlled reduction of activity after training or competition. Swimmers may swim slowly in a warm-down, while runners may jog and perform flexibility exercises. The warm-down helps the body to eliminate waste products such as *lactic acid and to reduce the risk of muscular stiffness.

warm-up A procedure, used prior to competition or hard training, by which an athlete attains the optimal body *core temperature and specific muscle temperature for performance, and prepares physically and mentally for the activity. A rise in temperature may be gained passively by taking a warm bath, but it more commonly involves taking light aerobic exercise. There is a lack of general agreement about the effects of the warm-up, but the possible advantages include an increased metabolic rate; increased heart rate with improved oxygen and fuel transport to the tissues; increased speed of nerve conduction; and increased speed of muscle contraction. The warm-up procedure usually involves *static stretching and callisthenics which reduces the risk of muscle and joint injury, and prepares the muscles for activity throughout their full range.

warm-up decrement The gradual loss of the effects of warm-up during a period of inactivity between the warm-up and competition. Warm-up is usually most effective immediately before competition. A warm-up decrement may occur after only a few minutes of inactivity.

wart A raised, brownish area of skin caused by a virus infection.

waste products Products of *metabolism which are eliminated from the body. Some waste products, such as *lactic acid, may be harmful if they accumulate in the body. *See also* **excretion**.

water A clear, colourless, tasteless liquid composed of hydrogen and oxygen. Despite having no value as an energy source, water is our most important nutrient. It constitutes about 60 per cent of the total adult body weight. Losses of as little as 9 to 10 per cent of body weight can be fatal. Smaller losses result in a significant impairment of physical performance. The speed of distance runners, for example, is reduced by about 2 per cent for each per cent of body weight lost by dehydration.

Among its important functions during exercise, water provides the main transport medium for nutrients and respiratory gases, regulates body temperature, and maintains blood pressure for efficient cardiovascular function.

water balance (fluid balance) The relationship between water taken into and lost from the body by all routes. Water balance is closely related to electrolyte balance. During exercise, water gains increase from the increased metabolic breakdown of food, but this is usually exceeded by water losses from sweating. When water losses exceed 2 per cent body weight, stamina is significantly impaired. *See also* **dehydration**.

water intoxication (dilutional hyponatraemia; hypotonic hydration) A condition of water imbalance which may result from a kidney disorder or from drinking extraordinary quantities of water very quickly. The extracellular fluid component is diluted, decreasing the sodium ion concentration causing a net osmotic inflow of water into the cells which consequently swell. This may cause metabolic disturbances, nausea, vomiting, muscular cramps, and in very extreme cases, death.

Extreme cases are rare, but mild cases do occur in athletes who replenish water losses by drinking too much, too quickly.

water potential The tendency of a system, usually a cell, to push water out through a semipermeable membrane. By convention, the water potential of distilled water at one atmosphere of pressure, is given a value of zero and all other solutions are compared to this level. Thus water potential usually has a negative value.

water replacement (rehydration) Replacement of water losses incurred during exercise, or lost from the body through urination, etc. Rehydration is of particular importance to athletes performing repeated bouts of exercise, and to those performing in sports lasting more than 50 minutes. Without adequate rehydration athletes become dehydrated and their ability to perform is diminished. Rehydration is best achieved by replacing electrolytes (especially sodium ions) as well as water. Drinking plain water reduces the thirst stimulus and increases urinary output, both of which delay rehydration. Replacement is best accomplished with a cold drink (8–13 °C), slightly hypotonic, and low in sugar (sugars retard *gastric

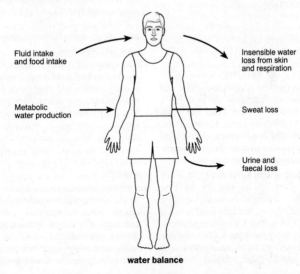

Fluid intake and food intake

Metabolic water production

Insensible water loss from skin and respiration

Sweat loss

Urine and faecal loss

water balance

emptying). Water replacement should not exceed the maximum absorption rate (about 800 ml per hour).

water-soluble vitamins Vitamins which dissolve in water. They include the *vitamin B complex and vitamin C. Water-soluble vitamins are generally not stored in significant amounts because they tend to be eliminated through the urine.

water tablets *See* **diuretic drugs**.

watt (W) A derived SI unit of power, equal to one joule per second.

wave 1 An energy-carrying disturbance, either continuous or transient, travelling through a medium as a progressive local disturbance of the medium without an overall movement of matter. **2** A graphical presentation of an energy-carrying disturbance, plotted as the magnitude of the disturbance against time.

wave drag A *drag force acting on a body that is moving at the interface of two fluids. A partly immersed swimmer, for example, is at the interface between air and water. Swimming movements create waves in the water and the reaction force exerted by the waves on the swimmer constitutes the wave drag.

wave summation The combination of responses from a *motor unit which has had two or more stimuli applied to it in quick succession. A motor unit of a muscle responds to a single stimulus with a simple twitch response. When a second stimulus is applied to the motor unit before the response to the first is completely lost, the two responses combine to produce a greater muscle tension than that produced by a single response. If stimulation continues, the combination of the individual responses may result in *tetanus. *See also* **temporal summation**.

Ways Of Coping with Sport (WOCS) A sport-related questionnaire initially used to measure *coping responses among basketball players, but now used across a range of sports. WOCS measures problem-focused coping, seeking social support, general emotionality, increased effort and resolve, detachment, denial, wishful thinking, and emphasizing positive coping styles.

WBGT *See* **wet bulb globe temperature**.

WBGT index *See* **wet bulb globe temperature index**.

WBT *See* **wet bulb thermometer index**.

weak-link rule A safety rule which states that if one member of an athletic team or group suffers a heat injury, other members are at risk and precautionary measures should be adopted.

weight The force of attraction exerted on an object by the gravitational pull of the Earth. Weight is often expressed in units of mass, but this is not scientifically correct. Being a force, weight should be measured in Newtons (N), and a body of mass will have a weight mg, where g is the acceleration of free fall ($9.80\,665\ ms^{-2}$).

weight-bearing exercise A physical activity, such as walking and running, in which the legs support the weight of the body.

weight control (weight management) The ability to control body weight by the appropriate balance of weight losses associated with the energy expended during exercise and weight gains associated with the intake of food. *See also* **energy balance**.

weight density The weight of an object expressed in terms of a given volume (e.g newtons per litre). *Compare* **density**.

weight-lifter's blackout A loss of consciousness experienced during weight-lifting or another strength training activity when the breath is held. The combination of breath-holding and isometric muscle action during a lift diverts blood suddenly to the head, resulting in a blackout. Weight-lifter's blackout is prevented easily by using a proper breathing technique and by contracting other muscles while executing the lift.

weight-lifter's headache An exercise-induced headache that occurs during strength-training when the breath is held, causing an increase in the intrathoracic and intracranial blood pressures. This type of headache can be avoided by using a proper breathing technique. *See also* **headache**.

weight-lifting strength Usually the heaviest weight that can be lifted once through a specified range of movement. Weight-lifting strength is a measure of the strength of *isotonic muscle actions.

weight-loss diet A diet which enables a person to lose weight. A weight loss of about 1 kg requires either a reduction in energy intake of 4200 kJ (1000 kcal) or an increase in energy expenditure of the same amount. Physically active people who are on low-energy diets (e.g. athletes trying to lose weight) have a high risk of nutrient deficiencies and should seek the advice of a sports dietitian. Of special risk are young women who reduce their energy intake so that they are not consuming enough iron or calcium-containing foods (*see* **osteoporosis**).

weight-loss maintenance Efforts to maintain weight after a successful weight loss programme. Methods of fat loss are often fairly successful, but the difficulty of maintaining weight is reflected by low success rate. Most dieters return to their original weight within a year. Efforts are now focusing on means of improving success in weight loss maintenance. Exercise, cognitive behaviour therapy, and education are increasingly involved in multidisciplinary approaches to the problem.

weight management *See* **weight control**.

weight-training A form of strength training or resistance training using either *free weights or a weight-training machine.

weight-training machine A specialized device which provides support while a person tries to overcome a resistance. Weight-training machines can be designed to produce resistances at a particular angle of pull for a specific muscle or to provide resistances for isokinetic exercises (*see* **isokinetic action**).

Weil's disease (leptospirosis) An infectious disease caused by bacteria belonging to the genus *Leptospira*. Stagnant water may be contaminated with this bacterium from rat or cattle urine. The disease begins with influenza-like symptoms 7–12 days after exposure. Complications, such as internal haemorrhaging, and inflammation of the liver and meninges, can be prevented by early diagnosis and treatment with penicillin, erythromycin, or tetracycline. Participants of inland water sports (e.g., canoeists) should minimize the risk of catching the disease by covering cuts before immersion and taking showers afterwards. They should also inform their doctors of the risk.

wellness A condition obtained when a person achieves a level of *health which minimizes the chances of becoming ill. Wellness is achieved by a combination of emotional, environmental, mental, physical, social, and spiritual health.

wet bulb globe temperature index (WBGT index) An index developed by the US armed forces and used by athletes as an indicator of the relative severity of environmental temperatures. It is computed using the following equation: WBGT index = 0.7(WBT) + 0.2(GT) + 0.1(DBT), where WBT is the wet bulb temperature (recorded from a thermometer with the bulb surrounded by gauze, moistened with distilled water, and ventilated by a fan or a whirling device), GT is the temperature recorded from a thermometer enclosed in a black or grey metal sphere and exposed to the full intensity of sunlight encountered by the athlete, and DBT is the dry bulb temperature recorded on a normal thermometer not exposed to direct sunlight. The temperature is measured in degrees Fahrenheit. The index takes no account of the *wind chill factor.

wet bulb thermometer An ordinary thermometer with a wetted wick wrapped around the bulb. The wet bulb's temperature is related to the amount of moisture in the air. When the wet bulb temperature and dry bulb temperature are equal, the air is completely saturated with water and the relative humidity is 100%. *See also* **WBT index**.

wet bulb thermometer index (WBT index) A simple measurement of environmental heat stress recorded by spinning an ordinary thermometer with a damp wick around the bulb. The temperature recorded is usually less than that for a dry bulb thermometer because of heat lost by evaporation. High wet bulb temperatures usually indicate high humidity when there is a greater danger of heat stress. Athletes wearing protective clothing may be at risk of overheating when the WBT exceeds 60 degrees Fahrenheit.

wheel and axle A simple machine consisting of a larger wheel-like device rotating about a smaller central device called an axle. The radius of the wheel corresponds to the force arm of a lever. When a force is applied to the wheel in order to turn the axle, the *mechanical advantage favours force; when the force is applied to the axle in order to turn the wheel, the mechanical advantage favours speed. Most wheel and axle arrangements in the human body, such as the *trunk rotating around the vertebral column, favour speed.

whiplash injury Damage to structures in the neck (usually the cervical vertebrae and its nerves and ligaments) caused by a sudden, uncontrolled abnormal movement of the head and neck (for example, when a forward moving body comes to a sudden stop). Rugby and American football players may sustain a whiplash injury when tackled simultaneously from the front and back. Rear-end motor vehicle collisions, particularly when a stationary vehicle is hit from the rear, are notorious for causing neck strains as the vulnerable *cervical spine is first extended, then fully flexed.

white blood cell *See* leucocyte.

white fibre A glistening white protein fibre made mainly of *collagen.

white fibrocartilage Flexible, tough, and elastic cartilage consisting of a dense mass of *collagen fibres in a solid matrix with cells spread thinly among the fibres. White fibrocartilage forms a thin coating on some grooves in bones through which tendons glide. It is also found between the bodies of vertebrae and in the menisci.

white matter Regions of the *central nervous system which contain mainly myelinated nerve fibres and few *cell bodies. *Compare* **grey matter**.

white muscle fibres *See* fast-twitch fibres.

whole method A method of *learning a skill in which the whole skill is repeatedly practised until its performance is perfected. It is usually adopted when the skill is relatively simple.

whole–part–whole method A method of *learning a skill in which the learner tries to perform the whole skill from time to time after practising parts of the skill, particularly those parts which are difficult.

Wilcoxon test A nonparametric statistical test for comparing two samples for overall significant differences. The test is performed on paired-data which is of the ordinal type so that the differences between the pairs can be ranked.

wind A movement of air horizontal in relation to the surface of the earth. In athletics, the wind is measured by an anemometer. If the velocity exceeds 2 m s^2 (i.e. 4.473 miles per hour) at a height 1.3 m (four feet) above ground level in a direction which would assist competitors, the performances are not valid for establishing records.

wind chill The effect of cold winds which can lead to a lowering of body *core temperature and the onset of *hypothermia. *See also* **sensible temperature**.

winding A common sport injury resulting from an abdominal blow causing a neurogenic shock due to overstimulation of the solar plexus. Typically, the winded person doubles up and has difficulty breathing because of a momentary paralysis of the diaphragm and spasm of the abdominal muscles. Drawing the sufferer's knees up to the abdomen is a popular treatment which may relax the abdominal muscles and assist return to normality, but even without special treatment the person usually recovers with no residual symptoms. Persistence of symptoms may indicate serious internal injury requiring expert medical attention.

wind pipe *See* trachea.

wind tunnel A chamber in which the motion of a current of air can be regulated for studying the aerodynamic properties of objects. Wind tunnels are based on the idea that the aerodynamic effects of an object moving in a fluid are identical to the effects of a fluid moving at the same velocity past a stationary object. Wind tunnels have been used to analyse the flight of a sports implements, such as the discus and javelin, and the flow of air over a human body (for example a cyclist or skier). The body (implement or person) is placed in the wind tunnel and the air flow is regulated so that the relative motion of the air and subject is the same as it would be in the natural environment.

Wingate anaerobic power test *See* Wingate 30-second test.

Wingate 30-second test A test of *intermediate anaerobic power in which a subject is instructed to pedal as fast as possible on a bicycle ergometer for 30 seconds with a resistance load for the leg test of either 45 or 75 g per kg body-weight depending on the type of ergometer.

withdrawal A discontinuation of interest in sport involvement. Factors causing withdrawal include loss of interest and injury. *See also* **noninvolvement**.

withdrawal symptoms Specific symptoms associated with discontinuation of the use of a drug on which a person has become physically dependent.

withdrawal syndrome A combination of symptoms and signs in an individual who is deprived of a drug on which the individual has become physically dependent.

wobble board An exercise device used during the rehabilitation of leg injuries, especially ankle sprains. Simple wobble boards consist of a circular board which, when placed on the ground, is supported by a central ball. The subject stands on the board and attempts to keep its edges off the ground. Wobble boards help re-train the balance mechanisms and restore coordination between the injured part and the areas around it.

WOCS *See* Ways Of Coping with Sport.

Wolff–Parkinson–White syndrome (WPW syndrome) An abnormal heart rhythm

giving specific *electrocardiogram changes and attacks of paroxysmal *tachycardia. It is a congenital condition caused by an accessory bundle between the atria and ventricles. There is no evidence that athletic exertion makes sudden death from WPW syndrome more likely. However, those with very low resting pulse rates, such as distance runners, may be more vulnerable to *ectopic beats.

Wolff's law A law which states that bone density changes in response to changes in the functional forces on the bone. Wolff (1836–1902) proposed that changes in the form and function of bones, or changes in function alone, are followed by changes in the internal structure and shape of the bone in accordance with mathematical laws. Thus, in mature bone where the general form is established, the bone elements place or displace themselves, and decrease or increase their mass, in response to the mechanical demands imposed on them. The theory is supported by the observation that bones atrophy when they are not mechanically stressed and hypertrophy when they are stressed. *See also* **bone remodelling**.

Wolpe's principle A principle of reciprocal inhibition which assumes that a detrimental response (e.g. muscle tension associated with a stressful situation) can be eliminated by the presence of an antagonistic response (e.g., relaxation). Wolpe's principle is applied when athletes relax in preparation for a potentially stressful event.

work The transfer of mechanical energy expressed as the product of force and the displacement of the resistance in the direction of the force; i.e. $W = Fd$, where W represents work (in Joules), F represents force (in Newtons), and d represents displacement of the resistance (in metres). *See also* **positive work**; and **negative work**.

work and family orientation questionnaire A questionnaire which uses *Likert-type scales to measure four components: work orientation (the desire to do one's best in whatever one undertakes); mastery (persistence in accomplishing difficult tasks);

competitiveness (enjoying challenging situations); and personal concern (lack of concern about what others think).

work ethic A code of conduct which emphasizes the value of being occupied. Those who adopt a work ethic generally view labour as a duty and regard leisure and the pursuit of pleasure with suspicion and feelings of guilt. Those who adopt the work ethic in sport tend to have a high regard for work rate, discipline, and team effort, and have less regard for flair, spontaneity, and individualism.

working hypothesis A suggested explanation of a group of facts or phenomena provisionally accepted as a basis for further investigation and testing. *See also* **hypothesis**.

work interval Portion of interval training consisting of the work effort.

work load The total amount of work completed in a specified period.

work rate *See* **power**.

work relief In *interval training, a type of relief period involving light exercise such as rapid walking or jogging.

work-relief ratio In interval training, a ratio relating the duration of the work interval to the duration of the relief interval. Thus, a work:relief ratio of 2:1 means that the duration of the work (e.g., high intensity exercise) is twice as much as the relief intervals (e.g. ,walking).

wormian bones Small irregular bones sometimes formed in the sutures of the *cranium.

wound A break in the continuity of an organ or tissue by an external agent. Wounds include cuts and lacerations.

WPW syndrome *See* **Wolff–Parkinson–White syndrome**.

wrestler's ear *See* **cauliflower ear**.

wrist The whole region in and around the wrist-joint, including the distal parts of the radius and ulna, and the carpus.

wrist abduction *See* **radial deviation**.

wrist abductor Muscle which effects abduction of the wrist (radial deviation). Wrist abductors include the flexor carpi radialis in the anterior compartment of the forearm, and the extensor carpi radialis longus, extensor carpi radialis brevis, and abductor pollicis longus in the posterior compartment.

wrist adduction *See* **ulnar deviation**.

wrist adductor Muscle involved in adduction of the wrist (ulnar deviation). Wrist adductors include the flexor carpi ulnaris in the anterior compartment of the forearm, and the extensor carpi ulnaris in the posterior compartment.

wrist drop An inability to raise the wrist resulting from damage to the radial nerve or from a tendon injury.

wrist extension Return of the hand to the *anatomical position after wrist flexion.

wrist extensor Muscle which effects *wrist extension and wrist hyperextension. Wrist extensors include the extensor carpi radialis longus, the extensor carpi radialis brevis, and the extensor carpi ulnaris.

wrist-finger speed A skill underlying tasks for which alternating movements of different fingers must be made as quickly as possible. Wrist-finger speed depends on the rapid coordination of muscles required for the up and down movements of the fingers and wrists.

wrist flexion Movement of the palmar surface of the hand towards the anterior forearm.

wrist flexor A muscle that effects *wrist flexion. Wrist flexors include the flexor carpi radialis and the flexor carpi ulnaris.

wrist fracture *See* **carpo-navicular fracture**.

wrist ganglion cyst A benign tenosynovitis cyst formed by a concentration of *synovial fluid just below the skin, usually just forward of the wrist crease on the top of the hand. It is most often caused by repetitive pressure (e.g., from rowing or gymnastics exercises) irritating one of the tendons that run along the top of the wrist. Asymptomatic ganglia are usually left, but those which are painful during activity may be treated with rest, ice, compression, and elevation (*see* **RICE**). Splinting may be prescribed to avoid worsening the condition. A persistent wrist ganglion may be drained. If recurrent, surgery may be necessary. Anyone with persistent wrist pain should consult a doctor.

wrist girth In anthropometry, the circumference of the right wrist distal to the styloid process.

wrist hyperextension Wrist movement which brings the dorsal surface of the hand closer to the posterior forearm.

wrist joint The *condyloid joint formed by the articulation of the radius with the three carpal bones, and articulations between the carpal bones.

wrist sprain *See* **carponavicular fracture**.

wryneck *See* **torticollis**.

 # X

 x-axis to **xylose**

x-axis 1 In anthropometry, the lateral axis formed by the intersection of the frontal plane and transverse plane. **2** A spatial axis parallel to the ground and directed to the observer's right and left, right being designated positive and left negative. **3** In mathematics, the horizontal axis of a graph.

X chromosome Sex chromosome present in both sexes. In males who have one X chromosome and one Y chromosome, the alleles carried on the X chromosomes are always expressed whether they are dominant or recessive.

xerophthalmia A disease characterized by drying and wrinkling of the cornea and conjunctiva, and caused by a deficiency of vitamin A.

xiphisternum *See* **xiphoid process**.

xiphoid process (xiphisternum) The inferior end of the *sternum which articulates with the sternal body and serves as an attachment point for the diaphragm and abdominal muscles.

X-rays (Roentgen rays) Electromagnetic radiation of very short wavelength which can penetrate body structures to varying degrees. X-rays are used in radiography to produce photographic images of the body structures, and they are used in some forms of radiotherapy.

xylose A pentose sugar involved in carbohydrate metabolism. It is found in some types of connective tissue and in small amounts in the urine.

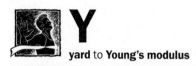

yard to **Young's modulus**

yard A unit of length equal to 0.9144 metres.

y-axis 1 In anthropometry, the longitudinal axis formed by the intersection of a *frontal plane and sagittal plane. **2** A spatial axis parallel to the ground and directed forwards and backwards from the observer; forward being positive and backward, negative. **3** In mathematics, the vertical axis of a graph.

Y chromosome The smaller of the two sex chromosomes. It is normally found in males only and seems to carry few genes. *See also* **gender verification**.

yaw 1 A movement in a fluid of a body, such as a swimmer, about the body's vertical axis. **2** The lateral deviation of an object moving in a fluid from a straight course.

yellow bone marrow The fatty tissue which occupies the internal cavities of long bones and begins to replace red bone marrow soon after birth.

yellow elastic cartilage (elastic tissue) Cartilage consisting of yellow elastic fibres (*see* **elastic fibre**) running through a relatively solid matrix with cells lying between the fibres. Yellow elastic cartilage occurs in the pinna, epiglottis, and Eustachian tube.

yellow elastic fibre *See* **elastic fibre**.

yellow fibre *See* **elastic fibre**.

Yerkes–Dodson curve An inverted U-shaped curve showing a proposed relationship between *arousal and performance. One end of the curve indicates an unaroused condition, such as sleep, while the other end shows overarousal. The curve suggests

that there is an optimum level of arousal between the two extremes which maximizes performance. *See also* **inverted-U principle**.

Yerkes–Dodson law A law which predicts an inverted U relationship between *arousal and performance (*see* **Yerkes–Dodson curve**) and that the optimal level of arousal for a beginner is considerably less than that for an expert performing the same task. It also suggests that easily acquired skills not requiring difficult discrimination or complex association can be readily learned under conditions of high arousal, whereas complex skills are more easily acquired under low levels of arousal.

yips An involuntary muscular disturbance that affects some golfers, characterized by jerking or muscle spasms in the arms during putting. Performance anxiety is believed to contribute to this disorder. Yips are notoriously difficult to treat. Some golfers change hand preference or position to alleviate symptoms, others have taken tranquillizers (e.g. benzodiazepines) to relieve the symptoms.

young runner's heel An *overuse injury of the growing points of the heel bone which results in pain as the heel strikes the ground. *See also* **Sever–Haglund disease**.

Young's modulus The *elastic modulus applied to tensional stress when the object concerned is not constrained. Young's modulus = applied load per unit area of cross section/increase in length per unit length.

Z

Zajonc's model to zygomatic bone

Zajonc's model A model of *social facilitation based on drive theory. According to the model, the presence of an audience increases the psychological arousal of performers. This increased *arousal (loosely called drive) tends to diminish performance on difficult tasks that are unlearned or incompletely learned, and enhances performance on well-learned tasks. The model has been criticized because it is based on 'sheer presence' of the audience with no interaction between audience and performer; this situation rarely occurs in competitive sport.

Zander apparatus Apparatus designed by the Swedish physician J.G.W. Zander to enable a person to perform, within a gymnasium, various exercises which are usually performed only out of doors. The apparatus includes machines for exercising specific muscles used in rowing, bicycling, and horseback riding. It also has components for moving joints to increase their suppleness after injury.

Zatopek phenomenon Beneficial effects associated with *tapering, named after Emil Zatopek. His intense training prior to the 1950 European Games was interrupted by illness which hospitalized him for two weeks. He came out of hospital just two days before competing in the 10 000 metres which he won convincingly. He went on to win the 5000 metres. His success has been attributed to the benefits of his enforced tapering.

z-axis 1 In anthropometry, the sagittal axis formed by the intersection of the sagittal plane and the transverse plane. **2** A spatial axis which is vertical to the ground and directed upward and downward from an observer, with upward being designated positive and downward, negative.

zeitgeber A word derived from German: *zeit*, time; *geber*, to give. A zeitgeber is a syn-chronizing agent, as in an environmental cue responsible for maintaining biological rhythms. For example, alternation of light and darkness between night and day acts as a zeitgeber for diurnal rhythms.

zeitgeist The spirit of the times; the dominant beliefs of a particular period. The term is usually applied to the study of literature, but it has also been applied to sport (for example, in connection with the current belief that winning is all that matters).

zero linear acceleration The acceleration of a body which is moving in a straight line at a constant speed or of a body which is at rest.

zero-sum competition A competition in which one participant wins totally and another loses without gaining any objectives. *Compare* **nonzero-sum competition**.

zinc An essential trace element that works in close association with vitamins and over one hundred enzymes. It is, therefore, involved in almost every physiological function in the body. It forms part of a protein (gustin) in saliva and plays a role in taste and smell. It helps the A and B vitamins to function effectively, and is thought to increase resistance against cold and some other infections. It also helps to heal wounds. Zinc deficiency may cause loss of taste and smell, and a reduction of appetite. A deficiency can slow down the healing of wounds (zinc oxide ointment is applied to abrasions to accelerate healing), retard growth in children, and reduce the sperm count of adult males (the concentration of zinc in semen is 100 times greater than in the blood plasma). In the USA, the Recommended Dietary Allowance (RDA) for adults is 15 mg for males and 12 mg for females. The UK Reference Nutrient Intake for adults is 9.5 mg for males and 7.0 mg for females (lactating mothers require higher amounts). Zinc can be obtained from seafood (especially oysters and other shellfish), cereal crops, legumes, wheat germ, and yeast products. Zinc may bind to some constituents of dietary fibre, interfering with its absorption from the gut. Consequently, vegetarians may require a higher than normal intake of this element. As zinc is lost in urine and sweat, exercisers (especially those who train intensively) may also need zinc supplementation. However, zinc supplementation should not exceed the RDA because excessive amounts can have harmful effects including inhibition of copper absorption, which may lead to anaemia.

zinc oxide ointment An ointment used as a skin protector to prevent ultraviolet light from reaching the skin, and to accelerate healing of burns and abrasions.

z-line (z-membrane; zwischen-line) A protein band which defines the boundary between one *sarcomere and the next in a *muscle fibre. The 'z' is an abbreviation for the German word *zwischen* which means between.

z-membrane *See* z-line.

zone of optimal functioning A narrow range of *arousal levels that produces the best performance in a particular activity. The zone of optimal arousal differs for different activities and even for different individuals performing the same activity. Weight-lifters, for example, benefit from high levels of arousal so they can generate maximum power during the lift. Golfers about to make a putt, on the other hand, benefit from low levels so that they can perform controlled, delicate movements. *See also* **catastrophe theory**.

Zwischen line *See* Z-line.

zwitterion An *amino acid or a protein at its isoelectric point which, although electrically neutral, has both positive and negative charges.

zygapophyseal joint *See* facet joint.

zygapophysis Any one of the facets of the *vertebrae which articulate with each other. The two prezygapophyses articulate with the two posterior zygapophyses.

zygomatic bone One of a pair of bones which run between the cheeks and the ear, forming the prominent part of the cheek and contributing to the orbits.

Appendix 1
Banned Substances

....

Performance-enhancing drugs and procedures subject to doping controls.

The International Olympic Committee Medical Commission list of doping classes and methods (September 1994), with representative examples.

I DOPING CLASSES

(A) *Stimulants

*adrenaline[1]
amiphenazole
*amphetamines
amineptine
benzphetamine (benzfetamine)
beta[2] agonists
*caffeine[2]
cathine
chlorphentermine
clobenzorex
clorprenaline
*cocaine
cropropamide
dextroamphetamine
dimetamfetamine
ephedrine
etafedrine
etamivan
etilamfetamine
fencamfamine
fenetyilline
fenproporex
furfenorex
mefenorex
mesocarb
methamphetamine
methylephedrine
methylphenidate
morazine
nikethamide
pemoline
pentetrazol
phendimetrazine
phenmetrazine
phentermine
phenylpropanolamine
pipradrol

prolintane
propylhexedrine
pyrovalerone
salbutamol[3]
*strychnine
terbutaline[3]
    ... and related compounds

Notes:
[1] Vasoconstrictors such as adrenaline are permitted if administered with local anaesthetic agents

[2] Urinary concentrations of less than 12 micrograms of caffeine per millilitre are permitted.

[3] Permitted by inhaler only, but must be declared to the relevant medical authority

(B) *Narcotics

alphaprodine
anileridene
buprenophine
dextromoramide
dextropropoxyphene
diamorphine (heroin)
dihydrocodeine
dipipanone
ethoheptazine
ethylmorphine
levorphanol
methadone
*morphine
nalbuphine
pentazocine
pethidine
phenazocine
trimeperidine
    ... and related compounds

Note: codeine, dextromethorphan, dihydrocodein, diphenoxylate, and pholcodine are permitted

(C) *Anabolic agents

androstane
androstenedione
androsterone
bolasterone
boldenone
chlordehydromethyltestosterone
clostebol
dihydrotestosterone
fluoxymesterone
metandienone
metenolone
methyltestosterone
nandrolone
oxandrolone
oxymetholone
stanozolol
*testosterone
   ... and related compounds

(D) *Diuretics

acetazolamide
amiloride
benzthiazide
bumetanide
canreonate potassium
chlorthalidone
ethacrynic acid
furosemide
hydrochlorothiazide
mannitol
spironolactone
triamterene
   ... and related compounds

(E) *Peptide hormones and analogues

*adrenocorticotrophic hormone (ACTH)
*erythropoietin
*growth hormone
*human chorionic gonadotrophin
*releasing factors
   ... and related compounds

II *Doping methods

(A) *Blood doping

(B) *Pharmacological, chemical, and physical manipulation

*probenecid

III Classes of drugs subject to certain restrictions

(A) *Alcohol

(B) *Marijuana

(C) *Local anaesthetics

(D) *Corticosteroids

cortisone
*hydrocortisone (cortisol)
corticosterone

(E) *Beta blockers

acebutolol
alprenolol
atenolol
betaxolol
bisopropol
cartelol
labetalol
metoprolol
nadolol
oxprenolol
propanolol
sotalol
   ... and related compounds

The above are *not* comprehensive lists of individual drugs. The IOC Medical Commission controls apply to all compounds related to those in the lists. This has the advantage that new drugs, some of which may be especially designed as ergogenic aids, are also banned. In addition, some sports federations have their own list of banned substances.

*See main text for individual entry.

Appendix 2

The Latin (L.) or Greek (Gk.) word from which the word element is derived is shown in italics and is followed by the original meaning.

a- *a* (Gk.), not; without.

A-, Ab- *ab* (L.), from, or away from.

acer- *acer* (L.), sharp.

acid- *acidus* (L.), sour.

actin- *aktis* (Gk.), ray.

ad- *ad* (L.), to, towards, at, or near.

adeno- *aden* (Gk.), gland.

adipo- *adeps* (L.), fat.

aer- *aer* (L.), air.

-aestehesia, -aesthetic *aisthesis* (Gk.), sensation.

albo-, albu-, *albus* (L.), white.

ambi- *ambo* (L.), both.

amphi- *amphi* (Gk.), on both sides, around, or double.

amylo- *amylum* (Gk.), starch.

A-, an- *an* (Gk.), without, or not.

ana- *ana* (Gk.) on, upward, again, or throughout.

andr-, andro- *andrikos* (Gk.), masculine.

aniso- *anisos* (Gk.), unequal.

ankylo- *agkylos* (Gk.), crooked.

ante- *ante* (L.), before.

anthropo- *anthropos* (Gk.), man.

anti- *anti* (Gk.), opposite, against.

apo- *apo* (Gk.), from.

arch-, archi- *archi* (Gk.), first, or chief

arthro- *arthron* (Gk.), joint.

-atomy, -otomy *tome* (Gk.), cutting.

auri-, *auricula* (L.), ear.

auto- *auto* (Gk.), self.

auxi-, auxo- *auxein* (Gk.), to increase.

axill- *axilla* (L.), armpit.

baro- *baros* (Gk.), pressure.

basi- *basis* (L.), footing or base.

bi- *bis* (L.), two, twice, or double.

bio-, -biotic *bios* (Gk.), life.

-blast *blastos* (Gk.), bud, or germ.

brachia- *brachium* (L.), arm.

brady- *bradys* (Gk.), slow.

brevi- *brevis* (L.), short.

calci- *calx* (Gk.), lime.

capit- *caput* (L.), head.

carbo- *carbo* (L.), coal.

cardio- *kardia* (Gk.), heart.

carpa- *carpal* (L.), wrist.

cata- *katalysis* (Gk.), down.

cauda- *cauda* (L.), tail.

centro-, -centric *kentron* (Gk.), centre.

cephal- *kephale* (Gk.), head.

-ceptor *capere* (L.), to take.

cerebr- *cerebrum* (L.), brain.

cervic- *cervix* (L.), neck.

-chord *chorde* (Gk.), string.

chondro- *chondros* (Gk.), cartilage.

chromo- *chroma* (Gk.), colour.

chrono- *chronos* (Gk.), time.

clav- *clava* (L.), club.

cleisto- *kleistos* (Gk.), closed.

-clinous *klinein* (Gk.), to bend.

costa- *costa* (L.), rib.

coxa-, coxo-, *coxa* (L.), hip.

crani- *kranion* (Gk.), skull.

cruci- *crux* (L.), cross.

cyano- *kyanos* (Gk.), dark blue.

cyst- *kystis* (Gk.), bladder.

de- *de* (L.), down, away from, or deprived of.

di- *dis* (Gk.), twice; hence, twofold or double.

di- dia- *dia* (Gk.), across, through, between, apart

digito- *digitus* (L.), finger.

diplo- *diploos* (Gk.), double.

dors- *dorsum* (L.), back.

-duct *ducere* (L.), to lead.

dynamo- *dynamis* (Gk.), power.

e- ex- *ex* (L.), out of.

ect- *ektos* (Gk.), outside, without.

endo- *endon* (Gk.), in, inside, within.

entero- *enteron* (Gk.), gut.

epi- *epi* (Gk.), upon, on.

equi- *equus* (Gk.), equal.

erg-, -ergic, -ergy *ergon* (Gk.), work.

erythro- *erythros* (Gk.), red.

eu- *eu* (Gk.), well.

exo- *exo* (Gk.), outside.

extra- *extra* (L.), beyond.

fibrino- *fibra* (L.), a band.

-**fid** *findere* (L.), to split.
-**fugal**, -**fuge** *fugere* (L.), to flee.
galacto- *gala* (Gk.), milk.
ganglio- *ganglion* (Gk.), swelling.
-**gen** -**genous** *genos* (Gk.), descent.
glia- *gloia* (Gk.), glue.
-**globin**, -**globulin** *globus* (L.), a sphere.
-**gluco**, -**glyco** *glykys* (Gk.), sweet.
-**gram**, -**graphy** *graphein* (Gk.), to write.
gyn- *gyne* (Gk.), female.
haem-, *haima* (Gk.), blood.
halo- *hals* (Gk.), salt, sea.
hemi- *hemi* (Gk.), half.
hepa-, **hepatico**- *hepar* (Gk.), liver.
hetero- *heteros* (Gk.), other.
hex- *hex* (Gk.), six.
holo- *holos* (Gk.), whole.
homeo- *homoios* (Gk.), alike.
homo- *homos* (Gk.), one and the same.
hormone *hormaein* (Gk.), to excite.
hydr-, **hydro**- *hydor* (Gk.), water.
hygro- *hygros* (Gk.), wet.
hyper- *hyper* (Gk.), above.
hypo- *hypo* (Gk.), under, below.
-**ific**, **ification** *facere* (L.), to make.
immuno- *immunis* (Gk.), free.
-**in**, **in**- *in* (L.), not; in, into, within, towrd.
infero- *inferus* (L.), beneath.
infra- *infra* (L.), below, or lower than.
inter- *inter* (L.), between.
intra- *intra* (L.), within.
iso- *isos* (Gk.), equal.
juxta- *juxta* (L.), close to.
-**kinesis**, -**kinetic** *kinesis* (Gk), movement.
lacto- *lac* (L.), milk.
lati- **latero**- *latus* (L.), wide.
leuco-, **leuko**- *leukos* (Gk.), white.
lipo- *lipos* (Gk.), fat.
-**lysin**, -**lysis** *lysis* (Gk.), breaking down.
macro- *makros* (Gk.), large.
medi- *medius* (L.), middle.
mega- *megas* (Gk.), large.
-**mere**, **mero**- *meros* (Gk.), a part.
mes- **meso**- *mesos* (Gk.), middle.
meta- *meta* (Gk), after.
metabolism *metabole* (Gk.), change.
-**metric**, -**metry** *metron* (Gk), measure.
micro- *mikros* (Gk.), small.
mono- *monos* (Gk.), single.
morpho-, -**morph** *morphe* (Gk.), form, shape.
multi-, *multus* (L.), many.
myo- *mys* (Gk.), muscle.

necro- *nekros* (Gk.), dead.
neuro- *neuron* (Gk.), nerve.
noci- *nocere* (L.), to hurt.
noto- *noton* (Gk.), back.
ob- *ob* (L.), against, reversely.
occipi- *occiput* (L.), back of head.
octa-, **octo**- *okta* (Gk.), octo (L.), eight.
oculo- *oculos* (L.), eye.
-**ology** *logos* (Gk.), discourse.
ophthal- *ophthalmos* (Gk.), eye.
ora-, **oro**- *oris* (L.), mouth.
ortho- *orthos* (Gk.), straight.
ost-, **osteo**- *osteon* (Gk.), bone.
oto- *otos* (Gk.), ear.
-**otomy** *temnein* (Gk.), to cut.
oxy- *oxys* (Gk.), acid.
palpi- *palpare* (L.), to stroke.
pan-, **panto**-, *pan* (Gk.), all.
para- *para* (Gk), beside.
patho-, **pathy**- *pathos* (Gk.), suffering.
ped-, -**peda** *pes* (L,.) foot.
penta-, **pento**- *pente* (Gk.), five.
per- *per* (L.), through.
peri- *peri* (Gk), around.
-**phage** *phagein* (Gk.), to eat.
-**phil** *philein* (Gk.), to love.
-**phobe**, -**phobic** *phobos* (Gk.), fear.
phospho- *phosphoros* (Gkl.), bringing light.
photo- *phos* (Gk.), light.
-**phylactic** *phylaktikos* (Gk.), fit for preserving.
physi-, *physis* (Gk.), growth.
-**plasm** *plasma* (Gk.), form.
pleura- *pleuros* (Gk.), side.
-**plicate** *plicare* (L.), to fold.
pneu- *pnein* (Gk.), to breathe.
-**pod**, *pous* (Gk.), foot.
-**poiesis**, -**poietic**, *poiesis* (Gk.), making.
polys-, *polys* (Gk.), many.
poro-, -**pore** *poros* (Gk.), channel.
post- *post* (L.), after.
pre- *prae* (L.), before.
pro- *pro* (Gk. or L.), before, in front of , or prior.
pseudo- *pseudes* (Gk.), false.
psycho- *psyche* (Gk.), mind.
pulmo- *pulmo* (L.), lung.
quadrato- *quadratus* (L.), squared.
quadri-, **quadru**- *quattuor* (L.), four.
quin- *quinque* (L.), five.
radio- *radius* (L.), ray, rod, or spoke.
rena-, **reni**- *renes* (Gk.), kidney.

reticulo- *reticulum* (L.), small net.
retro- *retro* (L.), backwards.
rhin- *rhis* (Gk.), nose.
sacchar- *sakchar* (Gk.), sugar.
-sarc, sarco- *sarx* (Gk.), flesh.
semi- *semi* (L.), half.
soma-, somato-, -some *soma* (Gk.), body.
spondyl- *sphondylos* (Gk.), verterbra.
-stat, -*static* (L.), to stand.
stern- *sternum* (L.), breast.
sub- *sub* (L.), under, beneath, or near.
super- *super* (L.), over.
supra- *supra* (L.), above.
sym-, syn-, *syn* (Gk.), with, or together.
synaps-, synapto- *synapsis, synaptos* (Gk.),
    union, joined.
synthesis *synthesis* (Gk.), composition.
tachy- *tachys* (Gk.), quick.
talo- *talus* (L.), ankle.
tarso- *tarsos* (Gk.), sole of foot.
tele- *tele* (Gk.), far.

tempor- *tempora* (L.), temples.
tetra- *tetras* (Gk.), four.
thermo- *therme* (Gk.), heat.
thrombo- *thrombos* (Gk.), clot.
trauma- *trauma* (Gk.), wound.
tri- *tres* (L.), three.
-type *typos* (Gk.), pattern.
ulna-, ulno- *ulna* (L.), elbow.
ultra- *ultra* (L.), beyond.
unci- *uncus* (L.), hook.
uni- *unus* (L.), one.
uro- *ouron* (Gk.), urine.
vagini- *vagina* (L.), sheath.
valv- *valvae* (L.), folding doors.
vasa-, vaso- *vas* (L.), vessel.
ventr- *venter* (L.), belly.
versi- *versare* (L.), to turn.
xantho- *xanthos* (Gk.), yellow.
xero- *xeros* (Gk.), dry.
-zoic, *zoikos* (Gk.), pertaining to life.

Appendix 3

International System of Units of Measurement (SI Units), and derived SI units commonly used in Sports Science and Medicine.

MEASUREMENT	NAME OF UNIT	ABBREVIATION OF UNIT NAME
acceleration	metre/second^2	ms^{-2}
amount of substance*	mole	mol
angular momentum	kilogramme metre^2/sec	kg m^2 s^{-1}
area	square metre	m^2
density	kilogramme/m^3	kg m^{-3}
electric current*	ampere	A
electric potential	volt	V
energy	joule	J
force	newton	N
heat	joule	J
kinetic energy	joule	J
length*	metre	m
luminous intensity*	candela	d
mass rate of flow	kilogramme/second	kg s^{-1}
moment of inertia	kilogramme per metre^2	kg m^{-2}
momentum	kilogramme metre/sec kg ms^{-1}	kgms^{-1}
potential energy	joule	J
power	watt	W
pressure	newton/metre^2	N m^{-2}
surface tension	newton/metre	N m^{-1}
temperature	degree Celsius	C
temperature*	kelvin	K
time*	second	s
torque (moment of force)	newton metre	n.m
velocity	metre/second	m s^{-1}
volume	cubic metre	m^3
volume rate of flow	cubic metre/sec	m^3 s^{-1}
work	joule	J

*Internationally agreed basic units.

Prefixes commonly used to denote decimultiples and submultiples of SI units

PREFIX	MULTIPLE	SIGN
atto	$\times 10^{-18}$	a
femto	$\times 10^{-15}$	f
pico-	$\times 10^{-12}$	p
nano-	$\times 10^{-9}$	n
micro-	$\times 10^{-6}$	u
milli-	$\times 10^{-3}$	m

centi-	$\times 10^{-2}$	c
deci-	$\times 10^{-1}$	d
deda-	$\times 10^{1}$	da
hecto-	$\times 10^{2}$	h
kilo-	$\times 10^{3}$	k
mega-	$\times 10^{6}$	M
giga-	$\times 10^{9}$	G
tera-	$\times 10^{12}$	T

Appendix 4
Units of Measurements and Conversions

....

DISTANCES

1 inch (in.) = 0.0254 m = 2.54 cm = 25.4 mm
1 foot (ft) = 30.48 cm = 304.8 mm = 0.304 m
1 mile = 5208 ft = 1760 yds = 1609.35 m =
1.62 km
1 kilometre (km) = 0.62 mile = 1000 m
1 metre = 39.37 in. = 3.28 ft = 1.09 yds
1 cm = 0.03937 in.

ENERGY

1 kilocalorie (kcal or Cal) = 1 000 cal = 4 184
J = 4.184 kJ
1 British Thermal Unit (BTU) = 0.2522 kcal =
1.055 kJ
1 erg = 10^{-7} J
1 hp h (horsepower hour) = 2.684 52 MJ
@Indent 1@

FORCE (OR WEIGHT)

1 dyne = 10^{-5} N
1 poundal (pdl) = 0.138 255 N

MASS

1 gram (g) = 1000 mg = 0.03527 oz = 0.001 kg
1 kilogram (kg) = 1000 g = 35.27 oz = 2.205 lb
1 ounce avoir. (oz) = 0.0625 lb = 28.3495 g
= 0.028 kg
1 ounce (troy or apoth.) = 31. 103 5 g = 0. 031
103 5 kg
1 pound (lb) = 16 oz = 453.6 g = 0.454 kg
1 sh cwt (US hundredweight) = 45.3592 kg
1 cwt (UK hundredweight) = 50.8023 kg
1 UK ton = 1016.05 kg = 1.016 05 tonne
1 short ton = 2000 lb = 907.185 kg = 0.907
tonne

POWER

1 horsepower (HP) = 33 000 ft-lbs/min = 4
5664 kg-m/min = 746 W
1 watt (W) = 44.22 ft-lbs/min = 6.118 kg-
m/min = 0.0013 HP
1 ft-lb per minute (ft-lb/min) = 0.1383 kg-
m/min = 0.00003 HP = 0.0226 W
1 kg-m/min = 7.23 ft-lbs/min = 0.00022 HP =
0.1635 W

TEMPERATURE

0 degrees Celsius (°C) = 32°F = 273°K
100°C = 212°F
°C = (°F −32) × 5/9
°F = (9/5 °C) + 32

VELOCITY

1 foot/sec (ft/s) = 0.3048 m/s = 18.3 m/min =
1.1 km/h = 0.68 mph
1 mph = 88 ft/min = 1.47 ft/s =0.45 m/s =
26.8 m/min = 1.61 km/h
1 km/h = 16.7 m/min = 0.28 m/s = 0.91 ft/s =
0.62 mph

VOLUME

1 UK fluid ounce = 28.413 cm^3
1 US fluid ounce = 29.5735 cm^3
1 US fluid ounce = 29.5735 cm^3
1 US liquid pint = 473.176 cm^3 = 0.4732
dm^3 (= litre)
1 Imperial pint = 568.261 cm^3 = 0.5682 dm^3
1 UK gallon = 1.201 US gallon = 4.546 09 dm^3
1 US gallon = 0.833 UK gallon = 3.785 41
dm^3